The Life Science Health System

by

T.C. Fry

VOL. 5

Lessons 81-101 of 101

Materials by The Life Science Institute

Cover Design by Rok Bernardic, © 2023
Book Interior Design by Rok Bernardic
Edited by Rok Bernardic

Publisher's Cataloging-ln-Publication Data
Imprint: Independently published 2023
Paperback: ISBN: 979-8-390458-90-7

Type Set in Calibri / Times New Roman

Rok Bernardic s.p
info@cooliee.com

Table of contents

Editors' preface

The Life Science Health System is the most exhaustive and comprehensive natural hygiene health system ever written, which has inspired and educated millions of Americans who were in need of the truth.

This valuable resource and knowledge is put together, written, and compiled by T.C. Fry between 1970-1994, offering one of the most complete explanations and guides to elementary human health and condition.

Originally, the materials of The Life Science Health System were used for T.C.'s students who participated in the teaching course for Natural Hygiene practitioners. The Life Science Institute, established by T.C. Fry himself, organized it.

Although T.C. Fry has written several works, very few are easily available nowadays, in a friendly, readable, or accessible format.

That is why I have decided to invest my time and resources in reviving some of his materials, the accumulated knowledge, such as The Life Science Health System script, which I was lucky to come across and read.

The complete course of 101 lessons is split into five book volumes in print and one e-book, totaling more than 3,000 pages.

I believe this work can readily serve as a valuable resource for many people to gain a true understanding of how our body works, how it is healed, and how to maintain good health and enjoy true wellness in our existence.

Whether one wishes to make smaller changes to their lifestyle, take back their health, or seek real answers regarding health, the information within these pages will provide the tools and universal knowledge for salvation and life.

I would like to express my sincere gratitude to Mr. T.C. Fry for the sacrifice he must have made to put all this knowledge together and write it down.

Also, my sincere invitation goes to the readers who have chosen to invest their time and energy to take this work and self-participate in their own health, and also to continue and preserve this essential knowledge of T.C. Fry for generations to come.

- Rok Bernardic, *the editor*

Lesson 81:

Socializing and Natural Hygiene

81.1. Introduction

Natural Hygienists, for the most part, are well aware of the truism that the mere fact that they are Hygienists causes them to live in foreign territory, captives within an environment that is polluted and mechanized beyond all rational reasoning, an environment that is an affront to unperverted senses and capable of almost unlimited assault on our physical being; and, most of all, captives of a social, economic and medical hierarchy which is capable of showing little or no mercy to those individuals who do not fully subscribe to its tenets.

We know that we are beset on all sides by a barrage of sights, sounds, and messages that are contrary to all organic reality and that we reside in the midst of a people apparently gone mad; people who, almost without exception, overeat on foods biologically and physiologically unfit for humans to eat, foods the virtues of which are extolled by powerful economic forces. There are people who are sexually and morally perverted. Unwillingly we find ourselves non-participants within a society which is mentally, morally, and spiritually decadent. We stand on the sidelines, so to speak, yet we are part of social and economic order which is not in the best interest of the people who, willingly or unwillingly, participate in it. People have come to seek after things and not ideals. They seem to know nothing of the values of life and lacking this knowledge, they have become manipulated puppets, apparently with little desire to learn or change.

Consequently, we Hygienists have had to choose. We have made a carefully thought-out choice to live as more-or-less isolated individuals living in society but nevertheless determined to survive in the very midst of multitudinous carefully controlled and orchestrated assaults of one kind or another on our mental, moral, and physical well-being.

If we are to survive under present conditions and circumstances, it is essential for us to have support from others of like mind, else we are likely to be felled prematurely as we attempt to wend our solitary way through life's maze.

Psychologists call this kind of supporting "stroking." Stroking refers to the giving to another person the assurance that he is loved that he is important to another person who really cares about him as an individual, this in spite of all possible foolishness and/or weakness on his part. All that the stroked one is called upon to do is to give evidence of a willingness to learn, to grow because, in time, he hopes himself to become capable of stroking others.

Hygienists have varying degrees of expertise in the principles put forth by Life Science, some more, others less, hygienists, for the most part, are thinkers, idealists, often in the upper ten percent of the population intellectually. All seek the higher road through knowledge. However, knowledge alone is rarely sufficient. We need the doing and to help us in this phase of our individual development, we often require the assistance of others; stroking, if you will. Socializing can provide such needed support.

Few among us comprehend the powers of the mind. A positive mind steeped in knowledge and fortified by conviction can often help a sick person to be restored to a far higher plateau of health so quickly as to confound the skeptics.

Let us give an example of what we mean. Jerry has a rare muscular disease. For three years he has been a student of Natural Hygiene. In these three years he has seen many of his former incapacitating symptoms either leave entirely or be remarkably reduced. Recently he had occasion to visit his former medical advisor. He had enthusiastically prepared himself to tell him all about his progress and how he had been able to bring about such remarkable improvement. However, his erstwhile respected advisor exclaimed, "Jerry, you are not 'cured.' You are just in remission. Don't be fooled. Your symptoms will all come back. Just wait. You'll see!"

This is an example of stroking in reverse, negativity. A sick mind, lacking both sufficient knowledge and perhaps conviction through lack of support and even because of negative strokes, can tarry overly long in the wall of depression, so burdened by toxic debris that he will fail to make any meaningful progress.

Socializing has a proper role to play in all healing. The right kind of socializing can help to restore and reinforce important mental values. If we have knowledge, conviction, and determination and, in addition, the support of caring from like-minded people, our forward progress cannot help but be accelerated. Socializing with other Hygienists can provide this kind of caring support.

81.2. On Being Sociable

81.2.1. Why This Lesson?

81.2.2. Start Where You Are

81.2.3. Our Student Hosts a Party

81.2.4. How to Have a Hygienic Party

Alexander the Great accomplished many things in his lifetime and on many occasions, he had cause to celebrate. And so, he did! Alexander was a master host.

Following his victory over Darius and his Persian army, Alexander the Great hosted a party to end all parties, a mass wedding feast. On this occasion, hundreds of his warriors took wives, even though most of them already had wives and family at home. Alexander did, too!

At this extravaganza there were thousands of gaudily attired dancers. Musicians strolled about serenading the guests. Flowers were everywhere and scores of servers brought in meats, wines, fruits, and an endless array of delectables to charm and delight the senses and tantalize the palate. Laughter, gaiety, happiness, and joy prevailed. The partakers gorged until the morning dawn found all having surcease in deep sleep.

We Hygienists, of course, don't condone such indulgence and gourmandizing but we also have cause to celebrate. We also have occasion for rejoicing even though presently we may not be in the best of health and even though we may be but novitiates and have barely made a beginning on the road to better health. We have cause to rejoice, to celebrate because we have found TRUTH. We know that we, at long last, possess knowledge of the only possible way to regain health if it has been lost, provided of course that sufficient vital force is yet resident within the body not only to instigate the healing process but also to energize it until the desired level of health is finally reached.

We rejoice also in the full realization that once we reach our ultimate goal of complete freedom from pain and full enjoyment of that euphoric state that only full health can bring (and we know that we will), that we now either possess knowledge of how to maintain our existing high level of health or we are aware of the essence of truth and are resolved to expand our knowledge of Hygienic principles so that we can attain our own individual goal(s), whatever they may be. We know that we possess great cause for rejoicing and celebrating because we are few among many. We are the lucky ones. The masses remain needlessly enmeshed in the throes of suffering and disease. Only we have escaped!

We fully realize that there are numerous and deep chasms of the unknown when it comes to full knowledge of the human body, but we also are aware that the fundamental truths of life have been established by centuries of correct living on the part of a few and that Hygienists of the past have set these forth for our acceptance and practice in the 19 requisites of organic existence, these having been learned in this course: fresh air, pure water, and all the others so important to our well-being.

Socializing, friendships—these are among the psychological plus factors of life. They are important to health. We have already noted that man is, by nature, a gregarious creature. We need to be part of a group, to be recognized, to be made to feel that we as individuals count, that each one of us is important.

A great healer knows that there are many things the average adult wants and yearns for and leading the list, before money and all the things money will buy, is health and the preservation of life. Socializing with other Natural Hygienists will not only expand our knowledge of Hygienic truths but will also underscore our conviction as to the rightness of our present course; or, if we err, it will serve as a medium to correct us.

81.2.1. Why This Lesson?

Learning how to contact other Hygienists for the purposes of socializing, having fun, expanding knowledge, underscoring our personal convictions, and giving mutual support to one another is, we believe, a legitimate part of this course. We have made it a part of our own practice and policy and have observed socializing in action. The rewards are endless.

The information contained in this lesson should help new Hygienists who may now feel set apart to find their own niche in life. It should show them how they can become a "best friend" to another or to many others.

Beginning practitioners should find in this lesson some ideas to correlate in their practice, ideas which will provide an outlet not only for their individual talents but also a release for their private cares and concerns. Socializing in a meaningful way can help to expand one's practice.

We should all remember that it is not wholesome to stay to oneself. We only reach the height of our own powers when we begin to reach out toward others. We have a real inner need to serve other people, to include them in our activities; and to be included in theirs.

We cannot, of course, cover in this lesson all methods of socializing possible or acceptable to Hygienists but, hopefully, we will offer a sufficient number of suggestions to enable practitioners and individual students alike to expand their contacts for the purposes herein set forth.

81.2.2. Start Where You Are

Common sense should guide us in our choices of where we shall go, what we shall do and with whom we shall socialize. Early in this discussion we pointed out that Hygienists have, by choice, removed themselves from the masses. However, this does not mean that we cannot make casual entrances into society at large. What it does say is that our strolls therein should be carefully chosen and formulated to fulfill a primary need.

For example, we personally go to church regularly. We attend both teaching classes and regular services. Generally speaking, the people we meet are individuals with whom we feel comfortable and from our contacts there we find a certain number with whom we can exchange thoughts and ideas in a social situation to our mutual benefit without feeling that we are being manipulated or reduced in any way.

One of our students enjoys painting in oils. She is a Hygienist. She could have chosen to paint in her own studio, or she might have set her lonely easel out on the floor of the desert and endlessly painted the beautiful mountains that surround the city of Tucson.

These mountains always intrigue artists—their colors and configurations change as the sun moves across the sky from east to west.

Instead, our student chose otherwise, at least for part of the time. She went to the Chamber of Commerce and learned where painting classes were being held and made her choice among the many beings offered: some by the city Parks and Recreation Department, others by churches; there were classes at local schools and colleges. She found many from which to choose.

Do you have a hobby? Undoubtedly similar classes having to do with your very own special interest can be found where you live or within a reasonable distance. Inquire around and find your niche.

81.2.3. Our Student Hosts a Party

Sometime later, after she had become better acquainted with her classmates, our student invited them all to join her for a fruit breakfast, this to be followed by a painting session in the desert overlooking the celebrated Pusch Ridge.

What did the party cost her? Nothing except the effort of extending the invitation. The whole class eagerly responded (everybody likes a party!) and, since this was to be a potluck occasion, they all brought their own food and their own service. And what is more, a fruit breakfast was a new experience which every single one found most enjoyable—a delightful change from the usual ham and eggs!

This same idea can be incorporated when one's interests lie in other directions. In every town and city these days there are clubs and group meetings, free lectures and seminars, classes to satisfy a wide range of interests. The Hygienist who feels set apart or lonely must learn to reach out toward that area of society in which s/he can feel comfortable.

Once you have become a part of the group, you must learn to reach out toward others. For some this reaching out to include others may be a new experience but remember our admonition: it is not wholesome to remain to ourselves too much.

Practice will expand our talents in reaching out. Margery Wilson, the charm lady, said it well, "When the mind dwells too deeply and too long on the self, it shrivels those tendrils of the heart that reach out from the warm and inclusive human being." So, strive to keep your own hospitality light bright and shining. Don't forget that you will begin to glow with an inner glow as you improve in health, so much so that your newly-found friends will soon begin to ask you questions. How rewarding that time will be. Then you will be given a golden opportunity to give to another human being the gift of life itself.

81.2.3.1. Parties Do Not Have to be Large

Two stories will serve to illustrate the point that parties do not have to be large to be happy occasions. They also demonstrate how easy it can be to make new friends when we are willing to make the first friendly gesture. We have told these stories elsewhere in other writings, but they deserve repeating here to emphasize the point that even small gatherings, indeed socializing with a single other person, can be rewarding.

One time we were aimlessly strolling around the streets of Rome in search of one of that city's famous fountains, since our knowledge of Italian is very limited, we had difficulty in communicating our needs to the passerby. So, there we were, lost in a foreign city, strangers among a people with whom we could not speak. What a hopeless feeling that can impart!

Suddenly, Dr. Elizabeth spied a tall, well-dressed gentleman standing on a nearby corner. Never bashful, she went up to him and, in her broken Italian asked for directions. The gentleman doffed his hat, bowed gracefully, and replied, "Madam, if you will but speak to me the American, so that I may practice the speaking of it, I will be honored to show you, my Roma!"

And so, he did. We spent a wonderful afternoon with our host. He showed us his Roma as few tourists have been privileged to see it. And, as the dusk was falling, he invited us to share refreshments with him at a little sidewalk cafe. Finally, to his obvious regret and ours, he bowed and, taking his leave, presented us with his card. To our astonishment, we found that we had spent this wonderful afternoon with a Count, a celebrated member of the Italian government.

On another occasion we were in Maxime's in Paris, that world-famous restaurant. We had been seated at a wall table overlooking the entire main room. Our eyes were wide with wonder as we watched "High Fashion" at lunch. A black gentleman was seated next to us at the adjacent table. Suddenly, he leaned over to Dr. Elizabeth and aid, "I beg Madame's pardon, but are you Americans?" Upon learning that indeed we were, we were asked to be his guests. For well over two hours, we received attention galore.

Our host proved to be witty, charming and a delightful conversationalist, a graduate of one of America's most elite universities. We had a wonderful time. Finally, our host said that he had to go to Geneva and, regretfully, must take his leave.

He, too, left behind his personal card. Only then did we learn that our friend was an official representative of an African country to the United Nations. He was a very important gentleman, indeed. And yet, he took time out to be kind to two strangers who, like him, were having luncheon alone in a foreign land. Why? Because Elizabeth had smiled at him as she was being seated!

81.2.4. How to Have a Hygienic Party

Let us first address the problem of the individual Hygienist, male or female, who knows no other Hygienists in the immediate community where s/he resides. However, he usually does have a circle of acquaintances that he has acquired from time to time during the years he has lived in the community or from among the population who live in the general geographical location.

The same format as detailed above for the painting class party can be used. Host a fruit breakfast, or a "brunch," or have a salad luncheon.

The Hygienist host or hostess may either supply the food and service for his guests or stipulate, "Let's have a potluck." You may decide on a salad potluck or a fruit potluck; or even make it a "bring your favorite dish" pot-luck; or just get together for an evening of fun.

If no food is to be served, you will, of course, have to provide a means of entertainment. Games of various kinds may be provided, tapes may be played (there are fun tapes to be had for just such occasions. These are tapes designed to make even the grouchiest listener smile once in a while.)

Invitations may be given orally, by telephone or in person, or they may be mailed on bright party-looking fun cards. They can be formal as for a sit-down luncheon or casual for a buffet-type gathering.

Potlucks are especially interesting, and they are easy on the person hosting the party. You need not be an Alexander the Great. We, of course, do not condone the gluttony and indulgence displayed by Alexander and his soldiers, but what we do wish to emphasize by that example and through this lesson is the fact that we all have a need to socialize. His party was a skillful way on his part of rewarding his soldiers for their excellent work. In the same way by having an occasional party we can reward ourselves for our good work and also give to other Hygienists an opportunity to share fun and friendship with others and thus in the doing enlarge our own happiness and our own social awareness and participation.

The "bring your favorite dish" potluck is always fun. Guests enjoy seeing and experimenting with the dishes brought by all the other guests.

81.2.4.1. Words to Ponder

Parties can be as expensive as your wish, or as inexpensive. The main ingredient of a happy party is hospitality, the offering of a friendly smile and the extending of a friendly hand in greeting. All people have a genuine need to be loved, to feel that they are important to someone.

Remember FDR? Franklin Delano Roosevelt, the thirty-second president of the United States, was a master host even upon small occasions having no particular significance either to him personally or to the country at large. One time a new car was presented to him as a gift by one of the large car makers, the car to be used on state occasions.

A chauffeur drove the car to the front of the White House and FDR with his entourage came down the steps for the formal presentation. There were many invited guests there for the occasion. FDR took it upon himself to learn the name of the man who drove the car to the White House and made it a point to thank the man not only personally but publicly. And he did even more, for a few days later, the chauffeur, who was obviously politically unimportant to the president, received a surprise in the mail: an autographed picture and a personal note of thanks signed by the president of the United States!

One time we were to act as host and hostess at a party for a well-known soprano. She is internationally famous and has sung before presidents and kings, frequently at our own White House. The party was given by an "important" musical group. Was it a formal black-tie affair? No, indeed! Just the opposite, as a matter of fact. So informal was it that no utensils were served and there were no chairs on which to sit. Our famous soprano and we sat on some boxes and delved into meringues and Hors D'Oeuvres with our fingers. After the party was over, she remarked that she couldn't recall when she had had such fun!

We can learn from these two examples. People are important, not the trappings of the party. Make your guests feel welcome and wanted and your party will be a success.

81.2.4.2. Some Party Ideas

If you are fortunate enough to have a pool at your home, your party plans are half made. Have a swimming party. If not, why not invite your new friends to meet you at a specified day and hour for a picnic at a public pool? Most communities have one.

On these occasions your guests provide their own food. Or, again, the potluck approach can be used. The main thing you will be required to do will be to arrange with the proper authorities ahead of time so that you and your guests will be expected, and a table set aside in an appropriate spot for your exclusive use. You should, of course, know just how many people to expect and have seating for all.

Occasionally, we host a "hiking breakfast." Our students or friends gather here at the ranch at an early hour and off we go on a specified route which covers anywhere from two to six miles, depending, of course, on the age and condition of individual guests. Brandy, our collie, particularly enjoys these parties. He's right up in front, tail wagging, leading the group.

Following our hike, we set out the fruit and usually sit quietly enjoying our fruit while we listen to a tape recording by some well-known Hygienist; or we simply enjoy each other's company discussing areas of mutual concern and interest. On these occasions, we ably support one another and that is our purpose, is it not?

81.2.4.3. You Need Not Be a Master of Ceremonies

Remember that on these occasions you need not be a master of ceremonies. It is better to be a casual host. Succeed with one guest at a time. Take it easy! All people, no matter how important or influential, like every other person who ever lived, need to be recognized. All people have a deep need to be loved, to feel that they are important to others.

81.2.4.4. Students in Rural Areas

If you live in a rural area and wish to make contact with other Hygienists for the express purpose of sharing thoughts on Life Science and your experiences with it but there are none within a radius of a few miles, you can still socialize in the manner stated with non-Hygienists, non-students of Life Science.

One way to do this is to put an advertisement in the local newspaper and on various bulletin boards that may be available in your area to the effect that you are interested in forming a group or club for the purpose of studying natural methods of keeping fit. Be sure to give your name and telephone number.

You may have many calls and perhaps only a few. The number is not important. The idea is to start a group and build numbers because the group is friendly, and the subjects discussed both interesting and informative. As the group becomes better acquainted, the other ideas suggested in this course may be introduced and implemented.

Additionally, each student has received a list of names and addresses of fellow students of Life Science. From this list, select a few names of persons who live in your part of the country or even elsewhere, if you choose. Introduce yourself by letter. Tell other students frankly that you would like to correspond with them so you can possibly support them and that you know they can help you. You may be fortunate and find a real friend, one who is eager to share knowledge, personal experiences and concerns.

After contact by letter has been made and you become better acquainted you may even wish to use the telephone for instant give and take of ideas and counsel.

For your mini groups you can use the information learned in this course to formulate your own basic course of instruction of Life Science for the benefit of your friends. You can purchase tapes by practitioners on various subjects. Each member of the group can be encouraged to participate by purchasing a tape of their own and sharing with the other members of the group.

81.3. Health and Fitness Clubs

Health and fitness clubs have sprung up across the nation like mushrooms after the rain. Many of these are quite expensive but they do provide an opportunity to socialize as you exercise if you can afford it. Some individuals we know pool resources to purchase such a membership and share the membership card from time to time on a regular schedule. At these clubs you can often find a willing ear and an opportunity to share the principles of Life Science.

One of our favorite students called recently to make an appointment for a friend. We were delighted because this particular student has a rare kind of muscular dystrophy which sets her apart from society. Two years ago, when we first saw her, her face was covered with black blotches. Her gait was unsteady, and she had a tendency to fall from time to time. Additionally, her hands were swollen, puffy-looking, and covered with red blotches. Having no understanding of her condition, people avoided her. She had no friends. On her first visit to the ranch, Dr. Elizabeth went up to her, put her arm around this young woman's shoulders and kissed her right on her blotchy black face. So, it was with pure delight that this young woman acquired a newly found friend. You see, thanks to the application of the principles you are learning in this course, this young woman no longer has those black clotches, she no longer stumbles and falls. She probably never will be "cured," but she IS presentable. People no longer stare at her or, the opposite, avoid looking at her.

Where did she find her new friend? At a health club! Her friend also needed a friend. She was far from her home in India. She knew not a single soul. She had a need is did our student. Today, they share meals together. Their silence, their resentment, many of their fears have gone. All because each one found a friend and they can socialize together.

The local Y.M.C.A. and the Y.W.C.A. usually have fitness classes which you may attend for a nominal fee. There are aerobic dance classes, jogging groups, hiking clubs. You can use various clubs, churches, hobby groups, and so on to "seed" a like-minded group. Again, advertising your desires is the key to success. Advertise that you will hold a "study session," or whatever, in your home and see what happens. In all likelihood, you will be agreeably surprised.

81.4. How to Advertise

Type up an announcement of your meeting (or party, or hike, or class, or whatever you have decided to host). Use old letters. You can acquire a set of transfer letters of many different styles from a local office supply store. Using these or the typewriter draw up an attractive announcement of the first meeting, let us say, of the SMALL-TOWN LIFE SCIENCE STUDY GROUP. Be sure to give time and place and include precise instructions as to how to get to your home or to the meeting room you have selected. Be sure also to include your telephone number so that interested parties can telephone for further details or directions. Use some intriguing phrase or information to encourage interest.

You may also be able to place an announcement of your meeting in a local newspaper. These are usually provided free of charge as a public service by newspapers.

Have several hundred flyers run off and place them in strategic spots throughout the community where you live. If the topic for discussion concerns health, you may find a welcome reception in health food stores. Sometimes librarians will post such notices. Ask various merchants to post them also. The idea is to contact as many people as possible over a sufficiently wide area. Exposure of the right kind will produce results.

81.5. Getting Prepared

81.5.1. Suggested Topics

81.5.2. Sealing Friendships within the Group

81.5.3. Don't Try Too Hard

81.5.4. Establish Certain Rules

81.5.5. When Your Group Becomes Too Large

81.5.6. The Practicing Hygienist

81.5.7. You Don't Always Have to "Wing It" Alone

81.5.8. Groups Have a Tendency to Grow

The first meeting is critical, so be well prepared with a topic of interest. Following is a list of suggested topics. The student will note that we have suggested ten, sufficient for a year's study, since most such groups disband for at least two months during the summer.

81.5.1. Suggested Topics

1. From Measles to What and How to Prevent the What? (The 7 stages.)

2. I Like Fruit!

3. The Zero-Calorie Diet.

4. I Like Being Skinny!

5. How to Lose 15 Years off My Face and Add 20 to My Life.

6. Body Burn-out and How to Prevent It.

7. Why Exercise?

8. Is Meat Good for Us?

9. Food Combining Demonstration

10. How to Plan Meals

You will probably have to carry the load for a while, perhaps for the first two or three meetings. After that, it is time to start assigning topics. Get lists of the available tapes from Life Science or from the American Natural Hygiene Society. These are valuable and can be used at your meetings to fill in gaps and to provide useful information to your guests. The tapes may be used to supplement presentations by yourself or by one of the guests who consents to make a presentation.

Throughout your many lessons there are numerous topics of interest and also discussions by experienced practitioners on specific subjects. These short articles often provide very valuable information. They can be reproduced, and a copy given to each guest or they can be read to the guests present. The idea is to choose subjects of general interest or of intrinsic worth, to line up articles and/or discussions which develop the theme, to have tapes that pertain to the topic; in general, to tie the whole meeting together in such a way that there are no awkward gaps. Your guests should leave well rewarded for their time. They should have enjoyed the fellowship and learned something of value.

When they do, they are only too eager to return again and again.

81.5.2. Sealing Friendships within the Group

Most people are lonely in some way or other. Many Hygienists feel lonely set apart. Meetings such as we have described provide an ideal setting for everyone to have an opportunity to find a friend or to make many friends. The host or hostess can play a useful role here.

At every meeting guests should be made to feel that, as host or hostess, you are delighted to see them. For this moment the idea is to make each guest the center of attention.

Dr. Elizabeth gives every person who comes to the ranch on these occasions a hug and a kiss. They love it. After one or two meetings, indeed, they expect it and so does she!

Both of us try to impart a sense of mutual love and respect. Not everyone is outgoing at first, but with practice, everyone can become more warm and outgoing. Within the group is one person, or even a whole group of persons, who think you are somebody and do not hesitate to show it.

Rid yourself of surface comparisons. Encourage yourself and your guests to be interested in life and each other. Learn to live through talking, listening, and sharing. Use your own loving talent. Plant the seed of love, of mutual caring and respect for others by your example—and watch your harvest grow.

81.5.3. Don't Try Too Hard

Strive to put your guests at ease, but don't strive too hard: avoid artificiality. Offer love, friendship, and knowledge to your guests. Don't be afraid to go more than half-way, especially at first and perhaps even the second meeting. Express sincere interest in your guests person and well-being.

Don't forget the round-the-room introductions at every gathering. Do this when your guests have settled. At times, or even every time, you can ask your guests to tell something about themselves as for example, how they learned about Life Science or how they became interested in learning about natural methods of health care, or about their hobbies, or special talents, or feelings, or whatever? Be sure to admire and inquire.

When we express interest in others, they become interested in us. The old adage, "If you want a friend, then be one" is very sound advice that is applicable to all of us.

81.5.4. Establish Certain Rules

We have certain rules at the ranch that hold for all guests without exception. You may like to adopt similar rules especially at the beginning when strangers join your group. Two of these rules are the "No Smoking" rule and the "Vegetarian Food Only" rule.

Any guest who wishes to smoke may do so outside and away from the house. We do not put out ash trays. If we see a guest with a cigarette in hand looking for an ashtray, we suggest to him that there are the other guests to consider but they can go outside on the porch or for a walk around the grounds if they wish.

No meat is ever brought or served. Even our meat-eating friends understand this and respect our wishes. At the beginning they usually bring a very complicated salad complete with a very elaborate and especially prepared dressing. They soon change their ways, and most become a cooperating part of the group—and willingly so.

We do not permit coffee, alcohol, or soft drinks. We always have distilled water available for our guests.

We do not make of parties and meetings a time for hurry-up, busy-ness and cleaning.

We try to keep everything casual and light so that we can enjoy them, too.

81.5.5. When Your Group Becomes Too Large

Sometimes a few friends can grow into many, and your group becomes so large that your home or the home of participants can no longer accommodate them. Then it is wise and timely either to divide into two or more splinter groups or to move to a public meeting place.

Community rooms are usually available in most areas, provided either by the city or town (for example, the town hall), by churches, lodges, by savings and loan companies, by the larger health food stores, and so on. The local chamber of commerce can often provide names and locations of such meeting rooms, as can the city or country recreation departments.

81.5.6. The Practicing Hygienist

It is true that health care is self-care but the practicing Hygienist, worthy of, the name, will realize that s/he has a moral obligation to students and clients to reinforce their understanding and conviction from time to time.

For economic reasons, most clients cannot be expected to keep paying in dollars and cents for repeated consultations. Unlike the medical doctor, the Hygienist will have an almost 100% recovery experience among clients. In fact, in many cases, recovery will be so spectacular that clients will be able to depart from guidance within a few months certain, in their minds at least, that they have acquired sufficient knowledge to enable them to continue their forward progress without further guidance from the practitioner.

For this reason, the practitioner must have some method or methods of providing a steady feeding-in of potential clients. Group meetings of clients, their families, and invited friends can provide such a pool.

In the beginning such meetings can take place either in the office setting or be hosted in your own home. These first meetings should be purely professional in intent, to provide reinforcement beyond individual counselling. These meetings are not open to the general public. They do provide a time, albeit brief, for some important socializing, for getting clients to understand that other persons exist who also have problems and, most importantly, that you as a practitioner care enough to give this extra time and without charge.

At times a practitioner who has speaking talents may wish to start a club or group similar to that which we have already discussed. These meetings should, of course, be open to the public. Again, at the discretion of the individual practitioner, they may be held either in his/her home, at the home of a willing client, or at a public community room.

The invitations may be on the personal level (telephone or mail), conveyed by flyers to the public (distributed by cooperative students), and also by notices placed in the public press: Sometimes local radio stations will provide time for a short announcement particularly when the topic to be discussed is of general interest.

Lecture groups of this kind also provide a pool of potential clients but, additionally, they provide an opportunity for socializing. Students and clients are often delighted to be asked to share their experiences with the public. Following the lecture, the practitioner should always provide a time for questions and answers. If you don't know the answer, say so frankly and then try to find the answer and communicate to the questioner. So, be sure to alert one of your students to write down the name and address of such inquirers. It is always well at public meetings to ask two students or two other interested people who have the gift of being able to greet people warmly, to be at the door to extend a "Welcome!" to everyone who attends. Always have a sign-up sheet on a table at the door which asks for the name of your attendee, address, and telephone number and even "How did you learn about this meeting?" This last information may help you to decide on your most effective means of advertising.

We suggest that between the time of the meeting and before your next meeting that you call your new attendees and thank them for coming. Also, when possible, answer any unanswered questions.

81.5.7. You Don't Always Have to "Wing It" Alone

The practitioner doesn't always have to "wing it" alone. Tapes may be used, or guest speakers invited. Don't be bashful about asking worthy speakers to come and address your group. Most of them will be most gracious and willing to come at their own expense. As a general rule we take our guest speakers out for dinner following the meeting. If a guest speaker is not available and you have been too busy to prepare a topic, do what we have done occasionally: have a "Show and Tell" party. For such occasions we like to meet at a home or at a community room with facilities for serving refreshments. Many people enjoy telling about their own experiences, about how sick they were, what they did to overcome their particular trouble and "Look at me now!" Potential clients always find such meetings of interest, as do your present clients.

81.5.8. Groups Have a Tendency to Grow

If those in attendance at your meetings experience warmth and togetherness, your groups will grow. When appropriate, then, a minimal fee may be charged. Just a dollar or two will suffice. Whatever sum is collected will be your reward for services rendered.

Volunteers can be asked to take over time-consuming chores, such as getting out the notices of meeting times, place, topics for discussion, collecting "dues," and similar tasks. There are always willing workers to be found in any group of any size. They only need to be asked. It helps them to feel important, a meaningful adjunct to you and to the group.

Certain people have special talents. If there is a good speaker in your group, request that s/he introduce you. Encourage volunteering among the participants. You will be agreeably surprised at how much help you will receive.

81.6. Entertaining

81.6.1. Special Parties

81.6.2. Entertaining Out of the Home

81.6.1. Special Parties

There are many occasions amenable to socializing. We hold parties to celebrate birthdays. We hold parties just to get together with friends. Last year we had a party on Christmas Day for our students. Most years we have our own private plans for the holidays but last year, we knew we would be at home on Christmas, so we decided to have a party!

We knew that some of our local students have no families. We knew also that those persons who do have families rarely extend the hand of hospitality to persons outside of the immediate family group. Personally, we feel that we have an extended family, one that consists of our students around the globe. So, we sent out the word: "Come to the ranch and spend Christmas day with us!" We made the occasion a pot-luck dinner, of course. We are not ones to seek after additional work!

On the happy day we had the Christmas tree lights glowing, Christmas candles, flowers, and tinsel everywhere. And even Brandy was all dressed up for the celebration with a big red bow attached to his collar.

Everybody was asked to bring an inexpensive gift and to mark it as being a gift for a man or a women's if applicable. Additionally, guests were asked to bring a gift suitable for an elderly person. We planned to present them to the elderly members of the Tucson Yaqui Indian tribe. We were overwhelmed!

We had fifteen guests that day but gifts for the Indians poured in from many unexpected sources. The manager of the produce department of a local Gemco store with the cooperation of the store manager brought us several large boxes of oranges, tangerines, and grapefruit. Students who could not attend sent or brought gifts of all kinds: food, clothing, nonsense gifts and practical gifts. In fact, the number of gifts was so large that one of the heads of the tribe had to bring a truck to carry it all back to the Yaqui Center. And what a time we all had. A Christmas to remember. The food was great. We sang Christmas carols. Dr. Robert played his violin, even though he was out of practice. We had all socialized!

Pick your occasion. Dr. Robert's birthday is on New Year's Day. Of course, that's an occasion to merit a party when we are in town. Why not a Halloween party? Thanksgiving time is a lonely occasion for many family-less people. Have a Senior Citizen Party. Guests must be 55 or over. There are ideas without end. You can come up with a few of your own. Partying is fun. Your clients are inclined, many of them, to have periods of depression. A party can be very therapeutic for such as these. A party can provide a time to relax, to have fun, to enjoy knowing your students as persons, to make friends out of faces and cases. And parties provide an opportunity for your clients to know you better, too, as a socially inclined person, as they meet you out of your office and in a friendly, warm setting.

81.6.2. Entertaining Out of the Home

Sometimes it's nice not to entertain in your home or in a public meeting room. At times it is pleasant to entertain an intimate, very special group of friends outside of your home. There is a trick to knowing just how to accomplish this satisfactorily. We find there are several ways to do this depending upon just how much you wish to spend for the occasion.

For elaborate entertaining, if you are not restricted economically, you may arrange for special dinners at a better restaurant, one of your choosing. For such an occasion, you must decide on a menu and make arrangements with the maître d'hotel of the restaurant or with the restaurant (or hotel) manager at the place chosen. In making such arrangements, you must spell out the menu you have selected item by item making sure that your contact understands that all food is to be fresh, neither frozen nor canned, if at all possible. The exact time at which dinner is to be served must also be understood by the party with whom you are making arrangements, by you and, of course, by your invited guests.

You may wish to have a little gift of flowers for the ladies. Arrangements for either home delivery or delivery to the table can be made; or simply bulk delivery to the restaurant in your name. If the latter, then the host makes the presentation to the ladies who are present at an appropriate time, preferably at the table just prior to the serving.

But you need not be so formal nor need you be so lavish in your entertaining. Inviting your friends to meet you at a restaurant of your choosing that normally features a well-stocked salad bar with a variety of salads can be fun, too. If the restaurant serves baked potatoes "on the side," you are doubly fortunate.

Many of the better steak houses boast excellent salad bars and almost all serve baked potatoes. Call ahead of time and choose your restaurant before issuing your invitations. Know precisely what kind of a menu is featured before you all get to the restaurant only to find nothing on the menu suitable for a practicing Hygienist to eat!

Some restaurants and even some cafeterias will set aside a special room or part of the restaurant if your group is large enough, just for you and your party. Many will be happy to make small changes in their menu or even to provide your choices of food if the number present warrants the extra work. They usually make no extra charge for this service and the cost of these meals is generally reasonable.

Some restaurants will be happy to provide your special choices for a small additional charge, too, so keep this in mind. Inquire around and be prepared for those occasions when you don't care to host a party in your own home. Then all that will be required of you is to put on your best smile and meet your friends at the place of choice. Because you have made the arrangements ahead of time, all you have to do at this kind of party is to enjoy yourself!

Of course, the food won't be strictly Hygienic. You and your guests are well aware of this fact. But, often the enjoyment of spending a few hours away from our daily responsibilities will more than offset any minor defects in a single meal.

81.7. Respecting Private Spacing

Every human likes his own space. Around each one of us is an invisible boundary which must not be rudely violated. We know one Hygienist whom everybody avoids. This person is lovely to look at, bright and eager to please and learn, but she has a major fault. She attempts to enter, without permission, into everybody's private space.

This woman is never content with a "No!" Nor is she rebuffed by other kinds of negative responses. When people turn away from her, she will make a point of loudly asking, "Why?" Why do you do this to me? Don't you want me around?" She will go on and on asking why, how, and where and keep on inquiring even though your answers may be evasive.

If she has a personal problem, she will contact every single one in the group to ask an opinion as to how to solve her particular problem, which is, more often than not, of a highly-personal nature. In short, this woman lacks finesse and common sense.

We must avoid becoming too inquisitive, hypercritical, or arrogant in our Hygienic contacting. We must learn just how far we can enter into another person's private space without becoming offensive.

It is far better to become a good listener than to talk too much, to let other people volunteer their thoughts and ideas rather than to attempt to cross that invisible line of privacy. Even practicing Hygienists should learn the art of listening. If you are a good listener, people will remark to others that you are a marvelous conversationalist! And so learned, too!

Remember that a sharp tongue is an asset to no one. A soft answer not only can turn away wrath, but it can charm the listener. Never be hypercritical of fellow Hygienists who may be but beginners, subject to error. Be gentle in discipline and slow to anger. It is important for Hygienists to pull together, not away from each other.

We should at all times in our social meetings avoid becoming arrogant and perhaps even rude. We have often observed this among certain individuals at large gatherings of Hygienists, by self-serving interests who are self-satisfied in their expertise about everything Hygienic. We have observed young people turned completely away from thoughtful consideration of Hygienic principles because a single person cut them off rudely as they asked a simple question.

This kind of arrogance has no place in Life Science. It can frighten off the more timid ones, the very ones who are perhaps most in need of bur concerned guidance and help. We need to be warm and outgoing, considerate of others and, above all, friendly in our contacts with other people. Who knows? They may know something that we don't know, some bit of knowledge that may prove to be of great value to us at some future time.

Socializing is a time for fun, for finding and making new friends, for stroking, for learning and for helping one another over the bad times. Only by a cooperative give and take in an atmosphere of sharing can e, as individuals, hope to realize the many multiple benefits possible through socializing, with our own kind. Only using socializing for this combined purpose can we hope :o convince others to join with us because we have something so valuable as to merit their attention.

81.8. Expanding Local Contacts

Quite often the number of students of Life Science who reside in a particular city is too small for gatherings to warrant the necessary expense of publishing and distributing flyer notices or the hours of thought and planning required to host and conduct a public meeting outside of the home.

If confronted by such a situation, it is often possible to enlarge one's horizons by including other health-oriented groups in your plans, such groups as vegetarians, vegans, members of a nearby health club and similar groups.

It is often interesting to learn just how many "hidden" vegetarians there are who do not belong to any well-known organization or club. At any rate, one should invite all interested parties to a general meeting for the purpose of hearing a talk on some subject of interest to all who might care to attend.

Various reasons for calling such a group together can also be put forth as, for example, to form a study club on vegetarianism in general; for the purpose of finding out whether or not there are sufficient numbers so inclined who might care to meet on a regular basis for potluck purposes or for dining at a public facility. One can think up various reasons for health-oriented groups to get together for purposes of socializing with likeminded individuals.

Sometimes these joint meetings can be in the form of a day-long seminar with a number of speakers being featured at two sessions, perhaps two speakers in the morning hours and a single speaker in the afternoon followed by general socializing.

Or if your choice is to make the meeting simple, present a single speaker on a topic of interest, topics such as the following:

1. How to keep your energy level high.
2. How to choose and use foods that burn clean.
3. How to keep fit in today's crazy world! And so on.

In other words, choose a topic of general interest, one that will attract and intrigue.

It is possible at such meetings to allow a certain amount of time for individuals to relate personal experiences, these being given, of course, on a volunteer basis. Questions may also be permitted if agreeable to these volunteers.

It is often fun to allow time after the lecture or seminar for socializing1 on a more intimate basis, both by groups and by individuals.

Occasionally, at meetings of this kind, it may be interesting to divide up into circle mini groups following the lecture presentation for the purpose of discussion of the topic of the day by those within each assigned circle. All such discussions should be preceded by round-the-circle introductions so that all may become better acquainted.

These meetings may become so popular that they can be repeated at frequent intervals. On subsequent meetings, circles should be regrouped so that, in time, everyone will become acquainted with those who choose to become regular participants. The same procedure of becoming better acquainted with each other as detailed earlier in this lesson, that off having individuals volunteer information about themselves, can be followed equally well here.

These circle meetings can prove to be the most interesting and informative way of socializing of all that we have presented. We have seen long-lasting friendships result from these casual meetings. They can prove both creative and supportive. Above all, they offer an opportunity for individuals to participate on an equal footing in groups, small enough to be nonthreatening, even to the most timid.

81.9. Good Public Relationship

Public relations is a phrase in common use these days. For the Hygienic practitioner and the individual Hygienist alike, good public relations can best be established through a continuing and on-going effort to promote satisfying social stroking.

While we should not work just for applause, achievement should always be rewarded. Becoming a bona fide working Life Scientist is an achievement of which we can all be proud. Let's advertise our pride in our knowledge of life's universal laws and our having come to appreciate the fact that there can be one penalty for error: premature death. We are few among many because we are so blessed.

Let's encourage getting together for all manner of healthful socializing: for dancing, either aerobic or your style; for calisthenics, eating, hiking, or painting; for study and learning; to offer support and to receive it. We all have such a great and wonderful gift to share. There can be no better way to share it than in a spirit of friendly love. The hand of friendship will draw all people closer to life's joy.

We hope you will try some of the ideas we have put forth in this lesson. We would enjoy hearing from you about your failures, which will be few, and especially about your successes, which will be many!

Article #1: How to Be Socially at Ease

Let us imagine that you are invited to a lovely party where you will meet strangers as well as people you know. I have decided to make this a tea, as the uncharted casual contacts of a tea party most nearly parallel those of everyday experience.

PLACE YOURSELF MENTALLY BEFORE YOU GO. Before you go to the party it will be well to study your attitude on your relation to other people generally. Right here your inferiority complex—everybody has one of sorts—begins to stir like a waking beast, doesn't it? So, our first task is to put him to sleep again until we can get rid of him permanently.

You can't have a good time at a party or be charming unless you feel on an equal footing with everyone present. Of course, it would be absurd and stupid to compare yourself with your hostess or host and each guest to see if you are an equal. So, we must rid ourselves of these surface comparisons. They are unprofitable and odious.

If a great singer is present, you can't honestly feel that your voice is as good as hers. If the richest woman in the community is there, gorgeously gowned, how could you feel that you are as well-dressed as she? Unless you are a striking beauty, you can't honestly feel that you are as good looking as the prettiest woman there. Unless you have a dynamic personality and are a witty conversationalist you can't even imagine that you are as entertaining as the cleverest woman present. The most popular and beloved woman may be none of these—but she is charming. So why bother with such comparisons?

There is another more important and deeper quality that you can feel which will enable you to mingle easily and enjoy yourself with people above you and below you on the social ladder. It is impossible to keep your social contacts on an even keel. If you lived in a palace and had six secretaries to protect your exclusiveness, you would still meet a number of undesirable people. So, you must reach a point in poise and charm where you remain the same regardless of what or whom you contact!

For this type of poise, we must have a little philosophy that supports our conviction of equality. There is a danger here that in striving too hard for a sense of equality with the highest types of people one may be a little belligerent and say with a chip on the shoulder, "I am as good as anybody in the world." The crudeness and bad taste that would prompt such a statement in that mood are sufficient proof that one is not!

FEEL A BASIC KINSHIP WITH EVERYONE. We are all travelling the same path. The only difference in people is that each has arrived at a different place on that same path—but we all have the same feelings and the same reactions somewhere along the way.

So, no matter how shy and small you feel, you may know that everyone present has experienced that same thing. If they have overcome it and seem assured, that should only prove to you that you, also, can conquer your self-consciousness. Try to understand that the other fellow has his problems of inferiority, perhaps not just the same as yours, but, nevertheless, just as real to him.

When you are meeting a new person, try to think of the stranger's problem of instantly adjusting to you—try to help him find familiar ground where he can be at ease. This will accomplish two things. It will take your mind off yourself, eliminating for the moment any possibility of your self-consciousness. (You know you can't be self-conscious unless you are thinking about yourself!) Then, too, your interest in the newcomer will make him think you are charming. Never be afraid to go more than halfway to establish social ease. Don't be afraid to walk up to people at a reception or party or tea to say or do something that will make them happier. A wallflower is usually self-elected. She slips through the door and slides into a side seat on the edge of the room as though she were clinging to the edge of a whirling disk and might be thrown off any minute.

NEVER, TAKE THE FIRST CHAIR IN A ROOM—walk calmly well inside and take the most inviting chair hat is vacant!

Pause before you enter the room, see where people are, locate your hostess or whoever is in charge of the affair. Go to her and shake hands. She will introduce you to those landing in her immediate group.

... "Remember that people put the same interpretation on us that we put on ourselves. They take their cue from is! We cannot control the smoothness of life from without— but we can control it from within—we can control our reactions to anything that happens to us. This is poise!

... WHEN WE REALIZE THAT THERE IS A STEADFAST, DIVINE PERSONALITY WITHIN US THAT IS BIGGER AND FINER THAN ANYTHING THAT CAN

HAPPEN TO IT, WE HAVE JUST BEGUN TO LIVE. This is when we get up on two feet from the all- "ours of animalism and bewildered ignorance and realize that we have souls. The experience passes but the experiencer remains to have other experiences.

When you realize the importance of this "experiencer" within you, then you are in a position to develop unshakeable poise. This is not a religious conception—it is an inalterable fact of life. The person that you really are is so basically a part of the harmony of the universe—so established in the world of reality—that you can afford to take our importance for granted and put your mind on others.

When you understand this basic truth, you will become socially unselfed and immersed in sociability. Just to refrain from talking about yourself, not to be patting your hair and clothes and not to patch your makeup in public—these do not guarantee charm. These are but the first baby steps toward charm in being socially unselfed. Charm demands that you be genuinely interested in your companions—you can't fake it!

YOU MUST SHOW GENUINE INTEREST. You must be so interested in other people that you understand their humanness, stand ready to smile at their arrogance, to fix up their failures, to admire their accomplishments and to ignore their errors. People are fascinating—the most fascinating study in the world!. ... If you can give humanity a mental handclasp of sympathy and at the same time a wink of tolerance, no king nor queen can throw you off poise!

... The desire to be capable of the best self-expression ... is a splendid motive that drives one to sharpen one's tools for the making of good conversation—but cold perfection will never warm the hearts of your hearers. You must strike the spark of animating warmth born of a pulsing human urge to share what you feel.

This spark comes from the fires of a burning desire to draw closer to the mind and heart of your neighbor, to give him solace when it is needed, encouragement and sympathy always, also laughter to brighten his spirits and to lighten his load. And when I say "neighbor" I do not merely mean that person whom you would like to cultivate for social or material reasons. I refer to every life that touches yours.

From The Woman You Want to Be by Margery Wilson. Published by J. B. Lippincott Co., Philadelphia, and New York. Copyright 1938.

Article #2: Real Houses Are Like Real People by Charles M. Simmons

Houses, REAL houses, that is, are very much like people. If you take a look at the houses in your community, you find quite an assortment, don't you? You see some old ones, some new ones, some shabby ones, and some "smart-looking" ones. There are some you wouldn't want to live in just because of their appearance on the outside. Others come closer to your choice, except that if they were YOURS, you would make a few changes. Some seem to have charm, while others lack it completely.

It is remarkable what a varied combination of houses makes up a community, yet they are all made of the same basic materials. However, keeping that observation in mind, take a second look at those houses, and you will realize that there is another factor that is causing your varied reactions.

It is the amount of love and caring found in the homes, or not found in them, that is evident the moment you step inside. It doesn't matter if the house is impeccably clean or has that "lived-in" look. These are only outward appearances and provide no real measure of the family that resides there. We can feel at once whether the house vibrates and radiates love or emptiness.

Article #3: An Excerpt from in Tune with the Infinite by Ralph Waldo Trine

... Many times, the struggles are greater than we can ever know. We need more gentleness and sympathy and compassion in our common human life when we will neither blame nor condemn. Instead of blaming or condemning we will sympathize, and all the more we will:

Comfort one another,
For the way is often dreary,
And the feet are often weary,
And the heart is very sad.
There is a heavy burden bearing.
When it seems that none are caring,
And we half forget that ever we were glad.
Comfort one another
With the handclasp close and tender,
With the sweetness love can render,
And the looks of friendly eyes.

Do not wait with grace unspoken, while life's daily bread is broken—

Gentle speech is oft like manna from the skies.

When we come to fully realize the great fact that all evil and error and sin with all their consequent sufferings come through ignorance, then wherever we see a manifestation of these in whatever form, if our hearts are right, we will have compassion and sympathy for the one in whom we see them.

Compassion will then change itself into love, and love will manifest itself in kindly service. Such is the divine method. And so instead of aiding in trampling and keeping a weaker one down, we will hold him up until he can stand alone and become the master. But all life growth is from within out, and one becomes a true master in the degree that the knowledge of the divinity of one's own nature dawns upon one's inner consciousness and so brings one to a knowledge of the higher laws; and in no way can we so effactually hasten this dawning in the inner consciousness of another, as by showing forth the divinity within ourselves simply by the way we live.

By example and not by precept. By living, not by preaching. By doing, not by professing. By living the life, not by dogmatizing as to how it should be lived. There is no contagion equal to the contagion of life. Whatever we sow, that shall we also reap, and each thing sown produces of its kind. We can kill not only by doing another bodily injury directly, but we can, and we do kill by every antagonistic thought. Not only do we thus kill, but while we kill, we commit suicide. Many a man has been made sick by having the ill thoughts of a number of people centered on him; some have been actually killed. Put hatred into the world and we make it a literal hell. Put love into the world and heaven with all its beauties and glories becomes a reality.

Not to live is not to live, or it is to live a living death. The life that goes out in love to all is the life that is full and rich, and continually expanding in beauty and in power. Such is the life that becomes ever more inclusive, and hence larger in its scope and influence. The larger the man and the woman, the more inclusive they are in their love and their friendships. The smaller the man and the woman, the more dwarfed and dwindling their natures, the more they pride themselves on their "exclusiveness." Anyone—a fool or an idiot—can be exclusive. It comes easy. It takes and it signifies a large nature to be universal, to be inclusive. Only the man or the woman of a small, personal, self-centered, self-seeking nature is exclusive. The man or the woman of a large, royal, unself-centered nature never is. The small nature is the one that continually strives for effect. The larger nature never does. The one goes here and there in order to gain recognition, in order to attach himself to the world. The other stays at home and draws the world to him. The one loves merely himself. The other loves all the world; but in his larger love for all the world he finds himself included.

Verily, then, the more one loves, the nearer he approaches to God, for God is the spirit of infinite love. And when we come into the realization of our oneness with this Infinite Spirit, then divine love so fills us that, enriching and enrapturing our own lives, from them it flows out to enrich the life of all the world.

In coming, into the realization of our oneness with the Infinite Life, we are brought at once into right relations with our fellow men. We are brought into harmony with the great law, that we find our own lives in losing them in the services of others. We are brought to a knowledge of the fact that all life is one, and so that we are all parts of the one great whole. We then realize that we can't do for another without at the same time doing for ourselves. We also realize that we cannot do harm to another without by that very act doing harm to ourselves. We realize that the man who lives to himself alone lives a little, dwarfed, and stunted life, because he has no part in this larger life of humanity. But the man who in service loses his own life in this larger life, has his own life increased and enriched a thousand or a millionfold, and every joy, every happiness, everything of value coming to each member of this greater whole comes as such to him, for he has a part in the life of each and all.

And here let a word be said in regard to true service. Peter and John were going up to the temple one day, and as they were entering the gate they were met by a poor cripple who asked them for alms. Instead of giving him something to supply the day's needs and then leaving him in the same dependent condition for the morrow and the morrow, Peter did him a real service, and a real service for all mankind by saying, "Silver and gold have I done, but such as I have I give unto thee." And then he made him whole. He thus brought him into the condition where he could help himself. In other words, the greatest service we can do for another is to help him to help himself. To help him directly might be weakening, though not necessarily. It depends entirely on circumstances. But to help a person to help himself is never weakening, but always encouraging and strengthening, because it leads him to a larger and stronger life.

There is no better way to help another to help himself than to bring him to a knowledge of himself. There is no better way to bring him to a knowledge of himself than to lead him to a knowledge of the powers that are lying dormant within his own soul. There is nothing that will enable him to come more readily or more completely into an awakened knowledge of the powers that are lying dormant within his own soul, than to bring him into the conscious, vital realization of his oneness with the Infinite Life and Power, so that he may open himself to it in order that it may work and manifest through him.

Originally printed and copyrighted in 1908. Bobbs-Merrill Co., Inc. NY. Last copyright 1970.

Article #4: Preparing a Dinner Party for Non-Hygienic Guests by Elizabeth D. McCarter, D.Sc.

So! You've decided to take that big step: to host a gala dinner party for some of your non-Hygienic friends. It can be done, you know, and without compromising your principles, too! And certainly, without all the hours and days of preparation required when hosting a more conventional dinner featuring the usual gourmet type of heterogeneous combinations.

Plan first of all to set a gala dinner table. Get out all your best silverware and fine china. Polish up the candlesticks and plan to dine by candlelight. Check your linens and, if need be, see that they are all freshly laundered, ready for the big day. All this routine work can be done days ahead of time.

Plan a centerpiece, of course. This can consist of flowers from your own yard or from the florist. In the fall or wintertime, lovely centerpieces can be made from a wide variety of gourds, pinecones, apples, or whatever. Women's magazines are filled with all kinds of ideas so go to the library and check a few of them to find an idea most appropriate to your circumstances.

Next, plan your menu. You will be a guest at this party, too, so plan your party with that in mind. Market a day or two before the big event and stock the refrigerator and ripening bowls with various kinds of fruit in season.

Purchase baking potatoes of good quality, several varieties of low starch and green vegetables, two or three kinds of lettuce, some sprouts (or better yet, grow your own) and two or three different kinds of nuts. Pecans are popular as are almonds and cashews, all unsalted and un-toasted. You might plan to have a casserole dish of some kind or even some lightly steamed ears of corn. Be sure to allow plenty of time for bananas and other fruits to ripen as well as the tomatoes and avocados.

The night before your party set your table. If you need some ideas on how properly to set a table, your local librarian can refer you to suitable books to obtain this information. Make it pretty and inviting. Set out the serving trays, dishes and appropriate ladles, tongs and so on.

The morning of your party make your food preparation. Wash and dry the lettuces. Carefully wrap the washed pieces in towels and put in the refrigerator. Scrub your fruits and rinse with pure water. I use a liquid soap that make using Ivory flakes for this purpose. Proceed the same with all the vegetables except, of course, the ears of corn. These should remain intact until dinnertime. All the vegetables can then be returned to the refrigerator.

I usually set up a buffet table, the longer the better, especially if you are hosting a fairly large party of fifteen or more guests. For smaller groups, a smaller buffet, perhaps comprising two card tables set side by side and covered with a single tablecloth would be sufficient.

You will want to have plenty of food available so that your guests will have a variety from which to choose.

Make several attractive fruit arrangements, each plate featuring compatible combinations of fruits. For example, you might place on one large round serving tray: an attractive assortment of strawberries, pineapple slices, kiwi fruit and oranges, all placed on a well-arranged bed of Bibb (limestone) lettuce.

On another dish arrange pieces of Romaine in a circle configuration and place a huge mound of assorted grapes on it, perhaps surrounded by schoolboy size red delicious brand apples or, in season, ripe apricots and nectarines or slices of papaya. On a third dish use dark leafy green lettuce and use it as a background for delectable, dried fruits: varieties of dates, dried figs, little paper cups of raisins with, perhaps, a star arrangement of bananas to separate the different kinds of dried fruits.

Always try to use the fruits which are readily available in your area. Persimmons in October and November often provide a wonderful treat as do the Bing cherries and apricots which are plentiful in the latter part of June. Some of your guests may have never eaten mangos or New Zealand kiwi fruit. And believe it or not, many may never have enjoyed the rich succulence of a Medjool date! All exotic fruits provide interesting conversation pieces. Place all the fruit dishes at one end of the table.

Next come the salad vegetables. Get the largest bowl you can find or dig out one of those huge long unused (we hope), but gleaming, pots that you may have used at one time for cooking. Fill it with a variety of lettuces which you have broken up into pieces. Add tiny slivers of carrots, red and green cabbage, chunks of green and red peppers, broccoli flowers, and strips of cucumber. (I always use the unwaxed pickling cucumbers). Place stalks of celery in a pitcher of your choice and place it near the salad bowl (or pot).

Or, let your guests make their own salads. This is always a good opportunity for questions and answers, too, although now we find more and more people are becoming salad oriented. If individual salad-making is your "thing," then place the salad vegetables in individual dishes and arrange them colorfully around a large lettuce bowl. Let your guests help themselves.

Make a salad dressing of lemon juice and olive oil sparked with a dash of walnut oil for flavor interest. Or make one of cucumbers, celery plus a little avocado—all of which are blended together with a little green onion. Put each dressing in an attractive decanter or in a small serving bowl with a ladle or large dipping spoon. Be sure to put out a salt-free seasoning mixture. Vegebase is an acceptable mixture.

Some guests may request salt and pepper. If so, you may purchase individual salt and pepper shakers at some gourmet or health food stores. The salad part of the meal often provides a time for friendly education in the making of healthful salads.

It is nice always to have quartered or sliced tomatoes and avocado strips on a side dish with either of the salad buffets so that guests who enjoy these fruit-vegetables may add them to their other choices.

If your choice or choices of main dish (dishes) has been baked potatoes or a casserole, or both, these should be timed for the proper cooking time and the oven lighted about 15 minutes before. The potatoes and casserole should be timed as exactly as possible so that they will be ready for your guests when needed. While neither the potatoes nor casserole will be strictly Hygienic, nevertheless some cooked dishes can often provide for your guests a most enjoyable finale to a very enjoyable repast.

There are numerous vegetarian casseroles that will delight the taste. Baked potatoes served with an avocado blend made from avocado, a little distilled water and some vegebase often prove to be a delightful treat. Why not bake your potatoes early in the day, scoop out the contents, mix with the avocado mixture, stuff, wrap in foil and keep in the refrigerator until your guests are ready to go to the table. At that time place the unwrapped stuffed potatoes in the preheated oven. They'll be heated and ready for your guests at the appropriate time.

If an eggplant tomato casserole is your choice, put it out on the serving table, surround it with an assortment of natural, undyed soft and hard cheeses plus a dish of sliced tomatoes and an assortment of nuts. Separate the nuts from the cheeses by using the tomato dish. (The nuts could also be placed with the salad, but we find it usually better to place them with an appropriate casserole.)

If fresh steamed corn or other steamed vegetables are to be served, they should, of course, be put out on the buffet along with other suggested main dishes. Steamed corn is always welcome. Most of your guests will want butter with their corn. Buy a quarter pound or so of raw unsalted butter if you can find it in your area. Place it by the steamed corn.

We serve baked corn gems in place of bread. I can make these several days before the party and keep them in the refrigerator. To make these, I purchase freshly ground corn and wheat at a local health food store plus some ground unsweetened dried coconut (or I grind my own). To four cups of corn meal, I add 1 cup of coconut and 1 cup of ground wheat. After a thorough mixing I add boiling water to make a dough-like consistency. I roll out the dough in a 4-inch-wide strip and cut into two-inch "gems." I put the gems on baking sheets which have been left to heat in an oven at 400°F. I bake these for about 15 minutes, then turn them over. I then turn off the oven and let the gems cook until the right consistency, about 10 more minutes.

Since the gems are cold when I take them out. of the refrigerator, I sprinkle them with a few drops of distilled water and remove them to the oven for 10 minutes or so before placing them on the buffet table. They are great when eaten with a salad of greens! For dessert, I usually prepare a frozen fruit delight which I make by pureeing a dried fruit (dates, apricots and apples are a good choice) with a little distilled water and then mixing it with banana "ice cream." This mixture can, then be placed in champagne glasses or in any kind of fancy glassy covered with plastic wrap, and then put in the freezer until dinner time. When your guests are seated at the table enjoying your stuffed potatoes or steamed corn or your tasty casserole, you can quietly set this wonderful desert out on the buffet.

Good friends, fine food, soothing music, fun, laughter and lively! conversation is boon to the soul. While many errors in eating will no doubt be made by your guests from time to time, nevertheless, they will welcome this kind of friendly introduction to natural foods for good eating. We need this kind of friendly rapport from time to time. There are many serving suggestions, ideas galore, to be found in various books written by hygienists and by almost-hygienists. Hannah Allen's Homemaker's Guide is a good one. Of course, we like our own, The Exciting World of Healthful Cookery! and Healthful Living always has some great ideas by Marti Fry. So, don't think you have to live to yourself. You really don't! Try some of our ideas and put a little fun into your life. Learn how to socialize Hygienically and even almost-hygienically once in a while. Watch your spirit's soar!

Lesson 82:

The Adolescent and Hygienic Living

82.1. Teenagers—An Endangered Species

82.1.1. The Question—To Leave Home or Commit Suicide?

82.1.2. Teenagers and Alcoholism

82.1.3. Other Drugs

82.1.1. The Question—To Leave Home or Commit Suicide?

Several million teenagers will leave home during the year 1984, either because their parents constantly "bug them" to be something other than what they are or want to be; or because they disagree with what they consider their parents' completely outdated ideas of morality and behavior. And, for a myriad of other reasons. If the present pattern continues, over 5,000 teenagers will commit suicide, either at home or away from home in some strange hotel room or other alien place.

Experts working in this field of social awareness tell us that adolescent suicide is underreported by a factor of from 25 to 100% and that, for each teen who is successful in taking his own life, there are 50 to 100 unsuccessful attempts. In other words, the potential exists "out there" for double 5,000 successful attempts and that 10,000 or possibly as many as one million teenagers are so emotionally torn that, at some time, they either seriously contemplate suicide or actually attempt to end their own lives.

82.1.2. Teenagers and Alcoholism

The problem of teenage alcoholism is widespread and serious, according to the National Institute of Alcohol abuse and Alcoholism, as the following statistics attest:

Almost 1 1/2 million young people between the ages of 12 and 17 years have a serious drinking problem.

One of every three high school students gets drunk at least once a month, sometimes more often.

One of every three high school students gets drunk at least once a week and some authorities claim that these figures are underreported and that more realistic studies show that as many as 30 to 50 out of every 100 teenagers get drunk every week.

Many 13and 14-year-olds sit half-stoned in school classrooms with the full knowledge of teachers and administrators, most of whom find themselves totally at a loss as to how to cope with a worsening situation.

Three times the number of teenagers are being arrested for drunken driving now than were arrested only 15 years ago.

Shockingly, too, drunkenness is now being observed in schools as early as eight and nine years of age.

Consumption of alcohol has increased in the U.S. by 40% since 1960, much of it among the college crowd, but also among adults. In fact, a statistical survey taken in

1950 of 17,000 college students who totally abstained from all liquor found that in 1976, 70% were now users with less than 4% now being abstainers.

Peggy Papp, a family therapist associated with The Center for Family Learning in New Rochelle, New York, is quoted by columnist Lew Koch as saying that alcoholism tends to relay itself from generation to generation. Youngsters see their parents drink and, as Dr. Morris E. Chafetz, M.D., Director of the National Institute of Alcohol Abuse and Alcoholism, says, "Youth drink to achieve a demonstrable measure of adulthood."

In other words, teenagers tend to emulate their parents, Ms. Papp contends that parents are largely responsible for teenage alcoholism, and they may have to admit "that the three-martini lunches and regular afternoon bar sojourns constitute drug abuse, just as surely as their teenager's tippling during baby-sitting jobs and stashing liquor in school lockers constitutes drug abuse."

Koch maintains that "teenage alcoholism is going to require honesty and vigilance on both sides of the generation gap." Dr. William Rader, well-known psychiatrist, says that alcoholic parent(s) give disturbing memories, anxieties, worries to a child that can haunt him for the rest of his life. "They just can't walk away from homes like that without scars."

It is scary to realize that some 250,000 infants will be born this year in the U.S. with congenital abnormalities and probably 6,000 of these will be due directly to fetal alcohol syndrome; that is, their mother's drinking problem is directly linked to the deformity. Many of these mothers will be teenage alcoholics.

The problem is not America's alone. According to Michael West, in an A.P. release dated April 2, 1979, in Russia, some children become bottle addicts before they reach the age of ten. It seems that 90% of Russia's alcoholics had their first drink before the age of 15 and fully one-third before the age of ten. It is noted that the greatest increase in alcohol addiction is seen in youngsters at schools and technical colleges.

In Britain there are almost twice as many teenage drunks as only 12 years ago. In 1982, in London alone, there were 4,805 convictions of drunkenness among teenagers and teachers say that alcohol is replacing hard drugs as a school problem.

In West Germany teenagers just ignore laws which ban the sale of liquor to minors and there are willing adults to be found everywhere who will sell alcoholic beverages to children for a profit, regardless of the cost to society at large.

It is said that Australia is becoming a nation of alcoholics with "the number of children with drinking problems increasing at an alarming rate," according to a press release.

Fifty-eight percent of all young women at Sydney University admitted to "a dangerous drinking level."

The Church of Scotland said 98% of boys and 96% of the girls in Glasgow regularly drink at age 17.

In all of Great Britain $132 million is spent each year on publicizing alcoholic beverages on television screens and elsewhere.

In Czechoslovakia alcohol advertising has been severely restricted in order to combat youth alcoholism which, according to authorities, was fast getting out of hand.

In wine-drinking France the problem among young people became so fierce that a government committee addressing the problem has banned serving alcohol at school lunches to those under 15. This is a radical departure for Frenchmen to take. We well recall taking a trip about eight years ago with a number of French children, ages perhaps four to eight years of age, and watching them all served a glass of sweet wine at lunchtime.

Ireland has taken a forward step to combat juvenile drunkenness by banning all advertising of alcoholic drinks on its state-run radio and television stations.

Here, in the general area of Tucson, there are an estimated 38,000 residents with serious drinking problems.

82.1.2.1. Alcohol Addiction

Alcohol addiction can create serious problems in the future for young people. Canadian findings indicate that chronic alcoholics who drink for ten years or more show significant signs of cerebral atrophy, according to Dr. Peter L. Carlen, investigator at the University of Toronto in Canada. X-ray scans of drinkers show loss of cerebral tissue and large cavities in the brain.

It was pointed out in the Toronto study that addiction becomes so ingrained that alcoholics will seek strange and bizarre ways to satisfy their cravings, going so far, for example, as John Barrymore, the famous actor, who is said to have in his early years "once sipped ethyl alcohol from his yacht's cooling system while the painter Maurice Utrillo reportedly imbibed lamp spirits, benzine, ether and cologne."

When Dr. Elizabeth was counseling at a reform school for juvenile criminals some years ago, she said that all flavorings, such as vanilla and almond, had to be kept under lock and key because the alcoholic inmates would drink a bottle at a sitting! Many became terribly sick after such indulgence, but this did not prevent their trying again the next time!

82.1.3. Other Drugs

We have spent considerable time presenting statistics on alcohol abuse because this is the single most widely-used drug among teenagers and alcoholism will, no doubt, become a matter of concern at times to practicing Hygienists.

However, teenagers are "into" other drugs, too. Marijuana is the most frequently used drug, after alcohol, among teenagers. A survey conducted at the Institute of Social Research showed that 51% of all teenagers surveyed used marijuana either at some time in their lives or consistently.

The active poison in this plant is cannabinol, a phenol aldehyde. The user "may have dreamlike experiences, with a free flow of ideas and distortions of time and space; a minute may seem like an hour. He may become talkative or pensive and quiet, or unsteady or drowsy." We observed this drowsiness in one teenage user who had confessed to "bombing out" the night before. He just dropped off into a sound sleep while we were talking to him.

Physical reactions may include rapid heartbeat, lowered body temperature, reddening of the eyes, and dehydration. In some cases, gastrointestinal reactions or increased frequency of urination may be experienced.

Prolonged use of marijuana may cause psychological (not physical) dependence. Investigators at the National Institute of Mental Health found that strong doses of marijuana brought on "strong reactions in every subject." Some experiments said the active ingredient in marijuana may destroy or deform the offspring of laboratory animals. Habitual users sometimes showed loss of memory and some difficulty in concentrating. A report issued by the U.S. Department of Health, Education and Welfare in 1974 seemed to suggest that:

1. Habitual male users of marijuana had been found to have depressed sex hormone levels.

2. Female users of the drug who smoked regularly during pregnancy might adversely affect the development of the fetus by decreased oxygen flow resulting from smoking.

3. Drivers of motor vehicles, when under the influence of marijuana, had slower than normal reactions and a reduced ability to concentrate.

4. Marijuana could interfere with the fundamental chemistry of the living cells of the human body.

Note: Researchers have often disagreed on the results of marijuana studies, and sometimes have come to conflicting conclusions. Not all of the side effects that are possible from a drug will necessarily occur in every individual—however, we still harm our bodies by abusing any substance, and certainly by smoking.

82.1.3.1. Cocaine

Jet Magazine for March 1981 states that in the two years from 1979 to 1981 cocaine use bad doubled. This is a truly remarkable statistic. Since that time, it has become the "in" drug and its use among teenagers who can afford it is on the rise.

The drug is believed to produce psychological dependence but not physical dependence. However, it can have certain alarming after-effects, such as the following: it can produce paralysis of the sensory nerve endings and nerve trunks, resulting in anesthesia (inability to feel pain); it stimulates the sympathetic nervous system, resulting in constriction of the blood vessels and dilatation of the pupils; it also stimulates the central nervous system, resulting in exhilaration and possibly in convulsions, followed by mental and physical depression, especially of respiration.

82.1.3.2. Heroin and Nicotine

Other drugs, such as heroin and nicotine, are not quite as common when it comes to working with teenagers. The Indiana Department of Health found (June 1982) that some 14% of the teens studied smoked cigarettes. Users of heroin are more rare. In fact, among most teens, heroin is known as a "bad trip," while drugs such as cocaine and marijuana are regarded as "fun" things.

However, nicotine addiction is established more rapidly than addiction to heroin and experiments by Dr. Michael A. H. Russell, psychiatrist at the Addiction Research Unit of Maudsley Hospital's Institute of Psychiatry in London has concluded that the smoking of just one pack of cigarettes provides some 200 successive nicotine "fixes," which is many times that received by a person first experimenting with heroin.

The frightening thing about teenagers and cigarettes is that their use is increasing and, apparently, no method of advertising about potential for harm appears to have had any impact either on teenagers or upon adults. The total number of cigarettes smoked per year rose 16% during the period from 1965 to 1978, this among all age groups including teenagers.

While some researchers in this field claim that smoking is not an addicting habit, that there are no withdrawal symptoms, no tolerance developed, and no antisocial behavior elicited upon stopping, others claim just the opposite. The Royal College of Physicians in London in a report entitled "Smoking or Health," said that there is evidence of a "nicotine-withdrawal syndrome" composed of "intense craving, tension, irritability, restlessness, depression, and difficulty with concentration" plus objective physical effects such as a fall in pulse rate and blood pressure, gastrointestinal changes such as constipation, disturbance of sleep, impaired performance at simulated driving and other tasks, and changes in the electrical impulses in the brain.

Any person who ever took his first draft of a cigarette and persists in smoking can attest to the fact that tolerance to this drug is developed and that rather quickly, too. And any person who has given up cigarette smoking after smoking for any length of time knows that the experience, to say the least, can be trying. Other nervous reactions are possible, including pronounced irritability, nausea, depression, and so on.

Most researchers agree that nicotine produces widespread effects on both the central nervous system and the cardiovascular and peripheral systems. We have observed that when several packs of cigarettes are smoked every day, that the complexion assumes a strange yellowish tinge which seems to underlie the overall effect. This is especially striking with teenagers.

It is interesting that in recent years researchers have become more concerned about "side stream" smoke rather than the smoke inhaled by the smoker. Two Danish investigators were the first to call the public's attention in 1974 to the fact that it is the carbon monoxide, and not the nicotine, which is the major toxin for the increased risk of smokers to develop atherosclerosis and heart disease. And, of even more interest, perhaps, is the study which shows that some low-nicotine, low-tar cigarettes actually yield more carbon monoxide than some of the more conventional cigarettes.

"Uppers" and "downers" are also in rather common use among teenagers but to a minor extent when compared to marijuana. These are the mood-altering drugs. They are capable of producing both psychological and physical dependence with prolonged use. These types of drugs were introduced by the medical profession to the public and thence to teenagers as early as the 1930s as a "treatment" for colds and hay fever. They were later found to be "useful" for nervous disorders of one kind or another.

Teenagers in the 1950s found that they could use amphetamine pills to supply an artificially high level of pep." Hence, they became known as "pep pills." Some youngsters and adults found they could get a real "high" injecting a solution of a pill directly into the veins. Amphetamines depress the appetite, cause digestive disorders of various kinds and eventually, with continued use, malnutrition with possible respiratory and circulatory problems to follow.

The tranquilizers which were introduced in the 1950s became a favorite with physicians who were called to "treat" cases of hyperkinetic behavior. Young children and teenagers alike are daily given these poisons by school nurses and sit half-aware of reality in the classrooms of America, just so the teachers and parents do not have to come to grips with the realities of incorrect living and eating practices.

However, those teenagers whose bodies have been thus violated must come to grips with the fact that these kinds of drugs do create physical dependence and that withdrawal can be difficult, indeed.

82.2. Teen Challenge—Enlightening Statistics

The following statistics have been obtained through the kind cooperation of the Teen Challenge Program for drug and alcohol abuse, a service which was first initiated in 1958 in New York City. The statistics are in a "Services Research Report-An Evaluation of the Teen Challenge Treatment Program" as issued by the U.S. Department of Health, Education, and Welfare; Public Health Service; Alcohol, Drug Abuse, and Mental Health Administration; and the National Institute on Drug Abuse.

We thank Greg Brewer, Tucson Director of Teen Challenge for his kind cooperation.

TABLE 1

Characteristics of Entrants into Teen Challenge Program

Characteristic	% or x (N=186)
Age	24
Ethnicity:	
% Hispanic	64.0
% Black	20.4
% White	15.6
Education:	
% 9th grade	23.5
% 9-11 grades	60.9
% 12 or more grades	15.6
% Married	29.6
% Admitted under legal pressure	22.5
% Ever arrested	79.0

%Arrested for drugs	47.9
Religion:	
% Catholic	43.6
% Protestant	29.5
% Jewish	1.6
% Muslim	2.7
% Other	0.5
% None	23.1
Heroin Use:	
% Heroin use at admission	87
% Using heroin at least daily	83
Age of first heroin use	17
% Reporting hospitalization for overdose	31
Other drug use at admission:	
% Tobacco	88
% Alcohol	39
% Marijuana	37
% Other drugs	44

TABLE 2

Characteristics of Entrants into Challenge Program at Age 12

Characteristic	% (N=186)
Type of residential community:	
City of 250,000 or more	59.1
City of 50,000-200,000	10.2
City of less than 50,000	15.6
Suburb	10.2
Farm or country	4.3
Don't know	0.5
Living with:	
Both father and mother	69.4
Mother	21.0
Father	3.X
Other person	5.4
In school	97.3
Attending religious services regularly	64.0

TABLE 3

Client Outcome 1975	Induction Center Dropouts (N=70)		Training Center Dropouts (N=52)		Training Center Graduates (N=64)	
Outcome Data	Pre-Teen Challenge %	Post-Teen Challenge %	Pre-Teen Challenge %	Post-Teen Challenge %	Pre-Teen Challenge %	Post-Teen Challenge %
Heroin Use *1	90.0	18.6	78.9	1.9	89.1	4.7
Alcohol Use	32.9	51.4	36.5	30.8	51.6	17.2
Tobacco Use	91.4	82.9	90.4	63.5	82.8	21.9
Marijuana Use	44.3	48.6	26.9	15.4	37.5	12.5
Obtaining money through illegal means	-	20.0	-	3.9	-	16
Employed/in school	-	57.1	-	61.5	-	75.0
Arrests	80.0	78.6	73.1	55.8	82.8	29.7
Any schooling post-teen challenge	-	28.6	-	21.2	-	40.6
Married/Living with	41.4	57.1	30.8	61.5	23.4	70.3

Health since Teen Challenge reported as good-excellent	-	58.6	-	75.0	-	92.2
Current nervous/ emotional problems	-	18.6	-	13.5	-	12.5
Any treatment other than Teen Challenge	40.0	80.0	38.5	63.5	54.7	26.5
Reporting self as:						
Very/ Somewhat religious	58.6	88.6	30.8	75.0	26.6	87.5
Not religious	41.4	11.4	69.2	25.0	73.4	12.5
Attending religious services *2	62.9	37.1		48.0	32.8	67.2

*1 An additional 18.6% of Induction Center dropouts, 15.4% of Training Center dropouts and 7.8% of Training Center graduates were using methadone, but it is unclear whether or not this was illicitly obtained.

*2 For Pre-Teen Challenge recorded as "church member."

* Not all the statistics are given here. Those persons wishing the complete report may request same from a local Teen Challenge office or from the National Institute for Drug and Alcohol Abuse, 5600 Fishers Lane, Rockville, Maryland 20857.

The entrants into the Teen Challenge Program considered in the report were largely from the Brooklyn-New York City area (about 90%) and may not be characteristic of all areas. However, they are interesting in that they show that drug usage is found among all races, all education levels, among both married and single. Our personal research shows that drug usage is common also in persons from all economic levels, affluent, economically depressed, in city dwellers and among those who live in rural settings. It is a problem which will come to the attention of the Hygienic practitioner sooner or later in his practice and one that must be appropriately addressed by him/her.

82.3. Working with Teenagers

82.3.1. A Health Class

82.3.2. The Drugging of Children

82.3.3. We Consult Our Attorney

82.3.4. We Do the Possible

82.3.5. The Younger Set

82.3.7. Methadone and Heroin

82.3.8. The Hygienist and the Addict

82.3.9. Teen-Clean Retreats

82.3.10. Other Characteristic Disorders

82.3.11. Emotions and the Teenager

82.3.12. Peer Pressure

82.3.13. School Support

82.3.1. A Health Class

Not too long ago we were asked by a high school health teacher to address his senior class on some topic we deemed appropriate. He had become mildly interested in Natural Hygiene after attending a lecture of ours some months before and thought the concept should be introduced to his students.

We decided to present the seven steps in the evolution of pathology, a concept we have found usually well accepted by young minds.

We had considerable difficulty in locating the lecture room but, after numerous inquiries, we finally found it hidden deep in the hollow of the earth! The "health" room was actually built underground. It had no windows, and all classes were conducted under incandescent lighting. A ventilation system apparently recycled the stale air throughout the building. We learned, on inquiry, that the heating and air-conditioning units were "self-contained," the introduction of outside air being deemed unnecessary except as directed through minimal vents.

It was in this underground dungeon that lectures on health were held. The various rooms in the facility were devoted to activities as diverse as lectures and discussions on hygiene, sex, biology and so on. We silently asked of ourselves, "How can health be taught where health cannot be found?"

Since we had arrived at the lecture hall some five minutes or so before the class was to convene, we had ample opportunity to observe the about-to-be-adults as they strolled into the room. And stroll and shuffle in they did! They seemed totally oblivious to the fact that guest instructors were present and kept up their loud chatter, their calling from one end of the room to the other as friends sauntered in.

As the students took their seats, some immediately laid their heads down on their folded arms, while others just kept desk hopping or from one part of the room to another. It was as if we were invisible.

Suddenly, a rather attractive girl entered the room. Loudly, and completely without hesitation, a male voice rang out and we heard, "Hi, June! Have you made out today, yet?" No one in the class seemed to pay much attention to the question, although a few did giggle. "No," came back the girl's reply. Then the young man said, "That's OK. Meet me after class and I'll take care of that!

No one in the whole class that we could see either looked up or stopped his chatter. Apparently, this open exchange was too common to cause excitement or comment. We had to assume that this kind of public sexual encounter was the "in-thing" among this particular age group.

When the teacher arrived, the chatter, the giggling, and the squirming, continued. We observed two or three students who were actually attempting to read. They sat hunched over their books and reclined well back in their seats, not on their buttocks but apparently on some portion of their spinal column. As far as we could see, there wasn't a single straight spine among either the boys or the girls in the entire room, rather a frightening thing when one considers that these young people represent the future fathers and mothers of the coming generation. The teacher was a tall, rather well-developed, young man, but neither his presence nor ours seemed to make any impact on the students. In fact, he had to call them to attention several times before the noise began to subside and some measure of attention was gained.

Since there were some matters of immediate concern to individual members of the class, the teacher took these up first and, while he was thus engaged, we had occasion to take a good look at the seated fifty or so young people, most of whom were between seventeen and eighteen years of age and, since this particular school was in one of the more affluent neighborhoods, we assumed that all the students probably came from upper middle-class homes and that most would probably go on to colleges of their choice throughout the country to continue their education.

As we took a critical look at these teenagers, we saw no health among them. Instead, we saw curved spines housing encapsulated lungs; pimply skins, some overly flushed, some pasty in color; lack-luster hair, overly crimped in the girls and many already thinning in the boys. A lack of vitality was evident in most, so much so that they slouched in their chairs or sat with head drooped to their chests; the hyperkinetic, of which there were many, twisted and squirmed in their seats. We saw not a single person sitting erect at his desk with feet firmly planted on the floor, with head held tall, resting on a well-formed neck. And not a single person appeared intellectually curious about the topic of the day which had been previously well advertised. They seemed just to be there because this class was part of a curriculum required for graduation.

Later that day, we both commented, "Can't they SEE"! Are their teachers, administrators, their parents and physicians, their coaches and health teachers all blind? Can they not see that this is all wrong? That this is not health? These are bodies saturated with poison. This is disease, rampant with foreboding terror for the future not only of these young people but of our nation. How can we, as a nation, hope to survive when these, the children of the most affluent of our people, have so little vitality, such a void of intellectual curiosity, when they look and act as these young people look and act? We asked of ourselves, "If this is the level of wellness displayed by the children of the affluent members of society, what can be said about the children of families less economically secure?"

82.3.2. The Drugging of Children

Another time Dr. Elizabeth was to speak before a group of sophomore students, tenth graders. We were requested to meet the teacher in the nurse's office. There we found a group of about ten teenagers lined up sitting in chairs along one wall. When the nurse saw us at the door, she left the group, made her apologies to us, and said that she would be with us in a few moments. "I have to give these kids their shots," she said, and off she went. We watched in horror as she went from youngster to youngster and either gave each one a pill or an injection.

After the children had all received their poisons for the day from her reluctant hands, the nurse came back to us and commented, "I really don't like to give these kids these drugs, but their doctors have prescribed them, so I have to!" Of course, we knew why they had been prescribed, but we asked anyway. The answer came back, "Oh! They're all so hyper. The medicine settles them down."

A few weeks ago, a mother consulted us about her daughter, age 15. She said she couldn't quite put her finger on what was wrong with the girl, but something was definitely out of character. She had always been a "healthy" child, never a problem but now the girl was too quiet sometimes and yet hyper at others. Also, she appeared to "leave the planet" on occasion and was just not "with it." Sometimes, too, she was just plain "moody" and often difficult to live with, crying for no particular reason.

We suggested to the worried mother that it would be advisable to have a comprehensive blood test made. We also requested and received a diet diary for one week and a rather complete medical history which revealed the customary childhood diseases and the usual complement of drugs which had been prescribed on numerous occasions.

Dr. Robert completed the Bursuk-McCarter Bionutritional Blood Test Analysis and Profile within the week. We were both astounded and dismayed by what this report revealed. This fifteen-year-old child's body was obviously revving in high gear. Out of the 33 required test readings, at least half were above the optimal level and eight were ready to jump off the chart. We recognized the signs of luxuriant metabolism that had gotten out of hand. Everything confirmed a body well saturated with poisons of one kind or another, poisons that were rapidly wasting this girl's substance.

We immediately notified the mother that we would like to meet with her daughter alone and inquired if the girl had a boyfriend. We learned that she did indeed have a boyfriend and that they were extremely close, almost inseparable. We suggested that he come with the girl, and this was satisfactorily arranged. You see, by this time, we were convinced that there might be more here than one would normally expect, and such proved to be the case.

We met with these two teenagers with their parents' consent, but without their, parents" presence. We told the youngsters that whatever they told us would be held in the strictest confidence. What we heard on that day was a tale of unbelievable destruction of both body and mind. We have no reason to doubt the authenticity of that confidence. In fact, everything we have heard since confirms it.

When shown the blood test Analysis and Profile and, after comparing her revealing Profile with that of another reasonably healthy young person, the girl confessed that she had been on drugs since she had been about twelve years of age. She had been introduced to them by her schoolteacher father, first to marijuana, and then later to cocaine.

The girl's boyfriend, who was seventeen years of age, was a heroin addict and it was he who had introduced her to that drug, although they both said they preferred cocaine. They smoked marijuana several times a week; drank alcoholic beverages including wine, beer, and whatever they could get their hands on. They admitted to being sexually active, having intercourse almost every day in cars, in the school basement, at either his or her home, or at the home of friends when the "gang" had their "sex" parties.

We inquired how they financed their habits and were bid that the young man was a pusher, that he sold drugs to all the other kids at school When we inquired how much he made, he simply replied, "Enough! Almost all the kids are on the stuff. It's easy money!"

By this time the young people were both talkative and so we let them talk while we sat back and listened. The girl told us that her mother was divorced, had legal custody of her for 6 months a year, and worked. The nature of her employment necessitated her being out of town quite frequently. On such occasions, a friend who lived nearby would look after the girl but the looking after amounted to telephoning every evening at about 10 p.m. to ascertain if the girl was at home. If she answered the phone, it was assumed that she was "safe," even though there was no responsible adult present in the house. On such occasions, with the mother safely out of town and the neighbor several streets removed, the girl and her boyfriend made a night of it, often having their friends in for sex exchange and drugs.

When the mother was in town, the daughter simply told her trusting mother that she was going to a girlfriend's house to study and spend the night. Apparently afraid of her daughter's possible wrath, the mother never checked on her whereabouts. In truth, on many of these occasions, the daughter would be at the boyfriend's house, drinking, and taking drugs. It seemed that the young man had been an unwanted child and his parents apparently didn't care what he did, just so long as he didn't bother them and didn't get into trouble with the "law!"

This was the picture of youth that we received that day: troubled in mind, filled with junk foods, chemicalized soft drinks and drugs; victims of irregular eating, of parents who either did, not care or were too occupied with their own concerns to worry about their children's well-being; children thrown into an adult world without any conscious awareness of the consequences of their own acts; children with immature bodies engaging in sex beyond the full understanding that they might bring children into the world.

82.3.3. We Consult Our Attorney

We felt obliged to consult our attorney on this case. In this day and age when practitioners of non-orthodox schools are often under close scrutiny, we keep in pretty close touch with him. We were, of course, righteously angry at the bold neglect and actual emotional abuse inflicted/on these young people by neglectful parents and by society at large. We had, of course, been aware of the fact that teenagers were "into" drugs, but this was right in our own backyard, among "our" kind of people, not in Detroit or New York or London, but right here. We had been dismayed at learning that almost every single teenager in their peer group was using drugs, some for years. Alcohol was commonplace. No one thought any more about drinking than about going to class. Almost all smoked, either marijuana or regular cigarettes. We felt like shouting to the world, to the parents, the school authorities and to the law about the means and methods being used to push drugs on the school premises, inside and outside of the classrooms. But we listened instead to the voice of caution which, as practitioners, we felt obliged to heed.

We were told that we should and could do absolutely nothing since we had received all this information in confidence. We could not even advise the parents as to their children's health-destroying behavior and practices. Our attorney pointed out to us that the children, if they so decided, could change their testimony, and leave us vulnerable. We could prove absolutely nothing.

82.3.4. We Do the Possible

Subsequently, we met with the parents of the girl in the presence of both young people, the parents expressing a wish for the boy to be at the consultation, something we do not ordinarily consider. We presented the parents with the results of the blood test and suggested that certain remedial steps should be given immediate consideration. We divulged no confidences. Nevertheless, we did strongly suggest that the proper course of action in this case would be for both teenagers to fast and to do so immediately; that, in the girl's case at least, the need was urgent. The fasting period over, then they should begin a well-planned Hygienic program which was to include the whole spectrum of organic requisites, especially exercise. The two young people thought the idea was "neat," and agreed to follow our instructions, whereupon everybody left quite pleased with themselves.

However, there was no follow-through. We had suggested that the girl should be sent to a Hygienic retreat and, indeed, inquiries were made by the parents as to prices, possible dates, and so on. However, as so often happens with this age group, these teenagers decided to take matters into their own hands because they didn't want to be separated and the boy could not go along with her to the fasting institution. So, without consulting with us, they decided to detoxify themselves! Foolishly, their parents agreed to let them try it.

Probably our students are way ahead of us in our story. Their fasting lasted one day! In that short a time, they began to experience so much pain, diarrhea and vomiting that they had to break the fast. They even began to hallucinate! The mother of the girl became so alarmed at the course of events that she refused all further advice.

We must assume, therefore, that both of these young people are still claiming that their parents, their teachers and all of us adults don't "dig it." Since we have not heard to the contrary, we must also assume that both teenagers are still confirmed drug users and that their bodies are becoming ever more saturated with poisons with every passing day. We know that the day of reckoning will come and that it will be a sad day, indeed, for all concerned, but especially for them.

82.3.5. The Younger Set

We bring you still a third example because it presents a situation which is somewhat similar, but also different, both in family involvement and in its legal ramifications.

A Hygienic mother brought her 13-year-old son to us. The boy lacked coordination. He could see a ball or other object clearly enough when it was coming toward him, but he could not control his muscles well enough to catch it. He was unable to maintain a proper balance when riding a bicycle, often bumping into his mother when he accompanied her on her morning rides.

The young lad's face was pimply, many of the sores oozing pus. We learned on questioning him that he was hooked on sugared foods—ice creams, chocolate candies, cakes, cokes, and other drugged foods. He had an almost insatiable craving for peanut butter and jelly sandwiches.

Stu was a very pleasant child, extremely good-looking if one looked behind the acne and, strangely, did not appear to be hyperkinetic. In fact, he was a rather quiet lad. The pimples, of course, betrayed a highly toxic inner state and it had been these and his lack of muscle coordination that had prompted his mother to bring him to us.

The father in this family was a very physical person. He liked football and other contact sports. The boy, however, seemed to take more after his mother than the father, being rather slight for his age and, as we have said, a quiet sort. However, Stu did want to please his father and had ambitions of becoming a professional soccer player. He said that he knew he was too small to play either football or basketball but thought he could qualify as a soccer player if he could just get his muscles under control. It seems the father was always after his son to "shape up" and be a "man."

Since the boy was well motivated, we set up a program which included a diet more Hygienic than his customary fare but one not so strict as to turn him completely off. The family physician cooperated with us and arranged an appointment for the boy with a physical therapist who designed an exercise program geared to his specific needs. The mother happily endorsed both programs as did the boy.

Apparently, Stu cooperated quite well for a time and showed considerable improvement but, some four years later, we were again contacted by the mother who said she had a "problem." Her son was now a young man, some 17 years of age, and was about ready to be graduated from high school. It seems that he had informed his mother that, at that time, he would be "taking off!"

We decided to meet the mother by herself before tackling the problem, to see if, indeed, it was soluble at this late stage. A very revealing story was hesitatingly imparted to us by the mother. It seems that, in the intervening years since we had last met, the husband and wife had slowly grown apart and were now totally estranged, coming, and going in the same house, but as strangers.

The young man, Stu, with the cooperation of his father was busy growing marijuana in the back yard! Stu harvested the weed and then sold it to his peers "at school." We later learned that Stu was actively selling the stuff at the local junior high school and that business was quite brisk, the demand steady. Again, we heard the story, "It's such easy money!"

We learned that both father and son were smoking marijuana and that, over the weekends, Stu, with is father's consent, had "parties" for his school "buddies," both male and female, in the family home.

All we could do in this case was to point out to the mother that both she and her husband were not only contributing to the delinquency of a minor child by consenting to illicit activities but also helping to destroy other parents' children.

It seems that the mother had become extremely weak-willed due to the fact that her husband, in order to protect his easy money, had actually used physical violence on her as a means of compelling her silence. We pointed out to her that because she did not actively protest and even go so far as to destroy the plantings or to forbid the drug parties in her house, that she could not be excused of culpability if the matter were brought to the attention of the authorities. We advised the woman to seek the advice of an attorney and to consult with a marriage counselor.

Again, we went back to our attorney and, as before, he pointed out that we were boxed into a corner. We could not divulge the confidence of consultation. He went on to make a further point. In this case, whatever knowledge we had was based solely on hearsay and, again lacking proof, we could make ourselves vulnerable to a legal suit for considerable damages if a false arrest followed our giving information to the police.

82.3.7. Methadone and Heroin

This last case was somewhat more successful. The client, a young man aged 19, was referred to us by a counselor at a local hospital who had heard about our work from a staff member at the hospital who had himself been a former client.

Jim had turned himself into the hospital admitting to heroin addiction. He was currently on methadone, a supposedly nonaddictive drug which is used as a "substitute" for heroin by physicians. Jim was a farmer who lived on a ranch near the Mexican border. It was easy for him to get all the heroin he wanted but he wanted desperately to get "clean" of all drugs and so willingly came to our office.

We learned that Jim's main interest was growing fruit trees and vegetables and said his farm was beautiful to behold. He was fully aware of the dangers involved in his continued use of heroin. We further briefed him on the systemic damage possible when any drug, even methadone, is used. Jim listened intently and being a highly-intelligent person, he agreed that no matter the cost, he would make valiant attempt to avoid all drugs but would do so on a "step-down" program since he had the responsibility for e care of an invalid mother and the farm and felt that he could not, at this time at least, enter a fasting institution.

We devised a program for Jim which included the Extended Detoxification Plan as given in Lesson 63 on "Hair", but the time intervals were expanded. At the same time, with the hospital's approval, Jim began to reduce the methadone intake—very gradually. He willingly cooperated with an 80% raw food diet since he could use all his own home-grown produce of which he was very proud. This approach was successful to the extent that the methadone dosage was cut in half within a relatively short time.

Jim is still fighting to win and we think he will soon approach his goal of once again being "clean!"

82.3.8. The Hygienist and the Addict

Addiction to any drug is amenable to fasting. The body saturated with poisons of any kind, including nicotine, heroin, marijuana, cocaine and all the mood-altering drugs, will give up its drugs while on a fast. The so-called "Withdrawal" symptoms of the drug addict are often very severe and include cramps, nausea, "spacing out," chills, violent sweating's, and others of lesser importance. The first few days are the most difficult from all accounts we have read, with symptoms continuing but lessening in intensity and usually concluding within a two-week period.

In drug addiction it is important to fast until the return hunger, the classic signal that the body fluids are clean." However, if the addiction has covered a period of some years, it may prove necessary for the once-addict to repeat the fast periodically, at least for from 10 days to two weeks simply because the "weakness," the tendency to yearn for the addicting poison, often remains.

Many will express willingness and a desire to become cleansed of drugs but only relatively few will be successful in following through. This is largely due to lack of willpower and/or sufficient motivation. One can preach all one wants to about the evils of drug usage. These are all well known to the addict. There has to be a higher motivation to keep him on his cleansing program and that is often difficult to find.

The National Courier of July 9, 1976, in an article by Bill Pennewill, claims that Teen Challenge (see previous reference) is the best drug rehabilitation program around. It apparently has a 70 percent "cure" rate. Its emphasis is on the spiritual and they encourage those who seek their help to become "born-again" Christians. No changes are made in their dietary practices except perhaps to avoid obvious "junk" foods.

Teen Challenge, like Natural Hygiene, requires a "tough, cold-turkey approach." Subjects just stop using drugs from the moment they seek the help of Teen Challenge.

The fasting approach recommended by Natural Hygienists has not as yet been properly promoted by those of us in Natural Hygiene. If it were more widely used, its success rate would approximate 100% and fewer former addicts would revert. Additionally, cleansing of the body fluids of drugs would occur much more completely and to rapidly than by any other method. Forty-three percent of those who get off drugs through Teen Challenge become addicted again. After a prolonged total fast, the use of any drug makes the taker on first use so violently sick that more often than not, he never tries a second time!

Obviously, those persons who "get into" drugs do so for a variety of reasons: peer pressure, emotional problems of one kind or another, undiagnosed illness, and so on. Following cleansing of the system by whatever means, the former addict requires help to solve the problems or situations which first caused him to use drugs. We suggest that professional counseling can be very useful. Teenagers need support even more than adult addicts. They should be encouraged to join groups of other like-minded teens. Probably this is a major reason for the proven success record of Teen Challenge, and it might be helpful to refer prospective clients to such an organization.

In our discussion we have, from time to time, put forth some signs that may indicate addiction of one kind of another, such signs as nervousness, hysteria, hyperkinetic behavior, drowsiness, inattention, looking away with reluctance to look directly at the practitioner, and other typical symptoms. When these are observed, it may be useful to suggest a private meeting with the young person. On ascertaining the true situation, then the practitioner must present the facts of Hygiene to his young client, telling him something about the realities of organic existence. He must point out that there are three avenues open and only three: 1. Continuing his present practice with the certainty that his life will either come to an abrupt end through overdosing or will be extended for an indefinite time with increasingly high dosages required and an uncertain future which will include an unknown number of afflictions of one kind or another, including but not limited to, brain and neural damage, atherosclerosis, malnutrition, kidney and liver disorders, many extremely painful, plus cancer; 2. An Extended Detoxification Program which is admittedly seldom successful in its entirety due mainly to lack of will power; and 3. Total Fasting, always at a fasting institution under the guidance of a practitioner experienced in fasting addicts, this to be followed by a carefully worked out regimen including a diet of raw fruits plus a few vegetables and nuts.

82.3.9. Teen-Clean Retreats

The problem of teenage drug abuse is admittedly out of hand. As we have already commented, Hygienists can play a constructive role in remedying this situation, not only through individual counseling, by means of lectures and by fostering public awareness programs but, in an even more meaningful way, by opening what we like to call Hygienic Teen-Clean Retreats where teenage addicts, regardless of the type of addiction, can come either to fast and/or to learn about how the full application of Hygienic principles in their lives which could produce dramatic results, positive results which could change their present empty lives into a future filled with promise.

We envisage the formation of nonprofit organizations complete with certain tax advantages at strategic places throughout the country, these expressly designed for the rehabilitation of America's youth so that the America of tomorrow can survive. Teen Clean Retreats, located in strategic areas and having the financial support of able adults, can prove to be competent performers in this field simply because it has been well demonstrated that the full application of the principles of Natural Hygiene can be 100% successful, even in difficult cases!

82.3.10. Other Characteristic Disorders

In our next Lesson, Number 83, we take a journey through an average lifespan, that of a person unfamiliar with the basic principles of Life Science. The journey is divided into nine stages, one of which covers the period from age 10 to age 20—the years during which the child becomes the adult—or almost an adult!

Since we will be reviewing the disorders so frequently observed at this stage in life at that time, we will simply comment there that the characteristic acute diseases of childhood become less frequently experienced generally after puberty, due (as Hygienists well know) to the fact that wrong habits have so dissipated the life force in this short a time that not sufficient vitality exists among many to power the exodus of a rapidly soaring toxicosis.

Thus, it is that we begin to see more serious conditions develop, some of these becoming chronic even at this early period in the life course. Inevitably in such cases, the life span is doomed to be seriously curtailed and, more often than not, the life span that remains, brief as it well may be, will be one filled with pain and suffering.

The acute conditions which do continue into the teen years are readily amenable to Hygienic care. We refer to diseases of the respiratory tract, the various catarrhal involvements; also, to those that afflict the gastrointestinal tract, such as colitis, ulcers, and so on; to the rheumatic pains wrongly associated with growth; to the bane of teens, troubling acne and other disfiguring and annoying skin eruptions. Usually, a few days, a week at most, of fasting followed by a carefully controlled diet will be sufficient to alleviate the conditions that trouble the young person, provided, of course, that the Hygienic regime is always coupled with constructive pursuits, including exercise.

Conditions associated with the emerging sexual awareness may prove more obstinate but not necessarily so. Several shorter fasts, for example, may be required to correct the female PMS Syndrome, the discomforts experienced by so many young girls prior to the menstrual period, discomforts which, if allowed to continue and worsen, may lead to emotional problems with the married scene.

82.3.11. Emotions and the Teenager

The teenage years are the years of maturing, of puberty and adolescence, and it is during these years that two general problems are usually presented: 1. Problems associated with sexual maturity, and 2. the many difficulties experienced relating to the approach to adulthood, independence, and self-assertiveness.

In order to successfully make the transition from childhood to full adulthood, teens need education, guidance and suitable role models to look up to and, possibly, even emulate. Without these factors and influences being available, many teenagers will flounder in their confusion, often becoming overwhelmed by fears, anxieties, worries and concerns.

These are the teens who are easily swayed and led into anti-social practices of minor and major dimensions.

Were it possible to measure all the impairment and inhibitions of systemic function caused by long-sustained deep emotions such as we have enumerated, we adults might be appalled at the amount of harm done to growing youth by our lack of awareness. It has long been known to Hygienists, especially since the pronouncements of J.H. Tilden, M.D., on the subject, that the maintenance of poise is one of the greatest conservators of nerve energy known and that fear is the greatest nerve energy annihilator of which we have any knowledge.

Many teenagers are afraid, afraid of the unknown world out there, afraid because they lack parental understanding, afraid because they lack a suitable male role model in a family split by divorce or in a family where the parents both work and there is no one immediately available to listen to and explain away frightening situations.

Young people become overly anxious when parents and/or others expect more from them than they are or ever will be capable of producing: the football-lover father who insists that his rather frail son participate actively in contact sports; the mother who failed herself to become the greatest dancer of her generation who pushes her young daughter into dance classes when the child has the secret ambition to become a classic pianist or to paint, or perhaps even to become a fine writer.

Intense feelings produce physiological changes which stimulate certain reactions such as either an accelerated or a retarded pulse rate, an increased or diminished endocrine hormonal secretive action which directly influences all cellular metabolism and/ or changes in body temperature.

It is well for us to understand that there are three primary emotions that are especially evident in the teen years: love, fear, and anger. Because of their youth and vitality, teen responses are usually more or less immediate—they often seem to come in a flash, almost for no reason. This is why so many adults have difficulty "understanding" the members of this age group. But we should comprehend that these fierce responses are in proportion to the individual's maturity. Handling our emotions is a learned experience.

Of importance to the Hygienist is the proven fact that when the fluids of the body have been cleansed, emotional control tends to improve. The energy forces of the body are thus directed toward intelligently coping with problem situations rather than buckling under to them either by expressing rage or by simply giving up.

Young people need to be given the opportunity to be successful in small projects, to be allowed to grow into more difficult challenges. Throwing an impossible at a teenager and then expecting perfection can so confuse a young person as to drive him to "show you!" with running away, rebellion, visible disease symptoms and possibly even suicide. Small successes, on the other hand, encourage greater performance because being successful provides pleasurable emotional responses, a more correct type of systemic stimulation.

All disorders which relate to the sexual maturation of the body become of paramount importance during the teen time-frame: anything which influences the appearance of the body or any single part of the body, such as the genitals in the male and the formation of the breasts in the female. If the sexual organs and the body as a whole mature and develop in size normally, the teen is generally happy provided, of course, that all other influencing factors are likewise normal. But, everything else in the teen's environment can be of the highest and most constructive order with some deficiency sex-wise and the teenager will be thrust into deep despair.

When plagued by emotional troubles, the health of the teenager, indeed, that of all humans, will diminish. The digestive system gives immediate response to emotional unrest and the stomach is generally the first organ to register protest. Digestion is inhibited; glandular secretion by all secreting glands can be either impaired or completely stopped. Even the muscular motions of the gastrointestinal tract can be suspended, sometimes for hours during severe emotional travail. This last is especially prevalent among badly enervated individuals with the result that ingested food simply lies in situ within the confines of the alimentary canal and is there subject to fermentation and putrefaction. Next to overeating and incorrect eating, mental influences cause most of the digestive upsets from which so many teenagers suffer.

The functional impairments caused by overeating, incorrect eating, and a wide variety of emotional disturbances eventually result in toxemic crises of one kind or another, some of which we have listed. If the causes are allowed to continue, organic changes will follow in due course, these according to inherited weaknesses and the intensity and nature of the toxic debris.

In working with teenagers, the practitioner must recognize that whatever the present condition may be that brings the youth to your office, it has been caused and that you, working with the parents or other responsible person and he teenager himself, must all do your best, first to ascertain that single cause or multiple causes and then either to remove it (them) completely or to reduce the impact.

Once cause has been ascertained and appropriately dealt with, then a workable plan of action should be presented to all concerned. This plan should provide for successful achievements to follow. For example, suppose the young man or woman is 50 pounds overweight and is greatly troubled by this. The practitioner must explain just how the obesity will be addressed and present reasonable goals to be achieved.

Young women can be driven to the point of hysteria by a bad complexion or drab looking hair. Young men who are acne-prone can be withdrawn and difficult to deal with. The Hygienist can point with pride to the fact that no one has better looking and finer-grained complexions and/or more luxuriant shiny hair than Hygienists. The fact that you have a plan of action to bring miraculous changes in a young person's appearance can often prove highly motivating.

Suppose the immediate problem is a lack of a suitable role model, either male or female. Then, group participation under the able direction of a well-motivated and suitable adult should be recommended. Group activity should always be directed toward an area of interest to the teenager himself, not to one of interest to someone else as, for example, an overly zealous parent.

Sometimes parents don't listen to their growing children, being overly concerned about economic and other problems affecting the family. Behavior modification needs to be encouraged in such cases. A first step is actually setting out both a time and a place for parent(s) to sit down and meet with the teenager for the purposes of listening, discussing and advising, all without condemnation, shock or criticism. In the absence of a willing parent, it may be necessary for the practitioner to become the confidant.

We remember well one 16-year-old girl who was brought to our attention because of severe digestive cramps, diarrhea, and so on. Her diet appeared to be above average. She was an excellent student in school and appeared to get along well with everybody. A previous physical examination had revealed nothing apparent to cause such a condition. We decided to have a confidential talk with the girl. We knew, of course, that her father was a minister representing a very strict fundamentalist group. The girl apparently had no quarrel whatsoever with the precepts expounded by her religious faith. However, we learned that recently a conflict had arisen between her and her parents with regard to the showing of a very fine movie which her whole biology class along with their teacher had been invited to attend.

The girls' parents had forbidden her to attend. This fact had proved a terrible blow to her pride. She was to be the only one in the whole lass who would not be present at the theater party. The particular movie was a fine clean presentation. Several teachers were to accompany the group and they would all be taken to and from the theater in the school bus. Neither we nor the girl could find a single valid reason for her not to attend the showing.

However, we presented her with some reasons we felt she shouldn't have to go to the movie. 1. Her parents felt obliged to set standards for their parishioners. 2. They obviously loved her and wanted only the best for her, 3. That so long as she was living with her parents she was in no position to force her will upon them, 4. She was presently unable to fend for herself, 5. In the future, when she was ready for college, it would be her loving parents who would continue to provide for her, and, 6. In return for all the financial support and loving care, she actually was being called upon to do a very simple thing, that being not to watch a few hours of flickering images pass across a screen, images that would be gone from memory within a few days or weeks at most.

We talked on and on that afternoon. We listened, we conversed. That was all that was necessary. Shortly thereafter, all the digestive troubles vanished like magic. Emotional poise had been restored.

All concerned within the family should be encouraged to develop family feelings of togetherness, of mutual understanding of concerns of both parents and child; feelings of joy, pleasantness, satisfaction and, most of all, of a shared love. In other words, they should be encouraged to explore the life adventure together, not separated by miles of misunderstandings.

We encourage new practitioners to study behavior modification techniques. We all need to learn how better to encourage our clients to take "baby steps," to accomplish those small successes which can lead to meaningful emotional development and stability, a state highly conducive to total well-being.

We should at all times remember that teenagers must have their vital needs appropriately met, such as suitable food, clothing and a friendly environment but, for them to reach their full health potential, we must be aware of the fact that they must also have their non-vital needs met as completely as existing circumstances warrant. Furthermore, if the present circumstances are unfavorable, then intelligent steps should be considered in the light of the possible to change them to the extent that they, will more favorably meet the needs of the maturing young man or woman.

82.3.12. Peer Pressure

In our discussion we have not directly addressed the subject of peer pressure. Since it is more often than not more powerful in the daily life of the youth of today than all the family's needs, desires and aspirations combined, it is important that this subject be considered, if only briefly.

Accordingly, when a youth has been brought to your office with any kind of physical or emotional problem which is adversely affecting his health, and peer pressure has been instrumental in causing the problem (as was true in the case of the minister's daughter), then the interview must be carried out in planned sequence.

First, the youth must be able to admit that he has a problem which needs to be solved. Second, that he should not be swayed by his peers when he knows he has the right solution to his problem; third, that the problem, if allowed to continue, will prove detrimental to him both now and probably also in the future; fourth, the problem must be identified and this as precisely as possible fifth, he must be convinced by the evidence that the problem is solvable and that you, his friend and practitioner, have the knowledge of how to solve the problem and that you will show him the ways and means whereby he can overcome the problem.

When the above steps have been taken, then the young person should be shown, by means of a diagram, that he is now HERE, of course, being in his present unfortunate and unhappy state, a condition of mind and/or body which restricts his forward progress, especially his social and interpersonal relationships with his peers of the opposite sex. A list of negatives should be set forth for due consideration.

Once the negatives have been addressed, then the positive potential should be presented, the going from HERE to THERE, there representing a time and place in which the troubling condition will have been entirely removed and the way laid open before the youth for whatever personal ambition or desires that s/he may have deep within the innermost self to be capable of fulfillment. This is the time to express and set forth the "Positivity's" which will challenge your young client.

The next step follows logically in sequence. The young client should then be asked, "What will you GIVE, what will you be willing to do, to reach the THERE in your life? To open up the doors that are now closed to you? Will you do THIS, and THIS, and perhaps even THAT?

In proper motivation lies the key to success. This kind of role-playing on paper can often overcome adverse and contrary peer pressure, provided the young person receives kindly and understanding support not only from the practitioner but also from the family. We must convince the teenager that he must do his own thing, not what the crowd wants!

82.3.13. School Support

While we have many quarrels with the public school system, sometimes support in certain difficult areas can be obtained through working with school counselors as, for example, when the teenager's interests lie in a definite direction, say in the arts, or in music, or in some particular kind of physical activity.

As a part of their extracurricular offerings, schools quite often provide a wide range of club activities: art clubs, bands, and orchestras, singing groups, newspapers, theatre groups and others. The counselor can often direct the student to activities with plenty of opportunities so that the student can enjoy success and the activities themselves.

When alerted to specific needs or desires of a student as for example, the yearning of a now spindly lad to develop his muscles, a physical education coach can often provide splendid advice. Teenage barbell sets are now available suitable for young people, girls, and boys, with less than average frames. They cost less than $20 and often are accompanied by an excellent instruction booklet. Sometimes this is all that is required to change tears into radiant smiles of determination.

We suggest that you explore what the schools in your area have to offer. They may provide just what you may need at some future time when you may be called upon to counsel a difficult emotional problem which adversely affects the health of a young client.

82.4. Questions & Answers

My 15-year-old son is sullen and depressed. His mother and I have just about reached the end of our patience. We are thinking of handing him over to the authorities. We have always tried to give him the best of everything but now we are losing our minds over this boy. His behavior is affecting his mother's health, too. Do you have any suggestions for us?

Do you think your wife's health would be any better if she were worried about where her son was and who was taking care of him or wondering if he were in trouble somewhere without any loving member of his family present to whom he might turn for advice or comfort? Again, let me reiterate. A healthy person is a happy person. Your son is sick, and this condition doesn't help his mind. Your son is emotionally troubled by inner hurts, by his toxic condition. You need to set up channels of communication with him, not shunt him off to some strange environment with strangers as companions. Don't ask "Why?" of him, but rather ask "What?" What can we do for you? And "How?" How can we help you to obtain your goals? Not ours, but yours? Then, begin to improve your family's eating habits, slowly if you must; immediately, if that is possible. Get interested in what he's doing or wants to do. Communicate! But, let HIM do most of the talking. Listen! Most teenagers complain that their parents don't listen to them. Let him open up his thoughts, his ideas, his heart to someone he knows really cares about him. That could be the beginning of a beautiful relationship between you and your son. But, most important of all, see to his nutrition. Get his body cleaned out and he should be just fine!

My daughter is 16. She has had asthma ever since she was 12 years of age. She has been to many doctors. They all just give her drugs, and they haven't helped at all. She just seems to be getting worse all the time. She is so unhappy. Can Life Science help her?

Indeed, it can! The full application of the principles and practices embodied in the science of life can. Your daughter's body is filled with poisons, and these are what is causing your daughter's unfortunate condition. I imagine your daughter had many colds as a youngster and probably experienced many healing crises in the form of some of the familiar "childhood diseases." She was probably vaccinated, too, perhaps several times. I see you are nodding your head. Let me tell you about a 17-year-old girl who was brought to our office by her parents. She also had been kept on various medications. In fact, longer than your daughter, because she had received her first dosing when she was a year-and-a-half old and, up to the day she first came to us, she had continued faithfully taking her pills every single day! During all this time, this girl had never been able to play with a puppy or cuddle a kitten. She had never been able to play ball or run with the other "children on the playground. Now, here she was, in her first year at college. She was still unable to be "one of the gang." Instead, she had to watch what she did and with whom she did it. She had to be careful where she went, too, because of her numerous "allergies." And, above all, she had to be careful to take her pills.

We presented to this girl and her parents the solution to her unfortunate condition: a complete Hygienic program which included a 100% raw diet of fruits, a few vegetables with occasional small amounts of nuts and seeds plus, of course, sunbathing, more rest and sleep, walking, etc. We asked the girl if she would be willing to give up her present haphazard way of eating for this new adventure in good eating so that she would have complete freedom from asthmatic "attacks" and her "allergies." We told her to take her time making up her mind, that this was an important decision and that the changes we were suggesting, this new way of living, would be for the rest of her life, from now on, not just for the next few weeks. The parents listened carefully to us and wisely kept silent, knowing full well that this had to be their daughter's decision. The girl thought it over—the time seemed long to us as we waited anxiously but quietly for her decision. Finally, she nodded her head. She was willing!

Three years have come and gone. Today this young woman has just about forgotten all about her asthma. She is no longer chained to her medications. Not too long ago, she brought her fiancé here to the ranch for us to meet. They are both into jogging, and the young man is learning all about Natural Hygiene. They have great plans for the future, including a family of no asthmatic babies! Yes! Your daughter can be helped, but it will take three things: 1. Knowledge of what to do, 2. Knowledge of how to do it, and 3. The DOING! We can impart to you all the knowledge you will need but it will be up to your daughter to complete the job. And you, her parents, can support her in the doing!

My son is 16. I know he is intelligent, but he is difficult to understand. His grades are terrible, his face is pimply, and he has very few friends. If he doesn't shape up soon, I don't know what will become of him. I want him to go on to the college where his mother and I went, but he'll never make the grade at this rate. Can you help us reach him?

I think so. The chances are that your son's moodiness, his poor grades, his lack of friends and his pimples are all caused by the same thing: a toxic condition of the body. The ideal thing would be to start out with a fast but, in his present state of mind, this might not be possible. I doubt if you'd get much cooperation from him. So, clean out the refrigerator and cupboards of all the junk foods—and I do mean ALL. Your wife can easily learn how to make delectable treats for him and his friends from natural fruits. She can easily learn, too, how to serve well-combined and more wholesome foods and perhaps you can, too! Make this a family project. Keep lots of fruit on hand. And nuts and sunflower seeds. If there's no junk food lying around, children will eat whatever is handy and they'll really learn to like fruit and vegetables, even if they won't admit it—out loud. Keep a plate of raw vegetables in the refrigerator, bits of carrots, celery, broccoli, etc. Teenagers will grab these, too, when they are hungry, and teenagers always seem to be hungry! I can almost guarantee that if you follow my advice, in about three months, or even less, he'll stop objecting to such "far-out" foods because, he secretly will have learned to like them! You'll find that his whole body, including his mind, will improve and his lethargy will disappear, as will the pimples.

You can help to motivate him in other ways, too. Find out what he wants out of life if he knows. If he won't cooperate, then it would seem you and your wife will have no other alternative than to take some "baby steps" but make these a family affair. Everybody in the family should participate. Make little changes at first, major changes as you and he adjust to them. Some suggestions. Perhaps you and your son can take up weightlifting. Compete with your son to see how fast you progress. Take him jogging with you and invite his pals to join you on the trip and for a watermelon feast afterwards. Get your wife into the act, too. The first thing you know, you'll all have stars in your eyes! Don't expect this all to be an easy trip, either for him, or for you and your wife. Just remember that the world can be terribly confusing place for teenagers. Their bodies are in a state of flux. One moment they are little children wanting to be held and comforted by their mother or father; the next, they are grown-ups struggling to make decisions about matters of vital importance to them. When young people have problems, but don't have a sufficient amount of knowledge to enable them to make judgmental decisions, then you, their parents, must become their mentor as well as their example. And, if they lack willpower and the ability to discipline themselves, then you must supply both the willpower and the discipline. They may not like it at the moment, but they'll respect you now and thank you for your efforts in their behalf as they grow older. But all this must be done without censure and in a kindly, loving manner. Communicate and explain the why's. It will help them immensely with their doing!

I am 19. I have stomach problems all the time it seems, no matter what I eat. I've been to one doctor after another and to several specialists. They tell me I don't have an ulcer, just a sensitive stomach. I take their pills and a lot of vitamins on my own, but I still have problems. I have a lot of diarrhea and cramps, too. I'm in my first year at college now and this condition is affecting my grades and my social life. Do you have any suggestions?

I sure do! Learn what foods you are physiologically designed to eat and then eat them! Learn about the kinds of food to which your body is best adapted and then learn how to combine those foods, when to eat them and how much and you'll soon find that your stomach will respond in perfect peace! There are many fine books on the subject. Stay after the class and we'll recommend a few but start with Dr. Shelton's Food Combining Made Easy. Applying the principles, you will learn in that little book should end your troubles.

Note: Shortly after the above exchange, this young man informed us that he felt "Just fine!" He enrolled in a course of study which taught Hygienic principles of eating and living. He says that getting into "people food" and taking this course changed his whole life around. All this happened just four years ago. We still hear from this young man quite regularly, even though his work calls for him to travel throughout the world. This "remembering" on the part of our students and clients is one of the more, important rewards of being a Hygienic practitioner!

Article #1: 57% of Teens Flunk Fitness Tests by Mike Feinsilber, A.P.

Fewer than half the youngsters in America are able to meet physical-fitness standards that should be attainable by the average healthy youngster, a study of test results showed yesterday.

Moreover, in some categories, the average older American teenager can't perform as well as he or she could at an earlier age, the analysis said.

For example, the average 15-year-old boy takes 13.3. seconds to sprint 100 yards while his 14-year-old counterpart can do it in 12.6. seconds. The typical 17-year-old girl can do only 38 modified pushups in two minutes, compared with 43 performed by an average 12-year-old girl.

Dr. Wynn F. Updyke, associate dean for graduate studies at Indiana University's School of Health, Physical Education and Recreation, attributed the fallout or leveling off after age 14 to the fact that many schools drop compulsory gym and physical education after the eighth grade.

The findings were based on a random sampling of 7,600 youngsters, taken from tests given tour million children during the last two school years.

The physical-fitness testing program is sponsored by the Amateur Athletic Union with underwriting from Nabisco Brands, Inc. Updyke said in future years the results would show whether American youngsters are becoming more or less physically fit.

"Although the basic standards are designed to be attainable by the average healthy youngster in each age and sex group, only 43 percent of participants were able to achieve them during the 1979-80 and 1980-81 academic years," according to a summary of the study.

Updyke said there were no significant differences in test results by geographic region and the scores in 1980-81 were no better or worse than those the previous year.

Updyke said the standards for what the average healthy youngster should be able to do in tests were based on AAU testing that goes back 39 years.

The results show that at age 14, the average boy does 43 bent-knee sit-ups in a minute, 38 pushups in two minutes, makes a 6-foot-3-inch standing long jump and a 3-foot-10-inch high jump, runs a mile in 9 minutes, 37 seconds and sprints 100 yards in

14.7. seconds.

Article #2: Beauty by Dr. Herbert M. Shelton

Hygiene of Beauty

Hygiene of Beauty

If there is any truth in the recapitulation hypothesis of the evolutionists, certainly the predominance of beauty in the young indicates that, primitively, the race was beautiful. Only as the child merges into adolescence and the adolescent merges into maturity do the evidences of his primitive beauty give way to the ugliness (deformity) that has overtaken the race. We watch a feature, or several features gradually become faulty and become more and more exaggerated until positive ugliness is produced. A nose remains flat or becomes too prominent; the cheek bones are sunken or too prominent; the chin either fails to develop or develops too much; the mouth becomes awry, the nose develops lopsidedly; the breasts either fail to develop normally or they become too large; spinal curvature shows up, one leg is longer than the other; defective vision or defective hearing develops.

Not all of these defects are due to heredity. Some are positively the outgrowths of faulty nutrition; others are the result of faulty use of the body, or a lack of exercise, sunshine, and other causes of disease. Failure of breast development is evidence of endocrine deficiency and this is probably most often due to nutritional inadequacies. Large, pendulous breasts represent the accumulation of fat in the breasts, and this grows out of food excesses. Heavy hips, heavy breasts and bulging abdomen are three of the most common figure faults of women and these represent physical indolence and nutritive redundancy. The woman who develops a moustache or a beard may, in most cases, perhaps rightly blame this development, not upon her ancestors, but. upon her own endocrine deficiencies growing out of her own wrong ways of life. Ugliness grows as much out of our unHygienic way of life as out of our dysgenic mating.

These deformities and defects cannot be corrected by any external applications. Paints and powders, nylons and silks, jewels, and showy objects of various sorts, are all vain and useless so far as the real beautification of the person is concerned. This object can be accomplished only by what Trail called the "cosmetics of the heart and daily life." He advised: "purify and elevate, and harmonize the affections, live nobly, justly, and generously, and observe all the physiological laws that govern the health of the body, and you will need no other cosmetics." So long as we attempt to substitute make-up and grooming for observance of the laws that govern life, we cannot hope to make any real progress towards genuine beauty. Drugs and operations do not remove the causes of ugliness; hence they can be of no value.

There are various reasons for associating ugliness with biological "inferiority;" the term "ugly" can also be understood, in its relations to plants, animals and man as meaning biologically abnormal and unfit. Lack of beauty can result from a lack of good health in the part and in the whole organism. Deformity of the lower limbs can indicate lack of health in the locomotive system; a bad complexion indicates no less a lack in the vital system. The highest degree of physiological excellence requires symmetry and coordination in every part, mirroring a wholesome balance of capacities. Deformities, deficiencies, and superfluities are not only incompatible with beauty, but with high efficiency in function.

Article #3: Living a Happy Life by F. Alexander Magoun

Not every gifted adolescent grows into an emotionally mature adult with a valid sense of who he is, or of his ability to live a happy productive life. Some wilt under an emotional blight which has nothing to do with economic status, social position, or education.

The wise youngster, with an eye on the long future, thoughtfully examines his aptitudes and his potentialities. He neither overestimates nor underestimates them. The one will lead to bitter disillusionment, the other to tragic, waste. As Frederick Karl says, each of us is born with a package, and we must discover with insight and clarity what the package contains before we can use its contents effectively.

Most young people expect either too much or too little in this world. To make it worse, they expect it too soon. We need time and patience to find ourselves and to reach our expectations achievement can be less at thirty-five than was hoped for and more at sixty than was anticipated.

In the rootless conditions of our industrial civilization, it is often difficult for a young person to determine where he is headed. He looks forward to success in business and love, but with no real criteria save the questionable ones of money, romance, authority (approached from the point of view of power instead of responsibility), prestige, and security. He has little realization of how life gets interfered with by the flux of fortune, unexpected death, economic upset, competition, loss of job, or the sudden duty to assume the obligations of a formidable task. The young people of today, seek what Harold Lasswell describes as "security, income, and deference." Fewer of them are looking for what my generation called opportunity. Nevertheless, like us, what they want more than anything else is happiness.

Youth has such obvious assets as vigor, curiosity, enthusiasm, anticipation, light heartedness, romance. There are also grave disadvantages, such as having to decide what to do for a living or whom to marry, without possessing the background wisdom of long experience.

The future is by no means entirely in our own hands. What we do about it is. To be able to stand up under adversity is largely to be able to keep our perspective, our courage, our faith in the future as worth living.

Article #4: Wit, Wisdom and Willpower by Edwin Flatto, N.D., D.O.

Once upon a time there was a wise man sitting on top of a mountain meditating over a jug of water. A villager, observing him, inquired of the Sage: "Tell me, what is the secret of your wisdom?"

The learned man replied, "I fast, meditate and sip this water when I am thirsty." The villager implored him: "Please, I must have some of that water... name your price!"

Reluctantly the pundit agreed to sell him a pitcherful of water for a piece of gold.

After paying the price the villager eagerly gulped down the water. A few moments later, upon reflecting over the transaction, the naive one complained to the sage, "Why did I have to pay for this water when I could have gone directly to the spring and obtained it for nothing?"

"See!" exclaimed the wise one triumphantly, "you're getting smarter already!"

Wisdom has been a quality most sought after throughout the ages, and fasting has long been one of the tools used to help acquire it. However, the principle underlying purpose of fasting is the development of self-discipline.

Nevertheless, few of us are willing to recognize the importance of developing this quality. Since time immemorial, wise men have constantly advocated employing this power as the only honest solution to many of our most serious problems. And the fools have never paid heed.

C.J. Van Fleet, in his provocative book, Conquest of the Serpent, shows that, throughout legend and folklore, the serpent or dragon has always symbolized lust. The famous allegory, St. George, and the Dragon, for example, portrays the seemingly invincible fire-breathing dragon as the destroyer of humanity. St. George, however, possesses a miraculous shining sword which alone can slay the dragon. The sword represents willpower and as soon as St. George learns to use it, the dragon of lust is doomed.

Self-discipline is like physical strength. In order to strengthen our muscles, they must be exercised. Every experienced weight-lifter knows he must start with light weights and by constant practice progress to heavier and harder tasks. Likewise, self-restraint must be diligently practiced by commencing with comparatively easy conquests and gradually progressing to the more difficult feats.

There are those who will not deny themselves the gratification of a single impulse regardless of the consequences. They will throw up their hands and say, "But learning self-discipline is impossible!"

Impossible, no. Difficult, yes!

Sending a man to the moon is difficult also. Nevertheless, we do not hesitate to make the effort. Yet learning self-discipline could well be more of an accomplishment.

Some of humanity's most perplexing problems could be speedily resolved by learning and applying methods to Strengthen this wondrous quality of self-control. For instance, an honest approach to the solution of the so-called "population explosion" would be teaching people the means of developing this attribute (self-control) instead of resorting to abortions, contraceptive drugs, and other dangerous devices. Another readily apparent example is given by the millions of overweight individuals who could become slender in short order by its development and application.

Narcotic and tobacco addiction, as well as alcoholism, could be conquered if this characteristic were generally practiced. Even a truly crimeless society might become a reality. This, of course, would mean a major step in evolution to a higher form of humanity. It entails higher ethical standards. It rules out gluttony and self-indulgence. It frees us from the coils of the serpent.

Unfortunately, the so-called "old-fashioned" virtues of self-control and self-restraint are no longer respected. Today we are living in an era of materialism and conspicuous consumption. Buy now—pay later! Enjoy now— suffer later! Gratify all your appetites instantly! Why bother to practice self-restraint or self-denial? This attitude shows up in our current moral codes and the growing crime rate. "Credit" may play an important part in keeping the wheels of our economy turning; however, for millions it has become symbolic of a self-indulgent way of life. We are never taught the most important quality in life—the art of mastering oneself.

As mentioned previously, fasting has long been recognized as a potent tool for the development of self-control, and for releasing the full potential of the human mind. Fasting, however, like exercise, is a means to an objective, not an objective in itself. One important purpose of fasting is to instill and reinforce self-discipline. Consequently, if this objective is not diligently followed after the fast, much of the benefit of the fast may be sadly wasted.

The pendulum has surely swung to the extreme in our hedonistic existence. Isn't it about time to re-examine our thinking, our attitudes, and practices? Or shall we continue the same approach as the fool in our parable who thought he could acquire wisdom by merely buying water with gold?

Article #5: Kids on the Run

Who Runs?

Why Do They Run?

After Running, What?

Who Runs?

Estimates of the current number of runaways range from 600,000 to two million. Many runaways are back home within a week. Of those who don't return, only a handful ever reach one of the 700 shelters set up for them across the country.

Technically, not all of them are runaways. Some are what youth workers call "throwaways"—youngsters forced out of their homes by abusive parents or made to feel unwelcome for economic reasons.

Officials of the Health and Human Services Administration says that more than half of all runaways have been physically abused, and that most are not reported missing by their parents.

An extensive survey of 14,000 households conducted by the Opinion Research Council of Princeton, N.J., revealed these facts about runaways aged 10 to 17:

1. About three percent of the households with children in that age bracket had a runaway child.

2. Most runaways are between the ages of 15 and 17.

3. Almost half (47 percent) of the runaways are girls.

4. The children of white-collar workers are as prone to leave home as those of blue-collar workers.

Why Do They Run?

The reasons for leaving home are as varied as the youngsters themselves. Sometimes there's no apparent reason.

For some running away is an act of self-preservation, even though it is fraught with danger. On a Christopher Closeup television program, William Treaner, founder of the National Youth Work Alliance and a former runaway himself, observed:

"In a number of cases, family life has deteriorated to such an extent that making a decision to leave can, in fact, be a fairly healthy decision."

Says William L. Pierce, president of the National Committee for Adoption: "Sexual activity is one of the major reasons why young people run. In a few cases there is sexual abuse in the home. Or it may be a young man who has fathered a child out of wedlock and is concerned about his situation. Mostly, it's a pregnant young woman caught in a situation where she feels she can't stay at home, can't talk to anyone."

A study undertaken in Boston uncovered these reasons for leaving home:

"I have no one to talk to at night." "My family did not want me." "It's better to get beat up by a stranger on the street than by someone you care about at home." Still others cite reasons such as these: "My teachers picked on me." "I got in with a bad crowd." "I was always getting in trouble."

After Running, What?

Sometimes the experience of running away brings a change of heart. Wendell Marthers ran away from his Pennsylvania home to find "movie stars, glamour and beach boys." Instead, he recalls being "scared just about every day I was gone, worrying about being arrested, about being killed or beaten up."

And he was beaten up—six times. He returned home five years after leaving.

However, one large shelter reports that only 10 to 12 percent of the youngsters it serves are successfully reunited with their families. The others?

Some of them "develop families on the street," according to Lois Lee, director of Children of the Night, a Los Angeles program to help youngsters break away from prostitution. "They'll form groups and look out for each other."

To survive, some youngsters turn to prostitution and crime. As Treaner observed on Christopher Closeup: "It's a very tiny minority—less than one-half of one percent, if that—who are able to run away from home, to find a place to live, to find a job, and to establish themselves independently.

A few reach a runaway house. Dr. James Gordon of the National Institute of Mental Health says such temporary refuges offer young people "a time and a place for themselves, a chance to take a critical and often compassionate look at the families with which they have been hopelessly struggling." The family discovers that impasses may be broken, that choices are possible and that differences do not necessarily spell disaster.

Lesson 83:

Senior Citizens Living Hygienically

83.1. Introduction

Most people who write about the elderly, their problems, and concerns, have never themselves been elderly. Nevertheless, they write profusely and give advice about what is, to them, an unknown dimension of life.

That certainly cannot be said about your authors! We have travelled life's road and experienced its turmoil and travail. We have known sickness and disease, suffered bereavement and sorrow, sustained life's defeats and also tasted the sweetness of success.

We have worked in the slums of large cities and counseled the children of migrant workers. We have travelled the highways of much of the world and have conversed and supped with both the great and the small. Throughout it all, life has been exciting and wondrously good to us. We count ourselves fortunate among humans because, when we had need, we learned about Natural Hygiene.

Life has taught us that living is itself a challenge. It represents, at birth, an unknown potential with goals to be won, an opportunity 10 change small dreams into large realities. In the end, life represents a parade of failures and successes. We are favored, indeed, when the successes of life out weight our defeats.

We ask you to remember that every senior citizen who seeks your advice will represent a person who has succeeded. Dr. Robert H. Schuller says that "Tough times don't last, but tough people do!" These are the tough ones! They have met life head on, they have successfully met the challenges and problems of life which felled many, if not most, of their peers. These older clients have survived while literally millions around them disappeared. They obviously entered life with a strong inheritance, and, unlike their felled peers, they took better care of themselves as they lived their years.

Each older person will represent a challenge to you, a personal challenge to become his friend, perhaps the only person he can truly call a friend. Melville H. Nahin in an article, "The Problem Solver" in New Age magazine, March 1983, compares life to a train ride. As we grow older and come to the end of our ride, the friends of yesteryear, the weaker ones who boarded the train with us at the same station, seem suddenly to have all disappeared. They got off the train here and there as the ride progressed. Suddenly, the older person looks around and sees that all the seats are empty: his friends are no more! Then it is that older people become consciously aware that they are devastatingly alone. The knowledgeable practitioner, the one with a social empathy, can often have the privilege of stepping in and filling this often unplanned-for void.

83.2. Older People Need Support

When health is our companion, the latter years of our living can be joyful years, indeed. The major challenges of life have been met. These should be the years of new adventure. However, if we are old and sick and filled with doubts about tomorrow, as so many of our elderly friends are, then we have a tendency to accept defeat before we should, largely because we are without family or friends to provide encouraging loving support. Every living person has the marvelous gift of vital force, some more, some less. But, whatever the amount, it gives opportunity, an opportunity to create, to accomplish, to give a part of oneself back to the world in exchange for the gift. This is true of the elderly ones as well as of the younger members of society. While life remains, there is also potential. When older people are taught how to live according to Hygienic principles, they often become enthusiastic, more so than they were for years, and begin to share their rich experiences with us and with others, to the enrichment of all.

As a rule, younger members of society have more vitality than most of the older people. They also have that idyllic vision of the future which inspires them to be problem solvers and doers. However, far too many of our senior citizens have lost their vision of the future. They are defeated at the beginning of each new day instead of being challenged by the rising sun. It is the purpose of this lesson to make the elderly ones who may seek your counsel as a Hygienic practitioner more real to you as individuals who have successfully coped with life's problems; they have overcome the stresses but now find the way weary. They ask of you some measure of support along the way.

With meaningful support, the elderly can often survive crisis periods which might otherwise serve to defeat them. Some four years or so ago, we were consulted about the condition of a 93-year-old gentleman who had recently suffered a mild stroke. He had difficulty in getting around, was somewhat senile, and had just about lost all interest in people, life and living. The prognosis was dim, indeed, considering his great age.

However, this man had a brother, not actually a brother by reason of birth but, nevertheless, a brother in spirit. The brother had been introduced to Natural Hygiene at one of our infrequent lectures. He studied and began to incorporate Hygienic practices into his own daily living. When his brother became ill, he introduced him to Natural Hygiene, too. At first, the way was rather unsteady. Habit patterns are deeply etched on the nerve pathways of the old. But the brother persisted, and it wasn't too long before this 93-year-old was busy every single day. He watered the many trees and shrubs which made his yard a veritable paradise of greenery. He set out seeds and seedlings and watched them grow as he administered his loving care.

We talked with him, and he told us how he had been a merchant seaman and about all the many countries of the world he had visited; about how he had jumped ship in San Francisco after the Russian revolution and had become an American navy man. What stories he told! It was exciting to watch his mind open up.

About a year ago, he presented Dr. Elizabeth with a young fan palm tree, just a little over a foot or so tall. He had grown the little tree from a seed. Unaided, the old man lifted the little tree in its container and placed it in the back of our station wagon, receiving a hug and a kiss in return!

Today that little palm tree grows just outside the entrance to our home. Every time we look out the window of our consulting room, we see that little tree. It is now more than four feet tall. Someday it will be a giant among giants. To us, that tree represents a love which will endure for generations to come, not just a tree to view and admire. That tree also represents hope. We point it out to the despairing ones and tell them its story. We often see their spines straighten and their eyes light up. They know that if this 93-year-old can do it, they can, too!

This wonderful friend recently celebrated his 97th birthday. To celebrate he went for a medical examination. The examining physician shook his head in wonder and told our friend, "The only thing we can find wrong with you is a little edema in your ankles. Other than that, you are fine!"

Was the old man content? After all, what's a little edema? We see that sort of thing all around us, don't we? No! He was not content. Our friend, you see, is a very determined man. He announced in a firm voice, "I will now give up bread!" We all sat back in astonishment. His brother had been trying to get him to give up bread from the very beginning, but to no avail. You see, he wasn't ready yet. But now he had made up his own mind: "No more bread!"

There is a lesson for all Hygienists to learn here, perhaps several. Sometimes the greatest gift we can give is the gift of hope and especially when it is given to the elderly ones in love. This is the gift that both directs and inspires. It is easy, of course, to present a plan of action; it takes love to inspire performance. Our 93-year-old friend also gives us another lesson: in working with our older clients, in addition to having the knowledge of what to do and the ability to offer love and support, we are also required to have patience.

Love is conveyed, of course, in many ways: in the way we look, in our manner of speaking, in our attitude toward the client. It shows in the patience we display when our client expresses ideas which may appear somewhat "peculiar" to us, but which are, nevertheless, important to the person before us—even if only for a passing moment. Our love shows in the way we greet and say goodbye, and in our acceptance of the fact that most of our elderly clients will require time, time to tell their story as they wish to tell it, and time to adjust rather slowly to a new and strange way of eating and living. Through the love you give to them, the older person comes to know and gratefully accept the fact that you have their best interests at heart. In other words, they have your much-needed support as they try to regain some better measure of health.

In order to prepare you to become more capable of giving this kind of support to your senior citizen clients, we ask you to retravel in your mind's eye the long road of life with us, to take the train ride, as it were, just as the average person living today in

America is doing. Much of what we have to say will, of course, pertain to persons living in all countries of the world, but we are all individuals. However, in this discussion we will be looking at gross details for the purpose of following a single common thread, the rising tide of toxicosis, and the wasting effect of the physiological and biological errors on the potential of the newly born as each person takes the train ride through life.

In presenting this overview of life we wish to emphasize that what we present is life as it is presently lived, not what it should or could be if Hygienic principles and practices were universally adopted.

When we have completed our imaginary ride through life, we will then present some case studies which will provide our students with some capsule glimpses of Natural Hygiene at work in the lives of some of our senior citizen clients.

83.3. The Path We Travel

83.3.1. The Nine Stages of Life

83.3.2. The Best in Institutional Care of the Elderly

With very few exceptions all of us are born capable of achieving a far greater potential in all areas of life than most persons presently achieve. Certainly, most of us desire to be happy in our old age and yet we are surrounded by a host of unhappy people, people who are filled with disease and despair. Most of us have a deep inner yearning to achieve something of real worth before we depart from this life but, obviously, few ever come close to a full realization of their earlier dreams.

We know that most people would prefer to be healthy and yet few among us can be held up as models of superior health—at any age. Indeed, most of us are gravely ill when we are compared to many more ideal specimens available for comparison. It would appear normal for us, as we grow older, to have our lives increasingly enriched by a growing number of friends and by enlarged familial relationship, but the exact opposite seems more often than not to occur as friends diminish in number, felled by accumulated poisons which were the fruits of incorrect habits of living and eating. Additionally, a more mobile population and a less-caring attitude of a commercially oriented society seems to gnaw away at family togetherness, the members of families refusing to accept responsibility one for the other and particularly between generations of the same family. There are exceptions, of course, and these families are to be commended for fulfilling a kinship trust.

From our position at the far end of the spectrum of life it seems that life tends to follow a pattern; that there appears to be a more or less regular sequence of events which may be characteristic of the times in which we live. Within certain very broad limits we can observe some definite patterns emerging, significant in various areas vital to self, to interpersonal relationships, to health, to family ties and obligations; and, of course, in the wider arena of life that is concerned with community and world spheres of influence. At no time in life do we or can we live in a vacuum. We leave our imprints on trees and shrubs and on the flowers we touch, but we also leave them on people, either directly or indirectly. Few among us fully understand our purpose for few know just what they want or can expect from, and far too many among us search frantically for an unknown that we cannot and will not find. Because of this many among us tend to fret and hence we do not accomplish. We wish for happiness, for monetary substance and even for health at times but we fall far short of the mark in almost every instance.

We are equally sure that most people would not have it thus if they were aware of the possibility of change. We live in a time of conflict and unrest, but that has probably been true in all ages and at all times. There is a "whisper in the minds of men" that all is not well. More than at any other time in history perhaps men and women, and even our young people, are wondering wherein they have been cheated and are beginning to ask important questions. Is this all there is to life? Are we born to enjoy but a few brief years of respite from care and trouble, disease, and suffering, experiencing but a tiny moment of a reasonable degree of health?

Must we undergo 30, 40 or more years of declining health wherein we are called upon necessarily to watch our ambitions fade away into a nothingness which yields only a deepening sense of emptiness, frustration, and loss of purpose in being? Must we experience a gradual erosion of our vitality, the stealthy degeneration of bodily and mental structure and function, an ever-deepening pathology of diminishing health which reaches out and destroys all vestiges of happiness and self-worth?

Rightfully, the questioning mind asks, must it necessarily then be the ultimate fulfillment of the life's course to descend from the heights of joy and the great vitality of the newly born into the whining depths of the frustrated, unhappy sick souls we observe in the harvest time of life, these being largely at the mercy of and dependent upon the whims of an uncaring society?

There is no doubt that man's most inner urge is, above all things, to be happy, to be wanted, to be recognized as a person, and, of course, to be healthy, but when we become elderly, we rarely are privileged to experience such emotional and spiritual nourishment even though it is as essential to life as physical nourishment. Indeed, the full acceptance of nutrients is impossible when we remain emotionally and spiritually vacant.

83.3.1. The Nine Stages of Life

We first began researching the aging process years ago. Interestingly enough, we began to distinguish nine fairly distinct stages in the average life course. We observed also that these stages had similarities as well as readily distinguishable differences. For example, certain stresses are more or less peculiar to adolescents, as was seen in Lesson 82, and yet these same stresses are perhaps of little concern in other stages.

There are some diseases which are characteristic of childhood which rarely, if ever, appear in the later years of life. We constantly observe how the errors in lifestyle and in nutrition seem to have a far-reaching and cumulative effect on health as the life course is traversed. Physiological insults of a myriad kind nibble away at health prevent the fulfillment of the birth potential of self. It is interesting to observe that in each of the nine stages, we find many of the same stresses, the same diseases, similar errors, and, of course, similar results. Our nine stages are arbitrary choices, of course, but our students can probably see the logic of the divisions chosen.

1. Period of Childhood
2. The Adolescent Years
3. The Emerging Adult
4. The Parenting Years
5. The Middle Years
6. The Late Middle Years
7. The Beginning of Retirement and Old Age
8. The Post-retirement Years
9. The Years of Custodial Care

Because we feel it is important to the understanding of the elderly, we are presenting a brief synopsis of the transition from Stage One to Stage Nine. We include some general observations to increase understanding, we note the types of diseases common to each stage, the determining factors as to the type(s) experienced and, finally, the most common errors made by individuals as they pass through each one of the nine stages.

It is important to note that young people are biologically very similar. This is true because their bodies have, as yet not sustained the vast numbers of physiological insults which can be experienced as the pattern of life is revealed. The changes continue slowly and inexorably, under present standards of living and eating, until the life force is exhausted, and the physiological point of no return is finally reached. This is why the elderly are so biologically different. Their bodies represent the sum total, the cumulative and final effect of multiple errors.

Each elderly person is different from every other elderly person because he has been imprinted by different stresses and to a greater or lesser degree. Also, because at birth he entered the world with a constitution, a collection of weak and strong organs which were strictly his own, his private legacy from the past. Persons with a strong inheritance survive the stresses of life far better than those less well endowed. Like strong trees that bend with the wind and grow stronger, persons with a strong constitution are able to survive relatively well the vicissitudes of life. The weaker ones seldom attain a great age.

However, it is the purpose of the Hygienic practitioner to teach both the weak and the strong to get the most out of life, to show them that life is a possible dream to be lived to the full and that this can be accomplished in full measure when we know and follow the principles you are learning in this course, the principles of Life Science. The student will observe in the following mini glimpses into the nine stages that we will, unfortunately, not be able to include all influences and/or conditions that could conceivably arise. Our purpose is to provide a broad index so that students can be aware of the evolving biological degeneration brought about through multiple physiological errors, these leading to the aging of people as customarily observed. The Hygienist, of course, has sufficient evidence to demonstrate epidemiologically and historically that such aging is contrary to organic law. However, by having knowledge of the progress of toxemia at work within the body, the Hygienic practitioner should, in the normal course of events, be better equipped to help his elderly clients to attain a far higher plateau of health than they presently experience.

As we progress through the nine stages, from birth to death, we will actually be watching the diverging paths of the chronological and biological clocks. We should bear in mind that humans are probably designed to live, on an average, about 150 years. Let us observe how the biological clock outpaces the chronological clock, and why!

83.3.1.1. Stage One—The Period of Childhood

In this first stage we cover the period of life from birth to about the tenth year. This is normally the time of childhood, a time of life when a person is more or less completely dependent upon parents and/or others for life's necessities:

- Custodial care both in sickness and in health.
- Housing.
- Cleanliness.
- Clothing.
- Education.
- Food.
- Environment including Social, emotional, physical, and spiritual.
- Other.

In Lesson 80 we paid some attention to child abuse and pointed out that there are many ways to abuse young children. Probably such abuse has existed throughout the history of mankind, but it remains, nevertheless, a troubling problem which must, in our view, be rightfully attributed to the inner turmoil which damages the nervous structures of the body and leads, more often than not, to erratic behavior.

We should remember that the various kinds of abuse are often difficult to detect and even more difficult, we are told, to prosecute since the child, either out of a sense of fear or love for the abusing parent, may refuse to testify or because of his young years, may be unable to do so.

In recent years still other multiple problems have arisen, these being most often associated with the single parent home. These are presently receiving some small attention, but they have certainly not, as yet, been resolved insofar as the possible psychological and other effects on the developing child are concerned.

In Lesson 80 we noted that the family unit, as traditionally constituted, is undergoing change. However, we must recognize, especially as we look forward to the problems of the elderly, that the long-range results of these changes, whatever they may turn out to be and however they may have been created, have yet to be evaluated. The evidence that is already "in," seems to indicate that the effects may be long-reaching and profoundly negative in kind. Many elderly clients are often greatly troubled by the fact that young children are being neglected by their parents and also by the fact that they themselves have apparently become almost "non people" in the eyes of their children.

The Types of Disease Commonly Experienced in Stage One:

1. Acute: Chickenpox, measles, eruptive fevers of all kinds, poliomyelitis, and similar "self-limiting" diseases.

2. "Allergies": Rashes, itches, various nasal and lung catarrhal disorders which may or may not exhibit periodicity, coming and going at intervals.

3. Others: Frequent colds, tonsilitis, glandular swellings, pinworms, and other fungus infections. (Don't forget, pinworms find a happy home in catarrhal victims!). Leukemia is the No. 1 killer of young children. Digestive disturbances, including diarrhea and/or constipation, infant colic, and irritability.

The State of Health Observed in Children is Determined by:

1. Inherited Diathesis—the child's legacy from generations of ancestors which have preceded him for hundreds of thousands of years; includes health of parents at conception.

2. The health and care of the mother during the prenatal period.

3. The care and feeding of the child following birth including, among other things, the following:

    a. The emotional environment and experiences.

    b. Physical care and nurture including protection from violence.

    c. Kind, quantity, and frequency of feedings.

The Most Common Errors Made in Child Care:

1. Overnutrition—Feeding too much food and/or feeding too frequently.

2. Poor Nutrition—Inability to nurse the infant. Poor quality food or too little food.

3. Too much handling or too little handling.

4. Failure to satisfy physiological and emotional needs. The "Empty House Stress" of children with working parents: "Latch-key children."

5. Too little exercise.

83.3.1.2. Stage Two—The Adolescent Years—Ages 10 to 20

In Lesson 82 we discussed the adolescent and Hygienic living and noted that this period of life is a period of transition from childhood to adulthood, one which begins with a more or less complete dependence upon others and evolves into a state of emerging independence.

We wish to call your attention to the bodily and health changes that gradually take place during this transition period, these changes illustrating, in many cases, the beginning of disorders which will trouble the elderly, but to a far greater degree. It is in these early years that we witness the alpha, beginning phases in the biological evolution which results, finally, in the elderly individuals as the omega, of life, when catastrophic diseases begin to take an ever-accelerating toll. When the foundation is faulty, the structure will eventually give away.

The Types of Disease Commonly Experienced in Stage Two:

- Acute: Note that the acute diseases of childhood become less frequent but other kinds of disorders develop, such as: Sinusitis, hay fever, bronchitis, and various other kinds of catarrhal involvements: frequent colds, influenza, etc.

- Digestive Disturbances including diarrhea, constipation, colitis, appendicitis, and ulcers. (Notice how the seriousness of the conditions is increasing.)

- New Disorders now often appear rheumatic disorders including neuritis and inflammation of the joints. (So-called "growing pains." Growth actually produces no pain. These pains are due to the increasing toxemia.)

- Eye Deterioration.

- Acne, boils, pimples, eczema, or similar skin eruptions.

- Mouth and body odors that prove annoying. In females, menstrual disorders: irregular menses, painful menses, vaginal discharges, edema, depression before and during period—the PMS or the Premenstrual Syndrome.

The State of Health Observed in Stage Two is Determined by:

1. All those cited in Stage One, plus the following:

2. The number, kind and frequency of physiological insults experienced during this stage in the life cycle: Emotional insults, poison insults (both exogenous and endogenous), Deficiencies, (either in lifestyle or in nutrition) and Excess insults (either in lifestyle or in nutrition); or a combination of these.

The Most Common Errors Made in Stage Two are:

1. Overnutrition—the "Eat All You Can" Syndrome.

2. Poor nutrition.

3. Failure to accept responsibility for one's acts, especially among males.

4. Emotional trauma: poor home environment, poor school environment, poor community environment, too much pressure to achieve on part of authority figure, usually parent.

5. Too little discipline in all aspects of life, but especially in the home and school. Creates the false sense that "I can get away with anything and the roof won't fall on me!"

6. Peer rejection or the converse, peer domination.

7. Failure to satisfy basic physiological, biological and/or emotional needs of the immature, but growing body.

83.3.1.3. Stage Three—The Emerging Adult

During these years, the chronological clock ticks on; the adolescent emerges into and becomes the adult. In the beginning of the period, there are varying degrees of dependence upon parents but, by the time this stage has been concluded, most persons have assumed full responsibility for their own care and well-being.

At about the halfway mark, that is, at about age 24 or 25, growth ceases and the body now begins to concentrate as best it can on health maintenance, on healing and repairing the wounded cells and, from this point on, it will be required to wage a constant war against sickness and death.

It is during this stage that mates are chosen, and new family units are established. In recent years, marriages have had a tendency to be postponed with many young people, for one reason or another, not seeking the responsibility for a family and opting, instead, for "live-in" partner either of the same sex or, more frequently, of the opposite sex. Almost without exception, however, the future beckons and is full of challenge, hopes are high, and all aspects of life are thought to be capable of a successful conclusion!

Those in the twenty to thirty age group, Stage Three, show considerable differences in emotional maturity, no doubt due to their current health status and different backgrounds. The imprinting of the years on their lives profoundly affects the manner in which they handle today.

Educational goals are usually achieved somewhere in this time frame and a wide divergence in aims and aspirations in life appear. Whether or not these are successfully consummated during the generally productive years of the twenties will certainly have a very noticeable influence following retirement, as we will soon see. In fact, it will color an older person's complete attitude toward life and living. It may also determine his health status. But, for now, the overall attitude among this age group can perhaps best be expressed in the words of a popular song: "Kiss Today goodbye. Point me towards Tomorrow!" To the 25-year-old the future is there to be conquered and he has no doubt that he will conquer it! Health maintenance is generally a matter of major concern only to those who do not have it.

The Types of Disease Commonly Experienced in Stage Three:

(Note: Observe the steady inroads made on the vital force, this being sapped by the adaptations required within the body in order to maintain life.)

1. Acute Diseases: the diseases of childhood are, for the most part, nonexistent. Colds and other respiratory disorders are common and more frequent. Asthmatic conditions, bronchial troubles and other similar disorders often become more severe.

2. The teenage "allergies" often disappear, and the young adult is said to have "grown out of them. The truth is that a higher level of tolerance to toxins has been attained with a commensurate and equal lowering of the health status.

   Some skin disorders now become more or less chronic: for example, chronic eczema or psoriasis.

3. Various other common disorders which are frequently experienced:

   a. Arteriosclerosis, multiple sclerosis, etc.

   b. Rheumatic and/or arthritic symptoms either now make their appearance or, if previously present, increase in severity.

   c. Heart irregularities and other disorders affecting (Note: These troubles seem to be appearing with more and more frequency also in Stage Two, especially within the last fifteen years or so).

   d. Digestive disturbances, especially ulcers, diarrhea, and colon constipation.

    e.   Kidney malfunctioning; especially frequent is nocturnal urination.

    f.   With females, the menstrual period continues to cause trouble and frequently increases in length.

    g.   Painful childbirth.

The State of Health Observed in Stage Three is Determined by:

1.   Care and nurture during prenatal period and during all the preceding years from birth to present.

2.   Inherited strengths and weaknesses.

3.   Frequency, number, and kind of physiological insults to which the body and mind have been subjected thus far during the life course.

The Most Common Errors Made in Stage Three are:

1.   Overnutrition.

2.   Poor nutrition.

3.   Indulgence in false stimulants: Condiments of all kinds, alcohol, nicotine; using palliating drugs to disguise symptoms; using prescribed, "social," hard or other drugs including herbs, synthetic vitamins, and/or other so-called "supplements."

4.   The emotional stresses incurred in trying to make a living and/or provide for a family in a very competitive business and social scene.

5.   The stresses caused by economic and other pressures as, for example, during a depression; the stresses of "keeping up with the Joneses;" trying to provide the "best" for one's children; competition for a suitable mate; the noise and fast pace of modern living, especially in large cities.

6.   Overindulgence in all aspects of living; sexual burnout.

7.   Failure to satisfy basic physiological and biological needs, especially two such needs: namely, sufficient exercise and rest.

83.3.1.4. Stage Four—The Parenting Years

In the normal course of events, those who have lived to this fourth stage in the life course have fully accepted their roles as adults and, as such, provide for their own requirements: physical, emotional, financial, and spiritual.

Families are usually established, children born, with parents now assuming the nurturing described in Stage One. By this time, the childhood home is no longer a factor except for the effect it may have had upon the individual in all phases of his life to this time.

Formal education has, for the most part, ended and the individual strives to establish himself in the business and social worlds of which s/he is now a part, although for a limited time. Efforts are still made to gain approval of one's peers, although peer pressure is not generally as important as in previous years. During this stage, which includes those between the ages of 30 and 40, both males and females tend to participate actively in the organized life of the community, joining several civic and service clubs, both professional and occupational, as well as participating socially and actively in all kinds of other organizations and activities. Church leadership is assumed by many while others play a more passive role. The over-riding concern of members of this age group is the welfare of the several members of the family unit but, particularly, that of the children they have brought into the world. There is now only a limited concern for the needs, financial and other, of their parents or for older generations still living; that is, for grandparents or great-grandparents. These have become almost non-persons in modern America. This is not true, however, in many other cultures.

During this stage, the future looks fairly secure. Stereotypes begin to emerge, especially in the business world as individuals find their "niche," as it were. This could well be called the period of "Individual Strategy" with the term "Individual" applying equally well to the individual, male or female, perse, or to the family as a unit.

The proliferation of this kind of activity is usually especially important among those with above average mental capacity and is limited only by the physical status of the individual and by his previous educational opportunities and/or achievements.

Sometimes the stress thus occasioned becomes an important factor in the downward decline in health so frequent and often so dramatic during this stage. The members of this group are often boxed into a corner by the times and are called up to develop strategies to compete, and to cope with all manner of situations and, importantly, they must now do all this on their own. The awareness of this fact can often assume major importance and have a profound effect on the nervous system, usually adverse in kind.

With females entering the business world more frequently now than in former years, they are now subject to the multiple stresses not previously experienced, and, in addition, they must often be concerned not only with the care and rearing of children but also with the maintenance of the household. Characteristically, few males contribute in this regard, although more seem to be doing so now. However, females are called upon to assume a multi-faceted role: giving birth to children; assuring that the emotional, physical, spiritual and education needs of the children are met; taking care of the physical home in which the family lives; assisting with the financial needs of the family unit; and, finally, participating more or less actively in community organizations such as the PTA, Boy and Girl Scouts and similar child-oriented groups. The stress factor can be enormous when the traditional maternal role is thus expanded and it is not unreasonable to expect a subtle erosion of the life force under such circumstances, one that will, no doubt, have an impact on women's later years.

The Types of Disease Commonly Experienced in Stage Four:

1. Acute diseases: Colds, influenza, and various other kinds of respiratory disorders of varying intensity according to previous history.

2. Chronic diseases now become increasingly evident and, when present, these can have a major impact on the family unit as well as upon the individual thus encumbered. As always, the conditions experienced are the fruits of the past.

The most common chronic diseases which emerge in Stage Four are:

1. Heart disease of one kind or another.

2. Liver complaints of varying severity.

3. Chronic prostatitis.

4. Ulcers (10% have either a stomach or duodenal ulcer).

5. Benign tumors.

6. Diabetes.

7. Various joint and bone diseases.

8. An assortment of the so-called "itis" diseases: cystitis, metritis, sinusitis, neuritis, colitis, etc.

9. Digestive disorders of one kind or another, including but not limited to: burning, constipation, diarrhea, gas emissions, fullness, anorexia, etc.

10. Varicose veins.

11. Sclerosis of arteries, poor circulation with cold extremities being a common complaint.

12. Most now wear glasses.

13. Irritability, extreme nervousness, tics, etc.

14. Female complaints worsen, with menstrual periods often extending from seven to ten days in length, indicative of extreme toxicity and causing many to opt for a hysterectomy.

15. Diseases commonly associated with the female sex organs.

State of Health Determined by:

We are sure our students can now begin to see where we are headed with the ticking of the biological clock, this, of course, under so-called "normal" living and eating habits.

1. All previous factors listed up to this point as they may be applicable to any one individual.

2. Whatever kind of disease or diseases which may have evolved will have been determined by the individual's own peculiar diathesis and by the number, kind, and frequency of the physiological insults—the multiple stressors—to which the individual has either subjected himself or to which he has been subjected, either knowingly or unknowingly. The stressors can be either mental or physical in kind, of internal or external origin, and multiple or single in number.

The Most Common Errors Made in Stage Four Are:

1. Overnutrition.

2. Lack of moderation in all aspects of life.

3. Failure to obtain a full quota of the organic requisites of life.

4. Failure to satisfy the individual's basic physiological, biological, or spiritual needs and/ or disobedience to any or all of the fundamental laws of life. Enervation, due to toxemia, of one or both partners results in the breakup of many marriages.

5. False stimulation: continuing to use condiments, alcohol, nicotine, drugs as detailed earlier; the wrong kind of sex life; snacking, using chemicalized soft drinks and other processed "food," generally poor nutrition.

6. Killing overstress in one or more areas of lifestyle.

7. A driving urge to achieve in one's career or profession, or in some other area of life in spite of demographic contrary evidence indicating possible failure.

83.3.1.5. Stage Five—The Middle Years

We include in this category those persons between the ages of forty to fifty, the period of mature adulthood. Persons in this age group are commonly referred to as being "middle-aged."

It is in this stage that individuals, both male and female, begin to question where they stand in the scheme of life. Many become extremely anxious and develop a sense of frustration and inadequacy. Many find that the problems and/or challenges they face seem increasingly more difficult to solve and/or meet successfully.

It is in this middle period of life that, perhaps for the very first time, a sense of foreboding failure produces a state of mind wherein the possibility of defeat becomes imprinted on the subconscious mind. Often people in middle-age begin to feel boxed-in, even hopeless at times. Many begin to make less and less of an effort to cope with daily matters of concern. Anxiety, worry and fear about the future replace planning and performance.

Many emotional peaks and valleys, destructive of health, are occasioned as children leave the home scene to pursue their own lives.

Sometimes the anxiety takes another line of defense with the three P's taking over:

An obsession with perfection, 2. Since perfection is either unlikely or impossible, the individual tends to procrastinate; and, finally, 3. The disturbed person simply settles for paralysis—non-performance—and often gets locked into life-destroying habits. This is especially true of men in the business world, but the same synopsis will, no doubt, appear in women attempting to cope with dual roles.

The more intelligent ones in this age group, the ones who have thus far fully coped with life, often begin to delegate responsibilities to younger employees, especially in those areas that require physical effort as well as mental. Some enter a new dimension of life successfully by developing a wide diversity of management skills, especially those concerned with decision-making and with long-term planning.

It is interesting to observe how physical activity begins to decrease as the middle aged, due to the mounting toxemic load within their stressed bodies, tend to lead a more sedentary lifestyle, this being due to the fact that they are increasingly plagued by muscular ailments, stiffening of muscles and joints.

The ranks begin to thin-drastically due to deaths caused mainly, in the male population, by heart attacks and, among females, by diseases associated with childbearing: uterine, tumors, kidney failure, breast tumors. Many females fall victims to surgical procedures such as hysterectomies and mastectomies or various drug-related (iatrogenic) diseases. The biological clock ticks rapidly during this period.

This is the period when both males and females become acutely aware of the fact that they are aging. They feel they have done all that could possibly be demanded of them and forget that when we stop producing, we are already old.

All the chronic diseases which previously annoyed become more so now. Many, indeed, become life-threatening. The vast majority develop what Dr. Virginia Vetrano calls, the "Run-to-the-Doctor Syndrome." Many also become addicted to the stimulant habit. These have been correctly termed, "The Critical Years."

The Types of Diseases Commonly Experienced in Stage Five:

1. Colds, bronchial and other respiratory disorders now tend to appear more frequently and last longer due to the diminishing vital force. Emphysema is now more frequently observed than in former years.

2. Arteriosclerosis and atherosclerosis with accompanying symptoms, such as cold hands and feet, sudden chills, and other indications of clogged circulatory channels.

3. Cirrhosis of the liver.

4. Heart disorders of all kinds; many fatalities.

5. Emphysema.

6. Rheumatoid arthritis. This disease was formerly considered to be a disease of old age. It is now common in this age group and even in much younger people. For example, there are at least 60,000 American children who are afflicted with juvenile varieties, according to Dr. John Baum, M.D., director of the Pediatric Arthritis Clinic at Strong Memorial Hospital in Rochester, N.Y. The medical community, of course, knows no "cure" other than palliation of pain and cannot understand why children often "recover" from arthritis while adults seldom do.

   Life Scientists know, however, that when cause is removed, the body wisdom takes over and tends to move toward perfection when basic organic needs are fully met.

7. Benign and malignant tumors, especially among the female members of the group. However, the medical community fails to recognize that these tumors represent the final link in the chain of errors both in lifestyle and eating.

8. Menstrual disorders with increased flow.

9. Cancer of the colon, especially among males.

10. Ulcerative colitis.

11. Obesity.

12. Alcoholism and/or addiction to other drugs, especially upon mood-altering drugs.

13. Lack of vitality—the "Fall on the Couch After Work" Syndrome.

14. Frequent headaches, especially among females but also among males, these being due, of course, to toxic overload.

The Stage of Health Determined by:

15. Failure to correct errors in diet and in lifestyle.

16. The type of counsel sought and obtained, whether knowledgeable or otherwise.

17. The inherited diathesis.

18. The number, kind, amount, and frequency of intake of drugs.

We note in this middle group that the ranks begin to thin as the indiscretions of a lifetime begin to take their toll/ The biological ticking now begins to accelerate.

The Most Common Errors:

1. Strangely enough, all of the former errors are usually continued largely because it is difficult to change long-established habits. This is especially so when education in the application of Hygienic principles has been nonexistent in the individual or in those persons consulted for advice in matters of health care.

2. Because of the errors noted in No. 1 above, "middle-aged" people as a rule tend to gravitate to an even greater dependence upon prescribed and over-the-counter drugs; and also, to cocaine, alcohol, nicotine, and so on. Many play Russian Roulette with themselves by using combinations of several drugs at one and the same time.

3. Overnutrition.

4. Increasing dependence upon sugar, tea, coffee, salt, pepper, etc.

5. Failure to seek suitable relief from stresses, many of which increase in number and intensity and seem to attack in various life spheres: at home, in business and in social contacts often due to the fact that younger people are striving for their own niche and so attempt to displace the older ones.

6. Failure to recognize and adjust appropriately to the subtle erosion of the life force which is now accelerating.

7. Reluctance to admit that parenting days are over and to find interests in new directions.

83.3.1.6. Stage Six— The Late Middle Years

Ages fifty to sixty represent the late middle years. The biological clock has far outpaced the chronological clock. Since the itinerary of life was not figured out in advance of the journey, and seldom is—we find that all the former symptoms of uneasiness about the future and all the diseased conditions usually continue and, indeed, become more intense.

There is an old saying to the effect that "you can't put an old head on a young man's shoulders!" This is true and perhaps fortunately so, but the Hygienic practitioner, if he wishes to be successful in working with patients, will necessarily have to come to grips with the realities of the aging process. This is so because the great majority of his clients will come from the older members of the general public. He should make himself familiar with the generalities noted as being characteristic of each age group, with the kinds of anxieties and hopes for the future, with the common errors in living and eating and, of course, with the kinds of disorders most commonly characteristic of each group. Only in so doing can he hope to develop the kind of empathy required for effective counseling.

Females

Females, in the late middle years, come to grips with the stresses customarily, but erroneously we believe, associated with the aging process, namely the "change of life."

Alexis Carrel, M.D., the Nobel Prize winner, in his book, Man, The Unknown, stated that herein lies a fundamental difference between men and women but comes to a rather abrupt conclusion in middle age among women. Carrel held that this single fact places women at a disadvantage to men.

Hygienists, of course, hold that toxemia and toxemia alone is responsible for the manifold discomforts endured by most women during this period of life, discomforts which are both physical and mental.

The hot flashes which at times seem about to consume the woman; menstrual flow which often lasts from ten days to over two weeks, often flowing so copiously that women are required to take to their beds; flow which returns at irregular times, sometimes after only a relatively short interval of a week or so. Such abnormal blood flow saps the body's energy reserves and aggravates a! » existing physical conditions.

We can but wonder at times that women in this age group survive as well as they do, although, of course, many do not. Hysterectomies are common. The concerns of women are a fertile hunting ground for money-hungry surgeons. In 1975 over 800,000 such operations were performed. In recent years we have heard of such operations being performed on gullible women as a "preventive" for uterine and other cancers. Such mindless butchering is a twin to the present trend to remove a woman's breasts, even in young women, as a preventive against the possibility of having cancer of the breast.

The Hygienic practitioner can often provide much comfort to older women in this time frame. Their physical discomforts lead to mental anxieties about their "worth" as women. Many believe they will no longer be attractive to men. They require assurance of their ability to play a meaningful role in the scheme of a well-planned life. They also require assurance that their physical discomforts can be alleviated provided they follow the teachings of Natural Hygiene. As we shall see when we come to our review of some actual case studies, the rewards for the Hygienist can prove highly satisfactory.

Males

When men finally attain this age, they start looking forward to their retirement. Then I'm going fishing. Then I'm going to take that trip. Then I will paint that painting, one worthy of the great masters. They spend many hours in their "magic moments." Their physical activity usually lessens. This is true of women also. Both sexes now prefer to be spectators at sports rather than active participants.

Many men begin to look around for groups to join service clubs, church-sponsored support groups, and so on. Both men and women tend to look around for "causes," much as young people do. This is often due to the fact that their children become more and more involved with their own family units and have less and less time or inclination to spend with their parents. They are forced into the realization that their parenting days are over. This is, for many, often a moment of cruel truth, particularly to those men and women who have devoted their time largely to their children and have forgotten to develop themselves as they travelled through life. Sometimes all the Hygienic practitioner is required to do to improve the mental health of clients is to suggest ways and means, to provide a list of ways in which the client may yet offer meaningful service to the community at large.

We suggest to the sincere practitioner that he contact the local chamber of commerce to obtain a list of clubs functioning in his particular community. Find out if the city or town has a recreational department. Interview the personnel and find out what is offered. Ask to be placed on their mailing lists. Contact local churches to see what group discussions are held regularly. For example, one local church this community of Tucson offers all kinds of classes from painting to aerobics. Additionally, the A.A., Al-anon and St. Luke's Healers meet there, as well as Over-eaters Anonymous. An individual well versed in Natural Hygiene can often provide meaningful input at these kinds of group meetings.

We should point out at this juncture that both the males and the females in this group normally become increasingly aware that there is a limit to the human life span which can reasonably be anticipated. With most people, this is like a thunderbolt out of the blue. Younger people seldom think about the end of life because they are deeply involved in life. However, even this acceptance of the fact that their days are numbered does not prevent their actively wanting to outlast all their peers!

This is why this age group is especially susceptible to spurious remedies which may be suggested by allopathic charlatans and other "quacks," this word being used in its commonly used sense and not especially in its original connotation as a reference to a medical doctor who overdosed his patients on mercurial remedies.

The use of tranquilizers becomes almost a way of life, particularly among the females, although as many as half the men may also become addicted to mood-altering drugs. Many begin to develop strategies to make themselves appear to belong to a younger age group as, for example, seeking for and submitting to suitable cosmetic surgery, dying the hair, taking up tennis or other physical exercises commonly associated more with those in a younger age group; not that there is anything essentially wrong with any of these pursuits except as they may prevent or hinder more correct age-deferring methods and practices. Coronary bypass operations and organ transplants, even though their effectiveness is open to Hygienic debate, are resorted to more and more frequently as sick men and women try vainly to stop the ticking of the chronological and biological clocks. We know one gentleman in this age group who has already had four heart bypass operations! In this age group many are actually reduced to medical servitude. Before they come to the Hygienic practitioner many will have had just about every expendable organ removed and will have poisoned their bodies for years. Many will expect, too, to be restored to health in a matter of days and weeks even though every single cell in their body has been severely damaged by the indiscretions and errors of a lifetime!

The Types of Diseases Most Commonly Experienced in Stage Six:

1. Loss of sexual drive or abnormal interest in same.

2. Breast cancer in females.

3. Cancer of the colon, especially among males.

4. Rheumatoid arthritis and, in women, menopausal arthritis.

5. Cirrhosis of the liver.

6. Cystitis and other kidney disorders.

7. Tuberculosis and other abnormal respiratory disorders.

8. Cancer of the larynx.

9. Strokes.

10. Heart attacks, angina pectoris.

11. Varicose veins, "grape" clusters.

12. Spine disorders and various bone diseases, especially osteoporosis or sponging of the bones.

13. Ulcerative colitis.

14. Chronic prostatitis.

15. Loss in vitality.

16. Depression as well as other nerve-related disorders ranging all the way from simple tics to Parkinson's disease.

17. Alcoholism.

18. Drug addiction. Many become victims of. polypharmacy, the indiscriminate prescribing and taking of drugs. This age group represents but 10% of the population but consumes over 25% of all prescription drugs as well as the larger proportion of other drugs, including social and nonprescription drugs.

We trust that our students are developing their understanding of how past errors can limit the quality of our present and future life unless suitable (Hygienic) remedial steps are taken and, of course, in time.

The State of Health Determined by:

1. As usual: the previous and continuing errors in the diet and lifestyle, the cumulative effect of which is now being seen in the rapid degeneration of all organs and systems. In many members of this age group, the biological clock is now racing even though they may be consciously unaware of this fact. As Dr. Robert W. McCarter, Sr. used to say, "Their inner parts are a foul mess!" They function, but barely.

2. The number and kind of operations to which the body has been subjected and the amount of adaptation and accommodation thus required, both mental and physical, and by all parts of the system. In many cases it becomes a matter of "Died at 36, buried at 60!"

The Most Common Errors Made in Stage Six Are:

1. All those previously stated, especially overnutrition, this in spite of the fact that both mental and physical activity has been curtailed, often greatly so because of one or more infirmities.

2. Drug dependence, especially on the mood-altering drugs and alcohol. Many of the elderly who live in mobile home parks, or other "Communities of the Aged," regularly go on alcoholic binges. The arthritic may take mood-altering drugs to relieve the depression so commonly associated with this painful condition as well as several highballs to impart a false sense of well-being. The arthritic often has recourse to one or more of such drugs as butazolidin alka, motrin, indocin, naprosyn and nalfon among the most common ones being presently prescribed in this senseless age of polypharmacy!

3. Surgical removal of ailing parts in a vain attempt to remedy past errors. We say "vain" because CAUSE remains.

4. Little or no effort is made to modify behavior to one more in keeping with the physiological and biological requirements of the living organism, largely because of a more or less complete ignorance of the same. Who is there on the present scene except the Hygienic practitioner to educate the public on the relation of cause to effect in body care?

5. Becoming increasingly out of the "mainstream" of life as more and more of the aging population moves into communities with their peers. They put themselves physically out of contact with other age groups and, by so doing, become the forgotten members of society, tolerated but not really wanted.

6. Overnutrition. Even though less active, physically, and mentally in most cases, they continue to eat as they always have.

7. Concern about the future becomes an added stress to all former stresses. Anxiety about one's health often becomes the major concern.

83.3.1.7. Stage Seven—The Beginning of Retirement and Old Age

In present-day thinking this age group arbitrarily includes all persons between ages sixty and seventy. These are the retirement years and the beginning of what is commonly recognized as "Old Age," although to the very young any person over the age of twenty-five is "old!"

Some few make this transition with flying colors. Usually, the more successful life travelers are the ones who possess a higher degree of health. The majority, however, because of numerous infirmities, begin to conserve and safeguard their constantly dwindling energy reserves. They walk slower, they think more slowly. They tend to make many attempts to retain their own image of the importance of SELF, husbanding the thought of their former status in life, their imagined or real prestige and even the authority and seniority they may have possessed in the work situation and, also, whatever, power, real or imagined, they may have had either in their own family group, at work or among community situations and groups. In other words, they tend to hold on to the past because of the emptiness of the present!

A relatively small percentage of the population managed to survive long enough to become a member of this age group. While there are conflicting reports in this regard, we have seen figures which state that only about 10 percent of the population at birth reaches the age of 65. These, as we have said, are the tough ones. They have either possessed a remarkable constitution, one that was able to withstand the multiple assaults of a lifetime or, possessing some lesser stamina, they knew enough to take good care of themselves.

Whichever may be the case, members of this group often become acutely aware of the fact that they are now old and this largely because of the fact that many of their financial and social expectations anticipated in their younger years have been shattered and also because many of the supports offered by the community at large to the more productive younger age groups are, in far too many instances, nonexistent. The media constantly presents the beautiful side of young life and the constant barrage of "that which might have been" becomes a physiological insult of major dimensions to the elderly. Too often, we fear, communities sadly neglect the social and other real needs of this age group and fail to offer or sustain beneficial activities for them, although we must say that there are exceptions. Tucson is such an exception. In general, this city provides well for the elderly.

In the previous age grouping both sexes generally look forward to retirement. They expect the future to be both enjoyable and rewarding. This often proves to be true provided three factors are in evidence: First, the individual possesses a higher degree of health than is experienced by the average person today who passes the sixty-year mark, secondly, his financial needs are well taken care of, and thirdly, both partners to a marriage survive and especially when both are physically and mentally well and-active.

Unfortunately, however, we find that shortly after retirement, far too many in this age group find that they suffer from this disease or that condition and that the ensuing rapid decline in physical vigor does not permit them to fulfill their former hopes and dreams. The vital force they do possess begins to decline even more rapidly and, during t the last five years of this stage, the loss in the ranks accelerates to a devastating degree, often due to an overwhelming depression occasioned by the loss of loved ones, friends, and relatives, and to a series of unanticipated happenings with which they have difficulty coping.

Of course, a few emerge from this decade relatively unscathed and in good mental and physical health, but the majority do not. They succumb to the pressures of financial and other worries and to their physical ailments. Many lose their life's mate and are overcome by loneliness and despair. Suicides become increasingly more common as life's problems become too great for effective coping.

The Types of Diseases Commonly Experienced in Stage Seven:

1. Cancer in its many forms.

2. Arthritis in its many forms but especially rheumatoid arthritis. Ankylosing (fusing of joints) is common, especially among the hardier ones. In the weaker, one or more organs may give way with death resulting. Deformed and painful joints often curtail participation in social events and can lead to social isolation.

3. Tuberculosis and severe bronchial disorders of all kinds.

4. Bright's disease.

5. Abnormal growths including benign and malignant tumors, these in various places within the body.

6. Digestive disturbances and associated diseased conditions.

7. Diabetes with organic degeneration as, for example, of the pancreas; extreme fatigue; failure to heal wounds, etc.

8. Bone diseases (brittle bones, sponging of bones, scoliosis of the spine).

9. Sclerosis.

10. Cataracts and other eye diseases.

11. Early signs of senility.

12. Extreme depression resulting in suicide. This age group represents 25% of all reported suicides!

13. Drug addiction.

14. Alcoholism is very pronounced.

15. Heart attacks and strokes.

Again, we suggest to our students that they go back to Stage Six and compare the disorders most frequently experienced in that age group with the above list. Note how the conditions have become pejoratively worse as the cause or causes remained operational.

The State of Health Is Determined by:

1. Those who have reached this advanced age (by present standards, of course, not by Hygienic standards), have demonstrated not only their good inheritance but also the fact that they have taken reasonably good care of themselves.

2. The frequency, number, and kind of physiological insults they have endured during their life course, including, of course, their prenatal care, their care during the dependent years of childhood and adolescence, and during the intervening years. An insult of major dimensions in this age group is the wasting of their resources by children who sponge off them, borrowing their substance and leaving the elderly parent "holding the sack," as the common saying goes.

The Most Common Errors Made in Stage Seven Are:

1. Overnutrition; often now a compensation for life's negatives.

2. Poor nutrition.

3. Lack of exercise.

4. Using drugs, including vitamins and other supplements.

5. Overstimulation and incorrect stimulation—especially alcohol.

6. Falling prey to charlatans and quacks who offer "quick" cures for a lifetime of errors.

7. Failure to seek help when needed from whatever sources are available in the community of residence. Such help is available from a wide variety of sources: churches or from community, federal, state, and private agencies which are to be found in almost every community either at no charge or for a very nominal fee. As we have stated, the Hygienic practitioner should become knowledgeable about these services. Many newspapers regularly list them.

8. Failure of the community to provide participatory and/or leadership roles for the retired. The government at the federal level does have a program for the retired in which they can share their wealth of experiences with younger members of society. This is especially available to persons with business expertise to share. Practitioners may make themselves more knowledgeable in this regard by visiting the offices of the Small Business Administration. Inquire about opportunities for the elderly.

83.3.1.8. Stage Eight—The Post-Retirement Years

We should like to point out at this juncture that the constant intake of drugs soon pushes the drug taker into new dimension of life in which all body cellular membranes suffer, nerve pathways become erratic and con fused, and the total metabolic routines become uncertain and inefficient. This fact no doubt has a profound effect on many facets of the life process, if not, in fact, on all.

This is the period of life, from ages 70 to 80, that is generally accepted by both the population at large and the individuals concerned as being "Old Age." It should be the "Period of Harvest," the time of life when men am women should enjoy the fruits of their lives of love and labor but, unfortunately, the contrary is more often true.

The post-retirement years are only too often the years of trial and tribulation, rather than a time to gather in the rewards of a life well lived. As we look around, we find very few persons in this age group who are still contributing members of society. This is, of course, both unfortunate and unnecessary. The members of this age group not only demonstrate their good inheritance but also the fact that they have generally, and more or less consistently, taken good care of their physical and mental bodies, at least according to the tenets popularly espoused, but certainly not by Hygienic standards.

This is the age that should be a time for oneself, a time to engage in one's very own thoughts and activities, in various hobbies, or in private work of one's choosing. I should perhaps be a time to go back to school for a higher level of "Re-creation," a renewal of soul and a reassessment of values. The world remains to be explored a does the mind and soul of humans. This could and should be the most challenging time of life.

Unfortunately, major emotional stresses often enter and intrude upon daily living: fear of further hurts, of financial insecurity, of disease, of loneliness, among a host of other possible stresses. Anxiety often comes from within and is sponsored by imagined or real states which prove unacceptable to the mind. When a loved one is lost through death as, for example, one's lifetime mate, an all-embracing grief takes over. Danger, loss, or injury, too, are often just imagined but these may, of course, prove to be real. The stresses occasioned by either state may prove devastating to poise and thus to life itself. Such individuals, even though threatened by an unreal threat, often withdraw into some inner world of their own, one which is more comfortable for them.

The more the physical body is beset by physical degeneration, the more intense the retreat into a personal kind of fantasyland. Ordinary griefs and anxieties become exaggerated and may then turn into deep depression, this being the most common psychological involvement among the aged.

With others, a deep sense of anger sometimes evolves, feeling that the entire world has placed itself in direct opposition to one's personal hopes, dreams, and ambitions. A scapegoat may then be sought in an attempt to find some person or something which can be blamed for whatever predicament the individual happens to find himself in Such an attitude, of course, tends to alienate those around him and the individual thus possessed finds himself re treating more and more from a society which is, in his view, antagonistic toward him. This kind of attitude is usually amenable to corrective changes in eating and living habits.

Some Types of Diseases Commonly Experienced in Stage Eight:

1. Organ degeneration throughout the entire body with all parts, organs and systems involved.

2. Heart failure.

3. Digestive disorders of all kinds, sometimes psychosomatic in origin; loss of appetite due to depression.

4. Bright's disease.

5. Tuberculosis.

6. Cancer, although with a lessening susceptibility, due no doubt to the fact that organs give way before the onset of true cancer, actually a rare disease.

7. Cataracts and other eye disorders.

8. Great loss of vitality; loss of sexual drive. Occasional increase in the interest in sex but often accompanied by the inability to perform, this latter often observed in nursing homes where patients of both sexes are watched constantly else, they intrude on other patients for the purpose of having sex; in other words, some develop an abnormal sexual interest, but it is not accompanied by sexual power.

9. Bone diseases, loss in hearing, nervous disorders, especially Parkinson's disease (the "shaking" disease).

10. Emotional disorders: schizophrenia, senility, organic brain syndrome (general deterioration) and other psychopathologies resulting in extensive disorganization of the personality; the suicidal tendency which is often demonstrated by a refusal to eat or to get out of bed when perfectly capable of doing so; and also, at times, an unexplainable loss in weight, or a total lack of appetite. Hygienists, of course, recognize that all these symptoms are indicative of the presence of an unusual complement of morbid waste within the body.

The State of Health Is Determined by:

1. All those errors, circumstances and situations previously cited.

2. The nature of the continuing care of Self, whether good or poor.

The Most Common Errors Made in Stage Eight Are:

1. Overnutrition.

2. Poor nutrition.

3. Lack of exercise.

4. Lack of challenging and purposeful mental activity.

5. Failure to enter into community and other affairs.

6. Failure to seek help as and when the need arises.

7. Failure to prepare properly for this time of life, financially and otherwise, including mental preparation.

8. Physical and psychological abuse by families and/or others; 2 1/2 million elderly are thus abused every year in the U.S.

83.3.1.9. Stage Nine—The Years of Custodial Care

In today's society when an individual reaches the ninth stage in life's journey, he is generally regarded as "having had it." We include in this grouping all those persons who have lived in excess of eighty years, ages eighty to ninety and beyond! Unfortunately, by far the greater number of persons in this category require more or less complete custodial care similar to that required at the other end of the spectrum of life—in the first stage.

There is another similarity to the very young, also. Sad to relate, the very old, like the very young, often suffer from family and/or institutional abuse—the battered grandparent syndrome, as it is termed. The abuse ranges all the way from the psychological to actual physical abuse. Family neglect is common with many in this age group being housed by their children in institutions of doubtful reputation. We have known of patients who have been placed in custodial care provided by second-rate and/or by good institutions and who have never thereafter been visited by their children or other caring members of their family. Often the desire for some small gesture of love and affection visibly evident in the older "inmates" is pitiful, indeed.

A very low profile is kept of these elder citizens, their public visibility being practically nonexistent and, since most of the members of this age group (in excess of 98%) have long since passed away, there are few physically and mentally able among them who are able or in a position to protest. So it is that this group is, more often than not, at the complete mercy of a noncaring society.

The crying need of our times is for loving homes for these citizens who have served us and our country so well throughout their lives, Hygienic homes in which correct diet and lifestyle are taught and encouraged; where meaningful, constructive activity is provided, both mental and physical; where all the biodynamics of life are employed according to the several capacities of individuals to utilize them.

Sad to say, most Americans simply don't like old people. They have an image, fostered by financial interests, that all the elderly are foolish and senile, a potential burden. Consequently, they do not wish to be reminded of their presence. In their childishness, they refuse to accept that they, too, are presently riding on the same train that these elderly once rode and that, by the very nature of life, if they too are tough, they will reach this station in life.

The Types of Diseases Commonly Experienced in Stage Nine:

1. Neuroses of all kinds, especially depression caused by ill health and extreme loneliness. The kinds of neuroses observed may range from sitting in complete silence to constant talking and even yelling, as if in pain; failure to connect the present with the past; loss of memory, unwarranted suspicion, etc.

2. Brain damage.

3. Loss of hearing.

4. Loss of some degree of sight; total blindness.

5. Various organic failures due to eruption of latent organic illnesses. Incontinence is a common disorder.

6. Digestive disorders, especially colon constipation, a condition which causes extreme emotional stress among the elderly.

7. Existing organic diseases and conditions become aggravated, due to lack of proper remedial steps, and these often prove fatal.

8. Fear of change. Even moving a bed-fast patient to another room may cause unwarranted distress.

The State of Health Determined by:

1. All factors, influences and conditions which have previously cited.

2. The present care and nurture.

3. The Most Common Errors Made in Stage Nine Are:

4. Overnutrition and/or poor nutrition, both in and out of an institution.

5. Lack of exercise.

6. Emotional uncase.

7. Lack of a meaningful purpose for living.

8. Extreme loneliness.

9. Loss of the "will to live."

83.3.2. The Best in Institutional Care of the Elderly

A short time ago we were invited by a newly found friend who is and will remain an active participant in life, to accompany him to a nursing home that had recently been built in Tucson. Since we had not, as yet, had the opportunity to look over this particular facility, we met both with him and the director and were escorted around.

Being new, this home for the elderly was shiny bright. The floors sparkled, assistants and nurses were everywhere. There were three sections, each designed to provide a certain predetermined level of "health" care for the guests.

The first section housed the elderly guests who were able, for the most part, to provide for their personal care. They could put on their own clothing, attend to their personal cleanliness, and even go shopping occasionally in a group setting accompanied by staff personnel, such excursions being arranged from time to time.

The guests in this section were able to wend their separate ways to the dining room at mealtimes and to go to a beautiful outdoor setting where there were tables and lawn chairs available. There was also a whirlpool bathing facility for those who cared to use it. A television set and mall library were at one end of the facility for the use of 'those who cared to do so. However, there was little else to do.

Consequently, the guests who care to, and there seemed to be many such, wandered the main hall; some eat in the circular lobby which served this and two other sections, and there they simply watched the comings and goings of other guests, visitors, and staff members. There were no crafts, no study groups, no organized exercise sessions, or sunbathing.

We were fortunate to be present at mealtime, so we observed the food which was served to the guests and staff. The day's main level, served at noon, consisted of either baked chicken or fish, baked potatoes, and a cooked mixed vegetable dish which looked to us like the familiar peas and carrots frozen mixture. The dessert was ice cream. White bread was on hand plus oleo margarine and, of course, plenty of coffee, tea or a popular chemicalized lemon mix. We must say that this meal was superior to many we have seen placed before the elderly in similar "homes."

We were given plenty of time to examine the facility. All of the guests were obviously suffering from chronic degenerative conditions of one kind or another. We observed signs of sclerosis, rheumatic disorders, forgetfulness, osteoporosis of the spine, etc. However, to us each and every person in this section appeared to have more than sufficient vitality to assure a reasonable degree of recovery, even at this advanced age, were they to be taken out of this kind of "care" center and then placed in a Hygienic institution where they could be taught the ways of health, rather than be subjected, as they presently are, to the ways of premature death. For example, when asked, the director told us that all guests were kept on some kind of medication, and most were required to take sleeping pills. Our students will recognize the fact that the meal served would in no way serve the cause of health.

We then returned to the circular main lobby and began our examination of the second facility, this being designed to house individuals who required more care. Most of the guests here required assistance in dressing, bathing, and for transportation, since many were confined to wheelchairs chiefly because of rheumatoid arthritis, heart conditions, and other advanced degenerative disorders. We were told that most of these guests were kept on medication more or less constantly.

The ages of the guests here in this section ranged from about fifty years of age to perhaps eighty years. None appeared to be older, and most were probably in their late sixties and early seventies. Their sad faces mirrored their multiple concerns, their constant pain, and their weariness.

These guests also went to the dining room for their meals. If they were unable to manage their wheelchairs by themselves, they were assisted either by other more mobile guests or by staff personnel. The same boring environment was evident here as in section one.

The director then told us that we were now about to enter the third and last section of this home for the aged, this "Health Care Center," as it is called. The guests here did not have free access to the central section or to the outdoors. Upon opening the large double doors leading into this restricted area, a loud bell clanged. The sound reverberated throughout the facility, from one end to the other. We heard it ring repeatedly as staff entered and left. The director explained that the guests here were not responsible mentally and therefore had to be restricted in their movements. Most were, of course, also severely impaired physically.

The director advised us to prepare ourselves emotionally before meeting the poor souls housed here. We, of course, had previously been in similar institutions but it is always a shock to see what can happen to humans who do not know or care about the ways of health or who, knowing what they should do, refuse to acknowledge in their mind's eye, the inevitable consequences of error: pain, suffering and eternal darkness of mind and consciousness.

Among the guests, we learned, were a former bank president, several retired schoolteachers, the wife of one of the wealthiest men in town, and the son of a deceased well known industrialist. All the guests came from the more affluent of society. The basic cost of housing in this third section is enormous by most standards and all extras are computed on a per item cost value.

We observed a television set and a small room or two where both the aides and guests sat. In one of these rooms smoking was permitted. The guests simply sat looking out into a nothingness. Some issued strange moaning sounds, others cried aloud, as if tortured by some inner demon.

A small courtyard opened to the outdoors from this section. It was surrounded by a high wire fence. Access to it was through a closed and locked door. Not a single guest was that day enjoying the sunshine and the cool fresh air. When we remarked how sad it was that the guests were inside instead of being outside, the director replied, "I know—but we're all just so busy!"

All the guests in the third section required maximum care. They had to be fed, clothed, and transported. They had to be put to bed and gotten up. Many suffered from incontinence and had to be kept in diapers. Like small infants, they required constant care and nurturing.

We were happy to have joined our friend on this excursion. This is one of the best "homes" we have thus far visited. The need to provide Hygienic facilities for the elderly is obvious. There should be many opportunities for our students, to enter into this field of true health care. We live in what amounts to a family-estranged society. So often the elderly are shunted away from the familiar environment of the past into a strange setting where they often lack the sight of family or friend for the duration. They are surrounded by the new, the strange, the unfamiliar. They miss the tranquility of their homes, the peace of the expected. They cope but only with great difficulty with the constant confusion stirring within and around them.

There are those in the medical community who do have compassion on these poor souls, but they lack the knowledge of how properly to serve them. Most facilities are, however, run strictly on the profit motive. There is nothing basically wrong about making money for work well done. But in most homes the foods are selected not for their nutritive value but rather with two criteria in mind: 1. Cost and 2. Palate pleasing.

We have yet to find a facility where Hygienic care or anything resembling Hygienic care is provided. Instead, we have seen the elderly lying in their own excreta and writhing in pain on their beds. We have heard them cry out to us, "Get me out of here!" and, sadly, we had to turn away. We have smelled the foul odor of decay that pervades the very air they breathe, the decay of their own sickened and poisoned bodies. This is the forgotten segment of society, the warehoused ones, stuck away so as not to haunt the eyes and minds of the young who do not yet comprehend that their own biological clock is ticking away, too, and that they, like these, will also dissipate their vital force prematurely because they have not learned how to live.

83.4. A Contrasting View

In America only about 0.4% of the total population is said to survive to age 90 or over and even this figure is suspect since older persons tend to make themselves older, for some strange reason! The majority of Americans in their sixties and seventies stare out of blank eyes at a nothingness. Their faces are lined with care, their bodies twisted by arthritis and sclerotic diseases, their minds are overcome by worry, anxiety, care. As a consequence, many relapse into early senility and withdraw into a world of their own making.

In contrast let us look at some other people. In the Caucasus region of the Soviet Union there are an estimated 4,500 to 5,000 over-100-year-old people. Nearly 50 out of every 100,000 people in that part of the world live to celebrate their 100th birthday and many just keep going on from there! In fact, most believe that youth end at about the age of eighty, but they just aren't quite sure about that! In 1977, the latest figures we have, the oldest Russian known was said to be a "hale and hearty 168 years old." Only three Americans in 100,000 ever reach 100 years of age and only a handful go much beyond.

Over 10% of the Vilcabambans of the Ecuadorian Andes customarily pass the century mark. The longevity of the Hunzas of Pakistan has been well publicized. The longevity of all we have mentioned has been well documented. But the intriguing part about the longevity of these various groups of people is not mainly that they have lived so long but rather that they have lived more or less constantly, throughout their lifetimes, always in a state of superb health. They seem to have stumbled onto the fountain of perpetual middle-age!" They remain vigorous in body and spirit all their lives. Their minds are alert, and they remain filled with a zest for living. At 140 years of age, and perhaps even beyond, they work in the fields beside their great grandchildren, and, in the upper regions of the Himalayans, it is said that the ninety-year-olds, after their hard days' work in the field, often join the "kids" for a game of volleyball. When was the last time you ever saw a ninety-year-old playing volleyball or any other physical game?

The head of the National Institute on Aging, Dr. Robert N. Butler, spent 17 days in Russia a few years ago at the invitation of his Russian counterpart, Dmitri Chebotarev. He concluded from his research in that country that the legendary long-lived Russians are indeed for real and that they don't do it by eating yogurt!

Dr. Butler found 1. That the Soviets are ahead of the U.S. in recognizing the intimate connection between nutrition and the aging process, and 2. That the U.S. has more equipment for research. He cited these reasons why, in his view, the people in the Caucasus lived so long:

1. They remain vigorous in body and spirit all their lives.

2. They keep their minds active.

3. They retain a zest for living, are fun-filled, family-oriented.

4. They work hard and are physically active all their lives.

5. They have a good inheritance. (He pointed at whole families, all the members of which live well over the century mark.)

6. They have good nutrition. They eat sparingly and do not snack.

Dr. Butler sounds like a Life Scientist when he says that he observed that the aged Russians ate mostly of fruits and vegetables and they consumed only modest amounts of protein, very little fat, no salt, and no butter. They garnish their food, he said, with nuts instead of using sauces and they do not eat just before going to bed.

Butler observed that the old people stayed active and participated fully in home and community life. In a Gannet News Service release Butler recounts how one of the very old men threw a party for him. "It appeared to be important to him to be a good host," commented Butler!"

In light of our present knowledge of what is required for us to live always in a high state of health, just as these Russians do, it is incumbent upon all Life Scientists to participate actively in educating all people in the principles and practices that will impart to our aged ones a far higher state of health than they presently enjoy.

Butler noted that the Russians are actively pursuing their research while at American facilities devoted to gerontological research he stated that, "The longest time we can get people to come in is for two or three days." The Soviets have even tracked down birthdates and histories put down in old Korans and retrieved passport data from border crossing records of centuries ago. It seems that the Soviets are learning what retards the ticking of the biological clock while Americans appear to, be quite content merely to pop their pills and, in their narcotized state, passively to catch the rising tides of catastrophic diseases and painful deaths as well as they skyrocketing costs of housing and caring for all the sick, diseased, the senile and the dying, the numbers of which seem ever on the increase.

83.5. The American Express

A total of 225 million prescriptions are written annually for older America. At least 80% of these prescriptions are for mood-altering substances. Sleeping pills are the most frequently taken drug of all.

As noted, the problems are augmented because of the resulting drug complications due to multiple drug usage. When drugs are taken, the elderly are far more likely to have visible adverse reactions which are long-standing than are the young. In the latter, drugs usually produce acute symptoms which are repressed by another drug and then forgotten.

However, in the elderly, pill taking often leads to unexpected death. In the U.S., it seems we are so obsessed with drugs that we fail to study the ways of health!

We recently attended a lecture by a prominent surgeon. The lecture was intended to inform those persons who were about to retire as to the proper course of action. We found that most of those in attendance had long since retired.

They had come to listen to the sage advice of this eminent man of medicine, words that would restore them to health.

The surgeon's first thesis was to assume that retirement comes with age and that with age comes disability. His first words of wisdom invited his guests to visit various nursing homes and to choose which one they thought would best suit their future needs. Why? Because this would be their final home!

Next, he began a long recitation of disorders and gave the medical solution. If you suffer from dropsy, why just take your pills. We have purified exact doses of digoxin. Retirement has a great salubrious effect, but you must continue the drug, and sometimes add a diuretic.

If you retire in the tropics, you must take your quinine regularly. Do you have a thyroid disorder? We have exact doses in tiny pills that aren't hard to swallow, and they are "curative" for myxedema or hypothyroid states. If diagnosed early enough, this physician noted, and then treated (with drugs was, of course, implied) regularly, mental, deterioration, weight gain, arteriosclerosis are prevented. Low thyroid states must be diagnosed early, before retirement, and the hormone continued through retirement. So, keep taking your pills.

If you haven't retired yet and you're having trouble with your gallbladder, get it out now. Don't wait until you're retired. We're really getting more skilled at this sort of thing all the time. And don't forget to take your aspirin every day to keep your blood pressure down! I take three myself.

In reference to pacemakers and heart blocks, he commented somewhat as follows: The block is an interruption in the electrical pathway making the heartbeat. It is temporary or permanent. Your pacemaker can be inserted safely to stand by and cut in if the pathway fails. No longer are you subject to the unexpected faints and falls as the heart stops, blood pressure increases, and brain fails. Moral: Keep checking the batteries. They last longer now.

Following the lecture, we introduced ourselves and requested a copy of the physician's notes. The above is only a part of the advice given to all those sick, worried, and suffering souls that day. Is this all-modern medicine has to offer: Take your pills and have that surgery now! At the end of his talk, this highly respected surgeon pulled out a long computer printout sheet. It extended for yards and yards. It represented the item-by-item billing for a single 28-day stay at a local hospital, at the end of which time, the patient had died. The total bill amounted to $28,950.00. His final words to the audience? Why, of course! "Don't forget to take your pills!"

83.6. The Hygienic Approach—Case Studies

83.6.1. The Case of Mrs. B.

83.6.2. The Case of Brother's Brother

83.6.3. Case Study—Mr. X

83.6.4. Case Study—Mrs. A

83.6.5. The Case of Mrs. R.

83.6.6. Case Study—Mrs. R. D.

83.6.1. The Case of Mrs. B.

We have told Mrs. B.'s story elsewhere in other writings but her story illustrates so well the kind of miracle that the full application of Natural Hygiene can produce that we feel it bears repeating here.

Mrs. B. was brought to our office by her daughter and son-in-law. She barely had sufficient energy to walk through the door even though supported on either side. She was 66 years of age. A large portion of her body was covered with ulcerated sores. She was obviously in pain and extremely weak. We were advised that her doctor had suggested that it might be necessary to amputate her right leg. That he had exhausted his resources.

Upon examination the leg appeared swollen, ulcerated and a reddish brown to almost black in color. In spite of the ulcers and grape-like veins on both legs, she had been advised by her physician to constantly wear a tightly fitting elastic garment which she put on like a pair of pantyhose. This was "for support," she told us.

Constipation, heart irregularity, lack of appetite, inability to eat any uncooked foods, gas, stomachache—all these symptoms and more were recited. This was, indeed, a woman in trouble. She was also a victim of the "poor me" complex. She was firmly convinced that nothing could be done for her, that she was doomed.

We decided to take "baby steps" with Mrs. B. We made no changes whatsoever in her eating program except to urge her to combine the foods she liked according to accepted Hygienic standards. We also told her to take off this restraining garment and to toss it in the ashcan. We carefully explained how it would serve only to restrict the circulation and how she needed a good blood flow to encourage healing of her leg.

Within two weeks, the stomach pains were gone, and she was having an occasional "normal" bowel movement. Gradually, but gradually, we improved her diet. Then came the sunbaths. This was a real adventure, but she decided she liked this, so they soon became a regular habit. We showed her a few simple stretching exercises. Dr. Robert lay on the floor and did them for her so she could see how to help herself when raising the legs up. She knew that if he at his age could do all that, perhaps she could, too! And she did.

Soon she began to walk. Walk she did around and around the mobile home park where she lives. Her doctor said it was a miracle. Today there is no talk of amputation, no drugs. Instead, there is hope. Mrs. B. knows that life can be beautiful. She is now over 70 years of age. We recently gave a lecture and guess who was there. Mrs. B., of course, there with a few friends. She blew a kiss. There was joy on her face but not a single ugly ulcer. For Mrs. B the past is history. She confided to Dr. Elizabeth that she has a boyfriend!

83.6.2. The Case of Brother's Brother

Our readers recall the story of our 97-year-old friend. Well, this story concerns the younger "brother." At age 73 he attended one of our lectures and subsequently enrolled in a class which consisted of seven sessions.

For 13 years Mr. M. had made regular visits to a local hospital to have his blood pressure checked and to get his prescriptions filled. For 13 years he had followed directions and taken his pills. His blood pressure reading was sky-high. Obviously, the danger of a stroke was very real to this man. However, he was an extremely intelligent man. He saw the rationale of the Garden of Eden diet and the grand sense of adhering to organic realities. He immediately shifted into high gear, as it were. Fruits, fruits, and more fruits. He bought watermelon and cantaloupes by the box. He complained at first because he had to get up at night, as many as ten times to urinate, but he persisted.

Mr. M. began to lose weight. He had to buy new clothes, but he kept on. He began to walk. He walked over all of Tucson! His complexion became beautifully smooth and clear, and his eyes sparkled with life. He began to fast on his own, first a single day at a time, and later extended the fasts first to three days and then to five. Each time he lost more weight which he did not regain. Now each time he fasts, he loses but very little weight. One of these days he will stabilize and then, perhaps, regain some of his lost pounds. But Mr. M. really doesn't much care about that. He is rejoicing in his new lease on life and, also, because his "brother" is doing so well and, especially, because brother will now give up bread!

83.6.3. Case Study—Mr. X

We include this brief news item to illustrate how abuse of the elderly can even be unintentional, simply perhaps a matter of negligence. Daily reports are made on local television as to the maximum sun exposure time before burning can be expected. Today, in the Arizona Daily Star there is an item which states, "The Medical Audit Committee for Pima County's Department for Improved Adult Living will hold an inquiry this morning into the circumstances surrounding the death of an 87-year-old man who may have been left out in the sun too long. This is the public program which oversees nursing homes. The man in question, it seems, was wheelchair bound. Left in the sun, he developed a temperature of 108° and died shortly thereafter."

83.6.4. Case Study—Mrs. A

Mrs. A. was aged 86 when she came under our care. Her husband, a few months older, was to come to us shortly thereafter. Mrs. A. was already senile, somewhat difficult to manage and suspicious.

However, she became greatly attached to Dr. Elizabeth who sometimes would just simply sit quietly by her side and hold her hand. Simple dietary changes were made with emphasis on food combining. Once each week, she was dressed and taken for a walk and out to dinner. She looked forward to these times. She responded well physically but the mind did not. In fact, she lost her own identity and that of her husband. One day she took out her false teeth and threw them at him exclaiming at the same time, "He just wants my money!" However, the physical improvement was remarkable, under the circumstances, considering the advanced state of deterioration present when Hygienic care was started. This woman lived to be 90 years of age. Her general disposition became loving and outgoing, but she became more and more childlike.

The husband had been diagnosed six years prior to our taking over his care as having leukemia. He told us his fecal matter had been so impacted that practitioners were compelled literally to dig into the colon to extract it. Apparently, he had been taking radioactive cobalt during these six years.

One day one of a pair of workmen who were doing some repairs at his house and also painting one of the ceilings was discharged by the old man who was highly dissatisfied with the work. Being very determined, he got up on the ladder to do the job himself and promptly fell off. The shock triggered an immediate and rapid deterioration, and it was necessary to place him in a nursing home since there was no one to care for him at home. He died shortly thereafter, and it is interesting to our study to note that an autopsy showed extensive organ deterioration and spinal bone sponging. He was 90 at the time of his death, also. This gentleman refused all dietary and other Hygienic suggestions. He continued taking his pills. He continued to suffer.

83.6.5. The Case of Mrs. R.

Mrs. R. came to us from another state. We bring her to your attention because she demonstrates how well the mind and body will respond when the full impact of the correctness of Natural Hygiene principles is immediate and causes radical changes in all aspects of living and eating.

At first meeting we learned that Mrs. R. had given birth to eight children and did not know what had happened to a single child. She was in her late 50s and the-children were all in the 20 to 35 age group. During the turbulent fifties and sixties, they had joined communes, and many had gotten caught up in the drug culture.

Her physician had diagnosed a severe liver disorder and given a dim prognosis. Our first meeting lasted two hours during which time she poured out all her misery, anxiety, her fears. We found out that she was very religious, so we urged her to concentrate on her faith and on the future. We gave her a course of study in Natural Hygiene and asked her to give it due consideration.

From time to time we corresponded and at such times answered questions. A year later she came for her second consultation. The change was remarkable. She was smiling, her attitude was positive. Her complexion was much improved but, best of all, she had developed an attitude that life's problems could be satisfactorily solved. She obviously had not as yet solved all of her problems, but she was certainly much more confident of herself and the future.

Three years have passed. She now knows where every single one of her children is. In fact, this last year, she, and her husband made a trip around the country and visited every single one of the young people. They have all, but one, entered the mainstream of life. The one exception is presently in a hospital under treatment for tuberculosis. But, best of all, this woman is herself a picture of radiant health. Her family doctor? Why, he has asked to borrow her study books! You see, even at her advanced age, her liver made a fantastic recovery, this in spite of his dim prognosis and, what is more, without his prescribed pills!

83.6.6. Case Study—Mrs. R. D.

Mrs. R. D. came to us after having experienced a limited hysterectomy, three massive heart attacks followed by a mastectomy and two years of severe angina "attacks." She had been advised that there were several coronary occlusions but that her body had partially corrected all but one of these. Mrs. R. D. expressed her willingness to place herself completely in our hands since she had finally come to the conclusion that her doctor of many years had nothing more to suggest. However, she was afraid to fast and, perhaps, it would not have been desirable in her case. We placed this woman on our Extended Rest Plan which involves the following:

First Three Weeks

1. A diet of raw foods only except for a single baked potato served twice a week.

   Breakfast—A single fruit, preferably melon.
   Luncheon—A simple vegetable salad with 3 T nuts or 1 medium avocado.
   Dinner—Fruit—2 varieties.

2. Ten hours rest at night.

3. During the day: 2 hours prone in a darkened room, 1 hour either sitting up in bed or, later on, in a chair.

4. Passive exercise: i.e., arms and legs being moved by an assistant.

5. Passive massage: Assistant using the flat side of three fingers lightly massages the skin and especially of the back.

Second Three Weeks

1. Diet same as above.

2. Night rest same as above.

3. One hour prone in a darkened room, 2 hours up, either sitting reading in a chair or listening to music, or about the third week, walking out of doors. Sun bath every day.

Seventh Week

1. Diet continued.

2. Client began simple exercises and extended walking to about one block.

3. Daily sunbathing when possible.

4. Up all morning. Two-hour nap after lunch. Got ready for bed immediately after third meal of day, at about 7 p.m.

Before the tenth week had passed, this client was able to walk a mile with ease. Almost three years have passed during which time she has taken no medication and has not had a single angina attack. Her physician requested her to go over her diet with the hospital dietitian and stated that he would like to try it on some other patients. Her EKG and other signs continue to stand up well under examination. Mrs. R. D. is now in her late sixties and travelling all over the country! The past is a closed book. This recovery is remarkable in that it took place in a cold, largely hostile climate. It shows the tremendous healing powers present within even a badly-abused body and how, when given the tools, the body will accomplish almost the impossible, restoring to even the very sick the opportunity to enjoy many more productive years of healthful living.

Article #1: Inward Time by Alexis Carrel, M.D.

The declining years of maturity and senescence have little physiological value. They are almost empty of organic and mental changes. They have to be filled with artificial activities. The aging man should neither stop working nor retire. Inaction further impoverishes the content of time. Leisure is even more dangerous for the old than for the young. To those whose forces are declining, appropriate work should be given. But not rest. Neither should physiological processes be stimulated at this moment. It is preferable to hide their slowness under a number of psychological events. If our days are filled with mental and spiritual adventures, they glide much less rapidly. They may even recover the plenitude of those of youth.

... So far, human beings are classified according to their chronological age. Children of the same age are placed in the same class. The date of retirement is also determined by the age of the worker. It is known, however, that the true condition of an individual does not depend on his chronological age. In certain types of occupation, individuals should be grouped according to physiological age. Puberty has been used as a way of classifying children in some New York schools. But there are still no means of ascertaining at what time a man should be pensioned. Neither is there any general method of measuring the rate of the organic and mental decline of a given individual. However, physiological tests have been developed by which the condition of a flyer can be accurately estimated. Pilots are retired according to their physiological, and not their chronological, age.

Young and old people, although in the same region of space, live in different temporal worlds. We are inexorably separated by age from one another. A mother never succeeds in being a sister to her daughter. It is "impossible" for children to understand their parents, and still less their grandparents. Obviously, the individuals belonging to four successive generations are profoundly heterochronic. An old man and his great-grandson can be complete strangers.

From the concept of physiological time derive certain rules of our action on human beings. Organic and mental developments are not inexorable. They can be modified, in some measure, according to our will, because we are a movement, a succession of superposed patterns in the frame of our identity.

Although man is a closed world, his outside and inside frontiers are open to many physical, chemical, and psychological agents. And those agents are capable of modifying our tissues and our mind. The moment, the mode, and the rhythm of our interventions depend on the structure of physiological time. Our temporal dimension extends chiefly during childhood when functional processes are most active.

Then, organs and mind are plastic. Their formation can effectively be aided. As organic events happen each day in great numbers, their growing mass can receive such shape as it seems proper to impress permanently upon the individual. The molding of the organism according to a selected pattern must take into account the nature of duration, the constitution of our temporal dimension. Our interventions have to be made in the cadence of inner time. Man is like a viscous liquid flowing into the physical continuum. He cannot instantaneously change his direction. We should not endeavor to modify his mental and structural form by rough procedures, as one shapes a statue of marble by blows of the hammer. Surgical operations alone produce in tissues sudden alterations. And recovery from the quick work of the knife is slow. No profound changes of the body as a whole can be obtained rapidly. Our action must blend with the physiological processes, substratum of inner time, by following their own rhythm.

... A child may be compared to a brook, which follows any change in its bed. The brook persists in its identity in spite of the diversity of its forms. It may become a lake or a torrent. Under the influence of environment, personality may spread and become very thin, or concentrate and acquire great strength. The growth of personality involves a constant trimming of our self. At the beginning of life, man is endowed with vast potentialities. He is limited in his development only by the extensible frontiers of his ancestral predispositions. But at each instant he has to make a choice. And each choice throws into nothingness one of his potentialities. He has of necessity to select one of the several roads open to the wanderings of his existence, to the exclusion of all others. Thus, he deprives himself of seeing the countries wherein he could have traveled along the other, roads. In our infancy we carry within ourselves numerous virtual beings, who die one by one. In our old age, we are surrounded by an escort of those we could have been, of all our aborted potentialities. Every man is a fluid that becomes solid, a treasure that grows poorer, a history in the making, a personality that is being created. And our progress, or our disintegration, depends on physical, chemical, and physiological factors, on viruses and bacteria, on psychological influences, and, finally, on our own will. We are constantly being made by our environment and by our self. And duration is the very material of organic and mental life, as it means "invention, creation of forms, continual elaboration of the absolutely new."

... There is a striking contrast between the durability of our body and the transitory character of its elements. Man is composed of a soft, alterable matter, susceptible of disintegrating in a few hours. However, he lasts longer than if made of steel. Not only does he last, but he ceaselessly overcomes the difficulties and dangers of the outside world. He accommodates himself, much better than the other animals do, to the changing conditions of his environment. He persists in living, despite physical, economic, and social upheavals. Such endurance is due to a very particular mode of activity of his tissues and humors. The body seems to mold itself on events. Instead of wearing out, it changes. Our organs always improvise means of meeting every new situation. And these means are such that they tend to give us a maximum duration. The physiological processes, which are the substratum of inner time, always incline in the direction leading to the longest survival of the individual. This strange function, this watchful automatism, makes possible human existence with its specific character. It is called adaptation.

All physiological activities are endowed with the property of being adaptive. Adaptation, therefore, assumes innumerable forms. However, its aspects may be grouped into two categories, intraorganic and extra organic. Intraorganic adaptation is responsible for the constancy of the organic medium and of the relations of tissues and humors. It determines the correlation of the organs. It brings about the automatic repair of tissues and the cure of diseases. Extra organic adaptation adjusts the individual to the physical, psychological, and economic world. It allows him to survive in spite of the unfavorable conditions of his environment. Under these two aspects, the adaptive functions are at work during each instant of our whole life. They are the indispensable basis of our duration.

Whatever our sufferings, our joys, and the agitation of the world may be, our organs do not modify their inward rhythm to any great extent. The chemical exchanges of the cells and the humors continue imperturbably. The blood pulsates in the arteries and flows at an almost constant speed in the innumerable capillaries of the tissues. There is an impressive difference between the regularity of the phenomena taking place within our body and the extreme variability of our environment. Our organic states are very steady. But this stability is not equivalent to a condition of rest, or equilibrium. It is due, on the contrary, to the unceasing activity of the entire organism. To maintain the constancy of the blood's composition and the regularity of its circulation, an immense number of physiological processes are required. The tranquility of the tissues is assured by the converging efforts of all the functional systems. And the more irregular and violent our life, the greater are these efforts. For the brutality of our relations with the cosmic world must never trouble the peace of the cells and humors of our inner world.

As extracted from his major work, Man, the Unknown. Out of Print.

Article #2: Overnutrition—All About Protein by The Doctors McCarter

Epidemiological And Historical Evidence

Epidemiological And Historical Evidence

In light of the continuing confusion existing not only among the public at large but also in many scientific circles with regard to the optimum amount of protein required to maintain superb health and especially because of the current media emphasis on our supposed need to eat a diet high in protein, it would appear of considerable importance to review some of the epidemiological and historical evidence that bears on this subject. It would appear that such evidence is the only really solid evidence to be had: how have people responded for thousands of years to whatever dietary practices they, as a tribe or people, have constantly pursued? It takes many generations to observe results that can be considered conclusive. Pottenger and his cohorts at Yale University demonstrated that it takes three to four generations to prove the validity or lack thereof, of a particular dietary regimen with cats. We must assume that the same would hold true with humans.

Throughout history, and in various parts of the world and in different climates and under diverse circumstances, millions and billions of people have lived exclusively on a simple vegetable protein dietary intake, rarely exceeding 30 to 35 grams per day. Some used animal flesh only occasionally, as on special feast days. Many have totally avoided all animal products, such as milk or eggs. In other words, they were vegans. Recorded history strongly suggests that they have as a rule, enjoyed far better health than the average meat-eating person or tribe of peoples.

Dr. Alan Walker of the Department of Cell Biology and Anatomy, The Johns Hopkins University School of Medicine, startled the scientific community when, in 1979, he announced that, according to extensive studies of fossil teeth performed by him and his associates, he had concluded that early man lived for millions of years on an exclusively fruit diet. (In a letter to your authors. Dr. Walker states that man was able to adapt successfully to progressive dietary changes. His paper on this research was published in Great Britain.)

It has been shown by many researchers that dietary habits powerfully determine the particular lifestyle and character of peoples. Walker, for example, quotes from research originally reported by R.A. Dart in 1953 as follows with regard to Australopithecus (an early man):

"... carnivorous creatures, that seized living quarries by violence, battered them to death, tore apart their broken bodies, disembodied them limb from limb, slaking their ravenous thirst with the hot blood of victims and greedily devouring livid writhing flesh."

Many modern studies have showed the relationship between diet and hyperkinetic behavior and how chemicals added to food can relate to adverse neurotic tendencies. Other studies have related depression, inability to sleep, loss of memory, moods in general to dietary insufficiencies or excesses of one kind or another. Dr. Brian Morgan, an assistant professor at Columbia University's Institute of Human Nutrition in New York City, is reported to have said that "You can affect your mood and behavior by the kinds of foods that you eat." Natural Hygiene has long held this view as have your authors.

Crime and cancer are rampant across America and in other parts of the world and especially in those parts where heavy meat eating is the custom; whereas among the rural Chinese, East Indians and among certain native peoples of Latin America, these scourges are almost nonexistent. These latter peoples all consume low-protein diets. The Hunzas of the Himalayas, for example, are well known for their emphasis on indigenous fruits in their diet and for the fact that they eat little, if any, animal protein. This tribe is also noted for the longevity of its individual members and for their superb health. It must be noted, of course, that these people live largely out of doors, work hard at their agricultural pursuits, do not consume processed and chemicalized food—all of which contributes also to their wellbeing. We hear that many modern "delights" are now finding their way into this area since the building of a road there. It should be interesting for future generations to observe the changes that may accrue in the health of these people.

Indians living at 13,000 feet in the Andes continue to eat their high natural carbohydrate, low-protein diets and continue to demonstrate amazing endurance and strength. The Tarahumara Indians of Mexico stick to a similar diet and are able to run 90 miles at seven miles per hour with no heart expansion or shortness of breath.

Perhaps we should contrast this ability with the condition of some marathon runners at the conclusion of a run of only 26 miles, runners considered by the press and the public at large to be in superb physical condition! Many collapse at the end of the run, some take weeks to recover.

The long-living and extremely healthy Georgians of Russia are living examples in our day of the correctness of a diet low in protein and high in carbohydrates. They are a hard-working, fun-loving, out-going people, family-oriented, who live, on an average, beyond the century. Most rarely eat meat. Many do consume Koumiss, a kind of fermented milk.

This is the kind of evidence that cannot be ignored. This is the kind of superb health which is the result of eating practices followed by hundreds of generations and for thousands of years. This is the kind of health and longevity which is in direct contrast to what can be observed among the tribes who consume a high-protein diet: the Eskimos, Laplanders and Masai being prime examples.

Both the Eskimos and Laplanders are gross in development and more or less dull mentally. They rarely live beyond the age of forty-five years. The Masai grow to great heights, often in excess of seven and even eight feet, but their life span is short. They live, on an average, to about the age of twenty-five years. The Masai are a tribe living in Africa. They are a sub-grouping of the Sudanese.

The Eskimos consume much fat and eat whale and other raw sea animals. At certain times of the year, they subsist on native plants of the far north. The Laplanders are reindeer-eaters, for the most part, while the Masai consume mare's milk and drain the blood from animals for sustenance. The Laplanders live beyond the Arctic Circle where vegetation is sparse. Those who live in coastal areas do have occasional access to fish. Gross of body and short lived they offer mute testimony to the long-term effects of their diet.

It is interesting to note that, for the most part, these meat-eating tribes maintain a high level of health during their short lives probably due to the fact that their lifestyle is basically correct: they live out of doors, the stresses of civilization are practically nonexistent, they are very supportive of one another, they do not have access to foodless foods and are not exposed to other factors known to be destructive of health.

The average person in America today probably consumes two to four times as much protein as he requires for optimum living with many consuming six to eight times as much. This latter figure would apply, in many instances, to executives on the "party-entertainment circuit," those who make a practice of consuming sixteen-ounce steak and lobster dinners and favor steak and egg breakfasts. (We recently heard about a restaurant that features steaks in excess of 40 ounces!)

It is the considered opinion of your authors that the nausea experienced so often by astronauts in space is due not only to the stress of the occasion but also to the emphasis placed on animal protein in their diets. They would be far better served to eat little or nothing prior to lift-off or to eat a meal high in carbohydrates, and especially if they ate a well-combined and properly constructed meal consisting of fresh ripe fruit plus, perhaps, some lettuce and celery. It has long been known that emotional stress can stop the digestive process for hours during which time all undigested foodstuffs ferment and putrefy giving rise to nausea, diarrhea, and other uncomfortable gastric and related disorders such as headaches, insomnia, as well as others. A meal such as we suggest would be largely pre-digested and pose no such problems. Additionally, it would tend to conserve body energy for the exacting tasks at hand. It would tend to "burn clean" and not add clutter to body channels.

A physiologically-correct dietary program such as we suggest would provide ample energy for performance, would conserve body resources, increase mental alertness, and permit normal metabolism. It would not occasion the four adverse responses of a high protein intake, nor would it waste energy resources—energy wasted during the required prolonged digestion and in combatting the fermentation and putrefaction forthcoming when poorly chosen and incorrect foods are eaten at any time, and most particularly, when they are eaten at times of great stress.

Article #3: Health

Extracted from The New American Encyclopedia published by Books, Inc. Copyright 1938, 1939. We include this extract for the purpose of showing our students that the requirements of the good life are both simple and well known. All that is lacking is the doing!

Health is the state in which the body functions normally. This condition finds the body free from disease, with all organs and component parts of its structure performing their functions properly and in correct balance.

Health is a normal and relatively constant state in wild animals, this condition prevailing from their heeding of instinctive guidance, and from the free operation of nature's laws of survival of the fittest which inexorably eliminates the weak.

Man's instinctive apparatus has become dulled by the exercise of his reasoning powers and by habits of civilization which lead him to rely upon others for guidance. Health to him represents a relative condition, in which he seldom enjoys a state of perfection.

With the development of medicine and surgery the weak are preserved, resulting in inherited defects or weaknesses. Hence a constantly increasing need for (1) Development of scientific treatment of disorders; (2) Understanding by man himself of the warnings and subsequent treatment of his ills.

It is an impressive fact that most ailments in persons can be, in part, prevented by properly regulating diet, by avoiding overindulgence in food and alcoholic beverages, by controlling the weight within normal limits, by taking mild physical exercise and leading a normal mental existence, free from excessive nervous strain or emotional disturbances. Our modern mode of living has much to do with involving us in what is known in medicine as a vicious cycle. At the age of thirty or so, a young person becomes deeply engrossed in his career. Exercise is soon curtailed, but since the nervous system craves some form of amusement and diversion, the pleasures of the table and the soothing action of tobacco or the stimulating influence of alcoholic beverages are substituted. In consequence, the weight increases, the appetite enlarges, and there is further disinclination to physical exercise, a deeper absorption in the business of and readier yielding to the temptations of food, tobacco, and wine; and so, endlessly, he whirls tighter with each revolution. As a result, at the age of fifty or sixty, he is likely to find himself the possessor of a fortune, a large abdomen, a bad heart, and a pair of damaged kidneys.

From the standpoint of health, the chief enemy of young people is tuberculosis; of the middle-aged, personal neglect. The middle age diseases such as chronic heart disease, high blood pressure, kidney disease, are painless, and their onset usually gradual and insidious. If one relies upon some signal from within to be warned of the impending danger, however, there is a risk of these conditions developing to the extent of causing irreparable damage before their presence is known. Good heredity and robust, constitutions are no guarantee of long life. The desire not to know if anything is wrong is cowardly and stupid.

The secret of good health is moderation in all things—in eating, work, mental effort, ambition, play, and exercise. The life of moderation is the simple life and, therefore, the healthy, long, and a happy one. Those who prefer speed and profess a contempt for the consequences, always change their views when, too late, nature demands payment.

After the age of 50, the thinner an individual is, the better is his chance of reaching old age, provided he does not have a tendency to develop tuberculosis or has not suffered from tuberculosis in earlier years, and provided, too, his light weight is not due to some organic disease.

You have no doubt been repeatedly told that persons who weigh too much past the age of 35 have poor prospects of attaining old age. Their particular enemy is heart disease. Statistics have abundantly demonstrated the truth of this statement. This does not mean that a very fat person cannot live to age 90 or even 100, but his chances of doing so are small.

Overweight is usually due to overeating, although stout persons nearly always insist that they are very sparce eaters; but they measure the amount of food that they eat by their appetites, and the appetite is a very flexible measuring rod, capable of being enormously stretched by hungry persons. With very few exceptions, any person who is too heavy can reduce if he will make an effort to do so. The effort is worthwhile. At the age of 50, for instance, every pound of weight in excess increases a man's likelihood of dying during the ensuing year by about one percent. In other words, if a man 50 years old weighs 50 pounds in excess of the standard figures, the likelihood of his dying is constantly 50 times greater than that of a man 50 years old who is of normal weight. (Hygienists generally hold that the standard figures are too high, possibly to the extent of 15 or more pounds. —The Authors).

In order to effect weight reduction intelligently, an elementary knowledge of food and food values is necessary. With regard to protein, this Encyclopedia comments, "The average person uses too much protein. If protein is taken to excess, the body is unable to split up this food completely into harmless end products; instead, certain irritating substances are produced which have a harmful action on vital organs of the body, particularly the kidneys." With regard to fats, "Fat is the most difficult food for the body to digest and consume. The energy of fat is released slowly and those who eat fats excessively become sluggish mentally and physically."

"If your work demands much physical effort, such as that of a laborer or farmer, this is not necessary except when you are not working. But the man doing office work must do some physical work daily to insure good health. Past the age of 40 the best exercise is walking. Five miles a day is not too much, provided you start out by walking a mile the first week and increasing it a mile a week until you are doing the five miles. Golf playing is good, not once a week, but daily. In the summertime, an hour or two in the garden, hoeing, etc., may be substituted for walking. Do not attempt the more strenuous exercises after the age of 40 and remember that outdoor exercise is better than indoor."

Article #4: Why Exercise?

Dr. Robert's Daily Exercises

"Why exercise?" We all want to keep the vigor of youth. Exercise is a means to that end, but we must exercise regularly to get the full benefits. Before the dawn of civilization mankind was not troubled by the need for exercise. Our forefathers, in the dim ages long passed, had to exercise to live—to get their food, to fight off enemies. Today we no longer depend on hunting and fishing for our food. Large numbers of us sit at desks or tend machines. We ride in automobiles, trains, elevators. The enemies of. primitive life do not bother us. And the result is that most of us do not get the amount and variety of physical activity which the human body needs.

The suppleness of limb and the untiring vigor developed in the play and sports of childhood soon tend to pass with advancing years. Our daily work often requires little or no muscular activity—or, perhaps, the use of only a limited number of muscles. And so, we must make up for this lack in our off-work hours. We must deliberately choose to exercise if we would enjoy its benefits. As we grow older it becomes all too easy to take us little exercise as possible, despite the fact that this is the time when a certain amount of exercise is very much needed. It is needed to keep the heart and lungs in prime condition—to keep the circulation active—to improve digestion and elimination—to preserve a healthful and attractive posture. In short, it helps to insure proper functioning of the whole body—to keep us full of vigor and feeling fit."

Dr. Robert's Daily Exercises

1. Twisting. Hands on hips. Turn to the right, then to the left. Up to 100 times.

2. Dr. Tilden's face and neck exercises.

   Turn headfirst to right, then to left. 10 times each.
   Move head backwards as far as it will comfortably go. Return to chest. 10 times.
   Move head to right shoulder, then to left shoulder. 10 times.

3. Rotate shoulders, first in one direction, then in opposite direction. 20 times.

4. Raise shoulders to ear level. 10 times.

5. Extend arms forward to horizontal position. Rotate hands as rapidly as possible until reasonably tired. Extend arms to full vertical position and repeat same exercise.

   Extend arms to horizontal position to side and repeat same exercise.

6. Shadow box for two to three minutes.

7. Rotate arms in full circle simultaneously crossing the chest. 25 times.

   Using dumbbells (start with 5 pounders and increase poundage as soon as ten Reps are comfortably achieved):

   Bend over at waist. Dumbbells in hand, bend arms at elbow. 10 reps. In standing position. Repeat.

8. Using both dumbbells elevate to overhead position and return to shoulder. 10 reps. Extend dumbbells out to side from hip position to shoulder position. 10 Reps. Shadow box with 10 pounders.

9. Windmill. Touch right toe with left hand, then left toe with right hand. 20 Reps.

10. Deep knee bends. 20 Reps.

11. Ride bicycle. 25 times. In bicycle position, 10 bending of knees and push up to extended vertical position. 25 times.

12. Aerobic dancing. Tap dancing to music. 5 to 10 minutes.

13. Running in place. 10 minutes.

14. Walking as time permits.

On January 1, 1984, Dr. Robert will be 83 years young. In addition to the physical activity, he spends 10 to 12 hours actively engaged in research, writing, and operating Bionomics Health Research Institute.

Lesson 84:

The Basic Four Diet

84.1. Introduction

There was a large wall chart, and the third-grade teacher was pointing to it as she taught me and my elementary school classmates our first lesson in nutrition.

There were four big pictures on the chart. One picture showed a cow surrounded by milk, butter, and cheese. Another picture had steaks, pork chops, and sausages piled high, with a few beans sprinkled around the different meats. At the bottom of the chart was a picture of loaves of bread and a bowl of cereal. Finally in the other corner of the poster was a head of lettuce, apples, oranges, and a yellow squash.

The teacher was pointing to each picture. "Now to grow up healthy and strong," she said, "you must eat different foods every day. You need milk and meat and bread and some vegetables or fruit at every meal." She pointed to the picture of the cow, and then to the steak (I didn't know at that time that the steak had come from the cow!) and then to the bowl of cereal and the yellow squash.

It sounded good to my eight-year-old ears. All you had to do to eat right and be healthy is just to remember to eat four types of food at every meal. It was logical and so neatly explained by that big food chart that had been supplied by the U.S. Department of Agriculture.

Twelve years later after following such a diet, I knew my third-grade teacher had lied to me. I wasn't healthy or strong or well. I studied nutrition on my own and discovered the real truth about diet and well-being—the truth that had been so carefully hidden from me and is still denied children in school today.

The Basic Four Food Group diet that was so vividly illustrated on that chart is still the most popular diet and nutrition plan in this country today. And it is dangerously incorrect.

84.2. What Is the Basic Four Diet?

84.2.1. Four Food Diet Plan

84.2.2. The Reasons for the Four Food Groups Diet Plan

84.2.3. The Advantages of the Four Food Group Diet Plan

The Basic Four Diet was created by the U.S. Department of Agriculture and is formally known as the USDA Four Food Group Plan.

This plan classifies all foods into four basic groups and recommends a minimum number of servings from each group in order to satisfy the Recommended Daily

Allowances (RDAs) of nutrients. The RDAs are a set of recommendations for daily intake of calories, protein, vitamins, and minerals made by the Food and Nutrition Board of the National Academy of Sciences. The amounts recommended by the board will, according to them, "provide for the maintenance of optimum nutrition in healthy persons in the United States."

In the Four Food Group Plan, foods are arranged into four categories:

1. Milk Group
2. Meat Group
3. Bread and Cereal Group
4. Fruit and Vegetable Group

Each group contains foods similar enough in nutrient content to be more or less interchangeable, or so the reasoning goes. The table below shows the four food groups, serving sizes for the group, and the alternative selections that may be chosen from when planning on a diet using the Four Food Group Plan:

84.2.1. Four Food Diet Plan

Food Groups Minimum Servings for Adults

1. Milk Group

    2 servings. (One serving is 8 ounces of milk or yogurt, or 1 slice of cheese.)

2. Meat arid Meat Alternatives

    2 servings. (One serving is 3 ounces of any of the following: lean meat, fish, shellfish, eggs, poultry, cheese with dry beans or dry peas or peanut butter.)

3. Bread and Cereal Group

    4 servings. (One serving is 1 slice of bread or 1 ounce of dry cereal or 2/3 cup of cooked cereal.)

4. Fruit and Vegetable Group

    4 servings. (One serving is 1/2 cup cooked fruit or vegetable, or 1 medium-size raw fruit or vegetable)

84.2.2. The Reasons for the Four Food Groups Diet Plan

The Four Food Group plan was basically devised to cover the foods predominantly produced by our agricultural and commercial enterprises. Ostensibly, it simplified meal planning, assured us of our nutrient needs, and was an easily understood approach to nutrition.

Here are the major nutrients in the diet that each food group was supposed to supply:

PROTEIN	Meat Group, Milk Group
CALCIUM	Milk Group
IRON	Meat Group
B VITAMINS	Bread and Cereal Group, Milk Group
VITAMIN A	Fruit and Vegetable Group
VITAMIN C	Fruit and Vegetable Group

84.2.3. The Advantages of the Four Food Group Diet Plan

There are two major advantages in using the Four Food Group plan to develop a diet:

1. The plan is relatively simple to understand. All foods are divided into four easily recognizable groups, and exact serving amounts of each food group are specified. Even those people entirely ignorant of nutrition can use the Four Food Group plan without any additional education.

Some nonfoods and junk foods such as soft drinks, candy, and other snacks are not included in any of the four categories. (You should notice, however, that many poor foods and processed foods are included in these groups— for example, nitrate-preserved meats, white bread, polished rice, pasteurized milk, etc.).

84.3. And Now for the Truth

84.3.1. One Man's Meat Is Everyone's Poison

84.3.2. If You Don't Eat the Cow, Why Drink the Juice?

84.3.3. The Staff of Whose Life?

84.3.4. And the Winner Is...

84.3.5. Second Helpings, Anyone?

The Basic Four diet plan is 75% incorrect. Three of the four food groups it uses (Meat, Milk and Bread) are inimical to human nutrition and well-being. The inclusion of foods from these three groups is the cause of most of the dietary ills suffered in this country today.

Only the group of Fruits and Vegetables can be considered essential for nutritional well-being. The Basic Four Food Group diet plan, then, has a batting average of 25%—perhaps not bad for major league baseball, but a deplorable percentage for your state of health.

Since the Basic Four Food Group plan is still the most popularly recommended and well-known diet plan in the country, you will need some hard facts to convince others that it is a dangerous and incorrect diet to follow. To help you understand why this diet plan cannot promote health or even supply basic nutrient needs, each of the four recommended food groups are examined in great detail in the following sections:

84.3.1. One Man's Meat Is Everyone's Poison

Meat is one of the most heavily-promoted food groups in the United States. We are told that we must eat meat every day in order to get the necessary "complete" protein that animal food products can supply.

In fact, the alleged need for meat-eating is based entirely on the need for protein in the human diet. Except for a few B-vitamins, protein is the only major nutrient that meat can supply. The meat group of foods that is included in the Basic Four Food Group diet is done so entirely because of an unhealthy obsession with protein foods that is common to American society.

Not only are protein foods heavily promoted, they are so intimately associated with meat that the two are almost synonymous. Tell someone that you do not eat meat, and he will almost assuredly ask, "But where do you get your protein?"

The Basic Four Food diet propagates this misconception that protein comes almost exclusively from meat by naming its first food category, "Meat and Meat Alternatives

Group." Notice that the category is not called "Protein Foods" or "Essential Amino Acids Foods" but "Meat." The other protein foods listed in the group which are not animal flesh (such as cheese, dry beans and peas, and peanut butter) are called "Meat Alternatives." An "alternative" is defined as a second choice or something that may be used in place of the first choice. In other words, according to the Basic Four diet plan, meat is the number one protein source. All other protein foods are called alternative (or "second rate") choices.

Dr. Herbert M. Shelton has stated that "the so-called scientific world is wedded to the carnivorous practice and all of its dietetic advice is designed to induce mankind to eat more flesh, eggs, and milk." Notice that the healthiest sources of concentrated protein, raw nuts, and seeds, are not even included in the protean or "Meat and Meat Alternatives" group!

The casual user of the Basic Four Food Group diet plan would probably conclude that the number one nutritional need is protein, and preferably animal protein. Of course, that conclusion suits the meat-packing, poultry, and dairy industries just fine. Please remember that the Four Food Group plan was devised by the U.S. Department of Agriculture which has a commitment to supporting and promoting cattle-raising, milk and egg production, and other livestock industries. In fact, the U.S.D.A. is staffed at the top by members of these industries.

Are protein needs so great that this nutrient should be our number one concern? The Basic Four Diet plan certainly places a strong emphasis on getting plenty of protein (or meat and meat alternatives) in our diet. Do we need concentrated protein sources or alternatives to this Meat group?

Dr. Shelton in his masterwork Human Life: Its Philosophy and Laws tells us that "the adult body requires only enough protein to maintain repairs and that this amount is extremely small if the body is rightly cared for. We can safely say, Dr. Shelton continues, "that if the adult person never touched any of the more concentrated protein foods s/he would never fail to secure all the protein, required by the body, to maintain repairs."

What can we say then about this first food group in the Basic Four Food diet plan? In a "nutshell," just this: Meat-eating is not only nonessential, but is a degenerative practice that leads to illness and disease. There is no need for "alternatives" to meat, and recommendations for other highly-concentrated protein foods are spurious.

If you eat a diet of natural and unprocessed foods, you will receive an abundance of amino acids, or "protein." You certainly do not need to eat two or more servings daily from a food group that consists chiefly of chemically-preserved, hormone-laden, and decomposing pieces of animal corpses.

Bypass the "Meat and Meat Alternative" group—there are biologically correct ways to meet your protein needs.

84.3.2. If You Don't Eat the Cow, Why Drink the Juice?

The next major food group in the Four Food Diet Plan is the "Milk and Milk Products" or dairy category. Before looking at the reasons for making dairy food items a separate category, you should know one fact:

Over 75% of the world's population—3 out of every 4 people on earth—cannot digest milk (or milk sugar-lactose) after the age of three.

For many people, indigestion, gas, cramping, and/or diarrhea occur after a single glass of milk is drunk. Does this sound like an "essential" food or food group when most people cannot tolerate dairy products, let alone digest, and appropriate them?

Let's ask another question. Do the government nutritionists sincerely believe that every human being must have two or more glasses of milk each day to survive in good health? Maybe or maybe not, but one thing is sure: The milk and dairy industries and similar vested interests would certainly like everyone to believe it.

"Milk has grown to become one of this country's staple businesses," Dr. Shelton notes, "and the profits of milk distributing are very high. This industry has fostered the idea that man should be a suckling—should never be weaned, and that he should suck at the teats of the cow even if he lives to be ninety to a hundred years old." Dr. Shelton concludes, "For adults, milk is both an inefficient and uneconomical food. It is certainly not an essential element of the human diet."

Over two-thirds of the world's population never have a single glass of cow's milk. They consume less milk in their, entire adult lives than is recommended for one day by the USDA. Only in the United States is milk-drinking so heavily promoted for adults.

Why, then, did milk-drinking and cheese-eating become so prominent in our society, and why are dairy products named as one of the four important food groups? Well, the obvious reason is money. The best way to get people to buy and consume more of a food item is to convince them that it is absolutely essential for their health.

And how are milk and other dairy products promoted as being essential for our wellbeing? The answer in one word: Calcium.

Calcium is to the dairy industry what protein is to the meat industry. If you can convince people that a nutrient which is abundant in a specific food category (such as calcium for dairy, or protein for meat) is required in large amounts for optimum health, then foods which contain those nutrients will be consumed in larger and larger quantities.

Except for a few B-vitamins and protein, calcium is the only major nutrient in milk products. Dairy producers try to "beef up" their products by adding vitamin D and fortifying them with other additives. Yet after all is said and done, even the highly-promoted calcium content of milk may be all for naught.

Studies have shown that the calcium in pasteurized and processed milk products is poorly digested and absorbed and used by the body. Indeed, the calcium in such products may be used more to form "stones" or inorganic deposits in the body instead of being used to build strong bones. Is it mere coincidence that patients prone to kidney stone formation no longer have this problem after eliminating dairy products from their diets? Still, calcium is an essential mineral for our well-being. In fact, it is the most abundant mineral in our body. Among the elderly, especially women, calcium loss is a real problem. Bones become osteoporotic and brittle. Hip injuries often occur due to demineralization and calcium loss. The solution, however, is not in using milk for calcium, but instead, to avoid those foods which increase our calcium requirements and to consume those foods that supply it in its finest form.

That's correct. A diet high in meat products and junk foods is the real culprit in calcium loss and calcium deficiencies.

Many foods eaten in the typical American diet are calcium-poor already, such as meat, starches, refined grains, and high-sugar foods. In addition, the majority of these foods are also acid-forming. To neutralize these acids formed by a poor diet, base minerals such as calcium are needed in excess of the body's normal requirements. Further, the body needs extra calcium and other minerals to metabolize these refined and deficient foods. Moreover, much calcium is deranged and thus unusable when foods are cooked.

When refined foods (already calcium-poor) that are high in acid residues are consumed, calcium needs increase. As a result, we are told to drink large amounts of milk to satisfy the calcium requirements of the twentieth-century diet.

When naturally alkaline foods such as a fresh fruits and vegetables are eaten, calcium needs are lowered because body acidity is lowered. Thus, the high calcium recommendations made by nutritionists are not valid for those who follow a natural and unprocessed diet of raw fruits and vegetables.

Writing in his book Superior Nutrition, Dr. Shelton states: "In a condition of markedly lowered alkalinity or so-called acidosis, calcium will not be utilized even though abundant in the diet. Increased alkalinity of the blood increases calcium utilization." A diet of fresh fruits and vegetables keeps the body in an optimum state of alkalinity for the most efficient use of calcium. Thus, although smaller amounts of calcium may exist in a diet that is free of milk and all animal products, the calcium is actually absorbed by the body at a much higher and efficient rate than in the body of the meat-eating and milk-drinking person.

And if you are a vegetarian that persists in using milk and other dairy products, you should ask yourself why. If there is no nutritional need for dairy foods, then why do you drink the juice (milk) if you refuse to eat the cow?

In fact, pity the poor cow. She is raised for both meat and milk and sold to consumers with a package of lies for the basest of reasons. And, like the cow, the consumers of this animal and its products are also kept in ignorance by the men who raise and promote the consumption of the beast.

Now ignorance is no excuse. You know that two of the four food groups (Meat and Milk) are never essential for our health and well-being and, in fact, are pathogenic. Protein and calcium needs are real, but these needs can be fully satisfied with a natural diet of fresh fruits and vegetables.

84.3.3. The Staff of Whose Life?

The third food group contains bread, cereals, and other grain products. Is this group just as nonessential as the meat and milk groups? Let's see why these foods are considered to be so important in the first place.

The chief reason for including grains arid breads as one of the major four food groups is that such foods are thought to furnish us with the B-vitamin complex, as well as vitamin E and (in the case of "fortified" bread) iron.

Whole, unprocessed, and unrefined grains do contain a significant amount of B vitamins. But are such foods otherwise health-promoting and beneficial to eat?

The truth is that whole grains and their derived products are at best "second-rate" foods. In times of famine or when fresh fruits and vegetables cannot be stored or not available, then grains may be used as a temporary food supply. Whole grains, however, are not a complete or optimum food and cannot support life when eaten cooked instead of sprouted.

"The only grain products that are permissible in the diet of an intelligent and informed individual are the whole grains in their natural state. However, grains are inferior articles of food, and they certainly form no normal part of the diet of man. Every man, woman, and child in the land would be better off by leaving them out of their diet."

If you have doubts about Dr. Shelton's statements, then please look at the case histories of those enthusiastic followers of a macrobiotic diet who have attempted unsuccessfully to live on a 100%-grain diet. Perhaps we should say "ex-followers" since all such attempts to live on a pure grain diet have resulted in poor health or death.

The Basic Four Food Group diet plan does not advocate a total grain diet. Still, why should we be told to eat four servings or more of bread or cereal each day? The reasoning for this recommendation is that the typical American diet consists heavily of sugar and white flour products. These nonfood items actually deplete the body of B vitamins. To get the vitamins back into the body, we are told to eat more breads and cereals.

But the very foods that are recommended, breads and cereals and other flour products, are usually so processed, refined, and cooked that all the B vitamins have been destroyed! The producers of these processed grain products then add artificial B vitamins to the breads and cereals. Of course, as a student of Life Science, you already know how terrible breads and cereals are.

The bread manufacturers also found another way to sell their worthless goods. They started adding iron to the flour so that their processed foods would then be eaten for the iron "content." Why stop there? Just add some calcium, protein, and vitamin C. Then you would supposedly obtain all of your nutritional needs from a delicious loaf of "fortified" white bread!

Unlike the Meat and Milk food groups, the Bread and Grain category of food is not totally worthless or destructive. When grains are sprouted and eaten raw, they are an acceptable addition to the optimum diet. If they are eaten fresh and raw from the field while still in their milky stage (as corn sometimes is), then they are digestible and usable food. Even if they are cooked and used whole and unrefined, the negative effects of these foods are still not as great as meat and milk. But if refined and processed flours and breads are introduced into the diet at four servings per day, they become as destructive to the health of the person as pasteurized milk and roasted flesh.

In summary, we should remember these four points that were made by Dr. Shelton in volume two of his book Orthotrophy:

1. Cereals (breads and grains) do not form any part of the natural diet of man and are not necessary to health and life. Man did not become a grain eater until late in his history.

2. Grain products are best omitted from the diet entirely, especially from the diets of infants and children.

3. When grains are eaten, only the whole and unprocessed grain should be used.

4. In any case, grains, breads, and cereals should form but a small amount of the diet and should be properly balanced and combined with an abundance of green vegetables.

84.3.4. And the Winner Is...

The last group of food items is Fruits and Vegetables. As a student of Life Science, you know that these food items should actually make up 90% to 100% of your daily diet. The Basic Four Food Group diet plan instructs its followers to eat four servings of fruits and vegetables daily. A serving is either one piece of fresh fruit or one fresh vegetable or one-half cup of cooked fruits or vegetables.

Fruits and vegetables are included in the Basic Four Food diet plan in order to supply the needed vitamin A and vitamin C requirements. The developers of the Basic Four Food Group diet plan also advise people to make sure that one of these servings is a dark green or dark yellow vegetable in order to get sufficient amounts of vitamin A into the diet.

There is nothing wrong with these suggestions, except that cooked vegetables or fruits are not healthful, nor are four servings of fresh fruits and vegetables a sufficient amount of food for a person following a healthy diet. Fruits and vegetables should not be merely eaten as vitamin insurance, or to get specific nutrients. They should be included in the diet because they are most suited to man's digestive physiology and have the highest health-promoting qualities of all foods.

Until only very recently, traditional nutritionists and government spokesmen have always downplayed the importance of fruits and vegetables in the diet. The only worthwhile qualities that these foods had, according to these people, were their vitamin C and vitamin A contents.

Vegetables were mere side-dressing to the bread and meat diet of so many people, and fruits were something for dessert or to bake into pies. For many people today, this attitude toward fresh vegetables and fruits as second-rate foods still exists. To suggest that a complete meal can be made on fruits alone, or upon only one fruit, brings raised eyebrows and disbelieving looks.

Yet students of Life Science and Natural Hygiene have long known that a diet that consists almost entirely of fresh, raw foods from this last food group (Fruits and Vegetables) is not only satisfying but conducive to the highest state of health.

Dr. Shelton strongly advises that "the bulk of each meal should consist of fresh fruits or fresh green vegetables." This is so for four reasons, according to Dr. Shelton:

1. It prevents the overeating of concentrated foods.
2. It assures an abundant supply of minerals.
3. It provides the highest quality of vitamins.
4. It insures the needed bulk that is necessary for normal peristalsis.

Of course, if your meals should consist chiefly of fresh fruits or vegetables, then the four serving amounts of this food group recommended by the Basic Four diet plan is an absurdly low amount. A person on a well-established all-fruit-and-vegetable diet might eat 20 or more such "servings instead of the four servings suggested by the USDA.

And this brings us to the next question about the Basic Four Food Group Diet plan: Are servings or measured amounts a good way to manage your diet?

84.3.5. Second Helpings, Anyone?

The woman was surrounded by notebooks, cookbooks, measuring cups, and food scales. She was chopping up a raw carrot and weighing the amounts on a scale and then looking at a diet chart.

"I know I'm supposed to have one serving of a yellow vegetable today, but I don't know if I should eat four ounces of carrots or a half-cup of cut carrots," she said to me as I visited her.

"Why don't you eat the whole carrot and just get it over with?" I joked.

She looked serious. "No, I'm going to do this by the book," she said. "Okay, what's next?" she asked as she reached for her diet plan. "Let's see ... four leaves of lettuce or two stalks of celery make one serving of green vegetables"

I left her with her charts and measuring cups. I wondered if she ever figured out what she was supposed to have for lunch before it got to be suppertime.

Do you also try to "eat by the book?" Many diets today, including the Basic Four Food Group diet plan, are arranged into groups and categories, and serving amounts. You can eat one serving of this and two servings of that, and three ounces of meat or eight ounces of milk.

Eating by serving amounts is like making love with a stopwatch, and just about as necessary.

If you are eating the proper and natural foods suited for our physiological constitution and biological heritage, then forget all about servings and helpings and quantities. Eat when you're hungry, eat until you're satisfied, and don't eat again until you're hungry again.

Eating by specified serving amounts is an artificial and meaningless practice. The Basic Four Food Group diet plan recommends these serving amounts so that the person will be "assured" of getting all the vitamins, minerals, and other nutrients needed. If you are eating a biologically correct diet, then such concerns are not needed.

According to Dr. Shelton, "Fresh, uncooked fruits, nuts, and vegetables will supply the body with a super abundance of the known and unknown vitamins, all the minerals, studied and unstudied, with fine sugars, easily-digested fats, and proteins of the highest grade." You don't need to eat one serving from this group or two servings from that group.

Just so long as all of your "servings" come from the fresh and wholesome fruit and vegetable group, then eat what you desire and don't be afraid to reach for "second helpings."

84.4. Does the Four Food Plan Work?

To complete our evaluation of the USDA Four Food Group diet plan, we should see how well or how poorly it delivers what it promises: a balanced and complete diet that satisfies our basic nutritional needs.

Here is one meal that supposedly furnishes "all of the serving amounts for one day," as recommended by this diet plan:

The "Complete" Nutritional Meal

1. Two cheeseburgers

2. A milkshake

3. One order of french-fried potatoes

4. A hot apple turnover

Here's how this meal breaks down into serving amounts and food groups:

1. Meat Group Two servings of hamburger patties

2. Milk Group One serving of cheese and one of milk

3. Bread Group Four servings of hamburger buns

4. Fruit and Vegetable Four servings, with one of potatoes, one of apple filling, and two for the lettuce, tomatoes, and onions on the cheeseburgers.

And there you have it. A fast-food meal that "meets" all he requirements for one day of nutrition as described by the Four Food Group diet plan.

Of course, the USDA did not actually mean that we should eat fast food and junk food to meet their serving requirements, but please note that they did not recommend that such foods not be eaten.

This is another major shortcoming of the Four Food Group Diet plan—there are no provisions for eliminating the really harmful and destructive foods (salt, sugar, cooked fats, white flour, etc.) that are such a large part of the typical diet, and no provisions are made for proper food combining.

Like so many other diets, the Four Food Group diet plan concentrates entirely on what we should eat and how much and ignores the harmful foods that we should avoid.

The best thing that can be said for the Four Food Group approach to nutrition is that it is simple and easy to understand. Even children can divide the foods they eat into basic categories and serving amounts.

But if the categories are all wrong. and, the serving amounts are totally meaningless, then what does it matter if anyone can understand the diet plan?

Let's look at an even easier-to-understand "Basic Four Food Group" diet plan that follows the rules for optimum nutrition.

84.5. The Life Science Basic Four Food Group Diet

If you want to divide your diet up into categories and serving amounts, let's apply your knowledge of an optimum diet to do so. Here are the four food groups that a Life Scientist should be concerned with:

1. Fresh and dried fruits.
2. Raw vegetables (excluding onions, garlic, hot peppers).
3. Raw nuts and seeds.
4. Sprouted grains and legumes.

For Group One (fresh and dried fruits), eat an abundance of servings. Remember that dried fruits are four-times as concentrated as fresh fruits and eat accordingly. Don't eat servings from this group with any servings from the other three food groups and combine fruits properly.

For Group Two (raw vegetables), eat a moderate amount of servings. Do not include the irritating vegetables from the onion or hot pepper families, and do not "overeat" from this lower calorie group so that you neglect servings of fresh fruit.

For Group Three (nuts and seeds), eat no more than three to four ounces daily. When eating a serving from this group, make sure you also include servings from Group Two (raw vegetables) as digestion, and assimilation and nutritional benefits are improved when nuts and leafy vegetables are eaten together.

For Group Four (sprouts), eat these at your option and to your taste. Eat other sprouts (lentil, wheat, and other legumes) in more moderate amounts if eaten at all.

Let true hunger dictate the number of "servings" you eat from each of these groups. I suggest you eat no foods that are not in these groups, and avoid all meat, dairy, and processed food products.

You will satisfy all of your nutritional needs if you eat a calorie-sufficient amount of foods from these four groups. Don't weigh or measure your food and don't be concerned with serving amounts. Eat food as it is packaged by nature and in amounts according to hunger. You will never make a mistake.

84.6. Questions & Answers

A simple question. If the Basic Four food group diet is as bad as you say, then just why is it so popular? It seems like that even with big business interests and government propaganda that people would discover the truth about nutrition.

That's a very interesting point. After all, we would like to think that the common man has the necessary intelligence and discrimination to know when he is being lied to.

It is a mistake to think that our country's dietary ills can be blamed entirely on the Basic Four Food Group diet plan. Actually, very few people follow any sort of diet plan—good or bad!

You'll notice that the Basic Four diet is very, very similar to what the average person eats anyway—a lot of meat and protein, dairy products, refined flours, and breads, and so on. Actually, if you just added a fifth group called Salt, Fats, and Junk Foods then you would have the twentieth-century United States diet pinpointed.

That is why the Basic Four diet approach to nutrition has held sway. There was already a strongly established base of support. People eat like that anyway, and so they think the government and the food industries are giving them good advice.

Everybody's the same: We all like to be told that what we are already doing is right and correct, even if it will eventually kill us in our relative youth.

You talk about the Basic Four diet plan as if everybody in the country knew about it. I'm sixty-three years old, and this is the first time I've ever had this concept explained to me. Aren't you exaggerating about how widespread this notion is?

At the age of sixty-three, you may never have been exposed to this nutritional scheme but ask your children and grandchildren. They will have heard about the Basic Four Food Groups because it is used as indoctrination for elementary school children. This is the standard, proscribed approach to teaching health and nutrition to school children.

What can we do then? Can we get our schools to teach another approach to nutrition?

Perhaps we are depending too much on public schools. It would probably be far better to leave nutrition teaching out of the curriculum entirely since the traditional and conservative approach to this subject that is always taken by schools simply perpetuates misinformation and institutionalizes error.

Don't forget that schools teach children what parents want them to know! What do you think the reaction would be if a teacher told a classroom of eight-year-olds that milk was not only unnecessary for health and growth, but actually harmful? The parents would have the teacher's scalp if their children were taught any nutritional information that conflicted with the family's normal eating practices.

That's why the Basic Four diet will be taught in our public school system for some time to come: It simply reflects the traditional diet eaten in this country. It doesn't "rock the boat" and it is a nonthreatening approach to nutrition.

Never mind that it is a completely wrong approach or that it perpetuates ignorance which will undermine the health of every person who follows its advice. It's what we're used to, and heaven help the person or teacher who is courageous enough to expose its fallacies, dangers, and lies.

As a parent, you can only work mightily to overcome the nutritional propaganda and nonsense thrown out in the name of education. Please teach your children and grandchildren the sensible alternatives to the Basic Four diet plan.

Article #1: Should We Drink Milk? by Dr. Alec Burton

Hygienists have always adopted the position that milk is for infants, mother's milk that is, and that this is the normal practice among all mammals. During the initial phase of life, it is the invariable practice of all mammalian species to take the milk of their mothers following which they are weaned. Then they spend the remainder of their life sustained by other foods. Man, on the contrary, teaches that milk is an ideal food, essentially cow's milk, and that after mother has performed her nursing, the cow should take over. In his feeding of infants, man has produced all types of formulae and means to usurp the natural habit of breast-feeding. Man even includes milk in the diet of his mammalian pets.

Many women regard breast-feeding as culturally regressive and primitive, something one should abandon as quickly as possible. They say it ruins their figure, that their breasts become atonic and pendulous. Such remarks are unfounded and other factors are responsible yet seldom considered.

It is normal in Nature for the mammal to breast-feed well past the time the infant obtains a mouth full of teeth, not just a few teeth but all teeth. Species of apes' nurse for six or seven months although their first teeth have appeared at the end of three months. With mammals there is a wide variation in the transition period and in many weaning takes place over a long period of time.

However, should milk constitute an integral part of the diet after weaning? Is milk a normal food for adults? The answer to both these questions is an unequivocal no!

Milk and milk products such as cheese and yogurt are viewed with suspicion by Hygienists. What are the unfavorable attributes of milk? Today milk is very much a processed product. It is pasteurized, homogenized, sterilized, and otherwise treated to render it "safe." All these processes greatly impair its nutritional value.

Besides all this, strong evidence indicates that gastric juice of adults does not contain rennin, an enzyme abundant in the stomach of infants which initiates the digestion of milk. The protein and fat of milk is constituted in such a way that enzymes of the human

151

digestive tract fail to digest it adequately—some of the elements are absorbed intact and cause trouble.

Milk also contains a high content of cholesterol and so has been a factor in the development of coronary artery disease. Many people observe the quick action taken by the body when milk is consumed; much mucus is secreted or diseases associated with the mucous membranes—asthma, sinusitis, bronchitis, etc.—are aggravated. Milk is said to be a "mucus forming" food. While I don't favor this description, I do suggest that the presence of milk and milk products in the body may occasion greater mucosal activity.

Milk is often considered a major source of the vital element calcium: the myth is that if we don't drink milk, our teeth will fall out and our bones collapse, or some such nonsense. The fact is that calcium is abundant in Nature. Most of the foods (fruits, vegetables, and nuts) we recommend are excellent sources of calcium. It would have to be a very poor diet indeed that did not supply half a gram of calcium daily. A good Hygienic diet provides over one gram.

It is extremely doubtful that we can utilize any of the calcium in milk in any event. The calcium in milk is bound to its protein complement, casein. Without the key enzyme, rennin, neither casein nor its nutrient complement, calcium, can be used in the digestive system.

Milk forms no part of the normal diet of man after the period of infancy and therefore our advice is—don't drink milk or eat milk products.

Reprinted from the Hygienic Review

Article #2: Hygienic Considerations in the Selections of Foods by Ralph C. Cinque, D.C.

84.1. The Superiority of Whole Foods

84.2. The Superiority of Raw Foods

84.3. The Superiority of Plant Foods

The selection of foods for optimum health requires that many factors be considered, including nutrient content, ease of mastication, deglutition, digestion, absorption and assimilation, presence or absence of irritants, the amount of vegetable fiber (which could be too little in the case of refined foods, or too much in the case of mature kale), gustatory satisfaction to the unperverted taste, and the effect on blood alkalinity. An ideal food would contain a broad array of nutrients, would be delicious, would contain a moderate amount of fiber, would be easy to eat and digest in the raw state, would possess no irritants or digestive antagonists, and would leave an alkaline ash after metabolism. Applying these criteria, we find that there are virtually no perfect foods. Most fruits and vegetables, for example, contain at least minute amounts of oxalic acid, which is a mild irritant, and which has a binding effect on calcium.

Tannic acid is contained in the skins of some nuts (particularly almonds) and this, too, is a mild irritant. Lettuce is said to contain lactucarium, a mildly toxic alkaloid with soporific effects. This is particularly true of head lettuce. Beans contain trypsin inhibitors, aflatoxins and purine bodies which raise serum uric acid levels. Grains contain much phytic acid which binds minerals like zinc and iron, impairing their utilization by the body. It should be obvious that perfect foods (like perfect health) are a theoretical ideal, not a reality.

From a Hygienic standpoint, there are three major tenets that guide us in the selection of foods. These tenets enable us to construct a diet that is philosophically and physiologically ideal for the human species. We will admit beforehand that due to various anatomical and physiological weaknesses and defects, not everyone can adhere to the philosophical dietary ideal with complete success. However, before alterations and deletions are made, it is important that we determine what constitutes an ideal diet, a truly natural diet, and then be guided accordingly. Our three major tenets are that:

1. Whole foods are superior to fragmented and refined foods.
2. Raw foods are superior to cooked foods.
3. Plant foods are superior to animal foods.

These three principles summarize Hygienic philosophy regarding food selection, and we will expound upon each in turn.

84.1. The Superiority of Whole Foods

The fact that whole natural foods are superior to refined foods such as white sugar, white flour, polished rice, requires no substantiation to the readers of this article. However, we must emphasize that any fragmenting of whole food destroys nutrients and lessens the suitability of that food as an article of diet. Whole carrots contain more complete nourishment than carrot juice. Brown rice is better food than rice polishings. Whole wheat is superior to wheat germ. Consider the following experiment conducted by Weston A. Price, D.D.S., the renowned author of Nutrition and Physical Degeneration.

"Three cages of rats were placed on wheat diets. The first cage received whole wheat, freshly ground, the second received a white flour product, and the third was given a mixture of bran and wheat germ. The amounts of each ash, of calcium as the oxide, and of phosphorus as the pentoxide and the amounts of iron and copper present in the diet were tabulated. Clinically, it was found that there was a marked difference in the physical developments of these rats. The rats in the first group, receiving the entire grain product, developed fully, and reproduced normally at three months of age. These rats had very mild dispositions and could be picked up by the ear or tail without danger of their biting. The rats fed upon white flour were markedly undersized. Their hair came out in large patches, and they had very ugly dispositions, so ugly that they threatened to spring through the cage wall at us when we came to look at them. These rats had tooth decay and they were unable to reproduce. The rats fed upon bran and wheat germ did not show tooth decay, but they were considerably undersized, and they lacked energy. The wheat germ was purchased from the miller and hence was not freshly ground. The wheat given to the first group was obtained whole and ground while fresh in a hand mill. It is of interest that notwithstanding the great increase in calcium, phosphorus, iron, and copper present in the foods of the last group, the rats did not mature normally, as did those in the first group. This may have been due in large part to the fact that the material was not freshly ground, and as a result they could not obtain a normal vitamin content from the embryo of the grain due to its oxidation. This is further indicated by the fact that the rats in this group did not reproduce, probably due in considerable part to a lack of vitamins B and E which were lost by oxidation of the embryo or germ fat."

This account demonstrates how important it is to distinguish between the nutrient content of a food and its overall biological effect. It has been shown repeatedly that eating wheat bran impedes iron absorption, despite the fact that it contains abundant iron. This may be the result of mechanical factors, or, perhaps it is the result of the high phytate content of the bran. In any case, it proves that foods cannot be evaluated solely on the basis of mathematical tables of nutrient analysis.

At first glance fragmented foods may seem to be more nourishing than whole foods. Dried apricots, for example, score much higher in calcium and iron than do fresh apricots. Quite obviously, if we extract the water from the apricots, we can triple or quadruple the number of fruits we are comparing, and thereby score higher nutrient values. This seeming enhancement is, of course, a figment of the mind. Whole foods offer the most complete nutrition. Powdered whey is a nutritional shadow of whole milk. Extracted chlorophyll is a lifeless fraction of green leaves. Lecithin granules are a denatured fragment of soybeans. These various extracts and concentrates are inferior to the whole natural foods they supposedly improve upon. Processing incurs drastic nutrient losses as a result of heat, oxidation, chemicals, and enzymatic destruction. It is correct to say that these foods have been devitalized. Only whole natural foods contain the amount and proportion of nutrients that the body requires. Only whole natural foods are acceptable in a Hygienic diet.

84.2. The Superiority of Raw Foods

Although some foods seem to be rendered more digestible by cooking, it is a fact that most foods are rendered less digestible. Furthermore, any food that is difficult to eat and digest uncooked is not a normal constituent of humanity's natural diet. Cooking partially or totally destroys the nutrient content of food. Water-soluble vitamins, like ascorbic acid and pantothenic acid, are particularly susceptible to thermal destruction, but it is to some extent true of all vitamins. What may be more important, however, is the fact that cooking alters the proportions of the various vitamins contained in foods. For example, cooking alters the natural ratio between thiamine and niacin in foods. This occurs because thiamine is readily destroyed by moist heat, whereas niacin is more resistant. Therefore, cooking not only lowers the vitamin content of foods, it also modifies vitamin ratios, which are a very important feature of whole foods.

Minerals may be rendered non-usable by the body as a result of cooking. A good example of this is the effect that pasteurization has upon milk. The complex organic salts of calcium and magnesium, in conjunction with carbon and phosphorus, are decomposed by heat, resulting in the precipitation of insoluble calcium phosphate salts. These inorganic salts are not assimilable by the body. This is one of the reasons why dental decay has reached epidemic proportions among milk-guzzling Americans.

Cooking tends to deaminize proteins and denature their secondary and tertiary configurations. With the exception of egg whites and certain dried legumes, they are rendered more difficult to digest by cooking. Subjecting fats to heat produces toxic cyclic hydrocarbons and free fatty acids, both of which are highly irritating. Heated fats and oils have been shown, by countless experiments, to be highly carcinogenic. No informed person will consume heated fats in any form.

Cooking causes a great loss of the soluble minerals in foods and drives off part of the food into the air as gases (this is particularly true of sulfur and iodine). Cooking softens vegetable fiber which may hamper intestinal motility and promote fermentation and putrefaction. Although cooking adds to the palatability of some foods (e.g., yams, asparagus, zucchini, grains), most foods are rendered less palatable by cooking, which gives rise to the use of unwholesome flavorings, condiments, dressings, etc.

On the basis of these considerations and others, a diet, in order to be considered Hygienic, would have to consist of at least predominantly uncooked foods.

84.3. The Superiority of Plant Foods

This category could also be designated the detrimental effects of animal foods. All animal products (with the exception of mother's milk) have certain negative features which make their dietary use questionable. Consider, first of all, the effect that animal foods have upon protein consumption. Even modest use of meat, fish, eggs, and dairy foods tends to create a protein overload, and this is one of the most dangerous dietary excesses. Research has shown that high-protein diets actually promote aging and early degeneration. Too much protein exerts a tremendous burden upon the liver and kidneys. It also leaves acid residues in the blood and tissues which must be neutralized by sacrificing indispensable alkaline mineral reserves. The process of aging is characterized by the transfer of calcium from the bones to the soft tissues, that is, to the arteries (arteriosclerosis), to the ureters (kidney stones), to the skin (wrinkles), to the joints (osteoarthritis), to the valves of the heart (producing frozen shoulder) and to other sites. This, course, leaves the skeleton osteoporotic, leading to the development of stooped posture, a kyphotic spine, spontaneous fractures, and other maladies that are so common to the elderly. High-protein diets (due to the accumulation of phosphoric, sulphuric, uric, and other acids) accelerate this demineralization of bone and bring about calcific deposits on the soft tissues.

One could argue that nuts and seeds contain as much protein as meats, eggs, etc., and therefore they are as likely to create an excess. However, most people are easily satisfied eating a few ounces of nuts or seeds every day, whereas few people will eat just a few ounces of yogurt. Restaurants serve up to a pound of meat at a sitting, along with other foods. Cottage and ricotta cheese is eaten in huge quantities, even by vegetarians. The simple truth is that animal proteins tend to promote overeating more so than do plant proteins.

The relationship between high-protein diets and cancer has been clearly established by studying both animal and human populations. Remember that cancerous cells are characterized by run-away protein synthesis and rapid cellular division. Protein synthesis is accelerated by increased protein intake, so it is not surprising to discover that cancer bears a close tie to excess protein. There is a direct correlation between the amount of protein in the diet and the incidence of cancer on a worldwide basis. Americans, Australians, and West Europeans, who ingest the largest amounts of protein, also have the greatest incidence of cancer, whereas the rural Chinese, the East Indians and native peoples of Latin America have the lowest cancer incidence. This is no causal relationship, and it cannot be written off by blaming it on the "stress of modern life."

Animal products are loaded with the worst kind of fat—saturated, cholesterol-laden animal fat. A mountain of evidence has been accumulated relating high animal fat intakes with the development of cardiovascular disease (which is characterized by the deposition of saturated fat and cholesterol in the intimal layer of arteries), and many different malignancies including breast cancer, colon and rectal cancers, and cancer of the liver. Even such diverse conditions as multiple sclerosis and diabetes have been related to the consumption of animal fats. As we have already stated, heated animal fats have been shown to be even more carcinogenic, and considering that Americans take all of their flesh, milk and eggs well cooked, it's no wonder that one in four eventually succumbs to cancer. Pandemically, those peoples who subsist on low-fat, low-protein, largely vegetarian, unrefined diets demonstrate the greatest resistance to cancer. The incidence of cancer and heart disease among the American Seventh Day Adventists is approximately half the national average. This is quite remarkable considering that only about half of this group are thought to be vegetarian.

Flesh, fish, yogurt, and cheese contain various putrefactive products resulting from their bacterial decomposition. Putting partially-spoiled food in the body can hardly be considered a Hygienic practice, despite the arguments of the fermented food enthusiasts. Flesh also contains considerable quantities of the end products of metabolism (like uric acid) which are held up in the tissues at the time of death. These wastes are poisonous, irritating, and burdensome to the body. Consider the fact that animal products tend to be reservoirs for pesticides, herbicides, and various other drugs and inorganic contaminants—there are many good reasons to avoid using them. Certainly, a Hygienic diet would contain no more than small amounts of animal food—better yet, none.

There are just five classes of foods that meet all the criteria established by our three, major, tenets. These are: fruits, vegetables, nuts, seeds, and sprouts. A diet comprised of these foods would abound in every nutrient known to be required by humans, with the exception of vitamin B-12, and most people apparently derive enough of this from bacterial synthesis in the intestines. However, we should note that soil bacteria also produces B-12 on the surface of roots so that adding stringy roots grown in organic soil (with abundant microbial activity) to the diet would constitute a pre-made plant source of B-12 that would be a perfectly acceptable addition to a Hygienic diet. Supermarket vegetables would not be adequate for this purpose.

We should note, in closing, that adding to the diet some cooked food (like baked potatoes and brown rice) or limited amounts of animal foods (such as uncooked, un-salted cheese), although not strictly Hygienic, may be required in some pathological conditions. Certain people would experience a drastic and undesirable weight loss were they to make an immediate transition to a 100% uncooked, all-plant food diet. For these people, eating a baked potato now and then represents not a mere compromise but rather a necessary modification of their Hygienic regimen.

Quoting Dr. Alec Burton, "We must adapt the system to the needs of the individual and not adapt the individual to the needs of the system." With this acknowledged let us state, in conclusion, that a diet, in order to be considered Hygienic, would have to consist predominantly (if not exclusively) of uncooked foods, of vegetable origin, eaten whole.

Reprinted from Dr. Shelton 's Hygienic Review.

Article #3: Eat Your Heart Out, Galloping Gourmet by Cary Fowler

Will an Apple a Day Keep the Doctor Away?

The Divorce of Food from Nutrition

Al Krebs of the Agribusiness Accountability Project tells a story about a scene from a popular TV show. "A Fernwood, Ohio, housewife is preparing a packaged pineapple filling pie for her family. As she pours the rather grotesque contents of a can of pineapple filling into the pie pan her sister Kathy, who is watching the process, wonders aloud where the pineapple is."

"The housewife reads the contents as they appear on the label. Amidst the various acids and flavorings and sugar, no mention is made of pineapple except in the advertising on the label."

"She pauses and, looking at her sister questioningly, remarks: 'I don't see any pineapple listed here.' Kathy replied: 'They don't make food out of food anymore.' The housewife asked: 'What do they do with food, if they don't make food out of it?'"

That's a good question! Eating is a personal activity all people share. At its core, eating is an emotional experience tying us to our home and upbringing and to the larger society and time in which we live. Yet today, control over nourishment is slipping from our fingers. Decisions about the type, form, and quality of food we eat are no longer ours to make.

Control over our nation's food system has shifted from people like you and me to an economically-concentrated food industry. The dazzling array of food products available at the modern supermarket gives the impression of a vibrant, competitive food industry. We naturally assume that such products as Wyler soup mixes, Borden cheeses, Drake's cookies, Wise potato chips, Cracker Jacks, Bama jellies, Rea Lemon and Kava coffee are made by separate companies, while in fact they are just a few of the many products made by one corporation—Borden.

Likewise, Maxwell House, Brim, Yuban and Sanka coffees, Post cereals, Stove-Top stuffing, Calumet baking powder, Bisquick, Shake 'n Bake, Jell-O, Cool-Whip, Baker's Chocolate and Kool-Aid are all made by General Foods, who also owns Burger Chef. Heinz's 57 varieties have mushroomed to over 1,200.

Of the 1,500 new items made available to the supermarket chains by such corporations each year only a few will reach your grocer's shelf—those that are highly advertised, those with fast turnover and those with the most attractive profit margins. Competition for shelf space is fierce. Initial decisions about what we will have to eat are made by the supermarket chains when they divvy up their shelf space. And these decisions are based on different values than we ourselves would apply to such a crucial matter as what we eat.

More often than not, the result is one row of fresh fruits and vegetables and ten or twelve rows of boxes and cans. The magazine of the world's largest agribusiness company, the Dutch-based Unilever Corporation (Lipton tea, Good Humor ice cream, Wish Bone salad dressing, Mrs. Butter-worth's syrup, Imperial margarine and others) bluntly sized things up when it conceded that "... the return on investment in the basic nutrition business isn't exactly promising." This goes a long way towards explaining why the airwaves are full of commercials for french fries and potato chips rather than raw potatoes for baking at home.

Will an Apple a Day Keep the Doctor Away?

As control over our food system has changed hands, alarming shifts in consumption patterns have occurred. From 1950 to 1970 per capita consumption of fresh fruit dropped 26%. Americans ate more sugar than vegetables by weight in 1970. Soft drink sales doubled. Fortunately, a recent study showed that salad bars are becoming increasingly popular, creating a new demand for fresh vegetables, but people still don't eat enough of them, considering that they usually cook those that aren't in their salads.

A Department of Agriculture study has concluded that better diets might reduce diabetes problems by 50 percent, heart disease by 20 percent, obesity by 80 percent, alcoholism by 33 percent and intestinal cancer by 20 percent. Recently studies have linked as much as 50 percent of the cases of hyperactivity in children to the heavy doses of synthetic colorings and flavorings in food.

The Divorce of Food from Nutrition

The individual should scarcely shoulder all the blame for the declining quality of the American diet. Few people with proper regard for "food the way Mother used to cook it" could be accused of having demanded the kinds of food they now eat. The deterioration of food and the divorce of food from nutrition parallels the growth in corporate control over food production and distribution. .Today nearly 75 percent of all food manufacturing assets are controlled by just 50 corporations.

Local, small farmers who once supplied our towns and cities with truly delicious produce have been pushed out of business. Today's supermarket produce, shipped-in from huge corporate farms in Florida or California, is a far cry in quality, taste and price from the locally-grown products we once had.

Our relation to food is no longer our relation to nature or even to local farmers and neighborhood grocery stores. We relate to food through the new suppliers. Food (most of it, that is) may still come from the good earthy but only after it has passed through the fingers of a General Foods or a Del Monte. Food has thus become just another commodity to be manufactured, altered, packaged, and sold like toothpaste or razor blades. Food is no longer simply food.

Manufacturers use television to teach us that certain foods, like other commodities, can "add life," make you an Olympic athlete or help your love life. By falsely attributing such capabilities to food in order to self-high-profit items, the crucial, age-old link between food and our true physical needs has been severed. Shall our food provide nutrition or shall it "add life?" Why should we make our own spaghetti sauce when we can buy the brand that will "take you back to old Italy?"

The modern American diet evidences a deep-seated frustration and no small degree of confusion about food and its proper place in our lives. The way in which people prepare and serve food says a lot about how they regard themselves and others. It tells us something about the spirit of a society and the quality of life, for food is life.

Golden arches, colonels, doughboys, and a host of other gimmicks have partially succeeded in distracting us from what is happening to our food. But for those of us who can remember what a truly good meal tasted like and can remember the warmth and intimacy which came with sitting down at the table to enjoy it with family or friends, a silent anger remains at the travesty. The, temple, we sense, has been profaned by the money changers.

Living and eating are forever a matter of politics. We can have any kind of food policy and any kind of agricultural program we want. We can decide to eat only hamburgers and sugar, throw our good food in the ocean, starve the poor and save one- or two-family farmers to use as museum exhibits.

Or we can decide that food, being a necessity, should also be a right, that we need family farmers to produce good food and we don't need the middle men engaged in destroying and polluting it. We might even decide we don't ed to have ourselves and our children indoctrinated by commercials which teach us "good" buying habits in the place of good eating habits.

Jim Hightower, author of Eat Your Heart Out, got right to the point when he said: "Food cannot be assembled like a telephone and there is no reason it should be. If anything ought to be real in our lives, ought to be left to nature rather than being simulated by corporate technicians, it is food. Monopolistic conglomerates cannot make our telephones work; why should they be arrogant enough to think that they can handle dinner? More to the point, why should we be dumb enough to let them?"

Reprinted from a pamphlet by Agricultural Marketing Project

Lesson 85:

The Dangers of a
High-Protein Diet

85.1. Introduction

85.2. The Problems with Protein

85.3. The True Needs of the Body

85.4. Questions & Answers

Article #1: The Enigma of Protein by T.C. Fry

Article #2: Proteins

Article #3: Protein Supplements by Hannah Allen

85.1. Introduction

85.1.1. A Case of Protein Poisoning

85.1.2. Too Much of a "Good Thing"?

85.1.1. A Case of Protein Poisoning

David looked really bad. His face was covered with red, rash-like bumps and his eyes were swollen. "My mouth and throat," he said, "feel like you poured burning chemicals down them. I woke up in the middle of the night and couldn't breathe," he gasped, "and my nose feels like a huge sore."

David thought he had an allergy, but there was another name for his condition— proteinosis or poisoning by protein foods.

It was the week after Thanksgiving and David had been to a family reunion. "I never ate so much turkey and ham in my life," he told me. "Everybody brought platters and platters of meat, and I had to sample them all. I also ate a lot of desserts. It must have been something in the food I was allergic to that made my face swell up like this."

It was indeed "something" in the food that had caused David's condition, but it wasn't some mysterious hidden allergen. No, what made David so sick, so miserable was simply an excessive amount of animal protein.

Protein in large amounts, and of the wrong type, can poison you as surely as any other substance taken in excess of the body's true needs. In fact, what many people call allergies are often symptoms of proteinosis. When you consider the super-high protein diet that most people in this country eat, it is no surprise that a majority of the population is suffering from a continual low-level of protein poisoning.

That's right—protein, the food item so widely hailed and promoted by nutritionists and meat industry spokesmen, can cause serious harm when ingested in amounts in excess of the body's needs.

85.1.2. Too Much of a "Good Thing"?

You've heard bad stories about fats in the diet, and even carbohydrate foods (especially refined sugars and starches) take a beating from weight-conscious individuals. But you probably never thought you would hear a bad word about protein.

Protein does the glamour jobs in the body. It builds muscle, hair, skin, and nails. Enzymes, hormones, hemoglobin, and antibodies are also made from protein, and everyone knows that protein (or amino acids) is essential for the healthy growth of the young.

All true. Protein does a vital job of keeping the body maintained, but it is required in far lower amounts than commonly consumed by the average person.

Well, so what? If protein is so vital for our well-being, then doesn't it make sense that a lot more protein would make you a lot more healthy? After all, you really can't get too much of a good thing, can you?

As with anything else taken into the body, the nutrient protein must either be used, stored, or eliminated by the body. If more protein than can be used is eaten, then it is converted into stored fuel for the body. Along with this converting of protein to stored fuel, toxins or nitrogenous waste products are produced from the extra protein. The toxins or by-products from this protein conversion consist of nitrogen or ammonia-like compounds and are eliminated from the body via the kidneys.

When protein is consumed in greater amounts than can be processed, toxicity of the blood will result from the excessive amount of nitrogen in the blood. Excessive nitrogen impairs working capacity, and the accumulation of a nitrogen product, kino toxin, in the muscles, causes fatigue.

Partially or incompletely digested proteins cannot be assimilated, and poisons are absorbed into the blood. Various symptoms of protein poisoning are experienced by different individuals, including burning of mouth, lips and throat, skin symptoms, nasal symptoms, and other signs of intolerance of certain foods and other substances, known as allergies.

In proteinosis, or acute protein poisoning, there is general aching and a bad headache. Hyperproteina is caused by incompletely digested protein due to impaired digestion or bad combination of foods and may be thrown off as mucus, and might also cause aching and headaches.

Can you get too much of a good thing? If the "thing" is protein, the answer is yes. High protein intake forces extra work on the body. It must convert the protein to fuel and eliminate the harmful acids created in the process of digestion. Acid saturation of the body cells, due to excessive protein intake, can quite simply cause death. Perhaps a better question is: how "good" a thing is protein anyway?

85.2. The Problems with Protein

85.2.1. Eat Your Meat, Lose Your Bones

85.2.2. Protein: A Kick in the Kidneys

85.2.3. Protein: Are Those Just Rumors About Tumors?

85.2.4. The High-Protein, Low-Health Weight-Loss Diet

85.2.5. You Can't Fool the Body!

85.2.6. The Ultimate High-Protein Diet

The following conditions may result from too much protein in the diet:

1. Heart disease
2. Kidney damage
3. Constipation
4. Tumors and cancerous growths
5. Biochemical imbalances in the tissues (overacidity)
6. Arthritis
7. Bone-loss (osteoporosis)

Let's look at some of these problems caused by an excessive protein diet in more detail.

85.2.1. Eat Your Meat, Lose Your Bones

As people on a traditional diet grow older, they often experience "bone loss" or osteoporosis. Bone loss usually occurs more often in elderly women than anyone else, but almost everyone who eats a high-meat and protein diet will suffer from some amount of bone loss, and this includes children as well as mature adults.

Bone loss, or osteoporosis, occurs when calcium is removed from the bones of the body in order to fulfill the body's metabolic requirements for this stored mineral. Why does the body need so much calcium that it must rob its own bones?

Quite simply, the answer, according to medical researcher Dr. Robert Heaney, is that "the more protein you take in, the more calcium you excrete." His studies have shown that a diet that contains 50% more protein than is needed may result in as much as one percent loss of bone per year.

Since almost every woman (and man) in this country exceeds the 50% excessive protein amount, bone loss does occur in about 98% of the population,. What are the dangers of the bone loss?

One of the most obvious signs of bone loss occurs around the teeth and under the gum lines of the mouth. As bone is lost or removed from the jaw, the teeth loosen and eventually decay or fall out. Most so-called gum disease in this country comes from bone loss.

Another very obvious danger of bone loss is the tendency of older people to crack their bones after a minor fall. The hips especially are susceptible to bone loss in elderly women, and there have been many instances where these women's hips have actually snapped under the body's own weight.

A high-protein diet can cause a total bone loss of 1 % or more per year. This means that a normally healthy woman of 25 years could lose up to half of her bone structure by the time she reaches 75 years, if she continues to eat the typical high-meat, high-protein diet of twentieth-century America.

85.2.2. Protein: A Kick in the Kidneys

If protein is not needed by the body for tissue synthesis (or rebuilding the body), it is returned to the liver. In the liver a process called deamination takes place which separates the amino acids into a nitrogenous residue and non-nitrogenous residue. The nitrogen portion undergoes a series of chemical changes and is converted into urea by the liver and excreted in the urine.

Intake of protein greatly in excess of the body's needs creates extra work for the liver. Excessive protein also creates extra work for the kidneys. Ideally, it is their job to remove excess acids, the deaminated group of chemicals being most suitably disposed of when excreted as urea.

When a high-protein diet is followed, the kidneys soon become overworked as they try to eliminate all the toxic by-products of protein metabolism.

David A. Phillips, a Hygienist author and lecturer from Australia, observes that: "The premature breakdown of kidneys in the Western world no longer surprises one when it is realized that the body's protein intake has risen all out of proportion to its needs." This condition is unfortunately compounded when the nature of the protein is more complex and more prone to create a high-acid residue, such as characterizes animal proteins.

Dr. Herbert M. Shelton, writing on the effects of a high-protein diet on the kidneys, states: "In middle-aged adults perfectly normal kidneys are the exception rather than the rule. By a careful selection of a low-nitrogen (low-protein) diet, it is possible to reduce the amount of work required of the kidneys to a level at which they are able to keep the waste products in the blood within normal limits."

Uric acid in the bloodstream, besides overworking the kidneys, is a preliminary to the later development of gout or arthritis, both conditions being invariably traceable to excessive, unsuitable protein in the diet.

85.2.3. Protein: Are Those Just Rumors About Tumors?

According to a recent popular survey, one of the things that Americans fear more than death itself is cancer and the painful, lingering death that ensues.

And no wonder. Cancer seems to creep up on us in the twilight of our lives—silent, unwarning, implacable, and uncontrollable. It is the death sentence that twentieth century man passes upon himself, and we fear it as much as any inevitable executioner or, faceless murderer.

Yet we create cancer in our own bodies with every bite we take of processed, refined, and preserved foods. And the biggest offenders are the traditional high-protein foods—cheese, eggs, and especially meat.

In 1982, the National Academy of Sciences suggested that there is a strong link between animal product foods high in protein and occurring cancers of the breast, prostrate, and colon. In fact, Dr. Colin Campbell, a member of the panel who studied the link between diet and cancer had this to say:

"The weight of the evidence certainly points to a link between high-protein foods and resultant cancers.

You don't hear too much about it because consumption of animal products is a big industry in this country. It's also a status symbol. But the result is that there's a higher level of breast cancer here than in countries where people eat fewer animal products."

By now it should be old news that cancer is related to the consumption of animal products high in fat (meat, dairy products, eggs, etc.). Heavy beef eating is directly related to the high incidence of colon and rectum cancer in this and other predominantly meat-eating populations. Almost ten years ago, Dr. Ernest Wynder announced to the Greater Boston Medical Society that dietary fat and animal protein combine with bacteria in the colon to form acids which are linked to tumor formations. He also said that evidence furthermore shows that such high-protein, high-fat foods are also implicated in tumors of the breast, pancreas, kidneys, ovaries, and prostrate.

Although animal protein is the biggest offender, all high and concentrated protein foods have the potential of becoming carcinogenic. Excessive protein, whether from animals or vegetable sources (seeds, nuts, beans, grains), decomposes or rots in the stomach and turns into poisonous ammonia. This ammonia in turn produces nitrosamines. Nitrosamines, according to biochemist Dr. Lijinsky, are "among the most potent cancer-causing chemicals known."

Malignant tumors require amino acids for growth that only protein foods can supply. The high-protein requirement for cancerous growths comes, as a rule, from eating animal carcasses (meat). Tumors have been described by some researchers as "traps" for excess nitrogen in the body. In controlled experiments, the rate of a tumorous growth increased twice as fast when concentrated protein was added to the diet.

Many recovered cancer patients must limit their protein intake so severely that they cannot eat even the vegetable foods high in protein. In her book How I Conquered Cancer Naturally, Eydie Mae Hunsberger described how fasting, and a raw food diet allowed her to overcome breast cancer. In the book, she states how she must avoid all high-protein foods, even peas and beans. "I go easy on the proteins," she said, "because cancer patients have a protein digestive problem. Soy products, for example, are too high in protein for me. If I want protein foods, I choose avocados, almonds, sunflower seeds, and sprouts."

The demand for protein by cancerous cells is almost ten times the amount as required by healthy tissues. Sufficient protein builds healthy bodies. Excessive protein builds tumors.

85.2.4. The High-Protein, Low-Health Weight-Loss Diet

By just following the typical United States diet of heavy animal foods, meat, and dairy, you will experience many problems associated with a high-protein diet. The average American woman consumes 50% more protein than the Recommended Daily Amount (RDA), while the typical male will eat almost 100% (twice as much) more protein than the RDA. Please remember that all RDAs are set intentionally "high" to make sure that people get all the nutrients they need. Even by these high standards, Americans are heavy protein eaters.

Yet there are some people who intentionally consume even more protein!

Athletes, weight-lifters, and body-builders are some of the people who consciously eat extra high-protein foods in a mistaken belief that such foods are needed for energy. Yet there are some people who increase their protein intake and reduce their carbohydrate intake in a bizarre effort to lose weight fast. On such a diet, weight-loss and a health-loss do occur.

The rationale of high-protein diets for weight loss, such as the Stillman high-protein diet or Dr. Linn's liquid protein diet, is based on the fact that protein requires much more body energy for digestion and metabolism than it supplies.

The body's first nutrient need is for fuel—carbohydrates. When excessive protein is eaten instead of needed carbohydrates, the body will try to convert the extra protein into a carbohydrate-type of fuel source. This conversion process is a difficult and energy-expending one for the body, and so a net-calorie or weight loss may occur.

The problem with this attempt at weight loss with a high-protein diet is that harmful by-products are produced in the protein to carbohydrate conversion process. Dr. Robert

R. Gross, Ph.D., New York professional Hygienist, stated the problem this way: "The hitch is the end products of protein digestion are acidic—urea, uric acids, adenine, etc., which, beyond a certain normal range, will cause degeneration of body tissues, producing gout, liver malfunctions, kidney disorders, digestive disturbances, arthritis and even hallucinations."

Dr. D. J. Scott, D.C., N.D., Ohio professional Hygienist, also agrees that weight-loss through high-protein diets is a dangerous practice. He says: "Too much protein solidifies (like coffee) and has the same stimulating effect, and a high-protein diet will eventually destroy the glandular system, and damage the liver, adrenals and kidneys."

85.2.5. You Can't Fool the Body!

High-protein diets for weight-loss are all based on fooling the body. Instead of giving it the carbohydrate fuel it needs, you fill the body with acid-forming protein that must be expensively converted into fuel within the body. It's like pouring water into your gasoline tank and hoping that your car will try to turn it into suitable fuel. Your body does try, but it really can't be fooled. Consider these latest research findings:

At the Massachusetts Institute of Technology, a husband-and-wife research team, Drs. Judith and Richard Wurtman, discovered that you simply cannot deny the body carbohydrates in preference to protein. In a controlled study, the researchers studied people who were denied carbohydrate foods (such as fruits, potatoes, etc.) and fed protein foods instead.

After a few days, the people on the no-carbohydrate diet did indeed lose weight. But they also developed such strong cravings for any kind of carbohydrates that they uncontrollably ate sugary and starchy foods in such amounts after the diet that they gained all their weight back.

In the January 1983 issue of the Journal of Nutrition, the MIT researchers concluded that carbohydrate-starvation caused by a high-protein weight-loss diet actually creates a chemical imbalance in the brain.

This imbalance drives people to seek out carbohydrates (which is only natural since carbohydrates are our most efficient fuel source). The desire for a predominantly carbohydrate, low-protein diet is inherent in the human make-up, and it cannot be fooled by a high protein diet.

The article in the journal also suggested that instead of a high-protein approach to weight loss, a more natural and healthy approach would be to eat small amounts of naturally occurring high-carbohydrate foods (such as fruits) and forget about the protein.

85.2.6. The Ultimate High-Protein Diet

What's worse than a high-protein, low-carbohydrate diet for losing weight? Answer: An all-protein diet.

Incredible as it may seem, there were thousands of people in the late 1970s who followed a high-protein, weight-loss diet that consisted of nothing more than highly processed animal protein, sugar, and artificial coloring.

Called "liquid protein," the only foods consumed in this diet were vials of animal extracts that contained hooves from cows and other animal waste products from slaughterhouses. This "protein" (actually the unusable by-products from meat-packing) was liquified or melted down and then artificially flavored and colored so that it would taste like a grape or cherry soda. You can imagine how melted cow hooves would taste—small wonder that they had to disguise the obnoxious odors and sickening taste of such a product.

Each day, a person would open a plastic tube of this pure protein "gunk" and squeeze it down the throat. The protein syrup would fill the person up at a low-calorie cost, and weight loss would follow.

Unfortunately, not only did weight loss occur, but so did vomiting, dehydration, muscle cramps, nausea, dry skin, and loss of hair.

In the late 1970s, the liquid protein diet craze was at its peak. Thousands and thousands of vile vials of grape and cherry-flavored protein were sold to gullible men and women who proceeded to wreck their health on a dangerous 100% protein diet.

To be certain, these people were also losing weight. And some even lost more.

In Dix Hills, New York, Donna Cochran began an eight-month Super Pro-Gest liquid protein diet. First Mrs. Cochran lost sixty pounds on the diet. Then she lost her life. She dieted because of heart complications brought about by the all-protein diet. Her husband and son sued and received $55,000—a small amount indeed for a loved one's life.

Liquid-protein diets can cause hard-to-detect, and possibly fatal, heart problems. The all-protein diet disrupts the body's mineral balance, and drastically reduces the potassium level. This dangerously reduced potassium level leads to arrhythmia, or the abnormal beating of the heart.

The liquid or all-protein diet was first developed by a doctor who got the idea from intravenous feeding. Just like intravenous feeding, the liquid-protein diet is an unnatural and debilitating practice. Fortunately, word has now gotten around about the dangers of this all-protein diet trick. Unfortunately, people still believe in the power of a high-protein, low-carbohydrate diet for weight loss, and think it is safe.

85.3. The True Needs of the Body

85.3.1. Carbohydrates—Not Protein

85.3.2. Sufficient Protein: It's Easy!

85.3.1. Carbohydrates—Not Protein

Carbohydrates in their natural forms of fresh and dried fruits and some vegetables should always be used in preference to concentrated protein foods. People who consciously reduce the amount of complex carbohydrates in the diet and eat more protein foods instead in an attempt to lose weight or "improve" their health are playing a dangerous game. Listen to what Dr. Helen C. Kiefer of the Northwestern University Medical School has to say about the relative importance of carbohydrates and proteins in a well-balanced diet:

"Carbohydrates must not fall below a certain limiting amount in any diet, or we run the risk of ending up in an unhealthy metabolic state; or, perhaps worse over the long run, we may waste the body's protein stores from tissues such as muscle to prevent this unhealthy metabolic state."

"Proteins, unlike carbohydrates or fats, contain the element nitrogen. When we strip this nitrogen from the amino acid components of proteins in order to convert them to carbohydrates for energy, we run the risk of building up ammonia in our bloodstreams. Ammonia is highly toxic.

After detailing the dangers of ammonia and other protein by-products in the bloodstream, Dr. Kiefer gives this unqualified endorsement of a predominantly carbohydrate based diet over the typical protein diet used for both weight loss and as a regular diet by so many people:

"An appropriate level of the oft-maligned carbohydrate is perhaps the best protection in any diet. It protects the need of the brain cells for carbohydrates; the need to metabolize fats for energy without increasing the acid load of the bloodstream; the protection of protein in tissue and the prevention of excess nitrogen excretion when protein components (amino acids) must be used for energy."

85.3.2. Sufficient Protein: It's Easy!

Protein needs and requirements are incredibly low for a healthy person. In fact, one measure of a person's health is how much protein they must consume to maintain their body weight. Sick and diseased people crave large amounts of protein for stimulation for their exhausted bodies. Healthy people, on the other hand, can function very well on about one-fifth of the protein the average American consumes.

How can we make sure that we get enough protein, but not too much? Easy. Just eliminate all substandard, harmful, and processed foods from the diet and eat an abundance of fresh fruits with some vegetables, sprouts, and nuts or seeds (if desired). All of these foods can be eaten in their raw state, and (with the exception of nuts and seeds) are low in concentrated protein. Yet these foods do supply all the essential amino acids that we need for a healthy life. More importantly, the foods of the Life Science diet supply us with an abundance of natural carbohydrates—our body's number one nutrient need. In addition, we receive a full array of vitamins, minerals, enzymes, and yet undiscovered elements from these fresh and wholesome foods packaged by nature.

A true protein deficiency on a calorie-sufficient diet is a rarity. Cancers from a high protein diet are all, too common. Say "No!" to the propaganda and misinformation that is circulating about any supposed benefits of a high-protein diet. Say "Yes!" to the health promoting and nutrient-abundant diet of fresh raw fruits, vegetables, sprouts, and seeds.

85.4. Questions & Answers

I feel so good after eating several high-protein meals. I feel like I could fight a tiger! How could that be bad?

There is a very good reason that you feel so "energetic" or stimulated after a high-protein meal. The chemical composition of uric acid, a by-product of protein metabolism, is remarkably similar to that of caffeine. You're not getting any energy from the high-protein meals, you're receiving chemical stimulation. Heavy protein eaters are always "high" on drugs—either from the stimulating effects of the uric acid by-products, or they may actually become intoxicated on the alcohol that forms in the body from protein fermentation. And please—don't go around fighting any tigers; they're almost as dangerous as those high-protein meals you're putting away.

Well, then, is protein bad? Should I just not eat any protein foods ever again?

Better not stop eating all protein foods, or you may go hungry! All our biologically-correct foods (such as fruits, sprouts, vegetables, etc.) contain ample protein in the form of easily assimilable amino acids. No, protein is not "bad." But protein from animal sources is harmful because of all the accompanying toxins, fats, etc. And excessive protein, whether from plants or animals, is always harmful.

Okay, so how much protein is too much? What do you mean by excessive?

If you eat any of the foods that are not suitable for our physiology (and this includes all meats, dairy products, eggs, and other animal products), then you will be getting too much protein. If you overeat the substandard foods such as legumes and grains, you will be getting more protein than is probably needed. To guard yourself against excessive protein intake, follow these simple rules: 1) Never eat any animal products. 2) If you eat concentrated protein foods from the plant kingdom, such as beans, peas, grains, soy products, then eat these no more than once every day or two. 3) Do not overeat on nuts and seeds. If you want more calories, or need to feel "full," then reach for some fruits, fresh or dried, instead of more nuts.

I was believing most of what you said until you told me that protein causes cancer. Come on! Everybody eats protein and we've eaten lots of it over the years. Why don't we all drop dead from cancer?

There is no single cause for cancer or any other illness. All such conditions take years of poor living, eating, and exercise habits to develop. The facts are this: Most cancer patients have a history of moderate to heavy meat-eating with liberal use of fatty animal products and processed protein foods. Dr. Frank Madden of the Egyptian School of Medicine in Cairo, Egypt, conducted an extensive study of cancer throughout Egypt. He found that the tribes in Egypt who lived on an almost exclusively vegetarian diet (the Sudanese and Berberines) never experience cancer. Never. On the other hand, cancer was very common among the Arabs and Copts who followed the traditional high-protein, high-meat European diet. You cannot say that protein "causes" cancer, nor can you even say that meat-eating causes cancer. But you can most assuredly state that the usual overall lifestyle and attitude that accompanies heavy meat and protein eating certainly seems to foster the development of all forms of cancer throughout the world.

One last question. My friends and I have tried the high-protein diet in the past for weight loss. We only stayed on the diet for about six weeks, and we lost ten to fifteen pounds. It does work! Shouldn't we judge only by the results?

This reminds me of a story about a salesman who went door to door, selling what he said was a guaranteed method of weight loss. He sold a small box that would take off pounds or your money back. Inside the box was a knife and the following instructions: "1) Sterilize knife. 2) Carve away unwanted pounds."

Hopefully, all of his customers took the package as a joke or novelty item. Unfortunately, it does illustrate how far some people will go to lose weight without changing the conditions that brought about the weight gain. Sure, a high-protein, low-carbohydrate diet will shed pounds, but you are not reducing—you're wasting away and wrecking your health. Are you sure these are the results you want?

Article #1: The Enigma of Protein by T.C. Fry

Even though the truth about protein as delineated in this article, and its role in human nutrition, have been known for nearly a century, there still rages a conflict and welter of confusion on the subject.

The misconceptions are primarily fostered by commercial businesses that are selling protein products, primarily meat and milk products. Even our American government serves these entrenched interests. The truth will not drown but ever keeps rising to fuel the fire of this controversy.

At the outset I would like to dispel some of the prevalent myths about protein.

MYTH NO. 1: We must have meat for best health. The argument goes that the best source for protein is meat inasmuch as it has all the requisite amino acids in a very assimilable form. Even the eminent (in so-called health food circles) Carlton Fredericks has gone on record as stating that the more nearly the composition of the flesh is to human flesh the more wholesome it is for us. Of course, there was never a better argument made for cannibalism than this!

The "we must have meat" argument is obviously good for the meat-packing industry, but it is patently absurd—the argument obviously destroys itself. If this were true every species could live from other animals but best of all from its own kind! The fact that almost all animals, including humans, do not have the anatomical and physiological equipment to make good use of any kind of meat is conveniently overlooked or denied. Cattle, rabbits, elephants, horses, etc., are herbivores and are equipped only for a leaf/grass diet. There are a class of graminivores, primarily birds, that thrive on the grains of various grasses. There are other animals that thrive on fruits. And so, it goes. Every animal has a class of food to which it is adapted.

Humans are anatomically and physiologically adapted to a diet of fruits, vegetables and nuts and can profitably use certain seeds and legumes under certain conditions. That this is true is denied by commercial interests and their "scientific" apologists. An educated populace would bring an end to their niche in the marketplace.

Not even carnivores thrive on an all-meat diet. For humans, meat is a pathogenic and deficient food.

MYTH NO. 2: We must have all the essential amino acids at every meal. This argument is based on two premises: (A) That the body does not store protein or amino acids and (B) that, in order to synthesize protein, no more protein can be created by the body than the amount creatable as determined by the least bountiful supply of the essential amino acids. Every protein link requires so much of such and such amino acids and if any are missing from the meal, no proteins requiring these amino acids can be synthesized. This argument, too, is absurd. It is not necessary to point out with detail that man and animals fast for lengthy periods and that, instead of suffering protein deficiency, the end of the fast finds them with restored protein balance!

MYTH NO. 3: A high-protein diet is healthful, and the body requires about one gram of protein for each two pounds of body weight. Obviously the body needs only what it needs and can use no more than what it needs. This "just right" amount of protein has been determined to be about one gram for each five pounds of body weight for mature humans of normal disposition. The one gram for each two pounds of body weight is about what a baby requires for maintenance and rapid growth. Obviously, adults do not require as much. The belief in a high-protein diet or that we cannot get too much of it is a source of highly pathological eating practices among Americans and other peoples of the world.

It is fitting that we have this little tome to set aright the attitude of those whom it touches in this most crucial aspect of human nutrition.

Article #2: Proteins

Proteins are organic compounds composed of amino acids. There are hundreds of types of proteins, each being identified by a combination of amino acids which constitutes it.

Amino acids usually contain nitrogen, hydrogen, oxygen, carbon, and sometimes sulfur and are synthesized by the body cells from the air and water or derived from food which is eaten.

The word "protein" signifies "of first importance."

Proteins form the principal elements of the skin, hair, nails, connective tissue, and all other organs. They exist everywhere in the body in cells which make up all the tissues, bones, cartilage, muscle, fibers, glands, and organs.

Among the most important proteins are substances called enzymes which are catalysts which accelerate the vital biochemical processes enabling a cell to do in one minute what would otherwise require many years.

Most hormones are proteins or derivatives of amino acids. Proteins are manufactured by cells.

Human proteins are different compounds than animal proteins and plant proteins. Thus, it is necessary to break down (digest) proteins entering the body into fundamental amino acids which are then recombined into human proteins. Complex animal proteins require a much greater expenditure of effort by the human body cells in the breaking down process than do the more simple plant proteins.

At the same time, a great quantity of wastes, toxins, and poisons accompanies the animal proteins.

These foreign substances are very harmful to the human body and contribute to progressive deterioration of the health, thus it is strongly recommended that all animal protein be excluded from the diet of humans.

A normal, healthy adult body, living in obedience to the rules of health requires very little or no solid food protein to maintain superb health. Since all of the elements constituting amino acids (nitrogen, oxygen, hydrogen, carbon, sulfur) are present in the air we breathe and in the body's storehouse, there is no need to burden the body with large quantities of food in an effort to supply protein. The body's processes easily produce the amino acids and proteins it needs from the constant supply of basic elements available to it.

It is wise to avoid eating all animal protein or too much vegetable protein to insure good health.

EAT SPARINGLY OF PROTEIN FOODS!

Article #3: Protein Supplements by Hannah Allen

Protein supplements should never be used. Dried and crystallized tablets, or protein powders, or various protein concoctions, are even more dangerous than other food supplements, because the consequences of protein overconsumption, especially as an isolated food element, may be disastrous.

To quote Dr. Alec Burton, N.D., D.O., D.C., eminent professional Hygienist in Australia: "A food element is a part of a complex food which, in the living plant or animal, almost invariably, contains some, even if only in minute quantities, of all the various food elements—proteins, carbohydrates, fats, minerals, and vitamins... The body is adapted to the use of food as a complex mixture of food elements. We do not eat food elements or nutrients in isolation when we consume a natural food. When we eat these items out of their natural contexts with other nutrients, ... the nutritional impact is different and can lead to unfavorable consequences."

The potential damage and artificial deficiencies that may be created through the use of protein supplements and other supplements are considerable. Just as an excess of nitrogen in the plant will create artificial deficiencies of other elements and prevent fruiting, so stimulation to the human organism produced by supplementation will disturb natural balance. This is the "Law of the Minimum": "The development of living beings is regulated by the supply of whichever element is least bountifully provided."

(This has been long known in plant life.) Using supplements, by creating an overabundance of some elements, creates an artificial shortage of other elements, known and unknown, and the element in shortest supply determines our development.

A very fine dentist and his charming wife, who are staunch advocates of so-called "natural" supplementation, told me that they know that supplements are beneficial and necessary, because "if they don't take their supplements, they just drag around."

What better proof could there be of the stimulating effect and addictive nature of supplementation? A Hygienist can skip meals, or eat fruit only for several days, or eat his regular diet of fruits, vegetables, and nuts, and continue to be his vital, sparkling, indomitable self, with no crutches and no pills.

Manufactured concentrates are sold by commercial interests who are determined, for their profit, to maintain the position that substitute and compensatory substances can provide superior nutrition. Supplements are unnecessary, expensive, stimulating, addictive, and create artificial deficiencies and pathological changes in the human organism.

The richest sources of protein and all other food elements are in living food: raw nuts and seeds, fruits, and vegetables, and it is here they are found in ideal combinations with other substances (known and unknown) essential to their full utilization. There is no better way: When you eat a variety of whole, raw foods, in accordance with Hygienic principles, you need not be concerned about amino acids or vitamins or minerals or anything else—everything will be adequately supplied.

Lesson 86:

The Supplement Approach to Nutrition

86.1. Introduction

One day in August, a thirty-three-year-old woman went to her doctor because she had a water retention problem. The family doctor advised the woman to take supplements of vitamin B-6 (also known as pyridoxine).

The doctor didn't say how much of the vitamin to take, so the woman started eating three or four vitamin tablets at each meal. "I started taking the vitamin in mega doses (large amounts)," she later told reporters. "I believed that was the way that vitamins are supposed to work. Taking large amounts seemed to be the in-thing for the 1980s."

After taking the B-6 supplements for two months, she still had a water retention problem. "My ankles were swelling, and I was still about twenty pounds overweight from all the water I was holding." So, she returned to her doctor who told her to just start taking larger doses of the vitamin.

"I didn't bother to ask him how large a dose," the woman said, "I just started taking more." By late October, she was taking between six to twelve grams of the vitamin each day. The minimum daily requirement for B-6 is about two to four milligrams per day. This woman was taking 3,000 to 4,000 times the amount needed.

By December, she started having a constant tingling in her feet and difficulty walking. "I couldn't get down the steps to my business," she told the newspapers, "and my feet felt like there were 50-pound weights tied to them."

She still persisted in taking huge doses of vitamin B-6, convinced that her doctor must be right.

Four months later, she could not even hold a fork in her hand or sign her name. The mega doses of vitamin B-6 had so severely disrupted her nervous system that the woman was incapable of performing even the simplest routine task.

"The vitamin ruined my health," she said, "and it forced me to sell my second business."

One of the neurologists who treated the woman had this to say: "There is an excellent chance that the large doses of the vitamin had a causative role in her illness. We must assume that mega doses of B-6 can injure both motor and sensory nerves."

In the same newspaper that this story appeared in, there was also an advertisement for the vitamin by a health food chain. "Vitamin B-6," the ad stated, "has been used to treat schizophrenia, water retention problems, and to build muscles by athletes. Shouldn't you add this wonder vitamin to your regular diet-supplementation program?"

Vitamins. Supplements. Minerals, enzymes, amino acids, brewer's yeast, dolomite— all are extracted, artificial, and fragmented dietary additions, and they have no place in health-promoting nutrition.

Yet the appeal and lure of dietary supplements is strong—so strong that a number of nutritionists and spokesmen have created an entire dietary school and philosophy that prescribes the regular use of potentially dangerous and utterly worthless nutritional additives and aids.

This lesson discusses the dangers of the supplementary approach to nutrition and why such a fragmented view of health is doomed to failure.

86.2. The Supplement Approach to Nutrition

86.2.1. The Supplement School and Its Beliefs

86.2.2. Who's to Blame?

Someone once said that there are as many approaches to nutrition as there are nutritionists. There is the "protein school" of nutrition which emphasizes a high-protein diet and protein foods over all else. One group tells us we must eat meat and drink milk; another group tells us we must base our diet on grains and seaweeds. There are vegetarians, fruitarians, sproutarians, and breatharians. There are nutritionists who defend junk foods and promote fast foods. Just about every conceivable approach to nutrition has its supporters and adherents.

This lesson is about one of the more bizarre cults of nutritionists: the supplementalists, or those who advocate powders, pills, capsules, and supplements of vitamins, minerals, and proteins. There have already been several lessons telling why we don't need nutritional supplements in the diet. You have already learned about the fallacies of using inorganic minerals, fragmented vitamins, and other worthless powders, pills, and potions. Yet the supplement approach to nutrition remains a trap for the unwary and uneducated. You need facts if you wish to educate your clients, friends, family, and patients about the folly of following the recommendations of the supplementalists. This lesson, then, focuses on the school of nutritional thought, and those spokesmen, that advocate the use of supplements as a normal part of a healthy diet.

86.2.1. The Supplement School and Its Beliefs

The supplementary approach to nutrition is based on these erroneous beliefs:

1. The human organism can utilize inorganic minerals, vitamins, amino acids, etc.
2. Elements of nutrition can be fragmented and employed in part instead of in total.
3. Nutritional needs have been accurately determined and totally analyzed.
4. More is better.

All of these beliefs are false. Let's briefly examine them one by one.

86.2.1.1. Fallacy #I: We Can Utilize Inorganic Minerals and Vitamins

When my grandfather was a young man, he plowed the clay fields each spring to prepare for planting cotton. He told me that every year one of the poor women who lived in the area would come to his fields with a spoon and a bucket. She would squat down near where he had plowed and start to spoon up some of the dark black clay into her bucket until it was full.

My grandfather thought that the woman was perhaps gathering clay from his particular field to use as a poultice, since the dirt in his fields was a darker color than other farms in the area. One day he noticed that the woman was putting spoonful's of the clay into her mouth and chewing it up. One spoonful would go into the bucket, and the next spoonful would go into her mouth.

He took his lunch pail over to the woman squatting in the field and offered her his sandwich, thinking that maybe the, woman was crazed from hunger and had taken to eating dirt.

The woman looked at my grandfather in embarrassment and refused the offered food. "I'm not hungry," she told him, "f just have a craving for this kind of clay. My body wants the salts in it."

Dirt of clay-eating was, and still is, a common practice in some parts of the poor rural South. It even has a name—pica, or the craving for unnatural nonfood substances. Many times the diet in poor regions of the country consists of, polished rice, grits, lard, white flour, and other totally demineralized foods. In a bizarre effort to compensate for their mineral-poor diet, the poor people (usually nursing mothers or older women) would develop "cravings" for clay or dirt.

Of course dirt-eating did not improve the health of these physically-deranged people; they could no more get minerals from the soil than they could get calories from the air.

Yet today there are still people who want us to eat inorganic minerals for health. The only difference is that these people have extracted the minerals from the dirt and just put them into a nice clean pill or capsule. But the approach to nutrition is the same. It doesn't matter if you eat clay with a spoon or swallow a pill from a bottle, you are still making a futile effort to get your mineral needs from a totally inappropriate nonfood substance.

We cannot utilize minerals, vitamins, and other elements of nutrition that are inorganic in nature. Our bodies are not meant to process such nonfood items. Many of the minerals and other nutritional elements that are packed into a pill originally came from rocks (dolomite), industrial wastes (fluoride), and even scrap metal (iron)! There are people today who would never consider sticking a spoonful of dirt into their mouths, yet they gulp an inorganic food supplement each day that is little more than dirt and soil that has been "prettied up."

Our mineral needs, and other nutrient needs, can only be satisfied by organic elements as found in plants. We cannot process dirt or soil into usable elements, nor can we metabolize extracts of these soils or chemicals that make up the supplement pills. We must eat plants (fruits, vegetables, nuts, seeds, etc.) that have elaborated inorganic mineral compounds into organic compounds and chains if we want to obtain real nutrition. Plants take minerals and nutrients from the soil; we take minerals and nutrients from the plants. We cannot bypass this all-important step as the supplementalists would have us believe.

86.2.1.2. Fallacy #2: Nutritional elements can be used in their fragmented form instead of in total.

Every nutritional supplement, no matter how complete, exists in an unnatural and fragmented form. To make a mineral, vitamin, or protein pill, you must first destroy the natural food source it occurs in and then refine and extract a specific element from that food. By so doing, you destroy and remove all the natural co-existing elements of nutrition that accompany the extracted element. As an example, consider the mineral iron.

Iron is present in a number of high-grade fruits and vegetables, such as the cherry or apricot. Suppose a chemist wants to make an iron pill. He could take raw inorganic iron and just stuff it into a capsule, as was once done with surplus nails, or he could take some natural source of iron (such as the cherry) and chemically extract it.

The mineral iron that is present in a cherry, for example, is readily absorbed and used by the body because the other necessary elements for the absorption of iron co-exist in the cherry or food itself. For instance, ascorbic acid aids the absorption of iron in the body by helping to convert ferric to ferrous iron. The cherry has the needed ascorbic acid present with the ferric iron compounds. If you swallowed a pill that had the iron extracted from the cherry but not the accompanying ascorbic acid, then your body would simply not have the needed co-existing elements to use the iron.

Nature packages our vitamins, minerals, and other nutritional needs in complete foods. There is no chemist smarter than nature; there is no laboratory as complex as the human body. Fragmented forms of minerals, vitamins, and other nutritional elements can never be as efficiently used (if used at all) as the total, complete array of nutrients that are abundantly present in every natural, wholesome food.

86.2.1.3. Fallacy #3: All of our nutritional needs have been determined and are accurately known.

The supplementalists base their nutritional approach on such concepts as Minimum Daily Requirements, Recommended Daily Amounts, and Therapeutic Dosages. They believe that they can determine how much of a specific nutrient a person may need, and the best dose of that substance to give. For example, let's look at vitamin A:

The Recommended Daily Allowance (RDA) for vitamin A is 5,000 IU (international units). Of course, the RDA for vitamin A, like most RDAs, is somewhat meaningless to begin with since it is based on averages, or a "typical" person. Vitamin A requirements increase or decrease depending upon the lifestyle we follow and the regular diet we follow. One of the nutritionists who strongly believes in using vitamin supplements states that for improved health, we should take 10,000 IUs and if we need a therapeutic or megadose of the vitamin, then we should increase our vitamin A supplementation to 35,000 IUs per day.

He also warns us that 75,000 IUs of vitamin A produce toxicosis in the body and that 200,000 IUs of vitamin A daily over a period of time can result in death.

The truth is that there is no one constant, standard, or safe amount of vitamin A to universally recommend. There has never been a way to experimentally determine the optimum dose of vitamin A a person should ingest each day. As long as you swallow pills containing vitamin A, you have little control or knowledge of how many IUs your body needs or can use. It is quite possible to take a continually excessive level of vitamin A for weeks or months before you realize the irreversible harm that has been done. If you want extra vitamin A, why not play it safe and get the vitamin from natural foods that it occurs in, such as cantaloupes, peaches, carrots, apricots, or most fresh fruits and vegetables?

The supplementalists will tell you that they know exactly to the last milligram how much of any specific nutrient that you need. You should remember, however, that new vitamins, minerals, enzymes, and other co-nutrients are being discovered all the time. No one really knows the full range of nutrients that the body requires to maintain perfect health, and you can be certain that there is no pill or supplement that can contain all of these life-preserving elements.

We do know, however, that fresh wholesome foods do contain all the nutrients we need for superior health and well-being. This has been proven beyond a doubt because millions of people for thousands of years have prospered very well on such a diet without ever swallowing one pill or one supplement. No chemist, no laboratory, and no nutritionist can make such an unequivocal statement nor replicate such a convincing experiment.

To repeat: We do not yet know what nutrients we need, or in what amounts, to produce radiant health. We do know that wholesome unprocessed fruits and vegetables do contain all of these elements, both known and unknown, and we would do well to rely on these alone to supply all of our nutrient needs.

86.2.1.4. Fallacy #4: More is better.

The "more is better" school of nutrition has been in control since the nineteenth century. These people believe that since a little is good for you, then a lot must be better. It is surprising that intelligent people will fall for this ruse. Suppose you run five miles per day for exercise. This amount of vigorous activity is enough to keep you in good health and promote a healthy metabolism. Suppose, however, that you decided since running five miles is great, then running fifty miles per day would help you ten times as much.

If you could even attempt to run fifty miles every day, you would quickly discover that you are in fact tearing down the body and totally exhausting its resources and reserves. The same way with good food. Since we have been told that a little protein is needed for good health, we think that a lot of protein would automatically mean much better health.

It's simply not so, and any excess whether in diet, exercise, or even relaxation, will have negative effects on your health.

Vitamins, minerals, protein, or any nutrient taken in excess of the body's needs become toxic and either must be eliminated by the body or stored, which may result in a toxic overdose.

With nutrition, "more" is not "better." Enough is enough is enough, so why burden your body or empty your pocketbook with needless nutritional overkill?

86.2.2. Who's to Blame?

Who are the people who are promoting the supplemental approach to nutrition and why are they so successful? The answer is that there is a willing, gullible public eager to take the easy way out when it comes to health and diet, and there are clever spokesmen and vested interests who do a superior job of selling hogwash to the people.

Let's see why the supplemental school of nutrition has such a strong appeal, and who its active supporters are.

86.3. The Appeal of the Supplement School

86.3.1. Eat Anything You Want!

You may wish to try an interesting experiment if you have a young child. When the child becomes hungry, offer him or her either a piece of fresh fruit or a large vitamin capsule to choose from. A silly experiment, right? Of course, the child or any adult who is truly hungry will select the easily identifiable food or fruit and bypass the colorless, odorless, and tasteless pill.

Yet Americans regularly gobble pills, capsules, and powders as a substitute for natural foods and wholesome nutrition. Why is that? Why would an adult put his faith and good health in an unidentifiable pill shaken out of a bottle? Why would anyone eat capsules, pills, vitamin supplements and mineral potions instead of fresh, delicious, succulent, and sweet fruits and vegetables?

There are several reasons why the "pill school of nutrition" holds such a powerful fascination for today's adults. Let's look at the reasons that people are fooled into buying and swallowing pills for nutrition instead of good wholesome food.

86.3.1. Eat Anything You Want!

One morning I found myself in a breakfast doughnut shop near an elementary school. I was getting change for a morning newspaper when I looked over to a table where a mother had her two school children.

The mother was handing the boy and girl a cup of frozen orange juice and a big sticky sweet roll for their breakfast before she dropped them off at the nearby school.

As the children ate the sugar-laden junk food for breakfast, the mother reached into her purse and carefully pulled out a piece of tissue paper that held two huge vitamin capsules.

In between bites of the doughnuts, she popped the pill into her son's and daughter's mouths. "Now swallow your vitamins so you'll be strong and healthy," she prompted. She absent-mindedly lit a cigarette and felt satisfied that she had discharged her motherly duties so well. In one fell swoop, she had neutralized the bad effects of a doughnut breakfast and assuaged her guilt by just sticking vitamin pills into her children's mouths.

Eat anything you like, but just take your magic vitamin pill and all is forgiven. All of your nutritional problems wiped out with just one swallow. Is there any wonder that there is such a strong appeal for a pill?

The public likes the "pill concept." It is a noncontroversial approach to nutrition that does not require any changes in diet or lifestyle. You can continue eating your favorite junk foods and you never have to question or face your bad living habits. Vitamin pills and dietary supplements are crutches for the nutritionally crippled. They are easy to standardize, profitable to promote, and give the appearance of effects without requiring any efforts.

Quite simply, the pill approach to nutrition is popular not because of what it does, but what it does not require us to do—change the poor eating and living habits that make us turn to supplements in the first place.

86.4. The Supplementalists

86.4.1. Writers That Aren't Right

86.4.2. A Supplement Proponent

86.4.3. A Catalog of Pills and Supplements

86.4.4. The Pill Store

The supplemental school of nutrition has three categories of supporters: 1) Vocal spokesmen who seek to attract a following; 2) Magazines and publications that cater to advertisers and the supplement industry; and 3) Health food stores and manufacturers of the supplements. While it is nonproductive to engage in name calling and finger pointing, you should be aware of the different approaches taken by these supporters of the supplement approach to good health.

86.4.1. Writers That Aren't Right

Every few years, a new spokesman for the supplement school of nutrition arrives at the newsstands with the same message for the masses: Swallow more pills for better health. The message may be worked differently; it may be couched in new seductive phrases such as "super-nutrition" or "therapeutic nutrients" or "mega nutrition," but the point is always the same: Continue with your poor dietary habits but take a magical supplement and your problems will disappear.

They write about "megavitamins," "magic minerals," and "longevity enzymes." They promise you salvation in a bottle and relief in a vitamin store. They quote miraculous cures effected by exotic nutritional additives and pills. And they make money selling their books and articles to an eager public that is nutritionally naive.

86.4.2. A Supplement Proponent

Perhaps no sadder testimony to the ineffectiveness and dangers of pill-gulping can be found than from the words of a woman known worldwide for her recommendations of daily supplements: Adelle Davis.

Mrs. Davis was a well-known and outspoken proponent of the supplemental school of nutrition. Her book Let's Eat Right to Keep Fit sold several million copies and it is full of recommendations for various supplements, pills, extracts, and other nonfood substances. When asked by an individual what her daily dietary routine is like, the woman responded:

"For years I have taken after breakfast a capsule containing 25,000 units of vitamin A and 2,500 units of vitamin D, both from fish-liver oil; 200 or 300 units of vitamin E or d-alpha tocopherol acetate distilled from soy oil; a tablet containing 5 milligrams of iodine taken daily, and 500 milligrams or more of vitamin C. With my other meals, I also take three tablets of calcium combined with magnesium, and sometimes another tablet of magnesium oxide alone to balance the calcium in the milk I drink. If I've eaten salty food, I add another three tablets or more of potassium chloride, 180 milligrams each. Besides yeast and liver, I also take with each meal two B-complex vitamins."

The woman was taking about 20 to 30 pills every day of her life. "People frequently asked me how long they should take supplements," Adelle Davis wrote. "I am tempted to tell them, 'Until you get tired of good health.'" The woman concluded her discussion of nutrition with the statement: "I expect to take supplements as long as I live, though I wish I might get all nutrients from foods."

Adelle Davis did indeed take supplements as long as she lived—until she died of cancer.

Adelle Davis was not alone; other active promoters and writers who have ballyhobed the marvelous effects to be gained from supplements, pills, and potions have also enjoyed poor health and premature death. Quite frankly, the success or failure of a nutritional school of thought should be gauged only by the health or sickness of its proponents and spokesmen. The supplement school of nutrition has had a dismal history in this respect.

86.4.3. A Catalog of Pills and Supplements

Today there are about a half dozen magazines and a score of popular periodicals that consistently promote the use of supplements in their pages. Their pages are so full of ads and come-ons for supplements that they appear to be nothing more than catalogs of wonder drugs. And these magazines exist for one reason:

Money. The majority of advertising in these "health" magazines comes from supplement and vitamin manufacturers. Do you expect to see an honest article that exposes the dangers and shortcomings of supplements in a magazine that is full of paid ads for these pills? Of course not. The truth is that for many of these health-oriented publications, their major financial support comes from companies who want to sell the public pills and capsules.

Quite often these magazines will publish articles that actively promote a specific nutrient, say zinc for example. You can be sure that in that same issue there will be full page ads offering zinc supplements and pills. Could this be merely coincidence?

These magazines work hand in hand with the supplement industry. They create the perceived need for supplements, and the manufacturers offer you the promised cure all—all in the same magazine and almost on the same page. If this doesn't strike you as a little too fortuitous, then you are indeed a great idealist.

86.4.4. The Pill Store

Have you been inside a typical "'health food" store lately? You'll probably see very little "food"' or indeed even "health," but you'll certainly get an eyeful of bottle after bottle of vitamins, minerals, supplements, and other exotic potions.

And that's not too surprising at all, especially when you consider that 40 to 50% of a health food store's profits comes from the sale of supplements.

"Vitamins, minerals, and other diet supplements are my bread and butter, an owner of a small health food store confided to me. "I can mark up each bottle about 250 to 300% over what I pay for it. They have an indefinite shelf life; they can't go bad like produce, and I can usually sell one person about $25 to $40 worth at one swoop."

"I can't really prescribe these pills and supplements to my customers—that's against the law—but I can tell them how Mrs. Such-and-Such bought a bottle and how it helped her. You know that kind of thing. I act people coming in here all the time looking for some miracle vitamin that's going to cure all their ills. I don't sell supplements: I sell hope to sick people. Maybe they help, maybe they don't. I don't think they're any worse off."

But of course, they are worse off. They've spent good money on useless products, and, even worse, they do nothing to change the conditions that brought about their health problems in the first place. Health food stores may not practice deception, but you could hardly call them a service to their customers who purchase the supplements and vitamin pills.

The health food stores are not the villains in this tale of supplements. The people who are really making money from the supplement scam are the manufacturers and suppliers of these pills and potions. Consider this: That $5.95 bottle of multiple vitamins that you bought probably has about 20 cents worth of chemicals in it. The huge profits from the sale of these pills are plowed back into advertising and promotion to get you to buy even more bottles of chemicals and supplements.

The supplement market operates on a tremendous profit margin and markup. The industry is unpoliced and relatively unregulated. For example, vitamins and mineral supplements marked "natural" and "organic" may legitimately contain only 10% of its elements from natural sources; the remaining 90% could be the selfsame chemicals sold in any other brand.

Be wary of any school of nutrition that promotes products for profit. You may be sold a false bill of goods.

86.5. The Only Safe Source of Nutrients

86.5.1. One-a-Day Multiple Vitamins and Other Lies

86.5.2. Safety in Nature

Dr. Herbert M. Shelton has studied the effects of food and nutrition on human health longer than almost anyone else in the world today. He has long detailed the dangers of depending upon supplements, pills, and powders for adequate nutrition. When asked about the use of nutritional supplements in the diet, Dr. Shelton replied with this list of four important facts:

1. We do not yet know how much of any food element the body needs.

2. We do not yet know all of the elements that are structural and functional constituents of the human body.

3. We do not know that all of the vitamins have been discovered.

4. We do not know that there are no other and hitherto unsuspected food factors in foods that are as essential as those that are known."

Since our knowledge of nutrition can never be complete, it is impossible to construct a pill or supplement that can most assuredly supply us with all of our needs. "These things being so," writes Dr. Shelton, "there can be only one safe source of nutriment, and only one source that is capable of supplying us with all known and unknown food elements. This source is natural foods."

There can never be a pill or supplement that will furnish a human being with all of the nutritional elements required for superior health. Our physiology has developed over hundreds of thousands of years on fresh, wholesome fruits and vegetables. Our entire system is geared toward extracting elements of life from plant foods alone. We cannot survive on pills; we cannot thrive on supplements.

We require and need only fresh foods from the plant kingdom and nothing else.

191

86.5.1. One-a-Day Multiple Vitamins and Other Lies

Still, there are people who are fascinated by pills. "Just to be safe," such a person says, "I always take a good, all-around multiple vitamin and mineral tablet." "Just to be we," such a person will say, "I swallow a tablespoonful f iron supplement each morning."

These people are not buying good nutrition; they are seeking peace of mind in a pill or tablet. Yet if they knew that they were swallowing lies along with the pills, they might seek peace of mind elsewhere. Consider this newspaper report which appeared only this month: "Survey Finds Multivitamins Dangerous."

In a survey of the 41 most commonly-purchased multi-vitamin pills, it was discovered that many of them contain either dangerously high or inadequate doses of vitamins and minerals. According to a clinical nutrition researcher, "Most vitamin supplements we looked at exceeded the 200 percent mark for the Recommended Daily Allowance, which makes the vitamins perhaps dangerous." The researcher further stated that these supplements often contain excessive amounts of fat-soluble vitamins such as A, D, E, and K which can be harmful since these vitamins are stored in the body when taken in amounts greater than the body's needs.

There have been many cases where people were found suffering from vitamin toxicosis due to the abnormally large amounts they were taking and retaining through supplements and pills. Well, what about wholesome foods such as carrots, melons, etc., that are naturally high in vitamins; Does this mean that we can get too many vitamins from these natural sources?

86.5.2. Safety in Nature

If you are eating fresh foods in their natural state, you cannot overdose on vitamins. Why is this? For one thing, the sheer bulk of the food alone prevents you from eating amounts that would contain excessive vitamins. Of course, if you juice all of your foods and drink quarts of carrot juice every day, then it might be possible to get too many natural vitamins. Yet even in these circumstances, there are built-in safeguards in natural foods.

For example, the vitamin A in plant foods comes from a compound called carotene. The carotene in these vegetable foods is converted to a form of vitamin A in the liver only if there is a need for the vitamin in the body. In other words, if you ate about ten large carrots, you could potentially be ingesting around 100,000 units of vitamin A. Yet if your body only needed say 20,000 units of vitamin A, then the carotene conversion to vitamin A would not occur for the other potential 80,000 vitamin A units.

The body has an innate wisdom and knowledge of its true needs. As long as we supply the body with its natural food and fuel, we need not fear the consequences. Any time vital elements are extracted from our foods and packaged as concentrated supplements and pills, then we are taking serious chances with our health. No scientist, no chemist, no nutritionist has the type of knowledge that the body possesses. No laboratory can duplicate the wonderous processes of the human body. No experiment can replicate the intricate life processes that occur during food digestion and assimilation. No pill or supplement can ever be labeled completely safe.

There is only one safe source for our nutritional needs: fresh, wholesome foods from the plant kingdom. All else is suspect and should be rigorously avoided.

86.6. Questions & Answers

I recently heard that the only way you can meet your recommended daily amounts for vitamins and minerals is to take a good all-around supplement. Are you saying that we don't need pills no matter what we eat?

What you are probably referring to is the recent study by a medical researcher who discovered this startling fact: Up to 80% of the typical American's diet consists almost entirely of products made up of sugar, fat, white flour, and alcohol. The study then stated that since so many calories are consumed in these nutritionally worthless foods, then we would have to take some type of pill to make up the difference if we don't want to increase our calorie intake. The researchers then speculated that if we tried to satisfy all of our nutritional needs from food alone hat we would have to nearly double our calorie intake.

This is pure nonsense. Of course, if you eat the typical junk food diet of most Americans, then your diet will most certainly be lacking in essential nutrients. The solution is not to eat more of the selfsame nutritionally worthless foods in order to get enough vitamins or minerals. And you already know that swallowing a few pills is not the right approach.

Wouldn't it make more sense if these people would eliminate the 80% of their diet that furnishes no nutrition, and instead eat only wholesome, unprocessed foods that are packed with all of our essential nutrients? In this way, they would not have to increase their calorie intake; in fact, they would lower it because they would have eliminated all the high-calorie, low-nutrient foods that make up over half of their diet.

You can argue all you want to, but here's one thing that proves you wrong. When I feel run-down, I take a good overall vitamin and mineral supplement for five to seven days. I feel great and all charged up at the end of the week. Now tell me that supplements are worthless!

Okay—supplements are worthless. Seriously, what you are experiencing is not at all uncommon. We have never said that supplements do not have an effect; we have only said that they cannot supply proper nutrition.

Some people will feel better no matter what kind of pill they swallow. This is called the placebo effect and it has been well-documented. However, supplements can often have an effect that is simply not illusory. They can provide a strong stimulus to the body just as any toxin or foreign agent can. This stimulus that accompanies the supplement is often mistaken for a beneficial effect; instead, it is the body's response to an unnatural and inorganic presence. There are some additional materials at the end of this lesson that examine this false side-effect of taking supplements. Just because you are "stimulated" do not assume that you are being helped.

Article #1: The Great Supplement Hoax! by T.C. Fry

One has but to delve into a little biology, biochemistry, and physiology to know that supplementation is not only impractical but a tragic commercially fostered hoax. There is no such thing as supplementation and there cannot be! There are foods and nonfoods. Supplements do not fill a single condition required of a food. That is the delusion of supplementation.

Under the "just to be safe" illusion we intoxicate our bodies with unusable substances. Fortunately, most supplements furnish only a placebo effect—their foremost benefit lies in the absurd belief that they will keep us from suffering deficiencies. But beliefs do not protect us from their ill effects. For instance, there are well authenticated cases of scurvy among supplement takers who were ingesting two or three grams of vitamin C daily, enough to suffice for a hundred days if it were usable.

Most supplements taken orally meet with a just fate-being indigestible (and therefore unabsorbed), they pass into the bowels. To the extent they are absorbed they create problems for the organism. As you'll discover in this issue there is no case for supplementation. There is a case against so-called supplementation. There is a case for eating whole ripe raw foods of our biological adaptation. That and only that is capable of furnishing our needs in a physiological manner.

For the most part supplements are synthetically derived, even if advertised as being of "organic" origin. This representation is an outright fraud, for a reading of the label will reveal that only a small percentage is from organic sources. Synthetic substances are neither digestible nor metabolizable. That's the best part about most supplements, for the body passes them through the intestinal tract. On the other hand, those parts that may be absorbed are treated like drugs, not nutrients. The body is stimulated by them just as if caffeine, nicotine, alcohol, or other drugs had been taken. That lends to the mistaken idea that vitamins give energy. That's false; If anything, they take body energy just as do other drugs. Only carbohydrates are raw materials for energy.

Mineral supplements are derived from inorganic sources. They are totally unusable. Though we have a heavy need for minerals, the very minerals we require are toxic if taken in an inorganic state. We need iron, selenium, iodine, fluorine, magnesium, and a host of other minerals, but if taken in supplements as derived from rocks, soils, sea water or ores, they are unusable and poisonous. One of the foremost characteristics of poisons is that they stimulate, that is prick or goad the body into a frenzy. The body steps up energy expenditure to cope with a heavy eliminative situation. Because this makes us feel "hyper" we are likely to mistake this squandering of energy as being derived from the toxic substance ingested rather than a draft on our energy stores. It bears repeating that the body derives its energies from carbohydrates, not vitamins, minerals, or supplements.

If you have any deficiencies, you can't make them good by supplementation. Only a few fractionated foods among the supplements can be appropriated. But, even so, eating refined fractionated foods is like taking refined sugar, refined white flour and so on. Almost anything derived by fractionating foods would be poor even if eaten in context with the whole food from which taken because the parent food is not of our biological adaptation. Many supplements are derived from bacterial and yeast fermentative and putrefactive processes. No matter how rich in nutrients, these substances are unusable. Taking these concentrated nutrients to supplement a depraved and deficient diet is like eating tobacco leaves for nutrients instead of fruits. The difference between eating fruits and deficient diets with supplements is fruits are something the body can use in a physiologic manner; and deficient diets including supplements are something the body expends its resources on needlessly for purposes of protection and excretion.

Eat whole foods to which you are biologically adapted, more specifically, fresh ripe fruits with dried fruits if an extraordinary requirements of caloric values exists. If this needs supplementing, and it doesn't for it is replete with more nutrients of every description than we require, then supplement it with super nutrient-rich vegetables like broccoli, lettuce, celery, cauliflower, carrots, etc.

Remove yourself from that army of victims of the commercial game called supplementation. You're wasting your money and your health! Wholesome foods suited to the human dietary are all that you need.

Article #2: Vitamins: A Quarter Billion Dollar Humbug by Dr. Herbert M. Shelton

Perhaps nothing has done more to confuse the man on the street and, all too often, the doctor in his office, about what constitutes nutrition than the ballyhoo about vitamins. The trouble, be it understood, is not with vitamins, but with the commercial exploitation to which they and their imitations are being subjected. It is estimated that the American people are now spending a quarter of a billion dollars a year for "vitamins." That's a

195

lot of money! America has become "vitamin conscious" and the gangsters who are responsible for thus duping the people are reaping rich harvests from the vitamin racket.

"Vitamins" are sold in the drugstores, department stores, grocery stores, five and ten cent stores, health food stores, and by mail. Every conceivable means of advertising them is employed and nobody seems to think that there can be any such thing as honesty in advertising. Anything goes in the advertising if it sells "vitamins."

The medical profession is not alone to blame for the exaggerations that are being peddled about vitamins. The manufacturers of the so-called vitamin preparations are chiefly to blame, while many medical men of high standing have dared to lift their voices in warning about the vitamin cure-all now being offered to the public.

Chiropractors, osteopaths, naprapaths, physiotherapists, naturopaths, dietitians, "health" lecturers, and similar cure-mongers and the "health food" stores have all played a very big part in promoting this vitamin racket. Various types of doctors prescribe and sell these things to their patients. It seems to be easier to prescribe (and sell) vitamin pills (perhaps, it is almost more profitable) than it is to find and remove cause.

Health food stores reap a rich harvest off the sale of vitamins. The men and women who run these stores, though rarely possessed of any knowledge of human ills and the proper care of the sick, and never making a proper inquiry into the conditions for which they prescribe, do not hesitate to prescribe vitamins for all who come into their stores looking for cures. The health food stores no longer sell healthful foods; they sell cures.

Vitamins have been promoted as cold preventives. Extensive experience together with careful tests have combined to show that vitamins do not prevent colds. What is the difference between taking vitamins to prevent colds and ignoring cause and taking cold vaccines to prevent colds and ignoring cause?

Vitamins have been promoted as cures for chronic fatigue. Chronic fatigue may result from any one, or any combination of a number of, causes and any effort to cure the fatigue without removing its cause can only fail. This use of vitamins is identical in principle with the use of drugs.

Vitamins have been promoted as cures for arthritis. The hundreds of thousands of arthritis patients who have taken large quantities of vitamins and watched themselves grow worse are living testimonials of the failure of vitamins as a cure for arthritis. Vitamin D has especially been bally-hooed as a cure for arthritis. It has been used in huge doses. These have often given rise to toxic symptoms. This probably always makes the arthritis worse.

Vitamins have been promoted both as preventives and as cures for gray hair. They do neither. Those who have used them have been disappointed.

In a recent issue of the Journal of the American Medical Association, Dr. Julian M. Ruffin, and David Cayer, of Duke University, record details of an investigation conducted to determine the value of adding vitamin supplements to the usual American diet.

I think it is significant that the "usual American diet," which is by no means an ideal diet, was used in this series of tests. Two hundred volunteer medical students and technicians were used in the tests. These volunteers were divided into five groups. They were all "in apparent good health" and were "consuming the usual American diet." The tests were run for thirty days "because that period is found sufficient for recovery under vitamin treatment" of patients actually ill from vitamin deficiency.

- One group was given vitamin tablets and liver extract tablets.
- A second group was given yeast extract tablets and vitamin pills.
- The third group was given vitamin pills and a sugar pill made to resemble the others.
- The fourth group was given vitamin pills only.
- The fifth group was given sugar pills only.

None of the volunteers were permitted to know what was in the pills they were taking.

Each man kept a daily record of his weight and of such symptoms as "gas" and indigestion, nausea, vomiting, abdominal pain and diarrhea. Also, he kept a daily record of his impressions of any effect on his appetite and on his "pep" or energy.

Ruffin and Cayer report that a "significant increase in diarrhea and a highly significant increase in abdominal pain and nausea and vomiting occurred in those receiving liver extract and yeast."

This effect of yeast is certainly no new find and I was not surprised that liver extract causes similar symptoms.

The experimenters at Duke University point out that "The use of vitamins is widespread throughout the country, not only in the treatment of disease, but also by apparently normal persons" and state, as a conclusion based on the results of their own and other tests: "It has been implied that even when no demonstrable deficiency exists, one's sense of well-being and ability to perform work can be improved greatly by the addition of vitamin supplements to the diet. There is at present no evidence to substantiate this point of view."

Medical men are, and long have been, prescribing vitamin preparations (cod-liver oil, yeast, etc.), vitamin extracts and synthetic vitamins in all types of conditions and standing around in groups and cursing because the expected results have not been forthcoming.

No one claims that present methods of determining vitamin deficiencies are sufficiently delicate to reveal the earliest stages of deficiency. There is no reason why correct use of real vitamins in these undetectable incipient stages will not result in definite improvement in health and increase in energy.

What, then, is the trouble? It is evident to the careful student of nutrition that the trouble is not simple or singular, but complex and multiple.

First, the "vitamins" are only imitations. They are not genuine. Only fools expect these synthetic make-believes to produce results.

Second, they are not properly used. Vitamins do not produce energy. They do not put on weight. They are enzymes that enable the body to utilize proteins, carbohydrates, fats, and minerals. The "usual American diet" is especially deficient in minerals. To add vitamins to such a diet and not add quantities of the deficient elements, and expect results, it to expect vitamins to work in a vacuum.

Results may be obtained by using real vitamins, as these exist in natural foods, and taking them along with the other food elements, as these, too, are found in these same natural foods. Better nutrition requires better food, not merely the addition of vitamins.

Need I describe the "usual American diet" of white bread, denatured cereals, white sugar, refined syrups, canned fruits and vegetables, jellies, jams, preserves, cakes, pies, candies, embalmed meats, pasteurized milk, coffee, beer, and cigarettes, taken by these "apparently normal students and technicians?" Only an ignoramus would expect vitamins, even if they were real, to do anything with a diet like that.

Vitamin salesmen, vitamin manufacturers, vitamin con men of all grades, types and sizes are encouraging people to buy and take vitamins. They do not encourage people to revolutionize their eating practices. "Science" in an illegitimate union with commercialism is responsible for flooding the world with the deluge of lies that bewilder, confuse, and mislead the poor man on the street and the ignorant doctor in his office.

Article #3: Are 90% or More of the Vitamins You Take Going Down the Drain? by T.C. Fry

The above headline is from an advertisement of, all things, a vitamin ad! It goes on as follows:

THE PROBLEM WITH TODAY'S VITAMINS

"It is an undeniable fact that so-called 'natural' vitamins are not truly natural. Actually, they are made from coal tar (a 'natural' source) but are not extracted from foods as is widely believed. They are artificial and synthetic, regardless of what certain vitamin manufacturers claim.

"Because so-called "natural" vitamins and minerals are synthetic chemicals rather than nutrients, they are biologically inactive or "dead." They can benefit you only if your body is capable of performing a little miracle, namely changing their molecular structure by complexing them with the essential absorption factors and nutrient carriers. If your body fails to do that, you will receive no benefit from the so-called 'natural' vitamins and minerals you take.

"Nutrition scientists believe that your body actually rejects, excretes and wastes as much as 90% or more of the vitamin and mineral supplements you take, receiving little or no health benefits from them!"

Now when a vitamin manufacturer tells the truth about the products of others you'd expect to get the truth about his product. Right? Well, I wouldn't tell you the truth in order to hook you on another commercial come on, would I now? I'm an honest Joe. I want you to buy my product, so I tell you the truth about your wasting money on your supplements. They're worthless—you're just feeding your bowels. Is that a way to waste your money?

What this vitamin company is advertising is a "historic breakthrough" with an exclusive formula that helps you absorb their vitamins.

Are their vitamins truly natural? Absolutely not. They're synthetic, too! But your body can absorb them. Is this a reason you should buy their vitamins? No! That's a better reason for NOT buying them. You're better off with the nonabsorbable vitamins, which go mostly into the kidneys and bowels.

Why should you be better off with vitamins and minerals that you don't absorb? Because, if you do absorb these vitamins, you'll be poisoning yourself, not nourishing yourself! Whether the supplements you take are derived from coal tar, petroleum stocks, fungal and bacterial fermentation, and putrefaction or from truly natural foods, you're not getting anything you can use! Only the vitamins contained in whole natural foods will not poison you.

That you can't use vitamin supplements, even if refined from natural sources, derives from one salutary fact: vitamins are proteins except for a very few. As such they are coenzymes that make the food you eat more available you. Nature puts her vitamins and enzymes within the context of a food package. Break down the package, according to the famed nutrition researcher, Roger Williams, and you destroy the teamwork (synergism) that nourishes you. Hence, even if the vitamins and minerals were, indeed, from natural sources, by their lonesome selves the body cannot use them! The body uses foods, not delusions!

Why not use ONLY whole foods? The only vitamins and minerals you're getting and using are from that source only regardless of what you believe—regardless of the bill of goods you've been sold by the slick propaganda from the manufacturers and peddlers.

If you eat anything other than the nutritious raw foods to which we are biologically adapted, you're cheating yourself. Of course, some of them may be grown on deficient soils but that's still the best bet you have! If they extracted vitamins from natural foods where do you think they'd get them from? Why, from the very same foods grown on deficient soils. Where else?

You destroy not only your body faculties but deny yourself vitamins and minerals a hundred times more by cooking your food, by making it partially or wholly indigestible with seasonings and condiments, by eating it with preservatives, synthetic vitamin/mineral additives, by eating it wrongly combined so that it is incompatible in digestive chemistry and befouls your digestion rather than nourishes you, by taking foods with oils (which coat foods and make them largely unavailable and indigestible), and by consuming alcoholic drinks, vinegars, etc.

Our truly natural foods eaten in a natural manner (raw) is the thin margin most of us survive on as well as we do. The true "miracle" is eating totally raw only the foods that you relish raw. This will supply your body with all the vitamins and minerals you will ever need.

Article #4: Resolving the Issue of Supplementation by Drs. Robert and Elizabeth McCarter

The best way to resolve the issue of the validity of supplementation of the diet with manmade supplements is to study the people who take them religiously. We see a constant parade of such people here at the ranch (the Bionomics Health Institute of Tucson). Almost every sick person who comes to us for help has been taking all manner of supplements for years, all the while watching their health fade away. Once they are taken off their drugs and supplements, detoxified and then taught how to live in a health-promoting manner, they are often amazed at how quickly their bodies respond; many coming to enjoy a state of health such as they have not known for 20, 30 or more years.

Just a few days ago a man and his wife stopped in to present us with a basket of freshly-picked peaches. They had arisen at five that morning and, along with another of our students, had driven to a peach orchard just outside of Tucson where they had picked the ripe fruit, luscious in its rich goodness. Their bodies were dripping with sweat from their labors but their faces were filled with joy as they gave us the fruit.

Why do we bring up this episode at this time? Because, by learning to live according to the laws of life these two remarkable people changed pain-wracked bodies into healthy bodies. For years pain was mirrored in their faces, now only joy. They are now living life as it should be lived—always in health. They have no need for pill or potion, for doctor or for surgeon. They are true Life Scientists relying for true nourishment on nature's food packages, many of which they grow themselves. They have learned well the secret of life.

When the dietary intake is correct according to human design, all of the organs will be properly and consistently nourished and perfectly capable of fulfilling their duties as required. However, the systemic mosaic of intertwining functions and structural activity can be disturbed, rendered less than fully effective, reduced perhaps by as much as one-half by an imbalance, by the presence of too much or too little of any one mineral or other nutrient because of the finely-tuned internal ecological relationships, the synergisms, and interdependencies, that exist among all.

Like a baseball team must have the pitcher, the catcher and all other players present and in tip-top physical and mental condition to become a winner, so must the human body have all of its required nutrients ready and available for action in the proper proportion, in the correct amounts and at the proper time if the individual is to be a winner in the arena of life.

Otto Carque was one of the first scientists to warn against creating any imbalance within the body; he pointed out that an imbalance of minerals, for example, can lead to obesity, asthma, rheumatism, and other serious disorders. Louis Kuhne, a Leipzig practitioner of great renown in his day, said it well, "Man is not a machine artificially put together by combining various pieces, like an automobile, but rather a living creature in the midst of a process of development." We are alive, not static; our bodies are constantly in a state of flux. Taking supplements can disrupt the flux by thrusting an unknown into the synergism, creating an imbalance which the body cannot tolerate.

It has not been determined to any exactness just how much of any one nutrient is required for maximum health, this undoubtedly being a variable from person to person and from time to time according to functional need as, for example, under great stress.

A momentary stress in and of itself can create a temporary imbalance recognized only by the monitoring agencies within the system itself.

The blood and lymph cannot be cleansed and made to flow through the 70,000 and more miles of channels throughout the body by the taking of any "magic" pill. Organs grossly deformed and malfunctioning cannot possibly be restored to health by therapeutic dosing.

One is a real student of health when he understands this one absolute of life: foods have been prepared for man, but only certain foods; man's natural food contains all that he requires to keep him living always in full health provided his lifestyle and environment are also conducive to health. Dr. Shelton reminds us that "nature ... is the author and ruler of all health and happiness, not the physician."

Many of the technological advances of science in this century are superb but, nevertheless and in spite of them, mankind would be best served by building up a store of vital funds through careful attention to his dietary needs, these being more than adequately furnished in the foods designed both to satisfy visual and palate pleasure as well as systemic need. We should look to field and forest and be content for there we will find nature's best. As Dr. Ralph Cinque has so well said, supplements are nutritional shadows, not the real thing.

The life-building forces of health are gentle, they are slow, but they are sure. They are gathered together and reinforced by a daily adherence to the principles of life, not by taking a daily recommended dose of any one isolated man-made nutrient or, indeed, by downing a bucketful of assorted supplements. If we would have abiding health through all of life, we must stop pill-popping. We must begin to live according to the principles which are sound, sure, and certain to give the desired results. Here lies the true elixir of life.

All supplementation is a "slap in the face to law and order," a crude attempt to treat and "cure" without removing the cause of the trouble in the first instance. Certainly, common sense negates the whole idea. Supplementation is a practice instituted and promoted by self-serving interests which foster the idea that man knows better than Nature what is needed for the maintenance of life. It is a bold-faced attempt to convince a gullible public that supplements are a simple way to prevent disease and heal hurts without making any attempt to discover and remove cause. In other words, it is a simple way for these self-serving interests to make a lot of money off of you!

Article #5: The Minerals of Life by Dr. Herbert M. Shelton

It seems quite clear that the vital importance of the organic salts of foods was established by men who were outside the regular folds. The older physiologists and physiological chemists gave no attention to them. In the tables of food analysis, they were regulated to the "ash" column and ignored.

At the present day, their importance is everywhere recognized. It is no longer thought that only the "nutritive values"—proteins, carbohydrates, fats—are important.

Animals fed on foods deprived of their salts (minerals) soon die. In the same manner, they die if, to these demineralized foods, are added inorganic salts in the same quantities and proportions as are found in the ashes of milk. The salts are not used except in the presence of vitamins.

Berg has pointed out that there does not exist one single complete analysis, either of the human organism or its excretions or of our foodstuffs. Not everything is known about the function of minerals in the body and of some of them almost nothing is known. Some, such as zinc and nickel, apparently serve functions similar to those of vitamins. Prof E. V. McVollum showed that animals deprived of manganese lose the maternal instinct, refuse to suckle their young, do not build a nest for them, and even eat their young. Their mammary glands do not develop properly, and they are unable to secrete proper milk for their young. Here are effects commonly attributed to vitamin deficiency.

This "ash" enters into the composition of every fluid and tissue in the plant and animal body and without even one of these minerals, life could not go on. They are of the utmost importance. They serve a number of purposes. They form an essential part of every tissue in the body and predominate in the harder structures such as bones, teeth, hair, nails, etc. The bones consist largely of calcium phosphate. They are the chief factors ill maintaining the normal alkalinity of the blood as well as its normal specific gravity. Salts are also abundant in the body's secretions, and a lack of them in the diet produces a lack of secretions. They are also used as detoxifying agents, by being combined with the acid waste from the cells. The wastes are thus neutralized and prepared for elimination. Their presence in the food eaten also aids in preventing it from decomposing. Acidosis produced by the fermentation of proteins and carbohydrates often comes because the mineral salts have been taken from the food, thus favoring fermentation.

In a simplified sense we may consider the blood and lymph as liquids in which solids are held in solution—much as salt is dissolved in water. The cells, which are bathed at all times in lymph, are also semi-fluid with dissolved matter in them. If the lymph outside the cells contain much dissolved solid, as compared to that within the cells, the cells shrink in size. If there is more dissolved solid within the cell than without, the cell expands and sometimes bursts. In either case the result is pathological.

If the amount of dissolved solids within and without the cell are equal, so that internal and external pressure are equalized, the cell remains normal. It falls very largely to the minerals of the food to maintain this state of osmotic equilibrium.

The waste formed in the body, due to its normal activities, is acid in reaction. The greater part of the work of neutralizing these acids is done by the mineral elements—the "ash."

These minerals enter into the composition of the secretions of the body. The hydrochloric acid in the gastric juice, for example, contains chlorine. Clotting of the blood does not take place without the aid of calcium or lime.

The mineral matters in food undergo no change in the process of digestion, prior to absorption, as do proteins, fats, and carbohydrates. They are separated from these other elements in the process of digestion and pass directly into the blood.

If our foods do not contain enough of the right kinds of mineral salts we simply starve to death. It does not matter how much "good nourishing food," as this is commonly understood, that we consume; if these salts are not present in sufficient quantities, we suffer from slow starvation with glandular imbalance or disfunction, more disease and other evidences of decay. McCarrison showed, definitely, that foods and combinations of foods that are inadequate and unsatisfactory in feeding animals are equally as inadequate and unsatisfactory in feeding man.

Life and health are so directly related to these salts, of which little enough is known, that we can never have satisfactory health without an adequate supply of them. We may be sure that each salt has its own separate function to serve, while certain combinations of them have long been known to serve vital services in the body.

No drug salts can be made to take the place of those found in food, As Dr. William

H. Hay, says: "Nature provides all her chemicals for restoration of the body in the form of colloids, organic forms, and man has for a long time sought to imitate her in this, but he has not been so very successful that we are now able to insure the recouping of the mineral losses of the body by any artificial means, arid must still depend on nature's colloids as found in plant and fruit." Well or sick, no compound of the chemist, druggist or "biochemist" can recoup your mineral losses.

Lesson 87:

Chiropractic, Homeopathy, and Osteopathy

87.1. Chiropractic

87.1.1. History

87.1.2. Chiropractic Philosophy

87.1.3. Determine the True Cause

87.1.4. Subluxation

87.1.1. History

In 1877, a man by the name of Harvey Lillard became deaf. He was in a stooped, cramped position, he heard something "pop" in his neck, and he was deaf for 18 years. One day in 1895, Dr. D. D. Palmer was called to examine Mr. Lillard. Upon examining the patient, he noticed a large visible bump. He reasoned that if the production of that bump produced deafness, reduction should restore hearing. He pushed the bump, three days in succession, the bump disappeared, and hearing was restored.

The more Dr. Palmer examined spines, the more he continued to find abnormal bumps. Some bumps were found on spines of people who were deaf, but most were found on spines of people with other illnesses. When he reduced these bumps, some illnesses, such as heart trouble, stomach trouble, etc., were relieved. Dr. D. D. Palmer believed that spinal bumps were caused by malposition's of vertebrae, called subluxations. It was believed that the subluxated vertebra occluded the neurocanal, or intervertebral foramen, and impinged on the spinal cord or spinal nerves. Since the nervous system controlled all systems, it was believed that any interference in the nerve impulse was the cause of disease.

Disease originally meant "uneasy, uncomfortable or disturbed." As medical men began to classify these feelings into symptoms called an illness, disease became an entity,

B. J. Palmer (Danial Palmer's son) liked the term disease. Dis-ease was used to mean "disorganized, or without organization," and Palmer believed that the cause had to be removed or corrected (adjusted). Chiropractic is defined by B. J. Palmer as follows: "Chiropractic is a philosophy, science and art of things natural; a system of adjusting the segments of the spinal column by hand only, for the correction of the cause of disease."

87.1.2. Chiropractic Philosophy

All parts of your body must work together properly to give you physical health. According to Chiropractic philosophy, the common denominator of life or health is proper transmission of nerve energy and the most damaging interference factors where nerve flow affects systems of organization must be corrected.

The primary system of organization is the nervous system. Our whole nervous system was developed to maintain our lives and make activity satisfyingly purposeful. Chiropractors reason that if we accept the premise that the nervous system causes organization, they draw a conclusion: any interference in the nervous system causes disorganization. They reason that any factor which abnormally adds or subtracts impulses to or from the nervous system acts as an interference and causes disorganization. Since the nervous system is so important to the survival of the human organism, they assume that the wisdom of adaptation provides good protection for it. To protect the most sensitive tissues (nerves), the hardest tissue of the body is used (bone).

87.1.3. Determine the True Cause

Chiropractic treatment is intended to eliminate the cause of a disorder. Upon correction, healing becomes easy. However, chiropractors take a rather narrow view of cause and effect. It is true that there are special cases where adjustments are necessary following injury or trauma. If nerves are being impinged upon due to abnormal pressures on the spinal column, chiropractic adjustments may be helpful.

Since disease is the result of an accumulation of toxins, chiropractic adjustments may bring temporary relief, but the underlying causes have not been corrected. If illness is caused by unhealthful living practices, then these habits must be corrected, and a more healthful lifestyle must be implemented. A straight spine will not produce health if you are eating junk food, smoking cigarettes, not getting enough rest and sleep, and doing other things that are wrong.

In some cases, Chiropractic treatment may be helpful, but such therapy will only result in health if all the conditions for health are provided simultaneously.

87.1.4. Subluxation

A subluxation is the condition of a vertebra that has lost its proper position with the one above or the one below or both. The chiropractor holds that a subluxation is the major nonpathological interference factor found in an unhealthy host that can be corrected by nonsurgical, nonmedical techniques, and is the most common cause of disorganization in the human body.

A rapidly increasing tendency on the part of the Chiropractic research and therapy is to seek the cause of disease in the spinal column and to correct that cause by correcting nerve interference. The spinal column, according to the chiropractor, is being recognized as the seat of more abnormalities than any other part of the body structure, and is being held accountable for an increasing number of manifestations of disease.

Dr. Andrew T. Still founded Osteopathy in 1874 based on the principle that disturbances of the musculoskeletal system may lead to disease and that the treatment of this problem should be manipulation. D. D. Palmer insisted that Chiropractic was different because the manipulation of the chiropractic method was a direct, specific thrust on the processes of the vertebrae for the purpose of correcting nerve interference.

Darald E. Bolin, D.C. states, "Neuromusculoskeletal conditions can be considered those disorders arising from the structural and/or functional alterations of the musculoskeletal connective tissues and their attendant neurological complications." The condition of a subluxation, he says, is a neuromusculoskeletal condition in itself. Strains or sprains almost always occur in the spinal column at the subluxations. He maintains that if the subluxation is preventing the natural healing of diseased conditions, the treatment of the subluxation is called for.

Chiropractic principle and practice is to adjust, to open occlusion, to release pressure, to restore normal quantity flow between brain and body, that innate intelligence can, does and will rebuild normal rhythmic energy wave flow to re-establish its normal rate of function, sensibility and cell activity, thus restoring a healthy level.

87.2. Homeopathy

87.2.1. History

87.2.2. A Little Poison Is Better Than a Lot

87.2.3. Similia Similibus Curentur

87.2.4. Requisites of Life Recognized

87.2.5. Vital Force

87.2.6. Nontherapy Is Best

87.2.1. History

In 1844, the first American Institute of Homeopathy was established. Homeopaths were much more popular than any other sect of the day during the epidemics of yellow fever and Asiatic cholera. Their practically drugless methods left the body comparatively unhampered in its healing efforts, while the drugging methods of the regular practitioners were destructive to health. Some other reasons for its wide popularity are that it attracted members of orthodox physicians, it appealed to middle and upper classes, and it offered a rationale for their practice—it was not purely empirical as were Thomsonian or Eclectic sects which preceded Homeopathy. In 1857, Homeopathy received strong public support, including that of Horace Greeley, editor of the New York Tribune.

Homeopathy was founded by Dr. Samuel C. F. Hahnemann. He stated that, if a physician is aware of the obstacles to recovery and how to remove them, then he understands how to treat judiciously, and is a true practitioner of the healing art. "He has become a preserver of health by knowing those things that derange health and cause disease; he knows how to keep a person in health."

Hahnemann always advocated prescribing the smallest possible dose necessary to help the patient. After the first dilution, one drop of a plant was diluted to 1/100 of its original strength; after the second, to 1/10,000 of its original strength; after the third to 1/100,000 of its original strength. This constituted the third dilution. Hahnemann recommended the thirtieth dilution.

He evolved a method of mixing, dilution and shaking which he called succession.

The result of this was a preparation which, because of its powers, he named potency.

The resulting medicine could be administered in either of two ways, according to Hahnemann. A globule of sugar the size of a mustard seed could be moistened with the thirtieth dilution of the liquid and taken internally. Or, where the patient was "very weak and irritable, one smelling of it is safer and more serviceable than when it is taken in substance."

87.2.2. A Little Poison Is Better Than a Lot

It was found that the greater the degree of dilution, the more effective the medicine. And although chemical analysis revealed hardly a trace of the original drug in the suspension, the preparation was found to produce a "symptom picture" corresponding to the proving made on a healthy subject.

This is a very crucial point for it really demonstrates that the most powerful healing agent which exists is that resident within the human body. The higher the dilution, the more unhampered is the body in its restorative efforts, hence the "cure" is the most effective. Thus, homeopathy is a happy delusion. The value of Hahnemann's practically drugless therapy is demonstrated in the successes that he achieved which were far greater than any of the other medical sects of his day.

87.2.3. Similia Similibus Curentur

The basis of Homeopathy is the most successful drug for administering to the ill is that very drug which produces the same symptoms in someone who is well. Thus the similium, the most resembling drug, should be given—"Like should be treated by like."

Hahnemann found that he was sensitive to quinine. He found that after taking a dose of quinine he was soon suffering from the symptoms of an illness similar to those he had frequently seen as a medical student in the marshlands of lower Hungary. In short, except for the fever, he was experiencing the symptoms of malaria. It then occurred to him that if this drug could produce symptoms similar to those of malaria, it then, might be the "cure" for malaria. It is then that he first applied the words to his theory, similia similibus curentur—like will be cured by like.

What Hahnemann was experiencing was a normal reaction of the body in eliminating poisons, be they quinine or others, but he misinterpreted these symptoms.

87.2.4. Requisites of Life Recognized

Hahnemann accepted the medically valid therapies of his time. He recommended the use of fresh air, bed rest, proper diet, sunshine, public hygiene, and numerous other beneficial measures at a time when many other physicians considered them of no value.

Hahnemann did not attribute his success to the real drug lessness of his therapy, but to his homeopathic doses. But there is no doubt that the "cures" which came about were due to the body's intrinsic power to heal itself which were assisted by the above recommendations of fresh air, bed rest, proper diet, etc. Also, the body was not interfered with in its healing process by large doses of drugs, blistering, blood-letting, etc., which were then used by the regular physicians.

87.2.5. Vital Force

But Hahnemann recognized that in the body there is a self-preserving, self-balancing mechanism that kept it in health in spite of the stress and strain to which man is subject. He used the term "vital force" to describe the balancing mechanism in every living body which promotes, or at, least maintains, health. He wrote that this "vital force" was stimulated by internal and external disorders to build up a reaction to counteract the disorders. The result of them interaction between the "vital force" and the conditions which set it in motion produced various symptoms in the body revealing that an imbalance has occurred, according to his theory.

We know that this vital force is the only true remedial agent that we possess and that the body will heal and repair when the conditions for health are provided.

87.2.6. Nontherapy Is Best

Hahnemann expected that regular physicians would not greet his system enthusiastically. He called them the "allopathic" schools because they used remedies whose action was opposed to the symptoms caused by the illness and described their practice by the maxim contraria contraris.

Hahnemann, despite the absurdity of his belief, really made one of the great discoveries of his time: he established that, given the existing state of medical knowledge, the absence of therapy was vastly superior to "heroic" therapy. The regular physicians' two basic objections to homeopathy was (1) that the doses prescribed by homeopaths were too small to have any physiological effect whatsoever; and (2) that the cures which homeopaths attributed to their drugs were actually brought about by the "recuperative effects of nature." Both of these statements were very true, and this is why Homeopathy was so successful. Regular physicians did admit that Homeopathy had produced a surprisingly large number of successes. In 1861, Dr. Oliver Wendell Holmes said, "Homeopathy has taught us a lesson of the healing faculty of Nature which was needed."

The homeopaths attacked the regular physicians' use of blood-letting, calomel, blisters, poisons, and the rest of "heroic" medicine as invalid, based on fallacies and speculative reasoning, and unsuccessful in treating illnesses. The regular physicians accused the homeopaths of chicanery in administering drugs which could have no possible therapeutic effects of any kind. From the point of view of the patient's well-being, it is easy to observe which was the superior system.

Homeopathy is still very popular today and widely practiced. However, we may conclude that if heavy use of drugs results in more illness and minute portions of drugs result in less illness, then no drugs at all result in health! It is thus demonstrated that nature is the most effective agent in the restoration of health.

87.3. Osteopathy

87.3.1. History

87.3.2. Modern Osteopathic Practice

87.3.1. History

Andrew Taylor Still, founder of Osteopathy, was born August 6, 1828. Dr. Still founded the first school of Osteopathy in the United States in 1874 and had apparently been developing ideas about the relation of certain diseases to disturbances of the vertebral column at least as far back as 1860.

Probably the first incident in the life of Dr. Still that had any bearing upon Osteopathy, was recorded on pages 31 and 32 of his autobiography.

"One day, when about ten years old, I suffered from a headache, I made a swing of my father's plow line between two trees; but my head hurt too much to make swinging comfortable, so I let the rope down to about eight or ten inches off the ground and stretched on my back with my neck across the rope. Soon I became easy and went to sleep, got up in a little while with the headache all gone. As I knew nothing of anatomy, I took no thought of how a rope could stop headache and the sick stomach which accompanied it. After that discovery I roped my neck whenever I felt those spells coming on. I followed that treatment for twenty years before the wedge of reason reached my brain, and I could see that I had suspended the action of the great occipital nerves and given harmony to the flow of the arterial blood to and through the veins, and ease was the effect, as the reader can see."

The power of nature (the body's intrinsic forces) began to be revealed to him and he devised a means by which nature would be permitted to exert her inherent powers. He considered nature as his laboratory. He said,

"I, who had had some experience in alleviating pain, found medicines a failure. Since early life I had been a student of nature's books. In my early days in windswept Kansas, I had devoted my attention to the study of anatomy."

The practice of allopathy had convinced him that the drug theory was radically wrong, and from his own researches he thought he saw the dawn of a better system. He determined to get closer to nature and learn from her the exact truth.

The first conclusion which he made was that an "all-wise Creator" was the designer of our bodies as well as the author of our spirits, and that the human body is, therefore, a perfect machine.

The second conclusion was the fundamental idea of the importance of the arteries and other tubular structures through which the nutritive elements are carried to their destination and the waste materials of the body are carried away to be expelled.

The third conclusion was that of the influence of the nerves and the part it plays, especially in the control of the fluids of the body.

"This year (1874) I began a more extended study of the drive-wheels, pinions, cups, arms, and shafts of life, with their forces and supplies, framework, attachments by ligaments, muscles, origin, and insertion. Nerves, origin and supplies, blood supply to and from the heart, and how and where the motor-nerves received their power and motion; how the sensory nerves acted in their function, their duties, the source of supplies and the work being done in health, in the obstructing parts, to perform their part of the functions of life; all awoke a new interest in me.

I believed that something abnormal could be found some place in some of the nerve divisions, which would tolerate a temporary or permanent suspension of the blood either in arteries or veins, which effect caused disease."

In the early years, Osteopathic practice consisted of (1) a physical examination to determine the condition of the mechanisms and function of all parts of the human body;

(2) a specific manipulation to restore the normal mechanism and re-establish the normal functions; and (3) the adoption of all hygienic measures conducive to the restoration and maintenance of health.

This method of practice laid stress upon correct diagnosis based upon a physical examination; removal of the supposed causes of disease through manipulation; and, as an important sequel, wholesome living. The Osteopaths differed markedly from the allopath's of their day by not prescribing drugs. They advocated removing causes of disease rather than treating symptoms. The early osteopaths reasoned that if a part is not doing its duty there must be a cause for it. They said that the cause may be a foreign substance, or a malposition, interfering with the free flow of fluids or the transmission of nerve force, interfering first with function and second with structure. The osteopath then proceeded at once to remove the supposed cause of the trouble, and in doing that set free all the forces of the body involved in combatting disease and maintaining health. The early osteopaths did not use germicides or antibiotics to kill germs on the theory that germs do not thrive in live tissue, and that every organ within the body as well as all other parts are supplied with nerves that are necessary to keep them alive. Surround the affected area with healthy tissue and the bacteria will soon die for want of suitable nourishment.

Internal cleanliness was said to be essential, but impossible without a perfect distribution of nerve force, nutritious blood, a free circulation of all the fluids of the body, and unimpeded excretion. These are the lines along which osteopaths had proven themselves to be knowledgeable.

87.3.2. Modern Osteopathic Practice

The osteopath of the present day still relies mainly on manipulative treatment for most diseases, but also dispenses drugs and utilizes all the other therapies of the medical physicians, such as surgery, X rays, etc. Still's emphasis on treating the whole person, however, has remained an ideal of the profession.

There are now 15,000 doctors of Osteopathy in the United States and others who receive their education here are now located in other countries. The profession maintains nearly 300 hospitals with a total of more than 20,000 beds.

Modern osteopathic medicine is a system of medical practice that emphasizes the importance of the muscles and bones of the body and their connecting tendons and ligaments. Osteopathy maintains that the musculoskeletal system, which makes up 60 percent of the body, has important interrelationships with all other body systems. Despite this, present-day osteopathic physicians use all the medical, surgical, immunological, pharmacological, psychological, and other harmful procedures of modern medicine that we, as Natural Hygienists, condemn as destructive of health.

Osteopathic physicians hold that a disturbance in the musculoskeletal system can lead to three main conditions. (1) It can produce symptoms that occur only in the musculoskeletal system itself. (2) It can cause symptoms resembling those diseases that affect other body systems. (3) It can affect the functioning of other body systems connected to the musculoskeletal systems through nerves and the action of hormones.

Osteopathic physicians are specially trained in the detection and treatment of musculoskeletal disturbances, and they use massages and other types of osteopathic manipulation to treat those disturbances.

In removing these supposed immediate causes, the real underlying causes are neglected. Therefore, health cannot be achieved. The massage and osteopathic manipulations increase the flow of blood and lymph and thereby may help initiate healing, but the wrong-doing that resulted in the disturbances in the first place must be discontinued before true health can be realized.

87.4. Naturopathy

87.4.1. History

87.4.2. Present-Day Naturopaths

87.4.3. Naturopathic Views on Health and Disease

87.4.4. Germ Theory Denied

87.4.5. A Healthful Lifestyle Advocated

87.4.6. Bach's Flower Remedies and Schuessler Cell Salts

87.4.1. History

As pointed out by Dr. J. M. Jassawalla, Naturopathy is not the invention of any one human mind. It does not place its origin at any given date but is the accumulation of knowledge and practices pertaining to the natural methods of living and healing throughout the centuries.

The history of "Nature Cure" is as old as the origin of man. All living beings know and practice "Nature Cure" by instinct. A sick dog will automatically fast; cats and many other animals know the importance of a sun bath. Among aboriginal races there were very few diseases in comparison with the diseases found in civilized societies.

Through his work on the subject of diet, Dr. Tilden (in conjunction with such dietetic pioneers as Otto Carque, Dr. Kellogg, Dr. Lindlahr, Bernarr MacFadden and Alfred McCann) considered wrong feeding to be one of the main causes of disease and wrote several books and pamphlets that are still very relevant today.

Dr. Henry Lindlahr was the first Naturopathic physician to combine in his practice various drugless methods in a systematic and scientific way. Now the school of "Nature Cure" covers not only the original basic philosophy and practice, but also includes other drugless therapies.

The first major development in Naturopathy came in the early nineteenth century in Europe with the pioneering work in hydrotherapy by Vincent Priessnitz and Father Sebastian Kneipp. Father Kneipp, a Bavarian who also went in for walking barefoot through the grass, is said to have cured many difficult cases by having patients bathe in fresh, cool "living water." Ideally, this was water in fast-flowing streams that had been irradiated by the sun. It was said that this water absorbed "curative solar energy." His water cures are still given in Woerishofen, Bavaria.

Then there was Louis Kuhne who advocated sun, steam baths, a vegetarian diet, and whole wheat bread. Heinrich Lahmann came along to stress no salt on foods and no water with meals, while Antonine Bechamp proposed the novel theory that it was disease conditions that occasioned bacterial presence and not the other way around. Dr. Benedict Lust called his health program "Nature's Path." In addition to being a naturopath he was also an M.D. and an osteopath. In the early 1900s he established health resorts and battled "the drug trusts." Some considered him the father of American Naturopathy.

One of the first American naturopaths was Dr. John H. Kellogg, a Seventh-Day Adventist. Adventists are a Protestant fundamentalist sect whose members follow a strict vegetarian diet. They adjure not only meat, but all stimulants, including liquor, wine, coffee, tea, and tobacco. In 1866, the Adventists founded the Health Reform Institute in

Battle Creek, Michigan. Ten years later, Kellogg reorganized the Institute into what was known as the Battle Creek Sanitorium.

Through the years the Adventists, who operate a number of hospitals and health institutions, have been in the forefront of nutritional research, particularly in the area of vegetarianism.

Henry Lindlahr is remembered for his convictions that disease did not represent an invasion of molecules, but the, body's way of healing something. In other words, he viewed symptoms as a positive physiological response—proof that the body is correcting whatever is wrong. Accordingly, a fever is a "healthy" sign, and one should let it be. The next naturopath after Kellogg was Bernarr MacFadden, the physical culturist who built a magazine-publishing empire. (His first magazine was Physical Culture founded in 1898.) He advocated exercise and fresh vegetables.

87.4.2. Present-Day Naturopaths

Today, naturopaths are licensed in seventeen states to diagnose, treat, and prescribe for any human ailment through the use of air, light, heat, herbs, nutrition, electrotherapy, physiotherapy, manipulations, and minor surgery. At present, one can earn a D.N. degree at the National College of Naturopathic Medicine in Seattle and Emporia, Kansas, or the new North American Naturopathic Institute in North Arlington, New Jersey. (There is also a school in Montreal, Canada.) The four-year curriculum covers many standard medical courses—anatomy, bacteriology, urology, pathology, physiology, x-ray reading, etc., but also includes botanical medicine, hydrotherapy, electrotherapy, and manipulative technique.

The basic philosophy of naturopaths and Natural Hygienists/Life Scientists are very similar but differ in that Natural Hygiene offers no cures or therapies. Life Science teaches that only the body can heal and does not endorse the use of herbs, manipulations, surgeries, or other therapies advocated by many naturopaths.

But Naturopathy also holds that the organism will heal itself, regardless of ailment, if given a chance to purge itself of the toxic materials that are the basis of the ailment. This is done by a detoxifying fast and correct life practices after that.

87.4.3. Naturopathic Views on Health and Disease

Naturopathic treatment aims at eliminating the symptom's, regardless of their diverse appearance, by total cleansing of the body from the inside out. All the different expressions of the body's efforts to expel uneliminated wastes or toxic materials, called symptoms, are encouraged, and utilized by Naturopathy. Diarrhea is seen as "nature's enemas," and enemas are considered an important part of body cleansing. This is another variance with Life Science philosophy. We do not advocate the use of enemas because they are enervating and usually result in weakening of the muscle wall of the colon due to stretched and detached musculature.

Sneezing and coughing are reflex reactions by the body to foreign materials or irritation, and are regarded as inconvenient but desirable. A runny nose or a rash is a sign that the body is ridding itself of waste. Since Naturopathy allows all of these symptoms to run, their course, it is not as comfortable at first as medical treatments which occasion immediate relief. Nature's course', however, is thoroughgoing and permanent if causes are discontinued.

According to naturopathic philosophy, the body is not an opponent to be battled against with drugs, but is an intelligent, immeasurably complex living system that will eek its own best good automatically. Given the conditions, your body will automatically heal itself. This is a fundamental of nature-cure. All naturopathic treatments are said to be designed to help the body, to give it the chance to heal itself. However, electrotherapy, hydrotherapy, manipulations, etc., are not natural and interfere with, rather than promote, healing.

Naturopaths hold that the healing power of nature is behind all cures, whether with the aid of natural therapies or in spite of medical ones. Your body will heal itself; again, this is the first rule of nature-cure.

Another principle of nature-cure, according to naturopath, Dr. Andrew W. Saul, is that all disease, all sickness, all illnesses are differing expressions of one root cause of disease which is termed systemic toxemia. (This is in line with Life Science doctrine.)

Systemic toxemia, according to Dr. Saul, means a "polluted body." The underlying factor, the common origin of sickness, is a body filled with wastes, chemicals, and poisons. Such a toxic body may express its plight as this disease or that illness, each with its particular set of symptoms according to the body's predilection. These are desperate measures on the part of the organism to throw off the accumulated wastes and toxins, or to cope with its impairing conditions. Toxic conditions result from wrong living, meaning eating wring foods or taking medicinal drugs and chemicals among other things. Over a period of time, often many years, the body's strength is sapped, and its natural defenses weakened such at it no longer seems capable of healing itself. The last thing that the organism needs is more pollutants and chemicals added to its toxic burden when it's attempting to cleanse itself. Naturopaths assert they assist the body in its cleansing and rebuilding work with rest, baths, mineral and vitamin therapy, and whole, unprocessed foods. A complete fast is used first to give the body the condition to clean house totally. Life Science agrees with the value of fasting, rest, and proper diet. However, vitamin and mineral therapy have a drug effect and therefore are deplored.

87.4.4. Germ Theory Denied

Naturopaths see germs as scavengers assisting in cleaning up wastes. With this in mind, they have confidence that nature heals and that the body will cleanse itself of the cause of illness. If your body is clean and healthy, they say, germs are irrelevant for "susceptibility" does not exist. Germs are not considered causes of disease.

Naturopathic treatment offers the following approach: first build health, and illness will automatically decrease. To let the body cleanse itself is to let the body cure itself. Dr. Andrew Saul defines Naturopathy as "a system of therapy in which the patient is treated without the use of medical remedies of any sort, but with correct dieting, exercises, baths, fasting, manipulations, etc." Dr. Saul states that the first and most fundamental principle of Nature Cure (Naturopathy) is that all forms of disease are due to the same cause, namely the accumulation in the system of uneliminated body wastes and toxic ingesta. The second principle of Nature Cure, he says, is that the body is always striving for its good no matter how ill-treated; and that all acute diseases are nothing more than self-initiated attempts on the part of the body to throw off the accumulations of impairing substances which interfere with its proper functioning; and that all chronic diseases are really the results of continued causes and suppression of acute diseases by devitalizing drugging and therapies.

The third principle of Nature Cure, according to Dr. Saul, is that the body contains within itself the power to bring about a return to a normal condition of well-being known as health, providing the right methods are employed to enable it to do so.

British naturopath Harry Benjamin, N.D. writes:

"Germs take part in all disease phenomena because these are processes requiring the breaking down or disintegration of accumulated refuse and toxic matter within the body which the system is endeavoring to throw off. But to assume, as our medical scientists do, that merely because the germs are present and active in all the decomposition processes connected with all dead organic matter, they are the cause of the death of the organic matter, is in question. Germs are part of the results of the disease, not its cause."

87.4.5. A Healthful Lifestyle Advocated

The view of naturopaths throughout the world is that we are the product of our dietary and lifestyle, that our ailments have basic causes, and that the way to eliminate disease is to establish the conditions of health. Fundamental causation of illness cannot be blamed on germs, bacteria, the weather, or even unsatisfactory medical treatment. We must look to ourselves for the reason—therein lie the causes of illness. We must look to ourselves for the answer to the problem.

Hunza people eat largely natural foods and are healthy. We eat largely unnatural foods and are not.

Naturopathy holds that a natural whole foods diet is of the highest importance in the maintenance and improvement of health, and that a scientifically-prescribed diet is of the proven method to cure disease. The scope of Naturopathy includes the total investigation and utilization of all Nature's vitamins and materials to promote health. They say that if your nutrition and lifestyle are truly natural, then illness will not be a part of your life. Sickness does not occur in a healthy body.

87.4.6. Bach's Flower Remedies and Schuessler Cell Salts

Bach's flower remedies are used by some naturopaths. Dr. Edward Bach was an English medical doctor and bacteriologist who left his practice to devote himself to studying the supposed healing properties of flowers. He claimed that flowers contain energies, which, when suitably prepared, appeared to heal an individual's disease on the level of the individual's temperament, attitude, and disposition. Dr. Bach was convinced that all disease ultimately stems from a person's wrong states of mind. If someone is chronically unhappy, or always worried, or constantly afraid, etc., then these states give rise to physical illness. According to Dr. Bach, by using a dilute flower extract, the person's temperament or attitude is healed, and therefore healing of the body follows.

There are 38 flower remedies, each prepared by floating the blossoms in spring water while exposed to sunlight for a few hours. The resulting solution is then extracted with alcohol and bottled. The extract is diluted again with pure water for use, and a few drops taken in a glass of water. The remedy is also taken dropped on the tongue or lips. This is reminiscent of homeopathic practices in many aspects.

Schuessler cell salts are also administered by some naturopaths. Twelve cell salts were recognized and categorized by a German biochemist, Dr. William H. Schuessler in 1873. He found that there are certain essential minerals that the body requires, in proper balance, in all of its cells. An imbalance or a lack of any of these minerals may lead to disease in the tissues so lacking. Providing the missing minerals to the tissues corrects that imbalance, it is said, to eliminate the illness.

Most Schuessler cell salts are in a homeopathic potency, which uses minute quantities of a substance. Schuessler remedies are commonly in a "6x" homeopathic potency.

The twelve Schuessler cell salts are as follows: Calcium Fluoride, Calcium Phosphate, Calcium Sulphate, Ferrum Phosphate, Potassium Chloride, Potassium Phosphate, Potassium Sulphate, Magnesium Phosphate, Sodium Chloride, Sodium Phosphate, Sodium Sulphate, and Silica.

Both the "flower remedies" and "cell salts" are only "valuable" in that they do relatively little harm when taken in such small homeopathic doses and they may give the patient a psychological "lift." They cannot, however, have any power to heal. Their only potential is harm for they do not attempt to remove causes—they fail to recognize real causes. Further, inorganic minerals are toxic in themselves.

87.5. Illusion and Disillusion

Many of the methods of treatment which were often advocated by physicians during the19th century and before are today considered useless, and, in fact, life-threatening. But the physicians during that time persisted in such practices as bleeding, blistering, purging and the use of heavy metals because they witnessed patients "recover" following such treatment. This, however, was an illusion. If the patient recovered at all, it was in spite of the treatment and certainly not because of it. Many people did die because of their treatment, but physicians did not recognize that the treatment itself was the direct cause of these deaths, attributing that to the disease. However, doubters soon began sounding objections, and the theories of the regular school began to crumble. Physicians fell victim to their delusion. Learned men of science and respected people in the community were practicing under the illusion that such "heroic" treatment would cure. Out of this illusion came disillusion to many, and thus there were cries of objection and new healing sects sprang up out of desperation.

The urge to make new discoveries along with preconceived ideas and autosuggestion, together with the desire to break new ground, drives men to make certain conclusions from observations which are deceiving. An example of such deceiving observations may lie in the supposed "healing power" of the homeopath's drugs, or the neuropath's Schuessler salts, or the manipulations of the osteopaths and chiropractors. General good reason tells us that there is no magic power in any homeopathic drug that could cure arthritis, or eliminate kidney stones, or heal a wound. We know that only our own body can do this by the methods described in earlier lessons. If we observe an individual being restored to health after a manipulative treatment, we must not be so quick to accept this illusion. One must investigate further into the history of the illness and the mode of treatment, and the conditions favoring restoration. If the patient was first taken off of medical drugs, placed on a better diet, and provided other requirements for health, and then given a treatment or cell salts, we must not immediately credit the treatment or cell salts for the cure. The fact that the homeopathic cell salts were far less harmful than the previous drugs that were taken and the fact that the conditions for healing were provided, gives the body an opportunity to heal itself. Keeping this in mind, the illusion becomes obvious.

Harm comes when people become so convinced of these illusions that a more rational approach is not sought. You must, therefore, strive to become independent thinkers. You must begin to question "cures" that do not sound reasonable to you and then seek the truth by seeing things from the rational perspective of Life Science.

If a certain drug is found by the medical community to be harmful and is taken off the market, you are told that you should not doubt the effectiveness of all of these agents. However, you should not allow yourselves to be deceived by them. You may feel better for a while after taking one of these symptom-suppressing agents, but your so-called "cure" is a deception. Your "cure" will not last. You must be alert to these deceptions and illusions.

Re-education is the key for recognizing misleading illusions. By constantly seeking the truth we will be led to the true cause of disease, and from this we may know how to maintain health.

Any violation of biological law, that is, physiological law, always results in impaired health. This would include any violation against sleep requirements, proper foods, air, water, sunshine, exercise, etc. The body's ability to adapt is remarkable, but health is a delusion when you attempt to produce it by drugs. Under such circumstances, the body will inevitably become exhausted and chronic illnesses will ensue.

Human conduct is affected by environmental factors which may be psychological or social as well as biological factors. Many types of mental deficiencies are considered congenital. Although such diathesis may be inherited, they will not necessarily develop, providing all the conditions for health—both physical and mental—are provided to the child.

The child's physical and mental health tendencies are implanted in his genes at the moment of conception. During the next nine months, the child's environment consists of the mother's womb. Here, the child may be affected by different influences, and it is imperative that the health and living habits of the mother be correct. We should not fool ourselves into believing that nothing can be done about hereditary traits because something can be done. But it must begin before conception and involve healthful living practices of both parents.

Alcoholism, drugs, X rays, wrong foods, etc., affect the fetus. It would be an error to dismiss any of these factors in the role of mental and physical health. You must not allow the delusion of these agents to affect your decision to utilize them, especially when the health of a future human being depends on your decision.

It is very easy to be deceived today concerning our health and well-being. The public media is flooded with advertising campaigns which involve a host of health-robbing agents. This would include coffee, alcohol, cigarettes, and "junk foods."

Our weapon against this misleading information is education so that we may learn the truth; so that we may eschew those things which destroy our health. Your health is your most valuable asset. In the world today, health is a commodity which requires a conscious effort to keep, but superior health is well within the grasp of every living being as long as they obey the "Laws of Life."

87.6. Questions & Answers

How can I eliminate my backache if I do not receive chiropractic adjustments?

In most cases, pain in the back is due to toxic accumulations. The most rational mode of action would be to fast, thus freeing the energies needed for detoxification, and then go on a normal Hygienic diet. When you feel better, begin a good exercise program and your back will mend.

Why do some naturopaths employ the use of herbs, electrotherapy, physiotherapy, manipulations, vitamins, minerals, etc.?

Many naturopaths are looking for "cures" to sell just as are the medical doctors. They do not fully realize that the so-called "disease" is the cure, and it is the body's way of eliminating toxins and initiating healing. If left alone, the disease will terminate itself.

How do you explain the success of the homeopaths and their popularity today?

The homeopaths prescribe drugs in such minute doses that the body can eliminate these poisons much easier than those prescribed in the regular large doses of the medical doctor. Therefore, the body is relatively unhampered in its healing efforts. So, it is still the body that heals and effects the "cure"—not any drug. The homeopaths would be even more successful if they prescribed no drugs at all and addressed themselves to removal of causes.

Is Osteopathy similar to that of regular medical practice?

Present-day osteopathic practices are similar to regular medical practices. Osteopaths prescribe drugs and all the other therapies used by the dominant school of medicine. The major difference is that the osteopath also uses manipulative therapy and the medical practitioners do not.

Article #1: What Is Naturopathy? by Dr. Herbert M. Shelton

Will the wonders never cease? Will the inventive ingenuity of the therapeutic dabblers never run out? Will the naturopaths ever "return to nature" and cease running after false gods?

Recently a four-page circular was deposited in our box at the Post Office. It was sent to us by the leading lay Naturopathic journal in the U.S. The first page is an ad for the magazine. The fourth page carries an ad of two Chiropractors in Missouri who say: "Natural methods approved by leading drugless doctors throughout the world are used in this office."

It is no secret to the readers of this magazine that chiropractors no longer believe in Chiropractic and are employing everything under the sun that any of the other schools of miscalled "healing" are employing. There are probably not more than three Chiropractic schools left in the world, although there are several that still call themselves schools or colleges of Chiropractic. Every "Chiropractic" magazine that comes to our desk is devoted more to physiotherapy, endocrine therapy, and "diet" than to Chiropractic.

It is unfortunate that when chiropractors abandoned Chiropractic they did not go forward to something better instead of following popular commercial trends into something worse.

But I did not set out to write this article for the benefit of the Chiropractic profession. I want to discuss the inventive ingenuity of the naturopaths. Naturopathy, as defined by its leaders and its schools, is being practiced, under one name or another, by practically the whole drugless world. Ninety-five percent of the chiropractors are practicing Naturopathy. And this reminds us that D. D. Palmer, alleged discoverer of Chiropractic, was a life member of the American Naturopathic Association; also, that here in Texas a large group of chiropractors have formed a Naturopathic Association and are seeking a law to license them as naturopaths.

On page three of the circular that "inspired" this article is an ad of a "health-building specialist and foot correctionist: Graduate Naturopathist, Masseur and Physiotherapist" of Iowa. He offers to the people of B. J. Palmer's hometown, the following cures:

223

• Complete Drugless Health Service

• Swedish Massage and Movements

• Vapor Baths and Hydrotherapy

• Ultraviolet Ray and Infra-Red

• Short-Wave Radio Therapy

• Arch Supports Built to Fit

• Personalized Notes on Health Building and Feet

Hereafter if anybody dies in Davenport, Iowa, it will be their own fault. This man certainly has enough machinery that he can push an electric button or turn a switch, or he can "use his hands" and get everybody well.

Why do so many naturopaths and chiropractors still advertise themselves as "foot correctionists"? Do they not know that Dr. Locke is dead and that his fake cure died before he did? Why not try twisting ears for a while? I guarantee that twisting the ears will cure as many diseases as twisting the feet.

Turning to page two of the circular I see an ad for 'Topeka's (Kansas) Naturopathic Physician." While he uses "no drugs, no serums, no surgery" he "is now using OCTOZONE OXYGEN, the new European treatment."

"OCTOZONE is an active form of pure oxygen—a natural element of the air discovered by Eugene Royer, the French physicist. A powerful germicide and detoxifying agent, it charges the red blood cells with oxygen, revitalizes the cells and tissues, and produces energy by strong oxidation. The function of oxygen in the blood is to convert nutrition into energy. These properties make OCTOZONE a valuable treatment in a wide variety of conditions and many cases receive benefit not otherwise obtainable.

"Arthritis, neuritis, sinusitis, colitis, sclerosis, catarrhal deafness, pelvic infections, and other conditions of infectious origin have responded to this treatment and in some cases have been astonishingly rapid. (It is not clear here whether it is the "condition" or the "treatment" that has been "astonishingly rapid." Ed.)

"Anyone sick and discouraged should investigate Dr. ...'s SYSTEM OF HEALTH BUILDING, which in addition to OCTOZONE includes all acceptable (acceptable to whom? Ed.) drugless and natural methods, such as short-wave diathermy, cold quartz ultraviolet rays, specific light waves, galvanism, colonic irrigation, natural foods, manipulative therapy, and personalized notes on health building."

Surely, here is a combination of machines and "use of ands" that will cure almost, if not quite, all the diseases in Topeka and the surrounding country.

There are plenty of naturopaths in the country who denounce these machine-shop methods and declare that they have no place in Naturopathy. There are plenty of naturopaths who scoff at these push-button doctors and refuse to recognize them as naturopaths. But how are we to decide what methods are Naturopathy and who are the real naturopaths?

The founder of Naturopathy defines it as "organized drugless healing." The above methods resemble chaos and do not seem to us to be very well organized, but they are drugless. As the naturopathic schools (the few that are left), are teaching these methods, hundreds of naturopaths are using them and the naturopathic journals carry articles about them, and ads urging them upon the practitioner and patient. I think we are safe in assuming that the new naturopath (neo-naturopathy) is a machine-shop operator. I assume that now that we have machines to give us "an active form of pure oxygen" we will no longer need our lungs and respiratory muscles. We can dispense with breathing and let the machine charge our red blood cells with oxygen, which we are surprised to learn, "is a natural element of the air."

But now that we have octozone and octozone machines, what are we going to do with our old stand-by, ozone and the ozone generators? What is to become of terpezone and the terpezone chambers? It will surely be heart-rending to have to discard those older loves for a new one.

I often wonder what the feeling of a patient must be when, upon first entering the office of a neo-naturopath, he sees there a vanload of Goldbergian gadgets designed to manufacture health. He hears the purr of the motors and the hum of the machinery; sees the vari-colored lights as these flash on and off and smells the odors of ozone, terpezone, octozone, and of other smelly things. Looking around on the shelves he sees various-size boxes and bottles wearing fancy labels and wrapped in cellophane, containing vitamin pills, food concentrates, gland extracts, laxatives, and various herb "remedies."

With credulous awe he must think to himself as he begins to disrobe for the ceremonials he is about to go through: "Surely now, I have found the right 'doctor.' This man certainly has enough machinery to manufacture all the health I need."

Some of the larger and better stocked of these machine shops have gone in for mass production. Health is turned out on the line like automobiles. They advertise that they treat three hundred patients a day—"each patient receives my personal attention."

It may amuse my readers; it may disgust them; they may react in various ways; but it is a curious fact that these push-button doctors all insist that their gadget-treatments are natural and that they are practicing "nature cure." Even their vitamin pills (often so-called synthetic "vitamins") and their food concentrates are "natural foods." Their thinking is as artificial as their methods: the machine age has run away with their feeble minds.

If Naturopathy did not change so much, so often and so rapidly, we might be able to find out what it is, but with its rapid kaleidoscopic changes it defies definition.

Reprinted from Dr. Shelton's Hygienic Review June 1942.

Article #2: Hygiene Vs. the Cures by Dr. Herbert M. Shelton

The medical dictionary defines cure to mean: "The course of treatment of any disease, or of a special case. The successful treatment of a disease or wound. A system of treating disease. A medicine effective in treating disease." Thus, do meanings of words change. From the Latin, cura, which is synonymous with our word care, cure was originally applied to the care of the healthy individual, then to the care of the sick; now it is defined as a method or means of treating disease or as a medicine effective in treating a disease. Once it also had the significance of a reinstatement of health in an organism that was recently sick, but even then, in both common and professional acceptance, it had reference to the means whereby this was supposed to be accomplished.

A drug was said to be a "cough cure," or a cure for constipation, or for some other disease. The present definition that it is "a medicine effective in treating disease" is ambiguous, in that it fails to define what the "medicine" is effective in doing. Few of medicine's "effective medicines" are claimed to do more than provide a little evanescent and doubtful palliation. Be this as it may, the sick would hardly be said to be cured, however perfect the recovery, without the employment of some drug or treatment. Cure is wrought by some foreign or external aid.

The sick are treated as they are clothed and physicked (drugged) as they are fed, in the confident assurance that, in either case, they are being fitted and burnished for new services. Hence it is that cure has reference to external rather than to an internal recourse. Call it a medicine or a course of treatment; the cure is the work of something outside the living organism, not the result of the body's own healing work.

Living things alone are subjects of the curative efforts of those who profess to be able to heal and it is the different estimates relatively that are credited to the vital, organic, or recuperative forces, and the part that treatment plays, that serves as the basis of the different views entertained of the subject. Apparently most members of the various schools of healing deem that disease is a destructive something that will inevitably consummate its malevolent work unless opposed by some counteracting and neutralizing power, the forces of life being little more than a spectator on the sidelines, until the disease is either vanquished, accepting the victory wrought in their behalf, or the patient dies. There are among these various practitioners, those (relatively few) who award some credit to the processes of life, if these forces are stimulated or goaded by measures capable of exciting or arousing their actions defensively.

Outside the schools of curing, there are those who place no dependence on any other means than those of organic recuperation and reconstruction, or in those all-efficient processes and means that continue the vital or organic changes in the healthy state. These hold that healing is a biological process, as much an activity of life as nutrition, respiration, excretion, etc., and that it requires no goads to action.

All the many schools of curing that have existed in the past and that exist now, with all their many and opposing theories, and their many and conflicting practices, have existed and acted under the assumption that all desirable ends in cases of disease have been and are affected by medical treatment.

Scarcely any reliance has been placed upon the intrinsic vital capacities. At all times, the big question in medical investigations and actions has revolved about the matter of the qualities, quantities and times in which medicines are useful.

Obviously there has been a mountain of error in all this theorizing and empirical practice. Schools of medicine and modes of treatment have followed each other into oblivion in a melancholy succession, leaving scarcely a trace behind. It has been assumed that what we call symptoms of disease are necessarily and invariably evidences of a destructive process; that a great variety of substances known to be inimical to health, are yet, also, antagonistic to disease; that on special occasions such substances may constitute special vivifying means, differing from those usually necessary, performing on local structures curative acts that differ from the ordinary nutritive and reproductive processes.

Writing in November 1954, George H. Taylor, M.D., said that the Hygienic or Physiological School "endeavors to show that these assumptions are to be taken, if at all, with many qualifications, and that the present state of science fails to warrant, or absolutely repudiates them." On this occasion he also pointed out that the Hygienic school "seeks to guide those liable to suffer from disease to a true knowledge of themselves, and to the probable causes of their physical miseries," and finds redemption "in the discipline and correction of faulty and perverted functional habits."

Taylor said that the Hygienic school abjures entirely the empirical or experimental practices of the curing schools, and refuses to admit, as untrustworthy, the ambiguous evidence in favor of such practices. Admitting that, even with the same data upon which to reason, there would be differences in judgement, he asserted that "life and its invariable phenomena, rather than medicine and its uses, should furnish the proper field of inquiry." From such a study is to be gained a knowledge of how the living organism behaves under different circumstances; we would learn what life ordinarily does, and how it will act under constraint and compulsion, and what are the proper conditions for its ascendency over the causes of disease.

As he pointed out on the occasion, we can never weigh or measure the vital principle, but we may observe the circumstances that attend its operations, its work, its invariable conditions, its laws, what it does, and that on our understanding of these we must base our actions in reference to it, both in health and in disease. All of this simply means that, whatever may be the essential nature of life, our behavior towards the body, whether well or sick, must be, if it is not to be harmful, consonant with human physiology.

A living organism grows, reproduces and multiplies its parts and, by this repetition extends itself. To do this, it selects from its environment such materials as it has the capacity to make into parts of its own structure, and as promptly rejects and refuses all other substances. These are necessary conditions to the maintenance of its vital integrity. In the one-celled organism, in the higher plant or animal, wherever we see life, selection and appropriation of food, assimilation and growth, and refusal and rejection are constant actions, and the energy of these actions must gear a constant relation to each other, for the living organism seeks its own welfare in all acts. As the constitution of the living unit is uniform and invariable, it necessarily follows that all external substances must be of three kinds, namely:

1. Materials that are identical with or are susceptible to being transformed into the same form as that of the living structure and are related to the organism as nutriment.

2. Substances that may be described as indifferent giving rise to no change upon contact, but may serve as a needed medium, for example, water.

3. Substances that cannot be transformed into cell substance, but the relation of which, to the vital structure, is one of antagonism, and in varying degrees of intensity, is destructive of the integrity of the vital organism, and are properly classed as poison.

We may properly think of water as belonging, essentially, to the first classification, as it is essential to all vital actions and vital syntheses. Viewing matter in this light, then, all substances with which the living organism comes into contact are either food materials or poisons. The class which we call poisons is very numerous and composed of a number of subdivisions—indeed, this class is almost as various as the number of elements and chemical compounds, after we have subtracted nutriments.

When non usable substances are brought into contact with the cells, they must be resisted, rejected, expelled. The actions by which these poisons are resisted and expelled have long been mistaken for actions of the poisons. In sober fact, the so-called actions of drugs (poisons) are actions of the living body. These actions are but phases of the primordial activities of the living organism in rejecting and casting off materials that cannot be normally appropriated into living structures.

Animal organisms are made up of parts and each of these parts is composed of lesser elements, each of which has a quasi-independent existence and exercises its own peculiar powers of action, and is capable of its own peculiar affections, hence the application of foreign substances to the general organism, through the circulation, gives rise to local effects in keeping with the characteristics of the parts affected, all of which are disturbances of the normal functions of the various parts, and this tends to impair and degrade and not to elevate the local function.

All this results inevitably from the invariableness that characterizes the constitution of living organisms as much as it does inanimate things. The same constituent elements and the same conditions of warmth, heat, activity, etc., are employed in the composition of each individual of each species, wherever produced or reproduced; the same laws ruling that are observed to rule other individuals. In the whole evolution of an organism and its activities, effects change in relation to changing conditions, but the laws governing these operations never vary.

Because of this invariableness, all attempts to impose materials or conditions upon the organism other than those that normally and naturally belong to it, are met with determined resistance, and can result only in a waste of its formative elements and actuating energies. The constant and orderly development of forms with which the forces of life are connected, and on which the functions and activities of life depend, is thus retarded, and even perverted.

The broad page of nature, with its infinite diversity, is but a statement of these principles. Organization, whether we regard it as something apart from the ordinary chemical and physical forms and forces or a special application of physical and chemical forces, is no less subject to fixed principles and invariable laws. It's almost infinite variety of manifestations are expressions of the values of the forces that inhere in particular organisms under special conditions. Matter itself undergoes no change in its intrinsic qualities.

All the importance that attaches to the effort to manage health and recovery by drugs, arises out of a failure to recognize the foregoing principles. They arise out of a mistake in the essential nature of the actions occasioned in the vital organism by the administration of drugs. The very liberality of man's constitutional endowments makes possible the great number and variety of actions that are and have been mistaken for the actions of "remedies."

Considering the nature of man, and his many constitutional capabilities, it should be evident that the variations in his health and the multitude of symptoms which occur, arise out of his complexity of structure and function as much as do the many actions that have, been mistaken for drug actions. It is the human organism, and not simple lifeless chemical substances, that is capable of such a wide variety of behavior patterns. Rightly considered, these many capacities for action are evidences of man's superiority, not of his defect.

Dr. Taylor thought that "the utmost reach of power demands the utmost freedom of its exercise," and pointed out, in this connection, that, the ends of man's intellectual existence "could not be attained by confining him to a fixed point of temperature, or locality, and a consequent uniform subsistence." To meet the requirements of his intellect, man requires a highly complex and plastic organism. The human organism is

229

capable of accommodating itself to a great variety of circumstances, making use, in so doing, of a variety of means of adjustment and adaptation.

Man is possessed of organs and systems of organs that, in their normal functions, act reciprocally to secrete and excrete, adopt and exclude, to the end that physiological equilibrium be maintained. With such marvelous means of adjustment at his command, man evolves no disease, so long as his needs (supplies) are filled and waste is rejected. Only when he has reduced his functioning powers so that waste is incompletely expelled, nutrition is impaired, secretion is checked and vital processes are hampered does he become sick, i.e., his body embarks on an emergency course of liberation and restoration.

If we exclude those "diseases" that result from poisoning by drugs or similar toxic substances taken in from without, disease is the result of impairments or imperfections in the functions of the body which permit the accumulation of endogenously generated toxin, the imperfection of function growing out of reduced functioning power (enervation) which, in turn, results from the dissipation of the energies of life. This is to say, disease is autogenerated. It is not an attack upon the body by an outside foe, but a consequence of violations of the conditions of a healthy existence.

Since the principles and conditions of vital as well as of chemical actions are fixed and do not change because the organism is sick, it becomes plain that the professionally induced "medicinal" disease cannot possess the intelligence or power to restore health. Recuperation and recovery are never the results of so-called medicines, but are always the results of the operation of the organic forces and of the conditions that usually maintain health. Health is to be restored, as it is to be preserved, by conforming to the healthful conditions laid down by nature.

This will be met with the assertion that good effects are seen to follow the administration of drugs; we will even be assured that drugs can and often do save life. The record of experience will be appealed to, to substantiate this position. Case histories and case records will be paraded in evidence. Such "evidence" takes no account of the self-healing powers and activities of the organism and, at the same time, assumes that the drug effect is additional to that of the healing work of the sick body. True, there is additional action—the activity needed to resist and expel the drug. The vital actions are changed, not helped.

Any benefit accruing to health must come, either through the ordinary physiological processes or through some temporary, even, perhaps dramatic modification of these to meet special occasions, and these can work only with the normal things of life: food instead of poison, rest instead of stimulation, sleep instead of narcosis, air instead of drug fumes, warmth instead of mustard plasters, etc., etc.

Those substances that the living structure cannot, appropriate and use, but must reject in a state of health are equally non usable and must be rejected in a state of disease when the powers of life are lowered.

Drugs can only further impair and depress vital powers. Drugs morbidly occasion the diversion of the very functions and processes upon which the body must rely for purgation and healing. This may so devitalize the body that it must suspend its healing efforts—symptoms are suppressed .

Finally, it must be observed that, in treating the sick with drugs, no lesson is taught, no discipline is enforced, and no condition is instituted that is of any value in health or in a subsequent state of illness. The intellect of the patient is left a blank, his body a scene of devastation. The patient does not know why he was sick, nor how he recovered, and he does not know how to avoid becoming sick again.

Reprinted from Dr. Shelton's Hygienic Review, August 1965.

Lesson 88:

The Vegetarian Diet

88.1. Introduction

88.1.1. History of Vegetarianism

88.1.2. Vegetarianism Defined

You can no longer cook and eat pet dogs in some parts of the country. Within the past year, a state (Texas) legislature passed a law which prohibits the sale of dogs for food. It seems that some people in this state were raising and selling special breeds of dogs to certain immigrants who were used to eating them as part of their national diet.

The pet lovers of this state raised such an outcry that a law was enacted to protect dogs from being used as food. Of course, in some parts of the world, household pets are still part of the evening meal. In these countries, leftovers are not fed to the family dog—the leftovers are likely to be the dog!

Almost no American would consider having Fido or Rover on the dinner plate, yet millions line up each day for a serving of old "Bossie" at the local hamburger joint.

And they think vegetarians are strange!

Vegetarianism is one of the most popular approaches to good health through better nutrition. It has been proven that ancient man was a vegetarian first and came to eat meat only much later in his development. The vegetarians were first, but the carnivores have gotten the upper hand in the past thousand years.

Because vegetarianism is such a proven method for improved health, and since it has a firm basis in historical fact and precedent, everyone who wishes to teach and practice healthful living should be eminently knowledgeable about the types of vegetarianism, its past, and its relationship to the Life Science diet. This lesson discusses vegetarianism in this light.

88.1.1. History of Vegetarianism

Vegetarianism is not new. It has been around as long as recorded history, and before. In the Far East, vegetarianism was devotedly practiced by the Hindus thousands of years before America was discovered. In the west, the ancient Greeks glorified and praised the virtues of vegetarianism. Plato, Socrates, Aristotle, Ovid, and Hippocrates were only a few of the great classical thinkers who strictly avoided meat and flesh.

The Romans gave us the word "vegetarian" from the Latin word vegetare. This word has nothing whatsoever to do with "vegetables." Instead, the word "vegetare" means "to enliven" or to fill with good spirits. When the Romans called someone a "vegetarian," they were not calling him a "vegetable eater," but instead were referring to him as a vigorous person, sound in mind and body.

88.1.2. Vegetarianism Defined

The original definition of vegetarian, then, is not someone who eats vegetables, but a person who possesses radiant health, a lively mind, and a sound spirit.

The common definition of a vegetarian is "someone who doesn't eat any meat." Meat includes chicken, fish, insects, and any living creature above the rudimentary cellular level. In other words, you can still consume small living microorganisms, or microscopic "animals," and still be considered a vegetarian. You cannot, however, eat tuna fish once a week or turkey at Thanksgiving and still be a vegetarian.

This is the loose definition of vegetarianism—the avoidance of animal flesh as part of the diet. The correct definition of a vegetarian, however, is this: A vegetarian is a person who practices living solely on plant products.

This means that not only is a vegetarian diet strictly from the plant kingdom (no eggs, no honey, no dairy products), but someone who practices true vegetarianism will not use or wear any products made from animals. This means no leather shoes, no fur coats, no purses, or billfolds made from cowhide, and so on. It also means that household products, such as soaps, glues, etc., made in part or whole from the remains of animals are not used.

Obviously, few people are total vegetarians. In our society, it is very difficult to avoid all products made from animals. It is, however, quite simple to avoid all foods derived from animals. Dietary vegetarianism is not only a practical reality, but an imperative one. We can no longer afford to exploit our resources to produce expensive meat for the select few.

88.2. The Two Approaches to Vegetarianism

88.2.1. The Moral and Ethical Aspects of Vegetarianism

88.2.2. The Dietary and Health Aspects of Vegetarianism

88.2.3. What Type of Vegetarian Are You?

88.2.4. How Many Vegetarians Are There?

Vegetarianism is both a moral and ethical issue, as well as a dietary and health practice. Although people may come to the vegetarian way of life for a variety of reasons, there are two major categories of vegetarianism: 1) Ethical Vegetarianism, and 2) Dietary Vegetarianism.

88.2.1. The Moral and Ethical Aspects of Vegetarianism

Some people practice vegetarianism because of their religious beliefs or personal morality. These people simply feel that it is "wrong" to kill and slaughter animals for food. Often, they also believe that animals should not be exploited, abused, or mistreated in any way. This means that an ethical vegetarian would object to vivisection, the skinning of animals for furs and leather, animal experimentation, hunting, fishing, and any other practice in which animals are hurt or murdered.

Vegetarianism is also a tenet of many religious teachings. The Hindus in India and various Christian sects in this country, such as the Seventh Day Adventists and Church of Latter-Day Saints, often avoid all meat eating. In these religions, the prohibition against the eating of animals is related to the taking of life. They simply believe that it is wrong to murder or kill anyone, whether it be a human, a cow, or chicken.

Many Buddhists who preach nonviolence generally practice vegetarianism, but they will also eat meat that is offered to them by their hosts. They do not kill animals for food but will often eat such animals that have already been killed by others. Buddha, the founder of Buddhism, was a strict vegetarian.

In fact, many founders of the world's greatest religions were originally vegetarians or became so after their period of enlightenment. There are a goodly number of serious Biblical scholars who also think that Jesus Christ was a vegetarian.

Vegetarianism as part of a religion has always existed and will always continue to do so as long as there are proscriptions against the taking of life.

Other ethical vegetarians, however, may refuse to eat meat on moral principles, yet not be associated with any religion or dogmatic belief. Percy Bysshe Shelley, an English poet of the nineteenth century, was both an atheist and an ethical vegetarian. In 1813, he stated in a treatise on diet that "man's digestive system was suited only to plant food" and that he abhorred the killing and slaughter that goes hand in hand with meat eating.

You may be considered an ethical vegetarian if you believe that all killing, including animals, is morally wrong. There are those who never eat any meat, not because they consider it unhealthy or even unnatural, but because the murder of any living creature is morally repugnant to them.

88.2.2. The Dietary and Health Aspects of Vegetarianism

Besides the ethical vegetarian, there is the dietary or health-minded vegetarian. This type of vegetarian may or may not believe it is morally wrong to take an animal's life. In fact, the question of morality or ethics really does not enter into this type of person's decision to eat meat or not.

Meat is avoided because of the health problems it creates. It is not included in the diet because of its past association with cancer, heart attacks, kidney failure, arthritis, and other debilitating diseases.

In the past, most vegetarians were so because of ethical or moral beliefs. Now with all the scientific findings about the harmful effects of meat and animal products, more people are becoming vegetarians for dietary or health reasons.

88.2.3. What Type of Vegetarian Are You?

Most people are vegetarians for both ethical and health reasons, and this is probably the best balance.

Ethical vegetarians, for example, often tend to be somewhat sickly and less healthy than those who are vegetarians for health reasons. Why is this?

Ethical vegetarians avoid meat for moral reasons; they may or may not be concerned with their health.

Consequently, they may indulge in white sugar, pastries, poor food combinations, and bizarrely concocted "meat substitutes." The one thing you can be sure of, however, is that those who are ethical vegetarians for moral reasons tend to be more consistent in their vegetarianism. They rarely revert back to meat eating because they have strong convictions.

On the other hand, those that come to vegetarianism for purely health reasons may go back to eating meat if their health does not improve or should fail. They are usually willing to try the vegetarian diet for a year or two, or maybe for five or six years. Yet all too often they may start including fish or chicken back into their diet. They see nothing "morally" wrong with eating meat.

The best approach to vegetarianism is both an ethical and health-minded one. If you are not only convinced that vegetarianism is a superior way to health, but that killing animals is morally unacceptable, then you are more likely to be steady in your practice. Vegetarianism without ethics cannot last; vegetarianism without a health-minded and rational attitude is ineffectual. We should imbue our vegetarian practice with both morality and a practical concern for health.

88.2.4. How Many Vegetarians Are There?

If you are a vegetarian, you are not alone. At least one out of three people in the world today are vegetarians. For some of these people, however, vegetarianism is not a moral or dietary choice: it is a practical necessity. Meat may not be available, or it may simply be too expensive to buy.

In America, there are a few people who are vegetarians for economic reasons, but the majority of people who avoid meat in the United States (second highest per capita of meat consumption in the world) do so out of ethical or health concerns.

In 1978, an extensive poll was conducted by the Roper organization to determine how many vegetarians there are in the United States. Here are their findings:

Class	Percent of the Total U.S. Population:
Strict vegetarians—those that never eat any meat, fish, or fowl	0.5%
Mainly vegetarians—those that eat meat less than once or twice a week	2.6%
People who say they are "careful" about how much meat they eat	17.0%
People who eat meat less often than they once did	75.0%

In other words, about one out of 200 people in this country practice vegetarianism or approximately 1,150,000 Americans do not eat meat. Of course a goodly number of these vegetarians also eat milk, eggs, cheese, honey, and other animal products. In fact, about nine out of ten vegetarians still eat dairy products and eggs, it is somewhat encouraging, however, that the great majority of Americans are at least consciously cutting back on their tremendous meat consumption.

The reasons that these vegetarians gave the Roper organization for becoming a vegetarian are also revealing. Over half of those people who practice vegetarianism do so purely for health reasons (56%). About one out of six vegetarians (16%) do not eat meat for humanitarian or moral reasons. Saving money and the high cost of meat are the main reasons that 25% of all vegetarians follow their diet, and the remaining two or three percent vegetarians avoid meat because of the wishes of their family, spouse, parents, or children.

88.3. The Types of Vegetarian Diets

88.3.1. The Unrestricted Vegetarian Diet

88.3.2. The Lacto-Ovo-Vegetarian Diet

88.3.3. The Lacto-Vegetarian Diet

88.3.4. Vegan Diet

88.3.5. The Macrobiotic Diet

88.3.6. Raw Food Diets

Although we can strictly define what a vegetarian is, there is not a standard vegetarian diet. Some vegetarians eat everything but meat; others eat cheese and eggs. There are vegetarians who eat only raw foods and vegetarians who eat strictly cooked foods. There are even vegetarians that never eat vegetables, and those that eat fish and still call themselves vegetarians.

Clearly, there is no one vegetarian diet and there are several dietary approaches to vegetarianism. The only thing common to all true vegetarian diets is a strict avoidance of flesh. Since vegetarian diets are so popular among health seekers, you should know the different types and the advantages and disadvantages of each.

For the sake of convenience, vegetarian diets have been divided into six general categories. Each category of diet is explained, and its strengths and weaknesses are noted.

88.3.1. The Unrestricted Vegetarian Diet

This particular form of vegetarianism is simple to describe: its adherents eat everything but meat. Vegetarians who follow an unrestricted diet consume dairy products, eggs, and even animal fat in the form of lard occasionally. They eat sugar, white flour, salt, fried foods, fast foods, and junk foods.

They eat just about anything that cannot crawl, swim, or run. And they are often very unhealthy.

I met a man and his wife who had been vegetarians for over ten years. They were both fighting a serious weight problem.

"I never thought I'd be an overweight vegetarian," the man joked with me, "but Susan and I each weigh nearly twenty-five pounds more than when we got married ten years ago."

I worked with the man and had a chance to see how he became a fat vegetarian. His diet was unrestricted to say the least. He continually drank soft drinks with sugar because he didn't want those "artificial sweeteners." He certainly enjoyed ice cream, and ate many of his lunches from vending machines in the form of snack cakes and cookies. His wife and himself enjoyed cooking gourmet vegetarian meals, and they used eggs, butter, and cream in all of their cooking for a rich taste.

One day he told me: "You know, I hate to say it, but I think Susan and I are going to have to start eating meat again."

I was astonished. After ten years, he and his wife were going back to eating animals.

Why, I asked him.

"Well, we read a book that said some people are probably not meant to be vegetarians. It has to do with the pituitary gland, and how it needs animal protein to be stimulated. When your gland is stimulated by eating meat, your metabolism increases, and you lose weight. We keep getting fat on a vegetarian diet, so I guess we'll try something new. Susan's fixing fish tonight, and it'll probably be pretty strange eating meat after all these years. Still," he said as he patted his stomach, "I'll eat anything to get rid of this."

Of course, that was exactly his problem. He had been eating "anything" and everything on his vegetarian diet. Listen to what Dr. Herbert M. Shelton has to say about vegetarians who follow such an unrestricted diet:

"Vegetarians often have the erroneous idea that the rejection of meat is all that is required to carry them into dietetic heaven. They do not know that a vegetarian diet may be even more dangerous than a properly-planned mixed diet. Indeed, the eating of most vegetarians is so abominable that one cannot blame people for not following them."

The unrestricted, eat-anything-you-like vegetarian diet is indeed poorer than the diet which includes meat but rejects other unnatural foods. Meat eating, for example, has been around much longer than white sugar, white flour, preservatives, and other junk foods. There is more in man's background that predisposes him to a raw hunk of meat than to a sugary ice cream cone.

This is not to say that we should consume meat in preference to vanilla ice cream; neither has a place in the healthful diet. Some vegetarians have only seen half the truth and remain "ice cream" vegetarians—addicted to junk foods and sugar, while proudly rejecting meat.

The unrestricted vegetarian diet has little to recommend it. It is certainly better than an unrestricted meal diet, yet it cannot be depended upon to build and maintain health. In summary, the unrestricted vegetarian diet can be evaluated as follows:

Advantages: All flesh and meat products are eschewed which reduces the level of toxicity in the diet.

Disadvantages: Old and poor diet habits are maintained. Junk foods are often substituted for the missing meat. The person is deluded into thinking that he has improved his diet, when in effect, only a small portion of the harmful foods has been removed.

Compared to the Life Science Diet: The only thing the unrestricted vegetarian diet has in common with the recommended Life Science diet is the mutual avoidance of meat. Other than that, the unrestricted vegetarian diet is more closely aligned with the traditional American diet than with the Life Science diet.

88.3.2. The Lacto-Ovo-Vegetarian Diet

Like the unrestricted vegetarian diet discussed, the lacto-ovo-vegetarian diet is a very liberal dietary approach. Both diets include all dairy products and eggs in the foods eaten. The lacto-ovo-vegetarian (abbreviated as LOV) eats cheese, drinks milk, and uses eggs as part of the regular diet.

Unlike the unrestricted vegetarian diet, the LOV diet generally excludes junk foods, white sugar, white flour and other widely-known debilitating foods. The LOV dietary approach, then, is a health-minded way to a better diet.

People who are lacto-ovo-vegetarians ("lacto" for milk, "ovo" for eggs) usually are former meat eaters who have decided to eliminate meat and, at the same time, substitute more whole and natural foods for processed foods. People follow a LOV diet for two reasons: 1) They are not yet confident enough or nutritionally educated enough to give up all animal foods and products. They continue to eat eggs and milk to "make sure they get plenty of protein," or whatever. 2) They do so for social and family convenience. A LOV diet allows a great deal of latitude in dining out, and it may be followed with a minimum of inconvenience.

Advantages: Meat is eliminated, and a gradual trend is started to a better, more wholesome diet. The LOV diet is socially convenient, nonthreatening. and requires a minimal amount of change in lifestyle.

Disadvantages: Milk, milk products, and eggs are totally unnecessary in the diet. These foods are constipating, acidic, and full of pesticides, hormones, and growth additives.

Compared to the Life Science Diet: The LOV diet has only two things in common with the Life Science diet—it too avoids all flesh, and it also emphasizes more whole and natural foods over processed and refined foods.

88.3.3. The Lacto-Vegetarian Diet

The lacto-vegetarian diet is the most popular vegetarian diet in the world. This diet avoids all animal products except for those made from milk. Eggs, lard, and the most blatant junk foods are avoided. Yogurt, butter, cheese, cream, and milk, however, are consumed in unrestricted amounts.

Many people follow a lacto-vegetarian diet for reasons convenience or nutritional "safety." Again, a lacto-vegetarian diet makes it easier to dine out and eat conventional foods. Some people use milk products in a vegetarian diet in order to meet the inflated Recommended Daily Allowance (RDA) calcium standards. Milk and cheeses are used in such a diet so that enough calcium may be consumed.

Calcium requirements, however, can be easily met and exceeded on a vegetarian diet that includes absolutely no dairy products. In fact, there is much doubt that calcium from pasteurized and heated milk products can be absorbed by the body at all. Calcium requirements on an alkaline vegetarian diet are far lower than for a meat-eating, acidic diet. In other words, meat-eaters need larger amounts of calcium than do vegetarians.

If you know vegetarians who use milk products as a matter of convenience, there is probably little you can do to enlighten them. If, however, they are adding dairy products to their diet solely to meet calcium requirements, then tell them the truth: It just isn't necessary.

Advantages: The healthy lacto-vegetarian diet does eliminate many of the harmful foods eaten today: meat, animal products, eggs, junk foods, white sugar. It is a relatively easy and simple diet to follow, and may be conveniently adhered to by those who do not wish to make major changes in their lifestyles.

Disadvantages: Most lacto-vegetarians greatly overeat on dairy products. It is a fact that lacto-vegetarians generally eat more cheese and drink more milk than many meat eaters and those on conventional diets. Dairy products are often used as a high-protein substitute for meat, yet they too are full of hormones, additives, and pesticides.

Compared to the Life Science Diet: Like the LOV diet, this diet has in common with the optimal Life Science diet the avoidance of meat and many substandard foods and junk foods. Eggs, too, are eliminated as in the Life Science diet. Yet the lacto-vegetarian diet still includes many, many foods not considered natural to our dietary heritage. Cooked grains, legumes, onions, garlic, spices, herbs, and foods eaten in poor combinations are all present in the lacto-vegetarian diet. Although another step in the right direction, the lacto-vegetarian diet still slops short of embracing the full principles of Natural Hygiene and Life Science.

88.3.4. Vegan Diet

All vegans are vegetarians—not all vegetarians are vegans. Life Scientists or Natural Hygienists are usually vegans—not all vegans are Natural Hygienists. Confusing? Let's explain:

A vegan is a vegetarian that does not consume any animal products whatsoever. A vegan diet does not include eggs, meat, milk, cheese, or any other animal products. The vegan diet even eliminates honey, an animal product used in many vegetarian diets. The vegan is the true vegetarian. Those vegetarians who continue to eat eggs or drink milk are really just nonmeat eaters. Estimates have placed the number of vegans at about 10% of the vegetarian population; in other words, only one out of ten vegetarians strictly avoids eggs, milk, and dairy products.

The vegan diet, like so many other vegetarian regimens, however, usually relies upon grains and beans for a large portion of its calories. Foods are often eaten in poor combinations and in large amounts. Vegans often substitute processed and refined soybean products in place of dairy and meat. Soy milk, tofu. tempeh, soy ice cream, and soy meat substitutes are the darlings of the vegan diet.

A heavy reliance on soy products, due in part to a misplaced concern about protein, is the major drawback to the vegan diet. Soy products cannot be completely digested due to enzymes present in the soybeans, and soy foods also inhibit iron absorption. Still, the soy foods are superior to the milk and eggs used by other vegetarians and to the meat consumed by flesh eaters.

Advantages: The vegan diet completely eliminates some of the worst foods in the American dietary—meat, milk, eggs, and junk foods. It also eschews honey, a food often abused and overused by vegetarians and other health seekers.

Disadvantages: Vegans still use sweeteners such as maple syrup or molasses. They consume too many soy products and eat a preponderance of grains and legumes. They often worry about "complete" protein combinations, and often eat a majority of the foods cooked or otherwise processed.

Compared to the Life Science Diet: The vegan diet can be easily adapted to the Life Science diet. All the vegan must do is to eliminate all processed foods, such as soy products, sweeteners, etc., eat more foods raw, and watch food combinations. If you follow the Life Science diet, you may also be considered a vegan, or "true" vegetarian, at well.

88.3.5. The Macrobiotic Diet

The macrobiotic diet is not strictly vegetarian, although most people regard it as such. Fish and seafood are often a small but frequent part of a macrobiotic diet.

Grains form the bulk of foods eaten by a person on a macrobiotic diet. In fact, most macrobiotic supporters recommend a diet that is at least 50% whole grains, and it is not at all uncommon for a macrobiotic diet to be 80% grain based.

The second most important foods on a macrobiotic diet are legumes (10 to 15% of the diet), followed by seaweeds and hard vegetables. Nuts and seeds are rarely eaten, and usually salted and roasted when consumed. Fresh fruits are almost never eaten by a person following such a diet; indeed, apples are about the only raw fruit eaten, and other fruits are usually cooked and sweetened as a dessert.

Salts, salted foods, pickles, tamari (soy sauce), and miso are used heavily in the diet. The Japanese, from whom the macrobiotic diet was chiefly imported, eat more salt than any other population in the world. Even their plums are preserved and heavily salted. Nothing escapes salting in a macrobiotic diet.

Strangely enough, the macrobiotic health seeker avoids most fresh fruit and vegetables. Citrus fruits, tomatoes, eggplant, potatoes, and other raw vegetables have no place in the macrobiotic diet. In fact, someone once said as a joke (but which is true) that a macrobiotic person is "someone who would rather eat a fish than an orange."

An avoidance of fresh fruits and vegetables occurs on a macrobiotic diet due to application of the mystical "yin-yang" outlook. Fresh fruits are considered too "yin" to eat, and they are often categorized in the same department as white sugar and artificial sweeteners. Most meat is considered too "yang" to eat, and grains (especially brown rice) are said to have the perfect combination of "yin and yang."

Besides the overuse of salt and the avoidance of fresh fruits and vegetables, the major drawback of the macrobiotic diet is that it is so heavily grain dependent. Dr. Shelton, when discussing grain diets, stated: "A cereal and pulse (legume) diet with a deficiency of green foods and fresh fruits is obviously inadequate. It is deficient in alkaline elements and Vitamins."

Another health pioneer, Dr. Densmore had this to say about the grain-based macrobiotic diet: "I object to bread, cereals, pulses and grains not only because of the predominant proportion of starch in them, but also because their nitrogen is distinctly difficult of digestion and the cause of unnecessary waste of vitality."

The macrobiotic diet has a strong appeal for those changing over from a conventional meat-based diet. Heavy grains tend to be as constipating and acidic as the meat that has been left behind. The heavily salted foods exceed the high-salt American diet. The avoidance of fresh fruits and vegetables in the diet certainly finds a kindred soul in the processed food diet of most Americans.

Yet it is an undisputed fact that people who follow a macrobiotic diet enjoy better health than those on a typical American diet. Why is that? Primarily because the macrobiotic diet is largely vegetarian. It avoids all dairy products and eschews white sugar. Simply the elimination of red meat, sugar, and dairy products will greatly increase one's health and vitality, and this is the strong point of the macrobiotic school.

Advantages: The macrobiotic diet is largely vegetarian. It eliminates many of the harmful foods present in the modern diet. It has a well-established history and provides an easily understandable dietary framework with specific recommendations and rules. It provides an easy transition for those breaking their addictions to white sugar, red meat, junk foods, and heavily-processed foods.

Disadvantages: The macrobiotic diet relies too much on grains and grain products which are third-rate foods. Salt is used in large amounts, and foods are almost always cooked. Fresh fruits, salads, sprouts, and nuts are rarely eaten, and never make up more than 5-10% of the overall diet.

Compared to the Life Science Diet: The macrobiotic diet is only similar to the Life Science approach in that junk foods, white sugar, red meat, and dairy products are eliminated. Other than that, 95% of the macrobiotic diet is unrelated to the optimum foods eaten on the Life Science diet—fresh, raw fruits, vegetables, nuts, seeds, and sprouts.

88.3.6. Raw Food Diets

A diet much closer to the Life Science regimen is the raw food vegetarian diet. People who are "raw fooders" eat a variety of foods, but all are eaten uncooked.

Some raw fooders eat uncooked grains, and others include raw milk, raw cheese, and raw cream in their diet. Many times, raw fooders will concoct entrees and main dishes that contain 15 to 20 ingredients, all chopped and mixed together. They often overeat on salads and raw vegetables and neglect fruits. They consume salad dressings, raw oils, and various nut butters with their plates of raw vegetables.

They rely heavily on avocados, dried fruits, and nuts, sometimes to excess. They are often enamored with raw juice therapy, and drink pints and quarts of fresh-squeezed juices each day.

One of the main problems with the raw food diet followed by most people is that its adherents eat far too little fruit and far too many nuts, fats, oils, and seeds for their fuel. Raw fooders who do not make fruit the major part of their diet will overeat on nuts, oils, salad dressings, or other concentrated foods.

They are on the right track but may fall short when it comes to food combining or avoiding inappropriate raw foods (such as onions, garlic, raw cheese, raw honey, etc.).

Advantages: The raw food diet, when it does not include dairy products or other relatively-indigestible foods, can promote the highest level of health. The diet is supers charged with vitamins, minerals, enzymes, and amino acids—all in an easily-digestible form. By eating foods raw, you avoid totally-inappropriate foods such as meats, junk foods, breads, and so forth.

Disadvantages: The raw food diet may still include certain noxious vegetables such as garlic and onions. Honey and raw dairy products may be included. An over-reliance on salads, salad dressings, and nuts is common. Weight loss may occur too rapidly if not enough fruits are included.

Compared to the Life Science Diet: The raw food diet comes very close to the Life Science diet. If all herbs, spices, and seasonings are avoided, as well as all animal products, the raw food diet can be said to be 90% similar to the Life Science diet. When raw foods are eaten in proper combinations and according to our fruitarian biological

247

heritage, then this diet closely approximates the Life Science diet of raw fruits, supplemented by vegetables, nuts, and seeds.

88.4. Pros and Cons of Vegetarianism

88.4.1. Should We Be Vegetarians at All?

88.3.2. The Beneficial Aspects of Vegetarianism

88.3.3. The Vegetarian Trap

88.3.4. Vegetarianism: Not Far Enough

88.3.5. Vegetarians People Love to Hate

88.4.1. Should We Be Vegetarians at All?

After all of this discussion of vegetarianism and the different types of vegetarians, we probably should ask the question: Is the vegetarian diet really that suited after all for optimum health?

If we consider the vegetarian diet to be chiefly based upon vegetables (greens, grains, stalks, tubers, roots, etc.), then we can answer: No, the vegetarian diet is not the best diet to promote health and well-being. The only diet that can truly insure the highest level of health is one that is based primarily on the foods of our biological heritage: Fruits.

Man is not suited to live on grasses, stalks, greens, and roughage that make up the greater part of the vegetable category. These may be additions to his natural diet, but such vegetables alone cannot give the highest-quality nutrients and fuel that we require. Fruits with their abundance of minerals, vitamins, natural sugars, and amino acids can furnish us with all of our needs. They are nontoxic (something that vegetables cannot make a claim to) and they may eaten with relish with no preparation (unlike grains, tubers, and hard roots).

Since T. C. Fry has addressed this question so well in the supplemental material following this lesson, we'll end this discussion by simply saying that the typical vegetarian diet as envisioned by the majority of people does not meet all the criteria for optimum well-being. We hasten to add that this is true not because a vegetarian diet is deficient or lacking, but because fruits alone should form the majority of foods eaten, and not vegetables.

Yet for its shortcomings, the vegetarian diet is vastly superior to the typical American diet and is unreservedly recommended as at least a first step for those seeking to improve their health. Let's look at just some of the more obvious benefits of a vegetarian diet.

88.3.2. The Beneficial Aspects of Vegetarianism

A recent study comparing diets and deaths from heart disease in seven countries showed that those people who ate the highest amounts of animal products (meat, dairy, eggs, etc.) also had the highest death rates. Finland, which had the highest amount of animal foods, topped the list in heart disease. The United States, second largest consumer of animal products, also took second place in death rate due to heart disease. The Japanese, which (had the lowest incidence of meat eating, also had the lowest amount of heart disease.

Vegetarians not only avoid heart disease, but also have lower blood pressure. A Boston study showed that vegetarians who ate little or no animal products (dairy, eggs) had lower blood pressure and cholesterol levels than their meat-eating counterparts.

In the Journal of the American Medical Association, a publication noted for its conservative position on the role of diet in health and disease, Dr. W. A. Thomas reported that "a vegetarian diet can prevent 90% of our thrombo-embolic disease (blood-clotting) and 97% of our coronary occlusions." In his book, Heart Attack, You Don't Have to Die, Dr. Christian Barnard cites several medical studies which prove that "people who eat a diet high in animal products (meat, eggs, milk, etc.) have a higher incidence of coronary heart disease than those who do not."

Not only do vegetarians suffer from fewer incidents of heart disease and high blood pressure, they fare much better when it comes to cancer. Several epidemiological studies and sources have shown a very strong correlation between the incidence of cancer of the colon and meat consumption.

One of these researchers says: "Because eating of vegetarian foods, free of animal fats, results in a shorter transit time and probably the production of less carcinogens, the incidence of cancer of the colon should be substantially less for vegetarians than for omnivores." He then goes on to make this very revealing statement: "At the present time, there have been no cases of such cancer among those who are total vegetarians (vegans)."

Cancer, heart disease, high blood pressure—the list of meat-related diseases and illnesses—grows and grows. The true health benefits of vegetarianism, however, must be experienced to be fully appreciated. Not only does physical well-being increase dramatically along with new energy levels on a vegetarian diet, but emotional stability and mental equanimity are much more likely to occur when meat is no longer eaten.

The vegetarian diet has so many benefits that few ever think that it could have pitfalls or disadvantages. Yet there are aspects of vegetarianism that you should avoid.

88.3.3. The Vegetarian Trap

Vegetarianism has been vigorously promoted by many health schools. And for good reason, when you consider the alternatives of blood-letting, murdering, and corpse-gorging that meat eating offers. Yet is vegetarianism without its drawbacks, shortcomings, or traps for the unwary? We must answer: No. There are pitfalls for the health seeker who turns only to vegetarianism for his answers. Let's look at some of the traps that vegetarians must avoid.

88.3.4. Vegetarianism: Not Far Enough

Whenever someone asks me what Natural Hygienists or Life Scientists believe, I jokingly answer that "we're somewhere to the left of vegetarianism." The point I try to make is that while some people consider vegetarians "radical" health seekers, Natural Hygienists view them as only beginners on the path to radiant health and well-being.

Vegetarianism is only the first step to a better diet, although it is an important step. The major trap for vegetarians is that since they have changed their daily diet so radically from the standard meat-centered American diet, they often feel complacent and self-satisfied. They feel that they have done enough to improve their diet simply because they have stopped eating meat.

Unless vegetarians give up all animal products, eat a majority of their food uncooked and unprocessed, and practice food combining rules, they will be doomed to a much lower level of health than those who follow the teachings of Natural Hygiene and Life Science. In addition, vegetarians must also embark upon a regular program of exercise and fasting to complete the detoxification process of their bodies.

Vegetarianism is unequivocally recommended and urged for every human being alive today, and the world will doubtless be a much better place if all gave up slaughtering and killing for food. But, becoming a vegetarian is only a very small step forward from the masses of sick and diseased meat eaters. To become truly well, truly healed, and firmly established on the road to total health, you must go beyond vegetarianism. Do not become smug, self-complacent, or self-satisfied simply because you no longer eat meat—you still have a long way to go before your lifestyle is in harmony with the universe. This is the first trap that vegetarians must avoid: the belief that vegetarianism alone is enough to insure health and well-being.

88.3.5. Vegetarians People Love to Hate

Another trap that vegetarians must avoid is the feeling of separateness and aloofness that sometimes accompanies a change in diet. Here's a conversation I overheard while shopping at a supermarket in California:

"Hey, look at all those idiots waiting at the meat counter for their poison," a smirking man said to his wife.

"Yuck. I can't believe people eat baby animals and feed them to their kids too. I can smell the blood from here. I've got to get out of here. I can't believe people are so stupid about eating decaying meat," his wife agreed with him.

I passed by them and asked, "You must be vegetarians. How long have you stopped eating meat?"

The smart smiled proudly. "I quit six months ago. My wife ate fish only for the last two years, but now she's a veggie, too."

The couple deserved a medal on the spot. Imagine—no meat for six months! No doubt they would continue to insult friends, alienate relatives, and give vegetarians a bad name for another six months, until they found some other fad they could indulge in and feel superior about.

This is the second trap of vegetarianism: us and them. When people first become vegetarians, they often act obnoxious and supercilious. They think of themselves as us against them—the meat eaters. They often forget that one, two, or even ten years ago, they were also lined up at fast food joints, wolfing down hamburgers and hotdogs with all the other "idiots."

Vegetarians need humility, patience, and understanding of those who have not yet become vegetarians. The majority of people who practice vegetarianism in this country also once ate meat, and probably even more meat than most people in the world. Yet as soon as they give up their foul habit, they immediately start to proselytize and seek unwilling converts.

Being humble, patient, understanding, and forgiving does not mean that we should tolerate or accept meat eating as a viable alternative to a vegetarian diet. Make no mistake about it: the willing and conscious consumption of animals is wrong—morally and physiologically wrong. Yet, we must not become self-righteous or hypercritical of those who still eat meat. Kind compassion, sterling examples, and extended help and support are the qualities that will win others to vegetarianism and better health practices. Avoid the trap of self-righteous vegetarianism. Don't become the vegetarian or health fanatic that everyone loves to hate.

88.5. Questions & Answers

I'm a little confused about lacto-vegetarians and lacto-ovo-vegetarians. What do you call a vegetarian who eats fish?

A hypocrite. You probably wanted a better answer than that. In the last few years, it has become fashionable to be a vegetarian or to be concerned about one's diet and health. As a result, many more people are cutting back on the amounts of meat they eat. As soon as they eliminate pork or beef from their diet, these people usually proudly proclaim that they are vegetarians. They may continue to eat chicken or fish or perhaps they may eat meat only once a week or even once a year. They really aren't too sure what to call themselves, yet they feel they must make some distinction between themselves and those people who continue to eat large quantities of meat.

Vegetarianism is already such an overused and misused word that it can scarcely afford any more bending or abusing by these well-meaning but misguided souls. Perhaps we should call these people who eat only fish or chicken or meat irregularly "half-vegetarians" or "reforming carnivores." Their goal is admirable, but their loose play with the term "vegetarian" only creates confusion in the public's mind and does a disservice to those who are stronger in their beliefs and will avoid all meat.

Is there any good book that teaches someone how to be a vegetarian? How can we teach others about vegetarianism?

You don't have to do anything to become a vegetarian. You just have to stop doing one thing: eating animals. Many books that conspire to help others become vegetarians are often full of meat-substitute recipes and devote far too much attention to the protein question. Some of the literature makes it sound like vegetarianism is a long and difficult transition, fraught with dietary perils. It is a fact: over 90% of all books on vegetarianism are bought by people who are already vegetarians.

A book or article may help a person make the final decision to give up meat once and for all. However, the desire to become a vegetarian must arise within the person himself. You cannot "argue" anyone into becoming a vegetarian. After the decision is made, however, you can offer your own support and provide an excellent example of the health-promoting effects of the vegetarian diet.

I want to become a vegetarian, but my husband is dead against it. The kids aren't too crazy about giving up hamburgers, either. Help! I don't want to start a family crisis, and I hate cooking two different meals all the time.

If you can't solve a problem head-on, be clever. Your mistake may be that you are trying to confront or convert your family. Nobody likes to think that they have been wrong all their life, especially when it comes to something so basic as the diet. Your actions are making your family uncomfortable because now they must also re-examine their dietary beliefs and habits. Be patient with them.

First, you do not have to eat meat to please any of your family. It is possible to be the only vegetarian in a family of meat eaters. My advice is to gradually phase meat out from your family's table. Don't do this by offering them unfamiliar substitutes or "weird health foods." Instead, try to have more and more of their favorite meatless dishes. Use meat more as a condiment or seasoning when you cook for them. Don't make it a point to tell them how bad meat is; eating is an emotional experience, and rational arguments rarely sway anyone. Arguing will only reinforce their mistaken beliefs.

Above all else, be happy, cheerful, and positive about your new lifestyle. Radiate health and well-being. Set a good example and keep a sense of humor about yourself and your diet. Your spouse and children must decide on their own to stop eating meat; otherwise, the change may be only temporary and be made grudgingly. The good health and happiness that a vegetarian diet will afford you will eventually win over your family to your side. Be patient, persevere, and remain confident that you are totally correct in your decision and that only good will come from it.

Article #1: Fruitarianism and Vegetarianism by Dr. Herbert M. Shelton

Prior writings have made clear the superiority of the all-plant diet over the flesh diet or over the conventional mixed diet. A few things, however, remain to be said. In nature it is obvious that in "temperate" climes, at least, animals that rely upon the surplus stores of plants for their winter food have infinitely greater chances of survival than do the predacious animals who must rely upon the kill for their sustenance. The plant feeding animals thus have a great advantage over the flesh eaters. This advantage extends to many other features of life which need not be discussed here.

I do not intend to enter into any lengthy discussion of comparative anatomy and physiology at this place, but will content myself with saying that every anatomical, physiological and embryological feature of man definitely places him in the class frugivore. The number and structure of his teeth, the length and structure of his digestive tract, the position of his eyes, the character of his nails, the functions of his skin, the character of his saliva, the relative size of his liver, the number and position of the milk glands, the position and structure of the sexual organs, the character of the human placenta and many other factors all bear witness to the fact that man is constitutionally a frugivore.

As there are no pure frugivores, in that all frugivores eat freely of green leaves and other parts of plants, man may, also, without violating his constitutional nature, partake of green plants. These parts of plants possess certain advantages, as has been previously pointed out, in which fruits are deficient. Actual tests have shown that the addition of green vegetables to the fruit and nut diet improves the diet.

The vast majority of the human race has at all times been wholly or largely fruit and plant eaters. Human tribes that have lived exclusively upon meat and other animal foods have been exceedingly rare or nonexistent and have shorter life spans. Even Eskimo tribes eat some 24 kinds of mosses and litchens, including cloudberry, barberry, crowberry, reindeer moss and other plants, that grow in the Arctic. It is probable that more meat is eaten by man today than at any previous period in history. Civilization is based on vegetarianism—on agriculture and horticulture. Tribes that depend on hunting and herding do not remain stationary and do not build civilizations.

"When I go back," says Higgins in Anacalypsis II, page 147, "to the most remote periods of antiquity which it is possible to penetrate, I find clear and positive evidence of several important facts: First, no animal food was eaten, no animals were sacrificed."

Origenes has left us the record that "the Egyptians would prefer to die, rather than become guilty of the crime of eating any kind of flesh."

Herodotus tells us that the Egyptians subsisted on fruits and vegetables, which they ate raw. Plinius confirms this statement. Harold Whitestone, in his The Private Lives of the Romans, says: "Of the Romans it may be said that during the early Republic perhaps almost through the second century B.C., they cared little for the pleasures of the table. They lived frugally and ate sparingly. They were almost strict vegetarians, much of their food was eaten cold, and the utmost simplicity characterized the cooking and the service of their meals."

It was only after the conquest of Greece that the Romans altered their table customs and became a luxury-loving, meat-eating people. Even then the poorer classes lived frugally and, as Whitestone says, "every schoolboy knows that the soldiers who won Caesar's battles for him lived on grain which they ground in their hand mills and baked at their campfires."

Isis, one of the best beloved of Egyptian goddesses, was thought by them to have taught the Egyptians the art of bread making from the cereals theretofore growing wild and unused, the earlier Egyptians having lived upon fruits, roots, and herbs. The worship of Isis was universal throughout Egypt and magnificent temples were dedicated to her. Her priests, consecrated to purity, were required to wear linen garments, unmixed with animal fiber, to abstain from all animal food and from those vegetables regarded as impure—beans, onions, garlic, and leeks.

Island tribes have existed who had no access to flesh food and there are several peoples who abstain from meat on religious grounds. We find this so in China, India, Turkey and among the Essenes in Ancient Palestine. The Spartans were forbidden to eat meat and, like the priests of Isis, were forbidden to eat beans. There are sects in India the members of which are still forbidden to eat beans.

Hindhede has shown that on the whole health and length of life are greater among vegetarians than among meat-eating peoples. McCarrison has shown that the better nourished fruit-eating Hunzas of North India are the equal in health, strength, freedom from disease and in length of life of any people on earth.

Vegetarian athletes have won honors in more than one field. Indeed, where great endurance is required they almost always win. Many thousands of invalids have turned from a mixed diet to a vegetarian or fruitarian diet and have, thereby, saved their lives, even where they were unable to restore themselves to vigorous health.

A surgeon on the staff of the Bone and Joint Hospital, New York City, who has had a wide experience among vegetarians, told me that vegetarian women give birth to their babies very quickly, "drop them like animals" with less pain, and recuperate very quickly. He added that when he gets a call to attend a childbirth in a vegetarian woman, he wastes no time, but rushes to her bedside and frequently arrives only to find the baby born before he gets there. He also stated that wounds heal more quickly in vegetarians than others. The surgeon himself is not a vegetarian.

A surgeon here in San Antonio, who has handled deliveries for several mothers that the writer has cared for through their pregnancies, once remarked to me: "When I am called to care for a parturient woman that you have fed I know there are going to be no complications and everything will go as it should, but when I am called to care for a woman who eats in the conventional way, I never know what will happen."

Professor Richet found that fruits and vegetables do not induce serum diseases (anaphylaxis), while flesh foods do and interprets his findings to mean that nature vetoes certain proteins, chiefly animal, as unsuitable. Certainly, no meat, meat juice or eggs should ever be fed to a child under seven or eight years of age. It has no power to neutralize the poisons from these until this time.

Auto-intoxication and liability to infection are less in vegetarian and fruitarian than in animal feeders: many of the latter scarcely defending themselves at all, but tamely submitting to parasitic imposition.

Tacitus tells us that the ancient Orientals refused to eat swine flesh because they were afraid of contracting leprosy if they consumed the animal that served them as a scavenger. Bacon is particularly resistant to the digestive secretions, its fat markedly slowing down gastric digestion. Bouchard found that solutions prepared from the stools of meat eaters are twice as toxic as those prepared from the stools of non-flesh eaters. Herter, of New York, observed that animals are killed quickly by solutions from the stools of carnivorous animals, but do not die of similar solutions prepared from stools of herbivorous animals.

It is quite evident that the greater toxicity of decomposed flesh foods would give rise to more severe types of diseases, should the putrefaction occur in the stomach and intestine, where absorption can occur. This perhaps accounts for the frequent development of cancer and other serious pathologies in meat eaters.

In his presidential address before Section 1 of the British Association, 1913, Professor Gowland Hopkins pointed out in connection with certain important protein reactions, that the carnivore behaves differently from the herbivore, the latter showing greater powers of synthesis and defense. As regards purity, stability and reliability, plant substances offer to man proteins and carbohydrates that are superior to those derived from flesh foods. It is known that in fruit and nut eating natives wounds heal much more rapidly than they do in flesh-eating Europeans.

There is evidence to show that vegetarians and fruitarians live longer than flesh eaters. Advocates of the flesh diet attempt to counter this evidence by pointing to the short life span of the peoples of India. In doing so they ignore all of the other factors of life that help to determine length of life. India is a land of immense wealth and the home of one-fifth of the world's population. She possesses natural resources rivaling those of the United States. But these resources are undeveloped, the wealth is in the hands of a very few, while her millions are poverty stricken. India has been ruled by foreign exploiters who take from her a great share of what should be used to clothe, feed, and house her teeming population. Ninety percent of her people are illiterate, only thirty-nine percent of her people are well nourished while 80,000,000 of them are perpetually hungry. Besides, many people don't have knowledge of, or access to, proper sanitation. Under similar conditions of filth, poverty, overcrowding, ignorance, hunger and malnutrition, meat-eating Europe during the Middle Ages had a much shorter life span. This contrast of meat eaters with vegetarians living under similar conditions presents a brighter picture for the vegetarians.

The unfitness of certain classes of substances as foods is evident from the frequency with which anaphylactic phenomena follow their use. The more closely these substances resemble the flesh of the body, the more unfit they are as foods. Thus, flesh is the worst offender, eggs are next, and milk is last. Cancer and anaphylaxis have much in common inasmuch as they are both due to protein poisoning. Indeed, chronic latent anaphylaxis may be the long-sought cancer virus.

Although cancer is a meat-eater's disease, we do occasionally hear of a vegetarian dying of cancer. In nearly all such cases the vegetarian is descended from meat eaters and became a vegetarian late in life. In such cases the inherited diathesis is simply too strong to be countered by the haphazard food reform so often resorted to. Many of these "vegetarians" are really so in name only, eating fish, chicken and other flesh "non meats" regularly.

The man or woman who becomes a haphazard or a partial vegetarian and then only after some serious impairment of health has forced the change, a kind of eleventh-hour repentance, will not always find salvation.

A pretty picture of how "vegetarians" are made to have cancer is presented in Dr. (M.D.) Louis Westerna Sanborn's account of cancer among the "vegetarian" Italians of Sambucci. Incidentally, in the course of his account, he makes it known that these "vegetarians" are pork eaters and wine bibbers—habits that have persisted since the days of ancient Rome. If the foes of vegetarianism are forced to hold up such examples of cancerous "vegetarians" in their efforts to show that vegetarians do have cancer, they are, indeed, driven into hiding.

I agree with Dr. John Round that (he vegetarian argument, like the cause of temperance has suffered from its friends. Pointing out that cancer increase synchronizes with the advance of meat eating, he says: "Amongst the Polynesians and Melanesians cancer is almost unknown, and these races are practically vegetarian; in Egypt cancer is seldom or never found amongst the black races; in South Africa the Boers and Europeans are largely meat eaters and suffer frequently from cancer, whilst the natives who are largely vegetarians seldom so suffer."

Article #2: Are Humans Meat-Eaters?

"Meat" is the dead flesh of animals, fish, or birds.

Putrefaction (decay) begins in all flesh from the moment of death.

This process of decomposition results in various poisons collecting in the dead animal tissue.

Most cases of food poisoning are the result of eating bad meat or meat products, i.e., canned meat, shellfish, etc.

The longer the time from the death of your meat to your mouth, the more dangerous it is to you.

Meat contains a high proportion of cholesterol (an important causative factor in thrombosis, high blood pressure etc.) with no lecithin (nature's antidote) to balance it. (All vegetable proteins, on the other hand, contain lecithin to naturally counterbalance it!)

Meat is not a suitable item of diet for the human being for the following anatomical and physiological reasons:

• Flesh-eating mammals have a short bowel to enable them to expel rapidly the putrefactive flesh, while man has a long and complicated alimentary tract to enable plant nutrients to be slowly and properly taken up.

• Flesh eaters have a different type of intestinal bacteria from the non-meat eaters. Man falls into the second category.

• Flesh eaters have long and sharp teeth. Man has the teeth of the grain eaters. (Fruit, cereals, vegetables, nuts.)

• Man can 'grind' with his jaws, flesh eaters cannot. Their jaws move up and down only.

• Man, the horse, cow, antelope, and monkey family all sweat through their skins. All flesh eaters sweat through their tongues.

• Man sucks his liquids—carnivores all lap.

• Man's saliva contains ptyalin (to commence starch digestion)—flesh-eating animals have no ptyalin.

• Carnivores have large livers, but man has only a comparatively small one.

• Flesh eaters secrete into their stomachs 10 times the hydrochloric acid as do non-flesh eaters, in order to cope with quantities of meat, bone, feathers, sinews, and so on.

The flesh eater takes nourishment from parts of the whole beast—not just muscle meat as man does.

Man, seldom eats raw meat. He has to cook it first so as to disguise it from the corpse it really is.

Meat eating is one of the links in the chains of addiction. Being a stimulating food (hence the sense of "strength" that meat eaters talk about so often) it demands complementary stimulation from such things as wine, brandy, cigars, drugs, tea, coffee, cigarettes, etc. Meat becomes 'dull' without alcohol and alcohol 'demands' meat— they go together.

Meat eating is also wasteful in that slaughter cattle live first upon a vegetable diet (grass, etc.) and their flesh is therefore only grass second-hand. Although the whole of their bodies are not consumed, they have still to be fed and grown upon land which might otherwise be growing food for starving humans.

Anyone who wishes to visit a slaughterhouse can decide for himself whether there is any pain, suffering or cruelty involved in the meat industry. This is perpetuated by eating meat.

The meat eater is directly responsible for the continued employment of fellow human beings in an ignoble occupation.

Most of the meat today is raised in pitiful, inhuman conditions. These unfortunate beasts are raised in tiny, cramped cells where they live in darkness and the stench of their own droppings from birth to the slaughterhouse.

Meat is acid-forming in the bloodstream and lays down the foundation for such degenerative conditions as arthritis; rheumatism, diabetes, arteriosclerosis and probably cancer.

In his book, How to Avoid Cancer, the well-known writer Fraser McKenzie quotes from eminent medical men who show that disease, in general, diminishes in those communities where there is little, or no flesh eaten. Also, that in the Western world, the disease rate rises in almost direct proportion to the amount of meat eaten. Vegetarian communities are free of such diseases as cancer, nephritis, arteriosclerosis, thrombosis, etc. The evidence is all there for the reading.

In this brief survey we have barely touched upon the 'humanitarian' aspect of this subject but defy anyone to show how meat eating is compatible with any doctrine of kindness, compassion, gentleness, and love.

Lesson 89:

Introducing Clients to the Need for a Lifestyle Change

89.1. What Do You Mean by "Change in Lifestyle?"

89.1.1. False Ideas Restrain

89.1.2. Where Life Exists, Possibility Is

In the context of this lesson, we will understand the concept of change in lifestyle to include those changes in both living and eating habits which are deemed by the practitioner as being essential for the restoration and maintenance of whatever level of health the present condition of the client will allow.

The client, guided by a knowledgeable practitioner, will be encouraged to leave the old ways that have failed him in the past and embark upon a new path, one designed especially for him but one which is based upon the known laws of life, so that he can more fully realize his birth potential.

The client must be given to understand that he will be required to make some changes; that he will have to discard many of his former familiar, but false, beliefs and habits which cumulatively and progressively were responsible for his present unfortunate condition, whatever these may have been; that he will now be required to adopt more scientifically accurate, biologically appropriate (but, perhaps to him, somewhat strange) ways of eating and living.

It is important at the very beginning of a new relationship with a client to establish the fact that superb health is normal and that any deviation therefrom is totally and perhaps even inexcusably abnormal, being the result of certain errors in living and eating. He should be given to understand that some changes will necessarily have to be made abruptly and quickly; others perhaps less so, depending on what degree of health he wishes to achieve, and how fast.

The client must be brought to an understanding that superb health is a possible goal, but one that can be achieved only as certain changes are made to meet the structural and functional needs of the living body, sick or well, these being dictated solely by the nature of the human body, the way it is put together; by its ability to adapt slowly or rapidly, to change; and by the fact that the present condition of the client, whatever that may be, is the result of how well, or how poorly, these needs have been met during his lifetime.

The client must develop an understanding that superb health is a possible goal, one that he can achieve just as surely as hundreds of thousands of persons equally ill have done in the past and are presently doing, once they came to realize that they had to make certain biologically approved changes and then proceeded, always with careful guidance, to make them as and when required and as rapidly as individual circumstances warranted.

We must be able to convince our clients that we have either ourselves witnessed and/ or learned about people just like them, through our research, who left the old ways of eating and living, the old ways of sickness, fatigue and premature death, and embarked on a new adventure which required certain adjustments on their part, new ways of thinking, definitive changes, some difficult to make but most actually quite easy and, in the doing, found to their great joy and personal satisfaction, that they had accomplished exactly what they had set out to do: they had attained their personal goal, they had even improved their health to an extent far beyond their earlier hopes.

Many began as physical wrecks and without hope but, before long, they had become eager participants in a manner of living and eating that they were now convinced, because of their happy results, would bring them full recuperation and regeneration of body, mind, and spirit. And, given sufficient time, they fulfilled their dream.

Those who intelligently recognized the need to make the necessary changes and then subsequently followed through in the doing, successfully overcame arthritis, depression, obesity, acne, breast tumors, asthma, and a whole dictionary of affections, many deemed by the "authorities" as being "incurable."

89.1.1. False Ideas Restrain

False ideas, old health-destroying habits, the disorders of life, drugs of all kinds, and all excess, these must all be cast aside in favor of new ways, new habits, new foods that encourage body building. Order and restraint must enter and become incorporated into the life plan, but there must come, also, a sense of adventure, of excitement, an awareness of one's living body, a deep inner conviction that, as the ways of health replace the ways of disease, suffering and death, superb health will follow as naturally as the stars come out at night to glow and grace the darkened sky after the day has been spent.

89.1.2. Where Life Exists, Possibility Is

The professional practitioner must remember and convey to his most seriously-ill clients that where life exists, possibility is and will remain. This attitude must place the despair that so often pervades the mind and restrains progress. Tell your clients, in advance, if need be, that it is possible to foretell or predict what an individual body is capable of achieving when it is provided with the necessary wherewithal of life. Change in attitude may well be the most important change the more seriously-ill person needs to make. So many have had all hope taken away£ from them by one person or another or by one defeat after another, and the future looks dark. Just as the carpenter requires the tools of his trade to build a worthy structure, so must they receive the necessary nutrients of life to restore them to health and, thereafter, to maintain it in full capacity. It must be made clear to all clients that, in order to reach that longed-for goal of full health, change must become a part of their daily living, and not a once-in-a-while thing.

The changes of which we speak are, of course, by the very nature of the life process, all based singly and separately on the basic requisites of organic existence already delineated in this course. Each and every one, without exception, must be incorporated into the lifestyle of the sick and the well, as need and capacity so indicate. These requisites should be set forth by the practitioner in a pattern for performance that is deemed appropriate for each client as his individual capacity to accept and utilize may warrant at the time, and adjusted as forward progress is made.

We must convey to the client that the body is a unitized whole and that we cannot neglect any single aspect of living unless we either completely destroy or limit the whole and that only as all the requisites of life, known and unknown, are incorporated into the life script in amounts appropriate to each individual, depending upon his present state of health, will wellness of one cell and all cells together, the totality, be achieved.

89.2. The Need to Inspire the Client

89.2.1. Establishing the Goals

89.2.2. Attitudes Are Contagious

89.2.3. Keeping on Target

89.2.4. Veras's Story

89.2.1. Establishing the Goals

In order to obtain maximum cooperation and subsequent performance, to say nothing of reaping the rewards of correct eating and living on the part of the client, it will be necessary for the practitioner to convince the client that following the regimen that you recommend to him will benefit him in ways which are, to a certain extent, predictable well in advance and, to a certain extent, with a fair degree of accuracy.

Predictability is so because we humans are basically the same. We possess gross details that are quite similar, it is only in the minor ones that we differ. Therefore, when we behave in a manner contrary to our fundamental needs, we can predict with surety that the health of the totality will diminish and in an exactly equal amount. But, the opposite is true, also for when we answer our body's fundamental needs, and do so in all respects, the body responds by discarding the old in favor of the new; in other words, like the contractor called to make repairs on a dilapidated building who must first tear down before he can rebuild with new and better materials so, too, must sick persons discard, before they can rebuild!

89.2.2. Attitudes Are Contagious

Attitudes are contagious, so it is important for the practitioner to present the possible benefits which can accrue to the client in an enthusiastic and convincing manner. In other words, as practitioners we should avoid the "pie in the sky" approach in favor of more reasonable immediate goals, one's attainable, in most instances, fairly easily and within a comparatively short time.

These goals can range from the physical (the elimination of certain rather minor digestive troubles, for example), the cosmetic (losing that look of utter fatigue that so many of our clients wear on their first visit), and even economic (no longer required to buy this or that drug or prosthetic gadget).

The list of possible benefits, of course, could be extensive, but several, comparatively easily attainable, immediate goals can and should be established initially and then, others advanced from time to time as the need for further encouragement may arise.

89.2.3. Keeping on Target

Sometimes clients require being reminded of where they have been, where they are now, and where they are going; kept on target, as it were. Presenting the little goals, the "baby steps" we so often talk about, can usually convey to the client sufficient inspiration to keep him following the straight path to complete freedom from disease and suffering.

The client should be told that you, the teacher, will provide him with the necessary training to enable him eventually to "go it alone," and this, too, in a relatively short period of time; that he will be able to overcome whatever problem is troubling him on his own without having recourse to his former "run-to-the-doctor syndrome."

It will be necessary from time to time to discuss with the client the importance of his becoming so knowledgeable about the science of life (Natural Hygiene) that he will feel confident to "go it alone," to take charge of his own Self. This concept, of course, should be discussed preferably before he experiences his first healing crisis, or else he may become completely confused or even disillusioned.

89.2.4. Veras's Story

The case of Vera illustrates this last point beautifully. Vera, a woman in her early 50s, was suffering from a very bad bronchial disorder which had troubled her for well over 15 years. In addition to the lung involvement, she experienced angina "attacks" from time to time. The doctor had told her she had a severely weakened heart muscle and must be careful not to "overdo."

Vera's medications consisted of nitroglycerine tablets, antibiotics, steroids from time to time (prednisone), and digoxin, all of which she took from time to time as directed by the family physician. Additionally, on her own, she took a multitude of vitamins and had done so for years. In spite of all her "treatments" and the various medications, prescription and nonprescription, her energy level remained dangerously low, and her ankles and legs remained swollen with edema. Vera was a very discouraged woman.

Vera had been referred to us by a pastoral counselor in whom she had much confidence and, since she was already seemingly convinced that the medical "treatments" offered had failed her in the past and were certainly not helping her now, she had agreed to "try" Natural Hygiene.

At our initial meeting, we reviewed Vera's eating diary which, as suggested, she had kept for the previous two weeks. It was obvious, of course, that most of this client's troubles were the result of a lifetime of incorrect feeding habits, and that a primary need was to detoxify her body.

However, we learned that her husband, Joe, was suffering from severe mental depression, caused no doubt from worry about his wife's condition. He had been forced to take a temporary leave of absence from his work. Under the circumstances, Vera felt that it would be inadvisable for her to go to a fasting retreat at this time.

Therefore, it was necessary to move in another direction. Accordingly, we explained to our client that we had no doubts that she could improve her health status and to a considerable extent by making some, at first rather simple, changes, these to be followed at a future time by other changes, as warranted from time to time. We sensed that Vera did not feel inclined to make any radical changes for fear of upsetting her already concerned husband and driving him, perhaps, into an even deeper depression. We emphasized, however, that doing it this way, making small changes slowly, would require considerably more time than it would if fasting had been the program of choice. Vera agreed that this was the way she must take. She would see what the future would bring.

We introduced our client to the seven stages in the biological evolution of pathology. She immediately saw the sequence of events as they had transpired in her own and in her husband's lives. She recounted for us some of her own past symptoms and history and we discussed how they seemed to suggest this or that stage. She enthusiastically grasped the concept that it was possible for her to retrace the various stages in this biological evolution and that, in so doing, her energy and general health would gradually improve. In passing, we commented that, during the retracement, it is often possible for certain persons to relive the past; that is, they may be called upon to experience some of their earlier symptoms as hidden pockets of poison are flushed out of their hiding places from time to time. Vera indicated that she understood this possibility and thought this might reasonably be expected.

However, apparently we failed to make a deep enough impression on Vera at this initial presentation and the subject did not immediately come up again. Things went along exceptionally well for some time. Vera was able consistently to reduce her drug intake, the nitroglycerine being completely set aside and the antibiotics, also. No steroids were now used, and the digoxin was considerably reduced. As for the vitamins, they became a thing of memory only.

The coughing up of mucus became less troublesome, her vitality level grew enabling her to participate in the activities of her beloved church, the digestive upsets that had plagued her for many years were all but forgotten and, all in all, both Vera and we were well pleased with ourselves.

Then it happened! A violent attack of coughing. Mucus poured out of Vera's throat gagging and choking her. She gasped for breath. She panicked. Dr. Ralph Cinque, in a lecture on June 27, 1979, reminded us that "The asthmatic often becomes terrified because of his wheezing and gasping for breath, sometimes feeling as though his life is at stake which naturally alarms anyone concerned. However, only occasionally is a person's respiratory obstruction so great that this is the case. Most of the time the attack is not nearly so bad as the victim might think." [From Overcoming Asthma by Beth Snodgrass. Available from Life Science.]

We had not prewarned Vera of this possibility. So, the "run-to-the-doctor syndrome" grasped ahold of Vera's mind and, almost instinctively, like a well-trained animal obeys its master, Vera trotted off to the very doctor who had failed her for over fifteen years!

She was immediately placed in the hospital where she was given a variety of tests, including X rays and scans, and plied with all manner of drugs.

The cough went away, and the mucus dried up, just as they had throughout the years past. The drugs accomplished their purpose: the nerves were narcotized, the symptoms suppressed. Vera remained in the hospital for nine days and then returned home, weak and spent. The "attack" had cost her well over $11,000!

Sometime later, a wan and weary Vera presented herself in our office once again. She recounted her story, exclaiming at the end, "What a fool I was!" She had finally remembered our telling her about what might occur as she retraced the former stages in the evolution of pathology on her journey back to health. She stated the events and the confirmation of knowledge simply. The conviction of truth was reflected both in her manner and in her eyes as she exclaimed, "I was just having a healing crisis, wasn't I?

Vera, you see, had not failed. We, her practitioners, had failed. We had failed to explain in simple terms BEFORE THE EVENT, and often from time to time as a reminder of what might possibly happen as retracement begins and accelerates.

There were other healing crises to follow, but now Vera was able to take them each in stride because she now fully understood the nature of a healing crisis and what, except in very exceptional circumstances, she could do on her own to remedy the situation. She understood now that her body was always in a state of flux, of change, and was so more now than ever before; that when a healing crisis came, she should keep warm and just stand aside and let the wisdom resident within her own body take charge and get on with the healing of hurting cells while she watched and waited and rested, confident in the final outcome.

We saw Vera not too long ago. She is still too thin but both she and Joe are on a clear path, a Hygiene path, that will lead them together to a life of great joy and boundless energy for living and extended and purposeful life. Vera and Joe are now "going it on their own." It has been some years now since Vera made her last trip to any doctor's office and she is confident now that she will never have to enter another hospital, unless compelled to do so by some unforeseen accidental injury that may require perhaps the services of an orthopedic surgeon. Changes were required in Vera's lifestyle, and she has successfully made all adjustments in philosophy and in practice. We are certain now that Vera will not panic again.

89.3. The Practitioner Presents the Plan

Clients must be convinced that the practitioner in charge is designing a program specifically tailored to meet their precise needs, one that will enable them to assume full responsibility for their own care and well-being, thus removing them from all necessity to depend any longer on the medical establishment for pills and potions that serve only to poison.

The capable practitioner must teach clients Natural Hygiene's rules of life and convince them that, by following the simple Hygienic ways of eating and living, they will gradually find their own aches and pains either considerably diminished or even no longer existent; that their impaired and troubled digestive and other afflictions will soon become but a memory. They must come to an understanding, by presentation of or the experiencing of evidential results, that it is possible for them to see their own energy levels soar to heights perhaps unknown since earliest childhood; that they may even experience once again the joy of sleeping undisturbed the whole night through and being able to awaken at dawn with vigor renewed, ready to meet the challenges and problems of each new day. But, for all this to happen, change is not only suggested, but mandatory.

89.4. The Client Must Be in Charge

89.4.1. Millie's Story

Clients must be responsible for making all changes. It must and should be made clear to them that they will be in charge of their own lives and that they will thus be designing their own future. Before they sought relief, but they gained no health. Now, they must make changes because they have a new goal, the attainment of a higher level of health. They must be brought to an understanding of the most important reality of life: that they can FREE THEMSELVES of all their sick cares and concerns as well as from the financial burden that being sick imposed upon them, a burden which kept them from enjoying many of the simpler pleasures of life; and that all this wonderful new world can be theirs by making some simple changes in their manner of eating and living, changes which have proved in the past throughout all of history to be health-building, changes which will replace their former health-destroying habits, changes which will soon bring them an abundantly rich life instead of their present half-life of sickness and suffering, one filled with the specter of premature death.

As a specialist in Life Science, this is what you have to offer and what they have to gain: a life without pain and complete freedom from all sickness and disease. But they must be made to understand that the new trip is not free, that no one can accomplish these promised and highly fortuitous results FOR them, that they must do it ALL ON THEIR OWN and that many changes may be required of them.

Furthermore, just as walking the sickness road can be a very lonely walk, indeed, just so, travelling the road to health must necessarily often cause one to desert the herd and be somewhat lonely, too. But, and this is what must be emphasized, WITH A HAPPY DIFFERENCE!

The sickness road is one filled with pain and suffering. It is a downward trek that" leads to more involved pathology and eventually, more often than not, to a life filled with untold agony and unpredictable pathologies. In contrast, the Hygienic life script unfolds like a happy drama and opens up a joy-filled road where there is no pain, no suffering. It is an upward path that can expand the mind, ripen the senses, open new doors, impart an expanded spiritual awareness of the meaning of life, and often provide an opportunity to help others to know the joys of living the Hygienic way. In other words, by proving himself amenable to change by the doing, the client can find a new purpose for living and, as always, with purpose comes performance and with performance in the arena of life, as contrasted with the lonely life of pain, all loneliness leaves, never to return.

Lastly, our clients must also comprehend that it has taken time and many mistakes, both known and unknown, to change the potential they possessed at birth to whatever state of diminished health they are presently experiencing, and that it will also take time to achieve whatever level of health is now possible considering the client's age, his present condition, his residual vitality and how well he follows the Hygienic road, and that sometimes the amount of time required will be more than we either like or anticipate.

However, clients should be assured, and this from time to time, that with each improvement, the speed of recovery will begin to accelerate, the healing crises will become less frequent and less severe, until finally they are no more. The ultimate goal will then have been reached and the, improved health level thereafter need only be maintained. The changes will, at that point, no longer be necessary, because they have become a part of one's natural life plan.

89.4.1. Millie's Story

Millie learned all of the foregoing the hard way. She came to us originally with a severely-impacted colon, diagnosed as a spastic colon. It had been years since she had had a normal movement. Enemas and cathartics, headaches and extreme lassitude were all a way of life with Millie.

She hated her life. She hated the constant fatigue that prevented her from doing so many of the things she wanted to do. A divorcee, she said that the constant enema-taking and the fatigue kept her from having any fun! She was only 42 years of age.

We explained to Millie that the enemas and the cathartics were her "crutches" and that, so long as she continued to use her crutches, she would never be able to "go it alone." She would always, forever after, require her crutches. The pills and potions were not removing the cause(s) of her trouble and, indeed, only served to add to them. These substances were all chemical poisons and, by using them, she was simply adding more poison to all the poisons resident within her own body. It was this poison that had caused and was continuing to cause her problems. Adding poison to poison would only serve further to kill more cells and to reduce even more the tone of the muscles of her digestive tract. If she continued their use, she might well never again be able to have a normal bowel movement. We told her that it would be necessary for her to make some changes in her manner of eating and living, that she must now, as one of our students from Kentucky recently remarked, "make getting the finest food her most important priority."

Like so many others, some successful, some not, Millie agreed to "try" Natural Hygiene. We explained why she should restrict her diet choices to the finest of natural raw foods, why she should now begin a regular and vigorous exercise program, why she should increase her rest and sleep periods, why she must now drink distilled water and when. In fact, we laid out a precise program for our client to follow, a step-by-step plan of action.

Millie took over and did extremely well. She followed the regimen laid out for her, making few mistakes. As a matter of fact, Millie became so imbued with enthusiasm about her program and her progress that she began to preach Natural Hygiene to all and sundry who would listen.

As her reward, within three months, Millie was having a natural bowel movement (bm) two and three times a week! This was like a miracle to her. After a year, all the digestive disorders of the past had practically disappeared; the heaviness, the excess gas, the occasional nausea, and belching, these were no longer any concern. Millie was once again going here and there, having the "good time" she had so yearned for. Rarely now did she have to have recourse to an enema.

At the end of the second year, the bms were coming almost every day. Once in a great while, but only rarely, Millie would have one of her former trying headaches. But, she wasn't satisfied, she wanted it all and NOW! She felt she needed two or more bms every single day and felt annoyed when such did not happen. She wanted to be rid of her headaches once and for all and forever. She wanted someone to wave the magic wand!

Without consulting us, Millie went to another practitioner, not a Hygienist, and enrolled in a "course of treatments" which were to take away all her cares in one magic moment. The cost of this series of muscle and bone adjustments, as we learned later, was

$1,500.00!

Well, a short time ago, Millie came back. The practitioner, at her request, provided us with his assessment of her progress. To Millie's chagrin and astonishment, the erstwhile waver of the magic wand was not $1,500.00 richer but, sadly, "disappointed" in Millie's "lack of progress." The "treatments" had failed.

We reminded a rather chastened Millie once again that there is no magic wand, that healing takes time; that not we, but our bodies are in charge. It is our inner wisdom, not we, that must be in control. We humans make too many mistakes when left on our own to be in charge of such responsibility. Our inner wisdom is so designed that it does not make mistakes and cannot just be diverted from its tasks by our whims and wishes. Just so long as we cooperate with that inner wisdom by supplying the correct tools, as and when required and in the proper amounts, meaningful progress will be made. Health will happen. Unhealthful ways of living always demand a toll of disease but abundant health follows in the wake of correct practices.

On its own, our inner wisdom will establish the necessary priorities, determine how these may best be addressed, lay out the plan, the ways and means, with exact directions and specifications; and then address each in its own manner and at the appropriate time. We are required only to provide the tools, then step aside and watch the magic within unfold.

Millie sat quietly, deep in thought as we quietly reminded her of this wisdom of the ages. She didn't have much to say, but we knew that Millie had learned a valuable lesson. Millie will wait now for time to bring its miracle.

Encouraging words help clients when the way gets tough. Knowledge and understanding can inspire the necessary changes both in practice and thinking. Clients must grasp the concept that health is, for them, indeed, a possible goal; that Natural Hygiene (Life Science) provides the ways and means of achieving superb health. We need to impart to our clients the confidence that you, as a practitioner, will teach the client how to live according to the laws of life and how to provide the tools for always living in health. If we can cause our clients to believe that they can be in complete charge of their own lives and that they can work this miracle, then we will be instrumental in bringing about the required changes. And then, too if we can bring to them full understanding of the fact that their former dependence on the medical community was not only totally nonproductive, but actually destructive of life, then we are to be commended for that is the first important change.

A client must realize, and deeply, that it will take time to accomplish the healing and to restore whatever level of health s/he is presently capable of achieving and that the results will depend on how well s/he follows directions. All diseased persons differ only in the degree of involvement and the site. All can respond favorably to health-building ways, but they must not wait beyond the physiological point of no return. In other words, there is a limit beyond which full recovery is impossible. This, too, is a change in thinking because, for so long, they have depended on that "magic" pill or, if that fails, upon some fantastic operation that they believe will remedy the hurt.

89.5. What Kinds of Changes Are Required

The kinds of changes which must be identified for the client will, of course, vary from individual to individual but, surprisingly, they almost always fall into the following categories:

1. Doing away with certain outmoded beliefs and superstitions that can only serve to hamper maintenance of full health or perhaps even to destroy it, if it is now present.

2. Causing a change in attitude through knowledge about the kinds of habits and practices in eating and lifestyle that are recognized as being destructive to health.

3. Developing a deep conviction about the need for the changes recommended by the practitioner, this obtained through knowledge of what is believed to be essential to health maintenance.

4. The introduction of positive action through practice, gradually or abruptly, as individual situations and conditions warrant, eliminating all destructive habits and replacing them with Hygienic, truly scientific, practices known to be instrumental in building health, not disease.

89.6. Outmoded Beliefs and Superstitions

89.6.1. Mike's Story

89.6.2. Other Superstitions

89.6.3. The Case of Rev. Kim

Most people today are mere puppets dangling at the end of strings, skillfully manipulated by self-serving corporate interests.

For example, there are few Americans today who are not complete and willing serfs to the medico-drug-insurance complex. As we look around at our own friends, relatives and neighbors, we find that everyone, almost without exception, goes regularly to a physician for a check-up, even though many physicians openly acknowledge that this is worthless. We recall years ago reading an article in the Long Beach newspaper, an article written by various physicians, which said, in effect, that such trips were a waste of money and meaningless, that nobody was perfect and that they were simply a means to an end, getting people to come on a regular basis to the physician of choice; and it did help to pay the rent!

Most people we know dutifully swallow their prescribed pills, submit to X rays at the slightest suggestion of "their" doctor, would never fail to keep their medical lifeline (their insurance policies) up to date, and grasp at the medical man every time they have the slightest ache or pain. Each one seems to be content with his "allergies" and his pills, having full confidence that somehow, in some way, "the doctors will find a 'cure' for whatever happens to ail him and the rest of suffering humankind."

Just last week a friend sat in our family room and told how he had gladly and willingly volunteered himself as a guinea-pig for a mass experiment to test certain drugs proposed as a possible "cure" for diabetes. The group sponsoring this mass experiment with other people's lives had apparently just received a multi-million-dollar grant.

We gasped in horror at his news. There he sat at least 50 pounds overweight, highly flushed of face, wheezing, and coughing as he talked—a prime candidate for a stroke, the mark of the needle plainly visible on his forearm. We inquired as to the nature of the injected drug. He didn't know, other than that it was some NEW drug that "they" hoped would soon prove its merit.

We asked our friend, "Why?" Why had he let himself be injected by any chemical, to say nothing of permitting an unknown and untried substance, about which he knew nothing, to be introduced into his bloodstream? Did he not realize that introducing any foreign substance into the blood could, almost instantaneously, lead to anaphylactic shock, with instant death a distinct possibility? Our friend nodded his head. He agreed that Yes, all that could happen but, "You see," he thoughtfully went on to say, "Unless all of us help these doctors, they never will find the cures for all these diseases." Like a puppet on a string, he had responded to the siren call of "Cure!"

Hygienists know that all this is pure hum-bug, anti-health, and anti-scientific nonsense. They also know that this trust in the medical community and in their drugs dies hard. In the back of the head of almost every new client who comes to you for help will remain the thought that if THIS (meaning you) fails, he can always hurry back to the known and familiar ways of medicine.

Thus, the Hygienist must point his client in a new direction. He must prove that all drugs are anti-health. He must remind his clients, when the issue arises, as it will, that the medical community has had over 30 centuries to prove that drugs and their methods are instrumental in curing disease and that, in every instance, they have failed. Drugs and surgery cure nothing.

Clients must change their minds and, accordingly, their practices in this respect. All drugs are anti-health and so acknowledged by the very persons who prescribe them. They are known to damage the nervous structure and actually to destroy cells. Drugs suppress symptoms but remove no cause. Clients must further understand that surgery removes an effect, but not the cause and unless, and until, the cause or causes are removed, the effect, the disease, will not only remain, even though temporarily abated, but will worsen. This, too, is an important change in thinking that every client must make before he can expect to improve his health.

It is true that most of the people who seek the help of a Life Scientist will be somewhat, if not totally, disillusioned about the effectiveness of medicines, at least in their case, even before they seek our help.

But, we should be aware of the fact that most of them know nothing whatsoever, or perhaps only a very little, about natural ways of healing. What you suggest to them is all foreign territory, a vast unknown, and like pioneers setting out for a new land, they have hope, but little else, because they presently lack knowledge.

It is the practitioner's job, if s/he, can, to drive the nail into the coffin, to bury all faith in medicines and surgery as the way to health. We must get across to our clients the relationship between cause and effect. Our clients must be brought by us into an understanding of the scientific sense of removing cause before they can reasonably expect once again to know health. They must be convinced by your attitude and by how you look and by what you say that YOU, the Hygienic practitioner, possess knowledge of what they must do to accomplish their objective.

Another false belief that grasps the American mind like the tentacles of an octopus holds fast to a tasty morsel is the need for enormous amounts of protein, this belief, of course, having been promoted now for almost a century, as Life Scientist well know, by the meat and dairy and other self-serving interests, particularly and knowingly or unknowingly, by the recipients of large research grants indebted to corporate interests for their research monies.

275

"But where do you get your protein?" becomes the plaintive cry of almost every new client when first faced by their new diets, so brainwashed have they been in this regard. One of our students in Sweden recently wrote us that "every adult male needs 250 grams of protein every day!" Where had he gotten this piece of information? Well, he had read it somewhere, he told us!

If a client has this or some similar idea etched in his mind, he must be deprogrammed. One can accomplish the required deprogramming only by substituting knowledge, an understanding of the scientific fact, for example, that the primary need of the human body is NOT for protein, but for single molecule carbohydrates, the kind abundantly supplied in fresh raw fruits. He must be instructed in the ways of catalysis and how the body recycles its discarded protein; about how the body, in fact, can change one kind of protein into another kind of protein as may be required for metabolic purposes; (that the body cannot and does not use protein, only amino acids, and that these are contained in fresh fruits which, when eaten, save the person who eats fruits all the energy wasted in processing concentrated protein and complex carbohydrates, energy which can then be diverted to more constructive tasks. Unless true Hygienic knowledge becomes incorporated into the client's subconscious, unless full perception on his part becomes a reality, all the doubt—the uneasiness which so limits progress—will remain.

Thousands of people, indeed millions, believe that herbs will restore a sick person to health. Health food stores stock their shelves with a wide variety of herbs. In fact, herb sales represent a major part of their income. Clients will surely ask you about this herb and that herb and why you do not recommend herbs? Or vitamins? Or brewer's yeast? Or a host of other magic substances. As a student of Life Science, of Natural Hygiene, you have learned about all these things, or will learn about them. This information has all been carefully documented and planned for your enrichment, to arm you well so that you will be enabled to meet the needs of clients for new knowledge to replace the old beliefs and superstitions. Without confidence in your knowledge and in the program proposed to a client by you, that client will make only limited progress, if any.

The horror of fasting is a prime example of beliefs that die hard. The average person, particularly here in America, the land of Surfeit Plus, is firmly convinced that missing a, single meal will cause him extreme anguish. School children MUST be "fortified with a good breakfast!" This is gospel truth, not open to debate. Fasting is what starving people do! He knows from watching the boob tube what starving can do to a person. You can't talk him into going without food!

Clients, therefore, must be given understanding of what the difference between fasting and starving is. Your new client will not understand that fasting, even for a short time, will allow the body to achieve a higher level of health and that prolonged fasting may well be the single most important way to be restored to a level of health such as s/ he has not been privileged to know in an entire lifetime.

Clients must be disabused of their antipathy, even horror, of fasting, and this can only be accomplished when one imparts to the client the known facts about fasting, that it is a biologically well-accepted modality which provides the physiological rest required for healing to happen and to happen with the fastest possible speed.

89.6.1. Mike's Story

Mike's story illustrates just how difficult it can be sometimes to remove from the subconscious mind this fear of fasting. Mike, age 56, has had rheumatoid arthritis for some 15 years. He had been referred to us by a former client. We were told that he would be unable to come to our office because he could not negotiate steps and also, because of his condition, if he did come, he would have to stand during the entire consultation. We agreed, therefore, to make a house call.

We were deeply moved at our first meeting with Mike. There he stood, emaciated, tall, and straight as an arrow, propped up on crutches, his face wreathed in smiles. You see, he had been given hope by his friend.

We immediately know that Mike was in the advanced, final stages of rheumatoid arthritis. He had to be suffering great pain. His fingers were twisted and curved. He could barely move his head; one area was completely motionless. With his one moveable arm, Mike gestured for us to be seated and then he swung over to his chair, one especially designed for arthritics. It lowered him slowly and gently to a sitting position. The smile remained fixed on Mike's face.

We knew that the only help for this man lay in fasting, but Mike knew nothing of Life Science. His housekeeper, herself terribly obese and obviously diseased, provided him for breakfast boxed cereals and milk, sometimes followed by two eggs. Occasionally, he told us, he also had a glass of canned orange juice and always several cups of coffee. Luncheon was a sandwich, usually made of white bread spread with either canned tuna and mayonnaise or with peanut butter and jelly. At this meal he also had coffee. His evening meal was provided by "Meals for Millions" and consisted of some combination of the four basic groups. At this meal, he drank either milk or coffee.

Mike lived alone except for his housekeeper. He was a veteran living on his veteran's pension. The housekeeper worked for room and board. She did the shopping, kept the premises reasonably clean and prepared two meals. It was obvious that Mike could not afford to go to a fasting institution if he had been able to get there in his condition. After discussing the matter with him, it was obvious, too, that he wouldn't have gone if he had been the wealthiest man in the world! Fasting, to Mike, was for those persons abandoned on a raft somewhere in mid-ocean, or for primitives living in some remote corner of far-off India or Africa, certainly not for him.

Obviously, here was a crying need for change, so how did we accomplish it? We took baby steps, making small changes count. The first important change we suggested to Mike was to forego his usual breakfast in favor of a fruit breakfast. He agreed that he could do this. Then, we suggested that he reduce his coffee intake. Mike was quite enthusiastic about our suggested changes.

We remained with Mike about an hour and then left, promising to return in two weeks. We left him with the first lesson in our Applied Nutrition Course, the one that recounts the stages in the evolution of pathology. We felt this was probably a good way to begin Mike's deprogramming and to establish in his mind the concept of change as it might apply to him, the idea that he might be able to retrace his own life script and someday return to health.

Before the two weeks were up, Mike was on the telephone. He had a special telephone hook-up which enabled him to talk into a speaker and thus did not have to hold a telephone. Otherwise, he would have had no way to communicate with the outside world. He complained of extreme weakness and said that he had felt it necessary to resume having his two eggs for breakfast, eating them after he finished his fruit.

We felt it was time to go back for another visit. This time we went armed with Lesson Two which explains, in simple terms, some basic information about carbohydrates, fats and proteins. We reviewed again with Mike the biological evolution of pathology and he said he understood about where he was presently in the evolution, that he had some real tough sledding ahead but he was confident he could make it. We felt that Mike had progressed extremely well. He had changed from a man filled with doubts into a possibility thinker; one filled, indeed, with "Positivities." Now, he was to acquire even more knowledge to fortify his conviction that change was possible. Old ideas and superstitions seem to fade and eventually disappear when replaced by knowledge and truth!

Within four months, Mike was eating two fruit meals a day, no longer ate his eggs every morning and was down to a single cup of coffee per meal. Of course, lacking his former stimulants, he became extremely weak, resting all day for the most part in his elevated bed. His bed was raised just high enough to permit Mike to slide out. You see, he cannot bend his legs, the knee joints have long since been removed surgically.

The housekeeper left to be replaced by a university student from mainland China, a fine young man who sets out sufficient fruit for two meals. He keeps the premises spotless. However, his school schedule leaves Mike alone all day.

By, this time, Mike had also eliminated all his vitamins, the steroids, and reduced his aspirin intake (or Tylenol) to 10 per day. Sometimes he had to grit his teeth to bear the pain, hut he did it. There was no need to suggest hot baths to relieve his agony. He was unable to get down into a tub. Then, Mike made a major decision. He was going to fast for one day. This was a banner day. We felt like firing the cannon and running up the flag of victory. Our man was to be wonderfully surprised. On his fast day, Mike found, to his amazement, that he had very little pain! However, he felt dizzy and even weaker, a rather scary experience for someone who had to remain all day in bed and alone.

Several weeks ago, we went on our monthly visit to Mike. As usual, he was in bed and, also as usual, smiling. He recounted for us how well he was doing. He was able now to walk 15 times every day back and forth down the long hall to the living room. He could now move his head more and, perhaps most wonderful of all, he had so much more energy than just a few weeks ago. Mike announced that he had decided to take still another step forward. He would now have his two fruit meals per day and, for his evening meal, a salad plus a baked potato and avocado! Mike would no longer now be dependent on "Meals for Millions," certainly a most worthy and commendable effort but one, unfortunately, which knows nothing about Natural Hygiene. Mike said he was convinced now that the principles of Natural Hygiene were correct principles which had already proved their worth to him. We encouraged him to go forward, that now his progress would accelerate. Mike's eyes shone!

Just a few days ago, Mike telephoned. He had made up his mind. On his own, he was planning to fast—this time for 36 hours. He said he felt wonderful and had reduced the pain pills down now to only four pills a day. Mike wants it all now. He has discarded the old ideas, the old superstitions. He is well on the road to better health. He is still studying about Natural Hygiene, the study lessons propped up before him. Knowledge, even though imparted slowly, has wrought the miracle of change in Mike. It has brought conviction. He now knows that there is only one possible way to improve one's health and that is by living healthfully.

89.6.2. Other Superstitions

Another superstition that is really hard to remove from the minds of clients is that in our meal planning, we have to adhere to the four basic food groups. My how some clients will argue about this totally erroneous concept. With such clients, it is well to be fortified with some good solid knowledge about how the human digestive system works. We always have ready a quart bottle, some vinegar, and some baking soda. We put some water in the bottle and then add a little vinegar followed by a teaspoonful or so of the baking soda and Voila! It fizzes! Most of our clients have experienced this fizzing in their own stomachs often enough to see the connection. They receive a study lesson on the digestive system, and they soon become disenchanted with the four basic groups concept, convinced that their own digestive disaster scene has been caused by incorrect food combinations. Understanding the digestive scene makes the idea of simple meals more understandable to them because, perhaps for the first time in their lives, they comprehend that the digestive process is a chemical, mechanical and electrical, very involved, process and that the more we add to the confusion by eating heterogeneous masses of foods, the less real nutrition will result. Why pay out all that money for food that never reaches the REAL you, the world of the cells!

Understanding how the digestive organs work, at least understanding this in gross terms, disabuses most clients of the idea that they can eat anything and everything, as and when they feel like eating, and still enjoy full health. It helps them to appreciate the scientifically-demonstrable fact that fruits are the foods to which we, by virtue of the structure and function of our digestive equipment, are best adapted and from which we humans will receive the finest nourishment. Making this adjustment in their thinking can change sick people into sturdy, strong, miraculously well people.

Clients must also disabuse their minds of the popular delusion, as Dr. Herbert M. Shelton terms it, that eating great quantities of food is necessary to health and strength. We used to believe that ourselves! We used to believe that it was necessary to provide great variety in order to enjoy our meals. Brandy, our collie, disabused us of that idea. Every morning, Brandy gets his dried figs and every evening his baked corn meal cakes, his pinto beans, lettuce and his egg. Every evening, he starts to drool at the same time. He doesn't need a clock! Every evening, he eats that same meal and then licks the bowl until it shines. Very rarely is his meal changed. Oh! Occasionally, we will substitute a piece of avocado for the egg, or a bit of cheese, but that is all. You see, Brandy doesn't even want variety!

We notice that our birds eat certain things at just about the same hour every day, as do the rabbits and the moles and the desert squirrels. The beans fall from the mesquite trees and soon are all gone, hidden in burrows for sustenance during the winter months. Humans don't require so much variety. They don't need so much food. They sicken on complex meals. Yes! Sometimes necessity forces change upon us.

Another popular idea that is around these days is the concept that our bodies are crying for protein, for enormous amounts of protein. Clients find that change here is vital. Again, knowledge of body happenings is the only way to bring about such change. They must learn that simple molecule carbohydrates are our primary need and that when these are in short supply, as happens on the usual protein-starch-fat-sugar diet of the average person in America today, energy levels fall, nerves become deranged, and health fails.

Our clients are victims of their own transgressions, transgressions fostered by superstitions, beliefs and the mores of the times in which all of us live. The list of possible erroneous ideas held by individual clients would probably fill a library. Many are of modern origin, inculcated in the minds of the average person by direct and subliminal advertising; others have their origins in cultural mores which have been handed down from one generation to the next, perhaps for thousands of years. Many false ideas have also been inculcated in the minds of the very teachers who are presently instructing our children today, when they themselves sat as little children in the classrooms of their time. The "need" to be vaccinated against this or that virus or germ is a classic example of this last superstition.

It is the happy task of the informed practitioner to impart the knowledge which will light the lamp of conviction, that will bring about changes in thinking and changes in doing; the kind of changes required to make sick people well again.

Probably the most health-destroying of all superstitions is the one that has been around the longest: the idea that drugs can be instrumental in "curing" this or that ailment. Hygienists marvel that humans can be so stupid as to believe that taking more poisons into an already poisoned body will restore health to a sick person when strong men, in the prime of life, can be felled by the very same poison as surely as if penetrated in a vital organ by a well-aimed bullet!

But that seems to be the perverseness of mankind. It is one of the great mysteries of the ages. Otherwise highly-intelligent men and women, all over the world, dutifully swallow their pills—Paul Erlich's "magic bullets!" And all because their "doctor" tells them to!

Our clients do not possess our knowledge. Natural Hygiene is a totally strange concept to them, one about which they have grave doubts. They must be motivated by us to learn that health must be built; that it follows change; that we cannot poison ourselves into health, only into the grave!

To accomplish whatever changes are desirable in a client's thinking and especially about the effectiveness of drugs in restoring health, we practitioners have to produce results! Our clients have to be shown by whatever means at our command that poisons kill, they do not and cannot become the instrument of health. We must show our clients that, when they continue to indulge the causes of disease, disease will happen; but when they choose to seek after health-promoting ways, then they will be enabled to stand aside in awe and watch their troubling disease replaced by health. This kind of change can only be brought about by education and, as Hygienists, we well know that it must come, or health will remain an elusive impossibility.

89.6.3. The Case of Rev. Kim

The Rev. Kim case illustrates how changing one's confidence in magic bullets into an understanding of the importance of living healthfully, of obtaining every day a full quota of all the biodynamic requisites of life, can also change sickness into health and even bind married couples together into an even closer relationship.

The Rev. had some kind of obscure disease that had been variously diagnosed. Nobody knew for sure what ailed him but, nevertheless, he had been prescribed numerous drugs, including a tranquilizing mood-altering drug. His condition had forced him to give up his pastoral duties and to go on a disability allowance. His wife had to work to support the two of them. There were several married children who lived out of state, so they were more or less on their own.

The Rev., it seems, was so depressed and frustrated by his inability to continue with his church work that he had actually become physically abusive as well as mentally so. In fact, his behavior and his treatment of his wife had become distinctly non-Christian!

Fortunately, someone called the Rev.'s attention to a course in Natural Hygiene that we were offering and both he and his wife enrolled. To this day, they say they don't know why they enrolled, just that they must have been "led."

This couple were both on drugs. In fact, they were swallowing pills "by the carload." At this time, obviously, the only thing they had going for them was hope.

As they progressed in their learning, studying their lessons together, they began to make some simple changes. It wasn't too long before they became private students and shortly thereafter the wife, and then the Rev., stopped taking their pills and adopted more Hygienic ways of eating and living. We will never forget how excited the Rev. was when he told us how "super" he felt on his daily breakfast of two bananas and 10 or 12 dates! Well, to make a long story short, the Rev. now has his church back and his wife is now in an executive position with an important company. She confided to Dr. Elizabeth not too long ago that the Rev. is now more loving than ever. Two of their married children, after observing the transformation wrought in their parents, are now also "into"

Natural Hygiene. Change can, indeed, be wonderful—and contagious!

89.7. I Can!

Applied nutrition represents the "I CAN" philosophy of living, a subtle psychological approach, using the psyche positively, which gradually does away with the old erroneous and negative concepts and ideas which limit and constrain the thinking of most clients on first meeting and replaces them with a sense of being in tune with the positive.

Once our clients are fortified with knowledge and provided with a well-marked road to follow, one furnished the start by the practitioner, then, more often than not, they come to see a bright light beckoning to them at the end of the tunnel of darkness and fear which formerly surrounded them.

Through knowledge comes conviction and once a person becomes convinced in his mind of the Tightness of what you teach, more often than not, the doubter becomes the positive thinker. He verbalizes to himself, "Yes I CAN do it! I can bring about these changes! I CAN live in such a way that health MUST happen. This is a way of life. I CAN be healthier than I now am. I CAN change. I REALLY CAN.

It is so important for clients to understand that, with you to guide them, they will be in charge of their own lives and no longer dependent upon a dispenser of pills nor will they, in their old age, require nurses to burp them and to change their diapers, so to speak. They begin to appreciate the immensity of the possible. They will no longer be required to take pills to elevate or to depress their vacillating moods because they understand that when health replaces sickness, they will feel euphoric with a natural high. They will no longer have to have recourse to hormones to make them into what they should not be.

Instead, the possible is theirs for the doing, for the changing. Through learning the ways of life and understanding the rules of life, they can find their own way, they can take charge of Self.

Understanding the potential behind the I CAN! will often make performers out of the helpless ones who are so because their cells are sick. The mind and the body are one and when the mind contains positive thoughts—thoughts that are capable, ready-to-go thoughts—then these thoughts replace the emotions of fear, anxiety and worry so miracles can indeed happen!

Clients must be given to understand that when we have problems, physical or otherwise, we must find solutions. If we do not, we simply cheat ourselves. If our problem is one of sickness and we do not find a solution, we can cheat ourselves out of life!

We have said elsewhere that attitudes are contagious, both the attitude that we, as practitioners display to the world, and the attitude cultivated in or by our students. We have an outer and an inner attitude. If our inner attitude is a conviction that we CAN attain better health, we WILL because our attitude strengthens our subconscious power and this power pervades the entire body, generating power in our endocrine glands, in our heart, in our brain stem and servicing nerves, in all organs, including our organs of digestion.

This is important, vitally so, for remember all that we are is dependent upon nerve power and upon the efficiency of our digestive powers.

If you believe you can, you will act. This is one of the great, not-well-understood laws of life.

If your inner self is powered by fear, it will soon pervade your being, too. If you fear that health will continue to elude you, fear that life will soon depart from you, you will remain in the sickness rut and more and more pain and suffering will be your unhappy lot simply because your inner fear-packed YOU will slowly, or rapidly, dissipate its power as it fears. Fear and worry are negative attitudes that steal away body power.

Far too many among us think and say, "if only." If only, I had this or that, I could be rich. If only I could find the right doctor, I could be well!"

Charles M. Simmons reminded us that we need to change that attitude to "if I do this, I will get what I want" attitude. This is a positive attitude which means you have a plan of action and that you will work your plan. When the plan is sound and we go into action, we will fulfill our every dream.

That's what the I CAN! concept is all about. The Hygienic practitioner who can get this philosophy across to his client and who gives him a workable plan to start him on his road to becoming a self-performer will be the successful practitioner. His clients will change from timid, doubtful, unhappy souls lacking power, souls filled with negative forces that are doomed to cheat and "to fail, into forward-looking, power-filled persons whose positive attitudes cannot help but bring to them the longed-for successful conclusion: the euphoria of superb health.

89.8. Questions & Answers

You maintain that health is normal and that being sick is abnormal. How can this be? Doesn't everyone have something wrong with him, even though it may be very minor?

You are correct when you say that I believe health to be our normal (natural) heritage. People become sick when they do not adequately answer the needs of their bodies, either through ignorance or because of other circumstances. Many people are sick today simply because they do not have knowledge of what these needs are. They simply follow the herd and do just as everybody else does. This is, of course, especially true when it comes to eating. We WANT to eat like everybody else, eats but the laws of life decree that eating that way is probably the most usual cause of disease. Therefore, if we desire health, we must eat foods to which we are biologically best adapted.

Scientists and dietitians have proved by laboratory experiments that we all need a variety of different kinds of food. Why do you claim that this idea is all wrong and that fruits are a perfect food?

It was determined many years ago by a Yale researcher, by the name of Pottenger, that with cats, it takes three to four generations to prove the adequacy or inadequacy of a particular diet. I suspect that this is true with humans, also, and perhaps even many more generations since humans take far longer than cats do to mature. Laboratory research is more often than not unreliable when it comes to feeding humans. We are not static test tubes, we are nutritive process which is ongoing and extremely complicated. Furthermore, many feeding experiments are performed on test animals who are biologically quite different from humans. We cannot, as true scientists, make a direct correlation as to compared results with two biologically different beings. That is not scientific. We have far more reliable evidence and that is the evidence observed in certain tribes and peoples who have lived in a certain manner and eaten certain foods for thousands of years. The health of the Hunzas and of many others who live on a largely fruitarian diet is incontrovertible proof of the correctness of their diet. In contrast, we see the short, pain-filled lives of the vast majority of those who eat in ways contrary to human physiological and biological requirements. We can eat a variety of fruits if need be. We can eat vegetables, fruits, and nuts if we crave variety. What we don't need is food and ideas concocted in a laboratory setting. We are feeding MAN, not a test tube or some other animal.

Your I CAN! concept sounds like a good plan in theory, but how do you know if it will work?

We have seen it work! Even in our own lives. When Dr. Elizabeth was so ill and wracked by rheumatic pains, she felt trapped. At holiday times she would say to herself, "I must make this an especially happy occasion because I probably won't be here next year!" This is negative thinking. This is the kind of thinking that destroys. She kept getting worse. It really wasn't until we went to Europe and saw that people DID recover from many different kinds of illnesses when they learned what and how to eat that we, and especially she, began to have the beginning of more positive thoughts. And when she first read Dr. Shelton's book, "Orthotrophy," Volume II of The Hygienic System, it was like magic. She KNEW she could get better and from then on it was clear sailing. I don't mean to imply that there were not healing crises. There were plenty of them, but she faced up to them and got over them because she continued doing what she knew was right to do! This is generally the case once people understand that nature not only revenges wrongdoing but also rewards correct practices. Their whole attitude changes. They become filled with "Positivities!"

Does a person always have to change abruptly, immediately? I can see where this might be very difficult for some people.

No. A person does not always have to change abruptly. Of course, nothing is to be gained by putting off making all the required changes and doing so immediately. Delay can sometimes make full recovery more difficult and prolonged. But bear in mind that any change for the better is health-promoting, even though it be but minor. With certain timid souls, radical change is scary and with such people, we encourage them initially to take "baby steps." As they succeed in conquering little goals, they can then move on to larger ones until, suddenly, they realize they have gone the distance, ran the mile, as it were. They have been successful. Then, usually, there's no stopping them!

Article #1: The Great Awakener by Dr. Herbert M. Shelton

Understanding has been defined as "the power to make experience more intelligible by analyzing it in the light of valid and appropriate general concepts."

The man who analyzes and understands may accept or reject on a basis of intelligence. He carefully considers and weighs all the facts and principals involved in a proposition and arrives at a decision.

Snap judgments and emotional acceptances or rejections do not grow out of a process of this kind. When we accept or reject a new idea or a new practice only because it disagrees or agrees or appears to disagree or agree with our prepossessions and preconceptions, we are guided, not by intelligence, but by prejudice and emotion.

Analysis is the sole guide for intelligent selection of alternative courses of action. If we lack sufficient data to make a full analysis, we do not accept or reject, but suspend judgment until more data can be obtained.

Mass media, so popular today, not alone with advertisers, but also with propagandists and pseudo-educators, make use of a form of hypnotic technique in their efforts to sway the popular mind.

By the constantly reiterated slogan, by frequent repetition of words and gestures, by holding the same image always before the minds of their intended victims, they seek to create a state of semi-somnambulism in which the poor victims of the mass media processes do exactly as they are told.

The people are said to be "conditioned" by such processes. Not merely the obvious, but also the hidden, persuaders are employed in this mass conditioning of the minds of the people.

Hitler's use of the "big lie" was made effective by the same process. In advertising and in much of the propaganda of various groups in our culture, the same effective use of the "big lie" is seen. No better example of this can be offered than the constant stream of false medical propaganda that pours from the presses.

Among a people who have been conditioned to "think" in slogans and to follow the crowd in all things, truth has rough sledding. When a revolutionary new truth that seems likely to disturb the status quo is presented to the herd mind, the owner is likely to quote some popular slogan and swing off into the jitterbug line.

In our mass-conditioned culture none of us are ourselves: We are faithful copies of what our masters want us to be.

Often arguing heatedly for or against this or that, we suffer a myopic inability to peer beneath the surface and discern the reality that lies below. We almost always miss tie fact that our acceptances and our rejections, as well as the receptors and rejectors, are all part of a very complex, persuasive cultural process.

It is disheartening to listen to the discussion of contemporary acceptances by the robot minds that constitute the product of our overworked mass media. But the case is not as hopeless as it seems.

Truth has a way of awakening sleepwalkers and clearing the conditioned cobwebs from their minds.

No man armed with the truth is ever welcome in any culture. He is spat upon and discredited by the masters of the culture and their robot underlings, in proportion to the extent that he is feared. But he never fails to dehypnotize many of the victims of the mass-cultural process.

Today we witness the gratifying sight of many sleepwalkers awakening from their fever-dream as a result of coming in contact with Hygienic truth.

We must bring this truth to more and more of the sleepers, that they also may awaken.

Article #2: Overcoming Compulsive Habits by Stanley Bass, D.C.

Habits determine success or failure. I don't care what you want to achieve in life, you can train yourself to be a success, or you can train yourself to be a failure. If you allow yourself to swim in bad habits, you are going to be trapped. Walker, one of the great early Hygienists had the ability to inspire people to right living, as did other early Hygienists. It seems that since the early days of the 1920's somehow the writers of Natural Hygiene took out the inspirational, the spiritual aspects of it. We were living in a scientific age, and everyone wanted to be scientific and Hygienic doctors did not want to be thought of as quacks or mystics or strange people, so they left out the inspirational part, but I have come to the conclusion that the only thing that makes people change is inspiration. You can give them all the facts in the world and convince them in black and white that this is the right way but that doesn't mean they will do it. The only way they will do it is if you get them emotionally excited.

Habits determine success or failure. If you are willing to go through these changes we have been talking about and get rid of the bad habits, reintroduce some new habits, you can do anything you want to do with your life. I don't care what you have done. As I mentioned before, for 15 years I failed. I tried to fast to the finish. I fasted 10 days, 12 days, 14 days, 17 days, and I would get caught with the wrong thought and I'd be pulled off. All my friends said to me, "Stanley, forget it; it can't be done." But I didn't give up; I kept doing it until I succeeded. The only failure, mark one thing well, is if you try to do something 1,000 times and you fail, then you quit trying. You are not a failure until you stop trying, and if you stop trying you are going to be a failure for sure. If you keep trying, eventually you're going to do it. So, the only failure is the person who stops trying, not the one who tries 1,000 times and doesn't do it. Remember that and don't get discouraged. Every time you fall back, remember this is normal in learning any new habits. Don't let it discourage you; keep going; never give up!

You shouldn't condemn yourself for failure. Some people have a bad habit of saying, when they try something and they don't succeed, "What a damn fool I am, what a louse." They start criticizing themselves and they tell all their friends about how stupid they are. "I'm so stupid, how could I do this?" They want everyone to know about it and by the time they get through they have lost all their energy and they can't do anything. They condemn themselves to the point that they lose all their drive. Don't do it, don't condemn yourself. You're divine. Everyone in this world is God-like but doesn't know it. Let it come out. Don't condemn yourself. Remember you can start all over again. Keep going.

Now, I must talk about procrastination. It's the worst thing you can do. It's the most vicious technique devised by the human brain since the beginning of time. That was my chief failing for a long time, so I am familiar with it and know all the tricks of it. What is procrastination? Procrastination is saying to yourself, "Oh, today is not a good day for me to do this; I'll start tomorrow." I'm a Natural Hygienist. When I opened up my institution a few summers ago in Woodridge, four out of five persons who checked in said, "I'm a Natural Hygienist." Do you know what they are doing? Two of them were bugging me for meat and chicken. I saw them eating bread, cake, and candy bars. When they left, we had to turn the mattresses over and found chewing gum wrappers and candy bar wrappers. They called themselves Natural Hygienists. What they mean by that is that they are procrastinators. They are telling themselves, "I ate well on Sunday. I'm really a Natural Hygienist, but today I'm under a lot of stress. It is not a good day for me, I'll start tomorrow." Then when tomorrow comes, "Oh! Gee I've got this problem. It's not good, I'll have to start next week. It will be easier. It's snowing out, or I have to meet people." You know the mind can rationalize anything. The mind is beautiful.

Hitler felt that he was a good man. Do you know that "Two-Gun" Crowley killed two policemen right before they sent him to the electric chair? He felt that he was a good man and a benefactor to humanity. You know people rationalize anything, even murder. If you can rationalize murder, if the greatest murderers that ever lived, the most famous ones felt that they were good human beings, what about a Natural Hygienist who is going to start tomorrow? How easy it is for him to rationalize if "Two-Gun" Crowley could do it. The mind will rationalize anything you want, but don't play that game, because it's too easy. I did that for 18 years.

What is procrastination? It's telling yourself that you are going to start tomorrow; that you are really doing what you think you are doing, but for some reason it is inconvenient. It's lying to yourself and saying you are going to postpone something. You don't say you're not going to do this; you say you're going to postpone it. "I'm really this but I'll start tomorrow." So, you see, you want to fool yourself.

I know a man who takes long fasts, lasting 30 days or more. After the fast he says, "Gee, I really purified my body so well." Then he starts with foods that are borderline and says, "Well, with a 30-day fast, I must have cleaned out six months of wrong living." Then he eats more and more garbage and before a few weeks go by he is eating the worst garbage in the world and he rationalizes that too. He says, "Well, I can eat meat and candy bars because the fasts will eliminate anything." So, he eats worse than the average person who is afraid to do that. He seesaws between fasting and bingeing. I know one man who has been doing it for 30 years. I did it for 18. I know how easy it is. So don't play the game of procrastination. It is the most insidious of all. It's a liar's game. It's a fool's game, and it is a failing game. Face up to it. If you are going to do something, do it this second. There is no tomorrow; only the present is real; the past is a memory, the future a hope. Only this second is real. If you are not doing it now, you are playing a game with yourself.

The law of vital accommodation needs a balance wheel. You can poison yourself but there is no true adaptation to these poisons. Your body only tolerates them. I explained that. It's stimulation first, then depression. All bad habits and addictions are expressed in stimulation and depression. You introduce poisons and you get "high." Then the body throws you down into a state of recuperation which is interpreted by the brain as depression, because the metabolism slows down to recuperate.

Why are bad habits hard to break? It's because they are stimulating, and the more stimulating the habit, the harder is to break because the lower down you go in depression to recuperate. That's ,all; that's the secret of habits explained. If you study all the addicts around you, you will find this true. The worse the habit, the more poisonous it is, the more difficult it is to break because of the greater "down" you go through when you try to stop it. But if you know that stopping it puts you into the recuperation phase, and when you are feeling "down," the body is trying to balance matters and rebuild to make you over again, and if you are willing to face it, you can give up any habit you desire. That is how I gave up tobacco. I took the depression "cure." I stayed in bed and slept through all the downs until my energy was recharged.

You see, energy comes, not from the thing that makes you feel good—that stimulated you—you can get high on fruit. If you get up in the morning feeling pretty good, and you start eating fruit and you eat more sugar and then more sugar, this will stimulate you and you will get your high. If you overeat fruit it may make you nervous, even restless, and if you eat enough of it, you are going to go down, because you overstimulated your pancreas, and your pancreas is burning up this deadly enemy of extra sugar and in so doing, it produces a temporary state of low blood sugar, which is interpreted as depression. The body intends for you to be depressed so you can recuperate. It can only do it by reducing your blood sugar to the point at it stops the excitation and allows you to recuperate. So, you see, there is a rationale in all of nature. Whenever you go down, it is because you have to go down to become normal again. If you know that, and you don't care—you're not afraid of being "depressed"—you can break any habit and then some.

Now I want to bring up the secret of changing anything in a second. This took me 30 years to learn through trial and error and suffering. When I discovered it, I could do anything I wanted to at any moment. I could give up anything, any object, or any possessive attachments of a person if I had to. This is a secret of learning to do without anything and changing anything.

The only suffering we can experience is due to the emotions. We experience suffering due to emotions and feelings and this comes from identification, from locking into something. In other words, if you are watching a movie and you see this little child and the child falls down and gets hurt, you may cry. You are identifying with the child—you are becoming the child—you are experiencing the child's problems so you are suffering. You're crying. If your broker calls and tells you that your $30,000 in A.T.&T. stock has collapsed and hit the skids and you are now worth $10.00, you either decide whether you want to continue living at that point, or try to get out of this somehow. You have just lost a fortune in the market, but then when you go to sleep there is no suffering. There is no stock market once you dream, and after your dream you go into a dreamless state of sleep and there is no suffering—there is no stock market—there are no more family problems—there are no problems—there is no more crime in the streets, there is nothing but peace. So, you see, suffering is related to identification with an idea.

At the time I was studying Yoga, there was something in a book that triggered me off. The author said, "Nothing exists that thinking makes it so" or "I, think, therefore I am," or "nothing exists but our thoughts." In other words, it doesn't mean that if you are unconscious that the world has no reality, it means that for you, if you are not thinking, there's no suffering for you. If you're asleep, there's no suffering for you because you're not in a state of identification with the object which evokes an emotion. So, I said to myself, "If that's the story, that's why I failed."

You see, every time I tried to fast, and I didn't lose my appetite, I'd look at the food and I'd smell it and I'd think of how good it smelled and how good it would taste going down and then before I realized it, I would get emotionally worked up. My juices began flowing and then I couldn't turn back anymore, I was finished. I had to eat and I'd wrestle or fight with anyone who'd try to stop me. Since I never lost my appetite, I knew that I had to master myself mentally. The average person loses his appetite after a few days of fasting. So, there is no struggle—no problem. I didn't lose my appetite, so I had to win the battle in the mental realm somewhere. I said, "It's got to be done on the battleground of thought."

At that time, I had finished college and I was called to go into town on a job. I was part of a band in a place that had a smorgasbord. Every day they put the food in front of the band. People would march up and down for hours and eat. I was on a fast and I fasted for 38 days, and I looked at the food and I said, "Ah ha, you're the culprit, you trapped me before and you are not going to trap me again." I looked at that food and refused to smell it, and I refused to see it. So, here I was, walking and playing, and the aromas were permeating my body, but I refused to acknowledge the existence of the food so there was no suffering. Even though I never lost my appetite and fasted for 38 days. I couldn't believe how easy it was. There was no pain at all. There was the secret of learning how to do anything immediately.

That's it. I wrote extensively on that in a book "Achieving Supreme Nutrition by Several Progressive Weekly Diets." You have to go through everything. Determine your goal. Expect to practice. These are long term concepts, but the immediate battleground is in the territory of thought. If you know that you are dealing with a thought and you decide who is going to be the boss, you can succeed. The secret is, when you get the desire or the temptation, at that moment you must not consider it at all, but simply move your mind to another subject. Transpose your thoughts at that point. You have got to move fast because it only takes a few second of emotions to get into the picture and the emotions are very strong. They are stronger than the intellect, and if you allow yourself to get emotionally involved, you can easily lose. So, you must win the battle before that happens. You have a couple of seconds to win the battle, and if you understand how thought works, you will win every time. You'll be in control.

Article #3: The Negative Power of "If" by Charles M. Simmons

There are many proven laws that govern the human relations and personal management of one's life. There are laws that govern negative effects as well as positive effects, but all of them are based on the actions of "cause and effect." When certain conscious thoughts and subconscious attitudes cause a person to do certain things a certain way, the end result will always be the same. In fact, the result can be predicted, even before the action starts. This "cause and effect" action in human living is inevitable.

The presence of the word "if," when applied negatively in your life, is an example of the power of such laws. When you say, "If I had certain abilities ..." or, "If I could be a certain kind of person ..." or, "If I could do what I want to ...," you are telling the world that you have a daydream with no plan for making it a reality. You are automatically letting a negative law affect you. A dream with no plan for action means that nothing will happen. Nothing can happen because you block out action through the power of a negative attitude. "If," when used this way, means "No," "Never," "Can't."

However, "If" can be changed from a black, gloomy word to a bright red-letter word by coupling it with the words, "I do." This puts you under the influence of a positive law. When you say, "If I do certain things, I will get what I want," you are expressing both a "dream" and a plan for making it come true.

Excerpt from Stop Cheating Yourself.

Article #4: Excerpt from "In Tune with the Infinite" by Ralph Waldo Trine

It is the people who have come into realization of their own true selves who carry this power with them and who radiate it wherever they go—they have, as we say, found their center. And in all the great universe there is but one center—the Infinite Power that is working in and through all. The ones who then have found a center are the ones who have come into the realization of their oneness with the Infinite Power, the ones who recognize themselves as spiritual beings, for the Infinite is spirit.

Such is the person of power. Centered in the Infinite, you have thereby, so to speak, connected yourself with, you have attached your belts to, the great powerhouse of the universe. You are constantly drawing power to yourself from all sources. For, thus centered, knowing yourself, conscious of your own power, the thoughts that go from your mind are thoughts of strength; and by virtue of the law that like attracts like, you by your thoughts are continually attracting to yourself from all quarters the aid of all whose thoughts are thoughts of strength, and in this way you are linking yourself with this order of thought in the universe.

And so, to those that have, to those shall be given. This is simply the working of a natural law. Your strong, positive, and hence constructive thought is continually working success for you along all lines and continually bringing to you help from all directions. The things that you see, that you create in the ideal, are through the agency of this strong constructive thought continually clothing themselves, taking form, manifesting themselves in the material. Silent, unseen forces are at work that eventually manifest in the visible.

Fear and all thought of failure never suggest themselves to you when you are such a person; or if they do, your mind expels them at once, so you aren't influenced by, and don't attract to you, this type of thought from without; you're in another current of thought. So, the weakening, failure-bringing thoughts of the fearing, vacillating or pessimistic about you have no influence on you. The one who is of the negative, fearing kind not only has his energies and his physical agents weakened or even paralyzed through the influence of this kind of thought that is born within him, but he also in this way connects himself with this order of thought in the world about him. And in the degree that he does this he becomes a victim to the weak, fearing, negative minds all around him. Instead of growing in power, he increases in weakness. He is in the same order of thought with those of, whom it is true, "and even that which they have shall be taken from them." This again is simply the working of a natural law, the same as is its opposite. Fearing lest I lose even what I have I hide it away in a napkin. Very well. I must then pay the price of my "fearing lest I lose."

Thoughts of strength both build strength from within and attract it from without. Thoughts of weakness actualize weakness from within and attract it from without. Courage begets strength, fear begets weakness. And so, courage begets success, fear begets failure. It is the man or the woman of faith, and hence of courage, who is the master of circumstances and who makes his or her power felt in the world. It is the man or the woman who lacks faith and who as a consequence is weakened and crippled by fears and forebodings who is the creature of all passing occurrences.

Within each one lies the cause of whatever comes to him. Each has it in his own hands to determine what comes. Everything in the visible, material world has its origin in the unseen, the spiritual, the thought world. This is the world of cause; the former is the world of effect. The nature of the effect is always in accordance with the nature of the cause. What one lives in his invisible thought world, he is continually actualizing in his visible material world. If he would have any conditions different in the latter, he must make the necessary change in the former. A clear realization of this great fact would bring success to thousands of men and women who all about us are now in the depths of despair. It would bring health, abounding health, and strength to thousands now diseased and suffering. It would bring peace and joy to thousands now unhappy and ill at ease.

And oh, the thousands all about us who are continually living in the slavery of fear. The spirits within that should be strong and powerful, are rendered weak and impotent. Their energies are crippled, their efforts are paralyzed. Fear is everywhere—fear of want, fear of starvation, fear public opinion, fear of private opinion, fear that what we own today may not be ours tomorrow, fear of sickness, fear of death. Fear has become with millions a fixed habit. The thought is everywhere. The thought is thrown upon us from every direction ... To live in continual dread, continual cringing, continual fear of anything, be it loss of love, loss of money, loss of position or situation, is to take the readiest means to lose what we fear we shall."

By fear nothing is to be gained but, on the contrary, everything is to be lost. "I know this is true," says one, "but I am given to fear; it's natural to me and I can't help it." Can't help it! In saying this you indicate one great reason for your fear by showing that you do not even know yourself as yet. You must know yourself in order to know your powers, and not until you know them can you use them wisely and fully. Don't say you can't help it. If you think you can't, the chances are that you can't. If you think you can and act in accordance with this thought, then not only are the chances that you can, but if you act fully in accordance with it, that you can and that you will is an absolute certainty. It was Virgil who in describing the crew which in his mind would win the race, said of them, "They can because they think they can." In other words, this very attitude of mind on their part will infuse a spiritual power into their bodies that will give them the strength and endurance which will enable them to win.

Then take the thought that you CAN—take it merely as a seed thought, if need be; plant it in your consciousness, tend it, cultivate it and it will gradually reach out and gather strength from all quarters. It will focus and make positive and active the spiritual force within you that is now scattered and of little avail. It will draw to itself force from without. It will draw to your aid, the influence of other minds of its own nature, minds that are fearless, strong, courageous. You will thus draw to yourself and connect yourself with this order of thought. If you are earnest and faithful, the time will soon come when all fear will lose its hold; and instead of being an embodiment of weakness and a creature of circumstances, you will find yourself a tower of strength and a master of circumstances.

Lesson 90:

Psychology and Practical Aspects Involved in Making a Change in Lifestyle

90.1. Introduction

Before we explore the psychology of the mind in this lesson, please review Lesson 16: Nutrition, Mind, and the Emotions, and refresh your memory on "a sound mind in a sound body."

Other lessons suggested for review are:

- Lesson 21 — Symptoms that Occur in Lifestyle Transition
- Lesson 38 — Sociological Benefits and Economic Ramifications of the Avoidance of Junk Foods
- Lesson 63 — Nutrition and the Hair The McCarter Extended Detoxification Regimen
- Lesson 69 — Nutritional Approach to Overcoming Addictions

90.2. The Psychology of Making a Lifestyle Change

90.2.1. The Psychology of Being

90.2.2. Collective Consciousness—The Universal Mind

90.2.3. Emotions—Releasing Mental and Emotional Toxins

90.2.1. The Psychology of Being

90.2.1.1. Nutrition and Mental Health

Usually when we think of the word psychology, a vision appears of couches and a "specialist" who collects impressive fees for talking to you about your life. Somehow the Indians in Mexico and fishermen in small Greek seaside villages, all struggling as we do to survive day by day, manage to get by in life without these "counsellors." In our rush to discover the space age, once again we have overlooked the wisdom of simplicity. Intuition and common sense help us to better understand the realms of our minds, just as they tell us how to care for our bodies. It is this common sense that tells us not to entrust our minds to a "professional" who includes all manner of drugs (from mood elevators to tranquilizers—all with their negative side effects—to shock treatment) in his treatment of patients. This "expert" seldom considers the obvious link between nutrition and mental health and will look instead for more esoteric causes for a person's mental state, all appropriately labelled and tagged with intellectual-sounding psychological terms to create an aura of mystique, terms such as parental upbringing, peer pressure and so on, all of which have their place, but none of which is so basic and all-encompassing as the person's everyday diet and regime.

Often the same people who run to doctors to ask them what is happening with their own bodies are the same types who run to an "analyst" to ask what is happening in their minds. These people apparently don't place much trust in their own faculties. We have seen time and time again in our studies of Natural Hygiene that our bodies have incredible self-healing powers, given the proper conditions for healing to take place. It is the same with the mind. People learn to work out their lives by solving each problem as it arises, so "people on the street" surely know as much about real life as the psychiatrist/ psychologist with his framed university degrees. If not more. If ever we feel confused, we'll do better to look inward and find out why and see what we can do to change. In some cases talking it out is the best form of help around—we can talk to friends or counsellors who don't prescribe drugs.

90.2.1.2. We Are What We Eat, Digest, Assimilate; and Think

Let's leave the psychology books on the, shelf for the moment and get straight to the point: we are what we digest and assimilate of what we eat, and we are what we think (our thoughts determine our actions and our lives) and these processes are totally interlinked. Health is threefold: physical, mental and of the spirit.

In the words of the poet/philosopher Kahlil Gibran:

"And tell me, people of Orphalese, what have you in these houses? And what is it you guard with fastened doors?

"Have you peace?

"Or have you only comfort, and the lust for comfort, that enters the house a guest, and then becomes a master?

Ay, and it becomes a tamer, and makes puppets of your larger desires.

"And though its hands are silken, its heart is of iron. It lulls you to sleep. Verily the lust for comfort murders the passion of the soul, and then walks grinning in the funeral."

90.2.2. Collective Consciousness—The Universal Mind

Since infancy, most people in this society have been more or less preoccupied with themselves. Now that they have discovered that they should "know themselves," they are more determined than ever to understand their minds. Where do all their thoughts come from? Sometimes they are self-originated, and others just seem to pop in from "nowhere in particular." There is also a universal mind, a collective consciousness, of which we are all a part. In an era where people are becoming increasingly self-aware, they realize that they do not exist completely separate from other human beings—we are all interdependent and part of a huge "aquarium" or microcosm in the sky: our planet earth. What we do and even what we think will leave its imprint someplace. Even if we feel "lonely" at times, we are never really alone.

Like children, we adults often continue to associate eating with gratification/satisfaction (Lesson 16). If ever there's a twinge of anxiety, whether it stems from this loneliness or general boredom, we tend to think of eating to bring us some form of "relief." If only we could fill the vague, cloudy, empty areas in our existence with something. Our goal is to find out just what to do with this energy. We create our reality, but just as we'd prefer to blame some mysterious "germs" for illness, rather than see that our lifestyle produces our state of health, we'd rather believe that "things just happen to us at random," with no control from within. That way we are relieved of any responsibility. Nothing could be further from the actuality.

Our normal, physiological functions take place on the subconscious level, without the conscious attention of the mind. We may or may not be aware of these processes, depending upon our sensitivity. Our conscious thoughts are woven with our subconscious mind in a blend that determines our existence. One may wonder at science fiction that likens our minds to computers—indeed, some do resemble busy information gathering and storage centers that workday and night. Perhaps some minds still resemble rivers, wherein the person can become fluid, relax, and "go with the flow," yet our compulsion for labels and categories in this day and age seems to grow. People want labels for disease, labels for their thoughts—they are constantly searching for data. When will they see that life is more than the bits and pieces? It is the whole. Every time people seek to define something, the something will change, as does every other thing on the planet, from instant to instant. Yet we insist on definitions, facts, labels, and data, and on externalizing what happens to us as being caused by coincidences or outside influences beyond our control. We're caught by the whirlwind propaganda of our times be somebody. How can we be somebody and at the same time not take ourselves too seriously? I guess we have to see that we must drink the water, but our lips don't have to touch the cup!

Life enjoys setting us up for learning these lessons. The more we learn, the sooner we'll be surprised at how few things are just happening to us at random.

Sometimes we'll find that the harder we work at something, the more progress we make in realizing our goal. At other times, mysteriously, it seems to be just the opposite. Sometimes the harder we want something and more attached we are to our particular desire, the less we succeed, and the farther we are from our goal. How can this be? This is especially hard for a work and goal-oriented society like ours to grasp. At times the conscious mind can interfere with the natural flow of events. When we stay only in the conscious mind and chatter on busily to ourselves, we may be missing intuitive subconscious messages trying to get through, just as it is difficult to listen and speak at the same time.

Let's look at an example. I once noticed that I often found something I had lost just at the point where I was about to give up looking, i.e., my conscious mind would detach itself from the search for a moment, maybe even just due to a momentary distraction. Somehow at the precise moment the conscious mind ceased to work, the subconscious mind would take over and I'd have an intuition to look under a particular book or in a drawer, and lo and behold, there was the missing object. It took me awhile to realize what principles were at work here: the conscious mind can "block" the subconscious.

Some people are almost completely unaware of their subconscious minds, just as some people are unaware of their body's innate capacity for self-healing and repair. They define the whole of their existence in terms of their conscious thoughts. This is very limiting, like trying to define the ocean in terms of the contents of a few of its drops of water.

Just as we can't watch two channels on TV at once, most of us can't tune in to both our conscious and subconscious minds at the same time. It can be done just as one can juggle and watch a distant object instead of the balls, but it takes some effort at first. Usually we spend most, if not all, of our waking time in our conscious minds, entertaining ourselves with various fantasies, plans and ideas, or tormenting ourselves with worries and what-if's, depending upon our moods. Often we don't slip into our subconscious minds until we are asleep.

Just where is this subconscious mind? Well, most of us can think of instances where we've been aware of two types of knowing—we may know something because we were told, or we read it in a book or saw it with our own eyes. Or we may say that we know something "by intuition." There is a fine line dividing these two types of knowledge, but most of us have had experiences of this "sixth sense." As evolution of human beings goes forward, more and more people are discovering heightened sensitivity. Many people consider it an upsurge of "spirituality"—not necessarily in the religious sense (though when some people are awakened they choose to define it as such). No matter what the name, it is clear that peoples' minds are expanding at an increasing rate to include more and more dimensions. The universal mind also expands and increases with every moment. There are thousands of books and words to fill our minds; we try to sort out the truth. Many things in the universe remain unexplained. We often hear of "paranormal" events or the ability to receive information from the universal mind. If we are tempted to be skeptical, we should wonder if people a thousand years ago would have laughed at someone who spoke of vehicles that could fly in the air. Before the invention of the microscope, no one would have imagined that there were thousands of tiny living creatures moving around in a piece of fingernail scrapings, but there are. People are notorious for believing "only what they can see," but obviously a lot exists whether they see it or not. The mind has more potential than we can, at this point in our evolution, know.

Some people receive messages or information from the universal mind when they are dreaming. I myself have dreamed dozens of times of people (some who'd been gone for months), and then seen them that day, enough times to finally realize that I was somehow knowing in my dream and subconscious mind that I would see them—I had no conscious clue that they'd be coming. Many people have these types of dreams. Some see a person in a dream and later find out they died; some have seen houses on fire or other events that later came to pass, or were happening at the time of, or before, the dream. The only explanation for such occurrences is that there is information accessible to people who can "tap into it," by whatever means may best suit their consciousness, whether in a waking or a sleeping state. (For some people, whose minds are always busily centered in the conscious when awake, the sleeping state is the time in which they can best "submerge" into their subconscious minds, with no interference from the conscious stream of thoughts usually present.) Dreams also seem to be a type of "re-sorting" of information and events of the day, or the past, and some seem to reflect (or "work out") our fears or anxieties, so we can't just classify all dreams into one category. There are different stages of consciousness even in sleep, because there are varying depths of sleep; so not all dreams are the "precognitive" type mentioned. After a while you'll be able to differentiate between your different types of dreams and whether they have any further significance for you. We shouldn't become unnecessarily preoccupied with our "average" dreams, any more than we would with any other part of our past. But we should learn to recognize any signals or any other information given to us if we feel intuitively that they are being given to us for a reason.

When thinking about knowledge, consider this. If you were to look at the ocean from a boat, you'd see the surface waves, but how would you ever imagine all the millions of fish under the water, and the ocean floor teeming with life, if you'd never been down there or known anyone who had? How would you then describe the sea, in terms of what you could see"! Your description would be a part of the truth, not the whole.

So, when talking about the subconscious mind, let's imagine a crystal-clear pool of water, so clear that you can see the bottom of the pool and even the reflection of yourself and the sky behind you. When the pond is still, you are seeing both sides, the inside and the outside, above and below the surface, into both dimensions. When you stop thinking and mind goes quiet, it becomes clear like the crystal pool, and you perceive more than one dimension, the subconscious as well. But if you drop a stone into the pond, the surface is broken and both images, above and below are distorted. Your thoughts are like the stones.

When the mind is clear and quiet, we may call this a state of meditation. The inner voice can be heard; this is somewhat different from the voice of regular conscious thought, but you can distinguish between the two if you are sensitive enough. Knowledge thus comes from the inside as well as the outside, from a place we cannot see or measure, and yet we know it is there. Inner space is, after all, as infinitely deep as outer space!

We must not forget to look inward in this busy outward world. There is much knowledge to be found there, and we must learn how to "let go" in order to open the channels in the mind. Constant thinking blocks intuition and saps our energy—the mind needs rest just as the body needs rest.

As we go toward a lighter diet of fresh, raw fruits, vegetables, nuts, and seeds, we will notice changes in our thoughts. We may find ourselves going through mental purgation as well as physical cleansing. Soon the mind will settle and become calm with the new healthy lifestyle, but whenever you feel an abundance of scattered thoughts, just let them go on by, don't repress them. Just as people suppress their cleansing symptoms with drugs and interfere with the body's natural healing process, so too do they sometimes hold in their real feelings. The result is a parallel to what happens when toxins are held in the body, only this time, wrong thoughts, attitudes, prejudices, etc., are the toxins: mental toxins.

90.2.3. Emotions—Releasing Mental and Emotional Toxins

Ever wonder why some people hold in their emotions? Some men are determined not to cry, for example. Women have traditionally been given more freedom in this area, fortunately for them. Children cry easily until they get the "message" to "grow up." Stop and ask yourself why we even have tears, tear ducts and emotions, if not for a reason? Some people plaster their pores shut with, underarm deodorants to "stop the wetness," somehow not bothering to realize that the body's natural eliminative sweat glands are there for a reason in the first place, to refrigerate the area and get toxins out. Who, in the name of wetness or dryness, wants to keep these toxins in their body? Who wants to keep others in their minds?

Those who have reached and kept to a 100% raw food diet say that they have gained health, peace of mind and serenity of soul that are literally indescribable. Our purpose in life is spiritual unfoldment (again, we use the term spiritual in speaking of the spirit, not in the purely "religious" sense). The body is a tool you use to work with, to carry you towards your goals in life. The better nourished the body is, the more clear the mind is, and the more beautiful the character becomes. The purer the body is, the more expansion of consciousness will take place. A live food diet of our biologically-correct foods will bring spiritual awareness and heightened powers of intellect and sensitivity.

90.3. Practical Aspects Involved in a Change in Lifestyle—Part I

90.3.1. Honesty with Ourselves

90.3.2. Habits—Breaking the Chain

90.3.3. Love Is a Basic Human Need

90.3.1. Honesty with Ourselves

Why does change come so easily for some people and so slowly for others? It all comes back to truth and honesty. How honest we are with ourselves determines the strength of our willpower. People who see the truth like a shining light and know a natural lifestyle is best for them, lose their false appetite for foodless foods, and change is easy. Other people choose to ignore the truth. Some of us find ourselves somewhere in between the two and see the truth even though we give in to our temptations at times. We have our excuses, but are we not also choosing to ignore the truth and look the other way?

Obviously the easiest way to lose all the "cravings" is to undergo a lengthy fast, after which a person will desire foods that are good for him instead. Some people say they don't have time to fast. Everyone has time for short fasts, one day a week, for example. Hopefully everyone has time, if they really look for it, for a longer one! How can they afford not to? We must find time for our health and well-being, for no one else is going to do it for us.

90.3.2. Habits—Breaking the Chain

"Humans are creatures of habits. Habits are conditioned responses—repeated performance of an action creates a mental pattern. We spend many years from infanthood in learning responses to many thousands of situations and circumstances. With set response patterns we don't have to go through time loss and trouble in solving problems anew every time we face them—once we have solved a problem, we develop a solution as a fixed, automatic response—a habit. When situations occur, we unconsciously use our habit patterns. We have more "conditioned responses" to carry us through more complexities than any other creatures in existence. However, sometimes these habits lock us into wrong conceptual frameworks, distorted outlooks, unwholesome practices, etc. Fortunately, like computers, we can be reprogrammed for better performance!" (T.C. Fry, How To Reprogram Yourself for Superlative Well-Being.)

Habits are made stronger by repetition, and many habits are self-perpetuating. Like the pendulum that swings to one extreme, the other extreme is the inevitable next swing. Some people live out the path of the pendulum quite literally in their lives, "awakening" in the morning with coffee and "relaxing" in the evening with alcohol. The law of dual effects states that stimulation is always followed by an equal amount of depression, and vice versa. People who are constantly altering their moods are swinging back and forth on the pendulum. Physical and mental balance and harmony must be restored to the body.

The following drugs and habits enervate the body with stimulation/depression cycles. At first the altered state seems "enjoyable"—once it becomes addictive, we crave its repetition more and more often. hard drugs: amphetamines, barbiturates, morphine, heroin, etc. soft drugs: coffee, tea, tobacco, marijuana, caffeinated carbonated beverages, sugar, chocolate, non-caffeinated carbonated beverages (full of chemicals, etc.), strong spices, vinegar, salt stimulating food: animal food such as meat, poultry, and fish, preserved foods, concentrated sweets and starches.

For example, meats stimulate the body; then a subsequent depression occurs that "requires" further stimulation. We must learn how to recognize and break bad patterns.

Food addiction is every bit as overwhelming, potent, and destructive of the human organism as a heroin addiction, when you look at its awesome short and long-term effects.

Yet many people cling to their culinary traditions in the face of all logic and reason, with mounting evidence (Hygienists have already been long-convinced) that many of their "favorite" habits are self-destructive. Why do they allow themselves to become puppets of fleeting desires, ignoring warning signs and playing a sort of Russian roulette with their health? There is an old expression that says, "if you want to dance, you have to pay the fiddler." Some people speak of karma: what goes around comes around. Others say you reap what you sow, or you are what you eat.

People have become brainwashed by the media. Commercials show steaming portions of spicy, heavy meals at dinner time, to the tune of "are you hungry?" How often do we see a commercial for fresh, raw fruits or vegetables? Probably never! We must wonder about the mental health of a nation that runs on cereals, milk, meat, sugar, caffeinated beverages, snacks, and processed foods, that washes off its natural skin layer with soaps and detergents, smothers itself in creams, lotions, perfumes, and as we said before, won't even sweat. Some people's eating habits are even regulated by time: they eat in a hurry and/or always eat at certain times, according to "convenience" rather than true hunger.

Are people truly becoming robots and prisoners of mechanical actions? What are they looking for in food? In Lesson 16, Mike Benton talks of food associations like sentimentality, security, family, rewards, friendships, childhood memories, and so on.

90.3.3. Love Is a Basic Human Need

People seek a sense of nurturing. They also search for shelter, a sense of belonging in a safe, secure, and trusted territory, and a sense of purpose. Yet the one most important need they have is for love. People must have love, touch, and contact with others. Let's not underestimate this for a moment.

If you travel to another country you're likely to notice that Americans (especially those who live in the cities) seem to be, for some reason, less tactile and more concerned with privacy and space than people of many other countries. This may sound like a generalization, but in the last decade here, there has been increased awareness of the need to "reach out," as evidenced by an upsurge in "encounter groups" and all sorts of "therapies" encouraging people to hug one another and express more of their feelings.

Is it possible that some people's isolationist tendencies stem from their unnatural birth experiences? Ever since doctors and hospitals took over, childbirth has become less and less natural. The traditional medical birthing ritual routinely separates newborn infants from their mothers and places them alone in cribs in the nursery, and one might ask what emotional price these children have paid. Did they "adapt" and, rather than become bonded in their first intimate relationship with another human being, adjust to their aloneness by becoming "more independent"? One can only wonder. In this society, families are also separated more often as people become increasingly mobile.

It's not difficult to see that many people make up for that restless, empty space inside by eating. Why isn't it obvious that we won't find love and affection in a double banana split? The conscious mind may be reaching for a bag of chips, but the subconscious mind isn't fooled. The person is no closer to his real desires, and the frustrations left behind because of unfulfillment are merely buried deeper, to be reckoned with at some later date.

Sound familiar? Just as we palliate symptoms of detoxification through drugging, so too do we resort to food for palliation of symptoms such as inertia, boredom, restlessness, thus leaving the mental toxins inside instead of dealing with our true feelings. Some people have difficulty admitting their true feelings to themselves. They may not see that it's love and contact they're after, deep down, but the subconscious knows, even if they don't see it in their conscious minds. The games people play with themselves far outnumber the games they play with others. They must first fool themselves before fooling others.

Some of us "cheat" when "no one's looking" (including ourselves, presumably) and eat something we've been trying to avoid. Trying to fool ourselves! We try to convince ourselves each time that it "doesn't matter" or that "next time it will be different." As long as our intentions are good, we are off the hook temporarily. But truth is truth, whether we like it or not. We must see ourselves as we really are, not as we should be. Again, our subconscious mind knows what is really going on. If we choose to let our conscious minds rule the subconscious, we will remain captives of our lower selves.

"Stuck here trying to figure out the price of having to go through all these things twice..."

—Bob Dylan

90.4. Practical Aspects Involved in Making a Lifestyle Change—Part II

90.4.1. Rule #1: See the truth

90.4.2. Rule #2: Live by the truth

90.4.3. Rule #3: Visualize the positive

90.4.4. Rule #4: Eat the optimum diet and live according to your natural mandate

90.4.5. Rule #5: Remember the Simple Joys of Life

90.4.6. Rule #6: Give of Yourself

90.4.8. Rule #7—Relax

90.4.9. Rule #8—Take your time

90.4.1. Rule #1: See the truth

The truth is all around you, free for the taking. Open your eyes and you will see that people are destroyed in their prime by wrongful living habits. The more they indulge and consume, the more vital energy is lost and dissipated.

90.4.2. Rule #2: Live by the truth

How many times have we heard the old saying "actions speak louder than words?" Or thought one thing and done another? Once we know the truth, we're only halfway home. We must teach our sometimes-reluctant ego (our smaller self) the true meaning of freedom, that of being as strong as our dreams, that of really being the most evolved, radiant soul possible. Why settle for second best?

Why, indeed? For that is what many people, possessing full free will and freedom of choice, end up doing.

The split second between desire and fulfillment of the desire is very crucial. The two can blend together into one before you know it. This is why it's been said that the best way to deal with temptation is to cast it out before even beginning to think about it, because once you give a thought "an audience" by letting it assert itself, you've given your emotional self the go-ahead. You'll need a will of iron now, for this is where some people give in, sometimes out of sheer frustration or irritation (and usually accompanied by some excuse to their higher selves).

When people have jaded taste buds, it becomes tricky to see the fine line between stimulation and enervation in foods. Some of them are so used to altering their moods that they may not remember what a "normal" mood is like, what it's like to be centered. It all sounds so logical, so why are we tempted? Is it because we're not really sure whether we should eat something? No, it is because we are sure deep down that we shouldn't, but we are still arguing with our physical self.

The mental self and the subconscious self-have already accepted the truth. Why do we sometimes refuse to listen to our inner voices? Only we ourselves know the answer to this question. We know how far we will go to follow truth. Either we will compromise and bend our principles (knowing full well that nature does not bend hers) or we'll choose freedom. We all choose our level of awareness and level of being.

Knowledge comes to those who should have it, those that seek it, those that see. Some people put as much energy into not changing by not doing it yet, doing it halfway or thinking of changing, as they could just as easily put into changing, and getting it over with!

I remember a Chinese expression saying, "much noise on the stairway, but no one comes through the door." Somewhere between the dreamers and the cynics are the actual doers. There is a quotation in Composition of Foods that says:

"Nothing in the world can take the place of persistence. Talent will not: nothing is more common than unsuccessful men with talent. Genius will not; unrewarded genius is almost a proverb. Education alone will not; the world is full of educated derelicts. Persistence and determination alone are omnipotent."

The truth may not seem easy at first glance, but it is simple. Change is easy when you want it. You have to love yourself enough to change. (No one else will do it for you).

90.4.2.1. Self-respect...self-esteem...self-love

Self-discipline is a positive force. Discipline does not diminish life—it increases it. When we decide to become true to our biological heritage, we are backed up by all the forces of nature and by life itself. We learn how to channel our energy flow and conserve our vital energy.

Those who are undisciplined waste their vital life force and spread themselves too thin. They drain their energy, making life harder for themselves. Life can be easier, and the choice is ours.

"He who has a firm will molds the world to himself..."

—Goethe

"People do not lack strength, they lack will..."

—Victor Hugo

Some say that 5% of the people in the world think for themselves and the other 95% don't.

When you get rid of a bad habit, feel glad. If you kick the drinking habit, don't think "now I can't drink anymore." Think "now I don't have to drink," or "now I am a free person." (Now I am saving money, now I am saving energy, etc.). True freedom is freedom from need. The less you need, the more free you are. You aren't denying yourself anything. You are giving yourself the greatest gift of all: life and freedom. You have chosen enlightenment.

"When you can control your tastes and appetites, you will be master of yourself." "You will be a soul in a body, not just a body with a soul."

—Stanley Bass

Poets, philosophers, and seers have written about this lofty state of being for centuries!

When you increase your willpower, you increase your self-confidence. You strengthen yourself to your highest potential.

Don't just break bad habits—cultivate good ones. Don't see your life as full of "restrictions." See that you are gaining all your power and energy, all your beauty and all your strength. You'll soon find that abstinence is easier than "moderation," and that it's easier to give something up than to indulge in it "just this once." More energy is saved. We should live with nature, not against it.

If we are tempted to "make exceptions," we must ask ourselves if we want to start the chain of habits again, giving reality anew to all the memories and obsessive compulsions attendant to them. We can't be on both sides of the fence. Once we give up a habit, its memory and hold will fade with time.

When we truly see that what we eat today walks and talks tomorrow, we may feel that we are one of a "chosen few." Once upon a time there lived a man who thought that the sun was the center of our solar system, and everyone knew he was crazy. They knew that the earth was the center, and it was flat!

In habit and thought you are different from the crowd but follow your instincts and do what you know to be right.

90.4.3. Rule #3: Visualize the positive

Please read the section on affirmations, Lesson 16, page 381. We must be aware of the subtle messages we may be giving our subconscious minds. Sometimes we don't realize we are expressing our positive hopes in a negative way:

We say:

I hope it won't rain I hope we're not late Don't slam the door We mean:

I hope it's a nice day I hope we're on time Close the door quietly

There is a certain power in the written and spoken mind, and there is a certain power in the way we formulate our thoughts. People with a strong will to live and a positive attitude live longer, other conditions being equal.

Smiling and laughing are healthy, both on the giving and on the receiving end. When we want to encourage the body's natural healing process when fasting or otherwise, we should not visualize the illness and the symptoms, which are a manifestation of the healing that is taking place. Instead, the body is to be imagined in its healthy state, visualized in the positive light, seen as we want it to be. Some people even speak of visualizing healing white light surrounding the sensitive area, protecting it. The idea is to focus positive energy on the body. This is vastly different from focusing negative energy on it; when we worry about symptoms we literally reinforce our "sick" state by lending strength to it with our thoughts.

A quick glance at the following two ways of life, the negative and the positive, will convince us at once to go with the life force, the positive!

Negativity	Positivity
narrow-mindedness	open-mindedness
evil, revenge	good, forgiveness
pettiness, prejudice, intolerance	tolerance
inflexibility	change, fluidity, flexibility
apathy, indifference, laziness	vigor, strength
gloom, morosity	positive outlook
negative conversation, gossip	positive conversation
dissipation of energy	focus of energy, centering
pride, self-righteousness, arrogance	humility, self-respect
self-pity	self-esteem

attachment, envy, jealousy	detachment
illness	health
anger	joy
hatred	love, touch, nurturing
anxiety, nervousness, tension	serenity, harmony, balance
dishonesty, deception	honesty, truth
self-deception, ignorance	vision, insight, wisdom, understanding, clarity
paranoia	trust, faith, hope
fear	courage
chaos	unity, simplicity
selfishness, greed	generosity
entrapment	freedom
violence, war	peace
regression	evolution, progress
destructiveness	creativeness
loss of powers, death	increasing abilities, life

90.4.3.1. "Mirror, mirror on the wall... who's the fairest of them all?"

The key to rule #3 is the positive image of ourselves that we keep in our minds. When we see this image, we will see that improper, compulsive eating in the past distorted our bodies and our minds and revealed a lack of love for ourselves, as well as an escapist lifestyle. We experience what we believe, so we must believe ourselves to be deserving, attractive, desirable, and lovable. We must create the image of our highest self. If we do, we will then become our highest selves.

If you look at anyone who is "successful," you will see their absolute faith in their ability to succeed. You must have faith in your inherent powers. You are not just a "victim of fate." Remember that what passes to the subconscious mind can be translated into action. As we said, negative thoughts build upon themselves. If you entertain thoughts of failure and if you doubt your ability to succeed, you will generate negative energy. Many of your anxieties become self-fulfilling. "As you thinketh, so shall ye be."

Let's not think negatively. Instead, let's cultivate positive thoughts, and create a constant flow of positive energy. We decide what mood will color our thoughts. It is best to choose friends, books, movies, and thoughts that nourish our minds and aspirations. When we look at any food or drink and cannot answer the simple question "what good will this do?" then we should let go at once. Old habits and crutches only stand in our way of our liberation. Soon the good, positive lifestyle will be habit, as strong a practice as the lifestyle it replaced.

90.4.4. Rule #4: Eat the optimum diet and live according to your natural mandate

We have discussed the diet of fresh, raw fruits, vegetables, nuts, and seeds, and getting plenty of exercise, fresh air, and sunshine, in earlier lessons.

90.4.5. Rule #5: Remember the Simple Joys of Life

Not only are they free, they're fun. In a positive lifestyle we will find an abundance of joy. Singing, dancing, music, artistic and creative expression of all kinds, gardening—these are but a few of the simple joys of life. When we sing and dance, we join with the universe in its larger song, the eternal fountain of life.

90.4.6. Rule #6: Give of Yourself

In a television documentary on the life of Mother Teresa in India, it was said that she sent new volunteers to work in her homes for the dying, where they received their first dose of reality. One such volunteer came to her, a middle-aged man given up to die of a heart condition by his physician. He'd apparently decided to put in some service to mankind before departing, but after working more and more with other people, and forgetting himself, his heart condition changed and he became well. (We know the role of diet in heart conditions, but some literature has also linked heart problems to people obsessed with themselves and with time, both of which will add stress to their lives.)

A person who doesn't give readily of himself suffers from a sort of poor sluggish disposition too. Giving of oneself is sometimes harder than giving of one's possessions. Either way, most people usually give to the persons of their choice, who are "worthy" to receive their generosity. We should give with the same readiness to strangers since they are the same as every living being.

Kahlil Gibran says of giving:

"It is when you give of yourself that you truly give.

For what are your possessions but things you keep and guard for fear you may need them tomorrow?

And what is fear of need but need itself?

Is not dread of thirst when your well is full, the thirst that is unquenchable?

There are those who give little of the much which they have—and they give it for recognition and their hidden desire makes their gifts unwholesome.

And there are those who have little and give it all.

These are the believers in life and the bounty of life, and their coffer is never empty. There are those who give with joy, and that joy is their reward.

And there are those who give with pain, and that pain is their baptism. And is there aught you would withhold?

All you have shall someday be given;

Therefore, give now, that the season of giving may be yours... You often say, "I would give, but only to the deserving."

The trees in your orchard say not so...they give that they may live, for to withhold is to perish.

Surely he who is worthy to receive his days and his nights, is worthy of all else from you.

And he who has deserved to drink from the ocean of life deserves to fill his cup from your little stream.

For in truth, it is life that gives unto life—while you, who deem yourself a giver, are but a witness."

90.4.6.1. Living in Excess of One's Needs

Wealth—who hasn't wondered what they'd do with a million dollars? In our search for "security" we should stop and reflect a moment. The easier it becomes for us, the more we should look to see what we can do for others.

Even when we feel the pinch financially, there's always room to stretch, and there's always someone with less.

Anyone living in excess of their basic needs is being self-indulgent if s/he doesn't share. Just as the body with excess food becomes saturated or bloated or toxic, the spirit of a person becomes cloudy when s/he has more than s/he needs to get by. If one has health, happiness comes naturally. Beyond these, what will money buy? It can't really even buy these, and this has been said in so many different ways by now that it seems we'd take it for granted. Yet we often lose sight of our perspective in the search for security.

Some of the most generous people I met travelling in foreign countries were people who had almost nothing.

If you can learn to be happy with nothing, think what you can do if something comes along!

90.4.8. Rule #7—Relax

If you want to keep pace with a world that is moving faster than ever, the best thing to do is relax. The younger generation is instinctively more open-minded and active because it has to keep up with constant change and expansion. We should be as fluid, tolerant and easy-going as possible at all times, and let go of our attachments. We don't hold our breath if we want to live, and must let go of one breath and flow into the next one. We should be this fluid in our deeper selves. We don't want our physical body or our minds to be rigid, contained or tied to one idea, rather they should be as changing, evolving and ongoing as life itself.

Negative emotions are only useful insofar as they can trigger us into positive action. A brief moment of anxiety makes us alert to something that needs attention. Adrenalin stimulates the body to action. Or negative emotions may serve as a release of pent-up feelings, a cleansing. Whatever their purpose, whenever they linger on and stretch into minutes and hours, we begin to drain our energy and enervate the body needlessly.

The anxiety (or whatever) alone, without action, is futile once its initial purpose, that of "warning," is fulfilled.

As long as we ignore stress, we are not in a state of mental well-being. Constant pressure injures us by interrupting the natural flow on a physical and mental level. Our brain becomes distracted and enervated. The autonomic nervous system gets out of control. We can feel the grip of stress in our necks, shoulders, facial muscles, feet, hands—we must break its grip.

The fear of failure can feel as threatening to us as an approaching train in whose path we stand. Your body can't tell the difference—it just feels the stress. In a chronic stress pattern, there is sometimes a crisis that arises to break the cycle. For example, illness will force the person to rest, for he'll have an excuse to stay in bed or do nothing.

If only doing nothing were that easy. Some people are afraid that it means they're apathetic or lazy. They've forgotten that one can creatively do "nothing." Clearing the mind space and letting the universe inside for a moment can hardly be called nothing! People should remember to relax simply.

The simple repetition of a sound can relax the body and the mind. In meditation, breathing slows. Heart rate diminishes. The sensation is calming and relaxing. Relaxation response is the result. We know that we must change to good dietary habits for health, but it is worth noting that meditation has been seen to effect changes on the physical level as well as the mental level. Studies have shown that it diminishes irregular cardiac contraction, particularly ventricular tachyarrhythmias, and that it can reduce the number and intensity of anxiety attacks. Insomnia, tension and migraine headaches, and certain other kinds of pain may be reduced. Meditation helps lower blood pressure in hypertensive people, and has helped drug, alcohol, and cigarette abusers too. It has been effective in treating speech problems such as stuttering. One study showed a significant reduction in serum cholesterol levels after eleven months of daily meditation. Yogis and serious meditators can learn to control their pulse, brain waves, blood pressure, heart rate, skin conductance, muscle tension, peripheral circulation and respiratory pattern and rate.

My purpose in mentioning this is certainly not to suggest that meditation should be a replacement for correction of dietary habits, but through meditation we may learn more about the powers of the mind, and this can help us on any level. We will be well-rewarded if we reach for both physical health and mental growth, for they go hand in hand. Meditation is a wonderful tool to employ in realizing self-knowledge.

Choose a quiet place where you will not be disturbed and get comfortable sitting or lying down. Close your eyes and let your mind drift. Let each thought go and quiet your mind. You'll be amazed at first how often your conscious mind will insist on asserting itself, accustomed as it is in preoccupying your normal waking state. But continue to let each thought go. Try to do this for fifteen to twenty minutes, twice a day, as a minimum. You may do it as often or as long as you like. With time you will see more and more changes in the quality of your meditative state. Some people read volumes on "psychic awareness," but these books can only describe various dimensions of thought and cannot of themselves bring the awareness to a person. Not all people gifted with sensitive minds are book-educated. Some of them are merely wise in their simplicity. Just as a fast (with temporary elimination of food) renews and revitalizes the entire organism, so too does meditation (temporary elimination of conscious thought) refresh the mind and elevate the spirit to new heights.

Pure diet, fresh air, sunshine, warm baths, swimming, dancing, hiking, camping, gardening, exercise, laughter (and crying) and humor are all possible ways of dealing with stress. Mild massage can help. Care should be taken to avoid rigorous massage with extremes of vigorous thumping, molding, and probing. This may result in over-stimulation, enervation, and possible harm. In mild massage, touch and the human factor are at work. There is something magnetic and caring about another person's touch that can do wonders. Love is truly healing.

Exercise should include some form of aerobics to get the heart pumping and circulation going. There was an inter-sting note in a book on longevity that said in one area with many old people the men seemed to live about 20 years longer than the women, with all lifestyle factors seemingly equal. Upon closer scrutiny, one difference was found: the women tended to walk around in their homes? on a flat surface, whereas the men climbed up and down the long, steep mountain trails for much of their days. They had well-developed, strong calf muscles which pumped the blood up to their hearts more vigorously—their circulation was better. So even when we walk and do housework and gardening, getting plenty of "old-fashioned" exercise, we must also do something with a bit more spark to it.

When I don't run or swim, I find dancing at home a good way to get the heart going and get a variety of movements done. It's my personal opinion that people miss a lot of fun when they reserve dancing just for special events or parties, or just for when they can find a partner.

90.4.9. Rule #8—Take your time

Time does not exist as we define it in our human terms. In fact, it even differs from individual to individual, from a child to a peasant in a field to a businessman checking his watch.

Before we are a year old, we live in an eternal present. At about 2, "today" appears, at 2 1/2, "tomorrow." "Afternoon" and "yesterday" come at 4 and "days" at 5.

Kahlil Gibran says of time:

"You would measure time the measureless and the immeasurable.

Yet the timeless in you is aware of life's timeless-ness and knows that yesterday is but today's memory and tomorrow is today's dream.

And that that which sings and contemplates in you is still dwelling within the bounds of that first moment which scattered the stars into space."

Quantum physics says that everything is one and time in not linear. Modern physics sees space and time existing together at once, as if they were a block, without separation in the block. It is we as individuals who divide it arbitrarily into seconds, minutes, hours, days, weeks, months and years, ad infinitum. While many people become more and more obsessed with and dominated by time, or bemoan their "lack" of it, it seems that children, primitive people, religious and mystical people all live in an eternal, continual present. When time ceases to flow in the fragments created by our words, we are enveloped by the stillness that all the great mystics have spoken about.

When you aren't living in the now, and you slip into the past or the future, you are alive in a time that is not the real time of the moment. Your focus changes, and you are no longer centered on balance.

When you think of time, does it seem that the last year has gone faster than the one before it? Do you often rush to get things done and fear that you'll never have enough time? What is enough time? Be assured that each of us has all the time we need.

If you let your mind jump ahead to the year 3000 you will see in perspective how important it is that the vase be dusted, or whatever. When you watch ants, some will get lost up on a twig for what seems like ages, doing who knows what. We are like these ants at times, distracted off in our corners, filling our time with all sorts of busy activity that seems important to us. We must survive and find our priorities in life. But in our rush to survive, we must not forget to LIVE. Once a day at least (if not more!), remember just to live, only to live, not to do. Stop listening only to your constant stream of thoughts; it's like looking in a mirror at yourself all day long—certainly most of us wouldn't consider that a thrill. Get outside yourself and listen to the birds, the wind, the silence, and you will hear other voices speak.

Feel the life force within yourself. Remind yourself to slow down for a moment, long enough to enjoy the miracle, for truly your participation in life in this grand universe is a miracle. Don't let life trickle through your fingers like the sand in an hourglass, so that once it's gone, it's too late and you never realized it. Don't wait to live. Feel it. Stop wasting your time worrying about time. An 81-year-old friend told me at 31, when I was lamenting about not having enough time: "don't worry, you'll have all the time you need when you're dead." Likewise, we have all the time we need to live. So, we must live our lives fully, for quality, not quantity.

John Lennon said,

"Life is what happens while we're busy making other plans.

90.5. Using Psychology on Others

90.5.1. Do's and Don'ts

90.5.2. "Am I My Brother's Keeper?"

Most of us have tried on one occasion or another to "convert" someone to a health regime or to use "reverse" psychology on children, all with varying degrees of success or failure. We all know at least one person so stubborn that we would be better off talking to a wall, too. We will have to know when to persist in hopes of turning a key in their minds, and when to let go of our need to change someone.

Everyone has the same opportunity to see the truth. Those who don't see it are like someone whose eyes are closed when a shooting star goes by...can they then say that it did not go by because they did not see it?

It is always sad for us when loved ones will not see what we see as true. We all know someone with an illness that we'd like to help if we only could, if they'd only listen, if they'd only understand, if...

It's hard to know what to say, but if you were to hold up a volume of cherished poetry in front of a person who cannot read and two people who can read, one will see words, one will read words and one will read between the lines of the words as well, beyond to another depth.

It would be difficult to make the book any more than a book to the one who didn't read at all. It might not be much more than a book to the one who can read but has less understanding. The third person, the one who sees more deeply, is really talking with the book's author.

How do you explain your ecstasy after listening to a musical piece to someone who doesn't feel it? How do you explain that the smell of lilacs is making you delirious with joy to a person suffering from a cold? How would you explain color to a person who is blind? In all of these instances, one can transcend words somewhat and get beyond them to another meaning, but different people will even respond differently to the same stimulus. We cannot expect everyone to see what we see even if they look in the same direction. Even if you hold up the same object, people see it differently.

This is what we must remember when faced with people who see and understand differently, and not become obsessed with changing their minds. We've seen parents try to change children, children trying to change parents, husbands and wives who try to change each other, friends who try to change friends, the list is endless. Someone always knows better. They beg and plead, or perhaps if these don't work, they try trickery, or, finally, give up or become angry.

It is up to us to decide in each individual situation how to handle conversations on lifestyle. After we make the truth known, each person will change only when ready to do so. Some of us have a hard enough time changing ourselves, so we should understand this quite well when we see it in others. Dr Albert Schweitzer said, "Example is not just the best way to teach: It is the only way!" Let us first change ourselves, and let others see for themselves what truth is, manifested in our example. Truth is self-evident. Each person decides whether to live by it. I am reminded of the words in a song of the last decade: "a man hears what he wants to hear and disregards the rest." Certainly true; but let's hope some of us can do better than that.

The following guidelines will help you in dealing with other people when the issues of diet/lifestyle come up:

90.5.1. Do's and Don'ts

DO	DON'T
relax	don't get tense
speak slowly, calmly	don't speak rapidly, nervously, or argumentatively
avoid obvious tender discussion topics at dinner	don't preach
suggest what you would do, mention what you do/or don't eat	don't tell others "do this/do that" in a dogmatic way, just because you do it
be patient	don't lose your patience
be subtle	don't be blunt or offensive
keep a sense of humor	don't alienate others with your seriousness
do what you believe in	don't try to prove yourself to others
be tolerant and understanding	don't be too judgmental

"catch flies with honey"	don't turn people off to Natural Hygiene
be humble	don't be self-righteous, know-it-all
know your limits	don't overdo your health "lectures"
be aware of others reactions; be sensitive to how much they want to hear. Does this person want your advice? Someone who does is more apt to listen and absorb what you say than someone who obviously isn't interested.	don't waste your breath
be optimistic and positive	don't approach a health discussion with a negative "fire and brimstone" attitude
be gracious even if antagonized	don't lose your temper or become angry when someone lacks understanding

90.5.2. "Am I My Brother's Keeper?"

To what extent are we responsible for spreading the truth? We already spoke of setting a good example. The power of collective thought is barely even recognized, let lone understood, by most of us. We are all busy travelling through space and time, like millions of voyagers on a journey towards the future, a future that waits for us with population growth, extinction of species, computers, robots, space travel, genetic engineering, prosthetic devices and implants, more drugs and the unknown. Where will we fit in? How can the children of nature keep a healthy perspective?

When the first settlers came to America they were full of passion in their beliefs, ready to make it in the next world. The planet is much smaller these days, and there aren't many new worlds left for us. What we do now affects one another more than ever before.

We might think that we are only responsible for ourselves, but it is this illusion that is responsible for destroying our life source: our planet. We must not let this happen. We are responsible for ourselves and others. The planet needs to be healed, and people need to live in peace.

Weapons have a way of being very unHygienic, even for people who eat raw fruits, vegetables, nuts and seeds. While we fret about the price of shoes and who's ahead in the World Series, or plan our perfect diets, there are people who are busy making decisions for us, very grave decisions. They hold our destiny in the palms of their hands. Those of us who see clearly, see that just as doctors mesmerize the public with verbal slight-of hand and drugs, our world leaders are trying to convince the masses that more weapons can "prevent" war. This continual addition of more complex and deadly weapons to our weapons arsenal has created such an over-kill potential (the planet can now be destroyed not once, but many times over) that it is like keeping a bottle of arsenic in the medicine cabinet to take to "prevent a cold."

There is a riddle going around that asks: "if we are in a closed room with a gas leak and have four matches, how many must you light for an explosion?" The answer obviously is only one. The nuclear freeze advocates have been trying to tell us something.

So, what kind of a lifestyle change shall we make? Shall we give up candy and pat ourselves on the back? Or shall we learn to weave our physical bodies, our minds, and our souls into the whole tapestry of life in the most beautiful way we can imagine? We will be our larger selves, linked to one another all over the planet.

Let us reach out to those who need help. The more love that goes out into the world, the more healing that can take place. There is no greater purpose in life than helping others as we would help ourselves.

90.6. Questions & Answers

There is so much suffering: having compassion, how can one be at peace?

Do you think you are different from the world? Are you not the world? The world that you have made with your ambition, with your greed, with your economic securities, with your wars—you made it. The torture of animals for your food, the wastage of money on war, the lack of right education—you have built this world, it is part of you. So, you are the world and the world is you; there is no division between you and the world. You ask, "How can you have peace when the world suffers?" How can you have peace when you are suffering? This is the question because you are the world. You can go all over the world, talk to human beings, whether they are clever, famous, or illiterate, they are all going through a terrible time—like you. So the question is not, "How can you have peace when the world is suffering?" You are suffering and therefore the world suffers; therefore put an end to your suffering, if you know how to end it. Suffering with its self-pity comes to an end only when there is self-knowing. (J. Krishnamurti)

What else can I do after I change my own lifestyle?

• Channel some of your energy into one of the following efforts to save our planet, our home and life source: clean up the environment recycle solar energy and other alternative energy forms help free animals from exploitation, in laboratories and livestock farming save seeds, especially open-pollinated seeds organic gardening plant trees, especially fruit trees, nut trees plant flowers educate others music, dance, beauty, art love others shelter those who need it help others

Article #1: Ahimsa Excerpts

Reverence for Life, and the Golden Rule

The phrase was originated by Dr. Albert Schweitzer to describe his belief that life has value; that life is a rich and rewarding experience for all who partake of it; and there is no such thing as worthless life. Probably the greatest of all is the Golden Rule: that we should act toward others as we would wish them to act toward ourselves.

The Golden Rule in Seven World Faiths Hinduism

"Men gifted with intelligence ... should always treat others as they themselves wish to be treated."

Buddhism

"In five ways should a clansman minister to his friends and familiars: by generosity, courtesy and benevolence, by treating them as he treats himself, and by being as good as his word."

Taoism

"Regard your neighbor's gain as your own gain and regard your neighbor's loss as your own loss."

Confucianism

"What you do not want done to yourself, do not do to others."

Judaism

"Thou shalt love thy neighbor as thyself."

Christianity

"All things whatsoever ye would that men should do to you, do ye even so unto them."

Islam

"No one of you is a believer until he loves for his brother what he loves for himself." The person who has a mind that is controlled and serene, a pleasant and calm disposition, and a ready and sincere smile for others, will find others smiling right back.

Good people instinctively are wary of someone who radiates fear and hatred, but one who shows universal love communicates this to others.

In this modern age of mass communication, a sweeping numbness has developed in many minds, a form of defense mechanism or reaction to the over-stimulation of our senses by visual and auditory gimmicks. The Golden Rule is still the real thing.

Man's insatiable curiosity has driven him to the conquest of Space and toward the stars, but man must master his lower self before he can realize his higher potential; and he must do both before he is fit to master the Earth, the sea, the skies and "outer space," let alone mastering other living beings such as animals, birds, and fish. Man claims absolute "dominion" over everything that breathes, crawls, runs, flies, or swims, but he has been ill-trained for such a royal position, and seems more like a petty tyrant instead. Without this first conquest of "inner space"—the conquest by man of himself at the individual level—we are only turning loose a monster with little restraining sense of morality, justice, fairness, and goodness. If only man would stop trying so hard to know and would make more effort to understand. If only we could understand that the universe is not malevolent, and that man can live in love and compassion without perishing. Indeed, it appears more likely that he will perish if he does NOT practice these virtuous attributes to a sufficient degree.

In any event, we cannot have it both ways: man cannot pretend to be higher in ethics, spirituality, advancement, or civilization than other creatures and at the same time live by a lower standard than the vulture or hyena. The truth of the matter is that it is high time for man to leave his lowest brute nature behind and bring his nobler self to the fore. Mankind has been in the jungle too long. As with a mole or owl viewing bright sunshine, we are presently so dazzled by the brilliance of what may lie ahead, that we prefer the comfort of our present position. We are possessed by a great inertia; we cling to that which we think we know, rather than attempting that which we do not yet fully understand. But the world is more than just a jungle; we might come out of the darkness into the lovely sunshine and become used to the bright light after a while.

We will never make real progress out of the jungle until we break off the chains we have forged for ourselves and which we so proudly wear and display: the fears and ignorance, and self-satisfied complacency.

322

Everyone has his own way to go—you have yours. Follow your conscience and your Inner Light; they are your greatest guides on the trek out of the jungle into a new and better tomorrow.

We may close with this gentle but firm cautionary note against ever mistaking the vessel for the contents, or the guide along the path for the path itself.

May you know Truth, Wisdom, and Peace.

Article #2: Excerpted from Live Foods by George & Doris Fathman

Even more fantastic are the cases of the Bavarian stigmatist, Therese Neumann, and Giri Bala of India. Miss Neumann's case is, of course, world famous, and has been carefully verified many times. Going through the agony of the crucifixion every Friday, she has lived her entire adult life on nothing but one communion wafer once a day. Giri Bala's case is practically unknown or was until it was first brought to the world's notice by Paramhansa Yogananda in his Autobiography of a Yogi. Her amazing story has been thoroughly verified. For fifty-five years she lived without eating! During all that time she prepared all the meals for her family, lived an active life, yet had no appetite for food. Both of these women maintain they live on God's light. When asked to explain, they say their secret cannot be revealed, that it is not for the mass of mankind, in this day, but only to prove that we are spirit, and that ultimately that spirit will rule the flesh.

Article #3: The Doctrine of the Memory of Cells by Stanley Bass

Man is constructed basically from the food and liquids which enter his body. When food is eaten, a profound effect is exerted upon the consumer in both the feeling and thinking nature, depending upon whether the origin of the food is from the vegetable or animal kingdom. The vegetable food induces a state of tranquility and inner peace in both feeling and thought with a disinclination to violence to either man or any living creature. The animal food induces a state of volatility and restlessness in the feeling, passional and mental nature with an inclination to anger and violence. The manifestation of these characteristics have their origin in two sources. First, from the intrinsic nature of the food itself.

For example, if the person eats flesh, the feelings, and emotions such as fear and terror which the animal experienced before it was slaughtered are transported along with its tissues to the consumer. Then again, according to many religions, the passion-exciting qualities associated with all animal products are said to reside in its blood. Also, we have here a protein which was once alive, but is now dead and filled with the products of decomposition, bacteria and added chemicals, etc. The tendencies produced by this are sluggishness, torpor, and inertia. All of this adds up to an assortment of disquieting characteristics of mental, feeling, and emotional stuff which is ingested along with the flesh which is consumed. The same corresponding interaction applies to all other food which is eaten. Any inorganic minerals, chemicals or preservatives which are added from the mineral kingdom are not directly usable by the body unless they have first been incorporated into the vegetable kingdom. Their presence in this inorganic form acts as an irritant to the body which manifests as thoughts and feelings of irritability, hyperactivity, restlessness, sensitivity, and feelings of insecurity.

The second source of origin of some mental and emotional tendencies relates to our state of mind when we eat. In some strange and as yet inexplicable manner, the thoughts and feelings we have at the moment we are eating enter and combine with the food. They are transported along with the food and are incorporated into the formation and fixation of the cells which are constantly being synthesized in all parts of the body. There they remain captive to exert either subconscious or conscious thought, feeling and behavior tendencies in the individual.

Now, when a person decides to undergo a process of detoxication, either by losing weight through restricting the food intake, or by upgrading the quality of food consumed, a very interesting process occurs. When the body intelligence sees that a higher quality of foods is coming in that is superior to the material that its tissues are made of, it immediately begins to disintegrate and eliminate its inferior tissues to make room for this better material in a new tissue formation. As these cells are dissolved, the memories, feelings and thought tendencies which were originally associated with the formation of these cells are released into the bloodstream. Therein, they circulate throughout the body and eventually are transported into the brain. When they enter the brain, there is a retracing of these memories and thoughts as the individual once again becomes conscious of them. A catharsis or washing out of these thoughts and feelings occurs and their hold upon the individual is broken from the subconscious fabric. A feeling of lightness, liberation and freedom from bondage is experienced and with it comes a feeling of release that one feels when a phase of life is completely finished with.

It takes 7 years to change and completely replace every cell of the body. When we detoxicate the body through fasting, for example, as cells which are 6 to 7 years old are disintegrated, we once again experience memories that existed at that time but have since been forgotten. As old fluids in the lymph spaces are discarded, their associated memories go with them. If a person hasn't eaten chocolate for say 20 years, but the chocolate has been retained in lymph spaces or fat cells, the taste and smell of the chocolate will leave the body and become evident to the individual and outsiders associated with the person—both will smell the chocolate. The memories associated with the time it was consumed will flash back into the person's consciousness.

Strange as this theory may sound, I have noticed the truth associated with it in my own life for more than 25 years and in the lives of hundreds of others who were puzzled about the buried subconscious memories which became released when they purified their bodies and bloodstreams.

The moral of this story is that it should teach us that: (a) there is more to food than just the chemistry of it (proteins, carbohydrates, minerals, vitamins, etc.); (b) the feelings, emotions, thoughts, and character of an individual are in some subtle manner closely associated to the quality of the food we eat. It makes one think about the character of the person who will be permitted to prepare the food of the household; and (c) it is important that the element of time be considered in the changeover of an individual from a lower to a higher quality of dietary. As the body changes, so will the quality of the feelings, emotions, thoughts, and goals change. The process is subtle and takes time. With change of blood and tissue chemistry comes change of character. Herein is the true alchemy of the "philosopher's stone," the changing of base metal into gold, so eagerly sought by the medieval alchemists. It behooves us all to become modern alchemists by learning to transmute the best food of nature into the best character-material, which is possible, which without fail will lead us to the highest happiness which is possible.

Excerpted from Overcoming Compulsive Habits

Article #4: The Green-Eyed Monster by Virginia Vetrano

Jealousy means an intolerance of rivalry or "unfaithfulness," and an apprehensiveness of the loss of another's exclusive devotion. It implies hostility toward a rival or one that is believed to enjoy an advantage. It implies vigilance in guarding a possession, person, or thing so that no one else can have it or enjoy it. Jealousy and envy can lead to evil actions. They become pathological when excessive and when the possessor and the object of the envy or jealousy are hurt. Not only does jealousy hurt others; it also hurts the one who is jealous because it impairs all the functions of the body. Jealousy consumes nerve energy at a rapid rate and hardens the features as few things will. Strong jealousy is a type of insanity, a combination of inferiority and selfishness. Jealousy is not merely the fear of losing the "beloved" one, for often there is no real love for the object of jealousy; it springs largely, often wholly, from wounded vanity. Wounded self-esteem, rather than undying love, characterizes the psychology of the deserted lover. This is forcibly illustrated by the well-known fact that the agony produced by a death, terrible as the shock may prove, generally more easily and in shorter time, and less often occasions suicide, than the pain and chagrin of a lover's "infidelity."

In cottages and luxurious palaces green-eyed jealousy takes all the joy out of domestic life, and plants thorns of strife. Jealousy is a vice, not a virtue. It poisons the wellspring of life. It kills love and respect and transforms human relationships into a hell.

There is every reason why we should learn to maintain emotional poise. There is every reason why we should avoid being, a green-eyed monster as long as we shall live, for you desire health, that spark of vitality and beauty, you will shun jealousy just as if it were a plague. It destroys everything.

Be ready to admit when someone can do something better than you. You are as good as your time and energy permits. There is no reason to be jealous or envious of others.

Jealousy and envy have their beginnings in childhood. Children should be taught to be happy with what they already have and not dwell on what they don't have. (In fact, we adults might do well to learn this lesson too). If you thrill with someone when they get something new, and enjoy it with them, you will share their blessings instead of sitting there envying them and being miserable. Early in life we must train our children not to be envious of the possessions of others. Our school system teaches competition: only one can win. Each child should be praised for his efforts and encouraged to develop his individual gifts, and not made to fit into a ready-made mold.

If you are lazy and can't discipline yourself to do anything, then admit it, and just be you. You may be happiest just doing little things, or just doing nothing all day long. This is just fine. This is what you desire out of life. Admit it and then enjoy the accomplishments of others. If you want to discipline yourself, you will. Often jealousy stems from a pathological fear of losing one's power.

If you harbor a green-eyed monster deep within yourself, then for your own sake turn it into an angel of love.

Article #5: Ridding the World of Violence by Arthur Andrews

"And at the root of it all..."

Almost at the beginning of it all is the violence we do to ourselves, not the violence others do to us or that we do to other humans or other animals.

If we could manage a microscopic existence, and join our own cells at their levels, and see their fears, their panic, the alarms they set off and the defense systems they throw up, the strategies they formulate, the communications, the cooperation and support they muster for each other and for the total good in the face of what we impose on them as we indulge ourselves; if we could be locked arm-in-arm with all our stomach cell brethren as gross amounts of gross food gets piled in upon us, forcing us out and out as we strive desperately to hold on to each other just to keep from bursting; if we could be part of those scenes at that level, we might feel and behave differently, because these are violent acts we commit upon our physical selves. What is required of our bodies in the face of a coffee or alcoholic dousing should be as embarrassing to us as it must be frightening to our nervous systems and befuddling to our other parts of the body. Really, think about it and recognize that we make our internal and external bodies into garbage bins and cesspools! How violent!

The very first form of violence, however, that no one ever considers (and it is the start of it all), is the violence we do to the food we eat before we take it into our bodies. We obtain quite live foods containing life force waiting for the opportunity to fulfill their intended purpose and thereby be rewarded by being incorporated into, becoming part of our higher form of life. But before they ever get that opportunity to gain their own evolution, we kill them, we cook them to death. The things we do to our foods would be considered the crudest of tortures were we to do them to things that could cry out, and especially so, were we to do them to humans. Few things are so violent as cooking is to live foods. And with very few exceptions, it is so unnecessary. What a price we pay for it!

That violence which we perpetuate upon our foods as we kill them goes into the food and then into our bodies where the violence is, in turn, heaped upon our cells, tissues, organs and systems. Then as it builds and compounds, growing all the while, it becomes incorporated into our beings. And in time, as we interact with other humans in the same state, we release the violence within us on each other ... from irritations, to anger, to hostility.

If violence is to be dealt with meaningfully and with finality, it must be dealt with at its beginning.

Lesson 91:

Methods for Inducing a Lifestyle Change

91.1. Introduction

91.1.1. The Gift of Potential

91.1.1. The Gift of Potential

At the moment of birth, all humans are endowed with a common gift, the gift of potential: potential to think, to solve problems, to dream, to accomplish.

Perhaps the greatest of all the potentials with which we are endowed is that of achieving a level of health and functional capacity far beyond our present knowledge, experience, and expectation.

Most of the data which gives us a glimpse into the enormous possibilities for superior health and achievement in our endowment is derived from gifted and highly trained individuals. Only rarely do we catch a glimmer of understanding of achievement of some aspects of the dimensions of human potential as it is revealed in a Leonardo da Vinci, the artist; or in a Socrates, the philosopher; or in an Owens, the Olympic gold medal winner; or in a Spitz, the swimmer, who captured seven gold medals; or in a Mozart, the child musician; or in a Buddha, the ethical leader of billions of people.

It has long been established that few achievements in any field of endeavor, except perhaps in the bizarre, are ever accomplished by persons sick of body or mind. It would appear reasonable to assume, therefore, that the basis for full achievement in any field or endeavor is to be found only on a base of perfect health, a commodity so rare in our day as to be practically nonexistent.

But the potential remains inherent. The potential for achieving perfect health lies in us all so long as we are not fundamentally deranged. We know that the possibility of a long, happy, productive, sickness-free life is there. Only the conditions for fulfillment must be established.

We also know that the organic requisites of life that sustain humans in perfect health are relatively few, very simple and easily possessed.

We have also learned that these fundamental needs of the living organism apply equally in sickness and health; that when a healthy individual satisfies all his basic needs adequately, but not in excess of need, he will retain his health; and, conversely, also, that when a sick person changes his attitude and lifestyle so that it now adequately answers these same needs, that sickness ceases. An ever-growing state of health then permeates the whole being. This is one of the miracles of life.

On a sliding scale of 0 to 100, we rarely, if ever, witness either extreme, most individuals falling somewhere within the middle, with some few failing greatly and, at the other end of the spectrum, some few achieving mightily. Some few dally on the

331

outskirts of life; some few are high achievers. Generally speaking, the individuals who seek the help of a Hygienist are on the outskirts because they suffer some degree of diminished health. However, while they may have lost some part of their health, they still have potential.

It is the purpose of this lesson to impart to you the ways and means of inducing clients to make whatever changes in their lifestyles that are necessary for the restoration of any possible higher level of health considering the potential they presently possess. Changes made, of course, must be based on established Hygienic principles.

91.2. The Three Requisites for Change

91.2.1. Inspiration

91.2.2. Motivation

91.2.3. Health and the Psyche

91.2.4. to Change, We Must Desert the Herd

91.2.5. The Hygienist's Knowledge

There are, of course, many ways to induce individuals to undertake change in their lifestyles so that they may enjoy a higher degree of health but basically they can all be categorized into three groupings:

1. Inspiration.
2. Motivation.
3. Knowledge of what to do and how to do it.

This last category implies the need for the client to have guidelines to follow, which are plainly marked, at least at the beginning of change.

In this lesson we will consider each category in sequence and see how we can employ it in our contacts with individual clients.

91.2.1. Inspiration

The "show-and-tell" technique is as old as history. Because it has proved to be an effective tool to inspire persons to increase performance in widely-diversified areas of interest and to induce change, among even the most reluctant, and has done so in all cultures throughout all of time, it merits our consideration in the context of this discussion.

The classic way for a Hygienic practitioner to use this very simple technique is by means of case histories.

To be most effective, the case histories should be of persons who have recovered from the kind of disease presently being experienced by the client who seeks your help. For example, if your client suffers from some rheumatic ailment, he will not be particularly moved or inspired to "go and do likewise" if you present him with a case study which relates how John Doe made a spectacular and complete recovery from asthma within a period of two days. He will not be motivated because he does not equate John Doe's recovery from asthma with his own aches and pains.

But, on the other hand, if he learns that Mary Williams who lives down the street from him and who he knows used to have rheumatoid arthritis so severely that it prevented her from ever leaving her own house, is now able to play golf two or three times a week down at the public golf course where he used to play, he will, all other things being equal, be inspired to believe that he can do the same. Hope is aroused.

If he also knows, because Mary Williams told him so, that you are the practitioner who taught Mary Williams what she had to do, how she had to .change, so that this miracle might be accomplished then, in all likelihood, he will have faith in you, so much so that he will follow your directions implicitly and without question.

And, similarly, if Ava Smith has psoriasis so badly that she sheds a cloud when she walks, she will hardly be persuaded to do as you suggest simply because you tell her (in words alone) that K. Singh living in far off Malaysia is now able to control his psoriasis to the extent that he is completely free of lesions except when he reverts to his former unhealthy ways of living. Not knowing K. Singh, she will not be inspired to follow his example, even though it be a truthful account and well presented by you. K. Singh is an unconvincing figure.

However, if Ava Smith were given a printed case history, even if it is about the same

K. Singh, and it is read aloud to her by you in her presence, the impact on her conscious mind will be fortified in two respects: by the sensation of sight and by the sensation of sound. This is a common technique which is more effective than using either one in isolation from the other. If it were possible also to present before and after photographs of

K. Singh showing full recovery, this would, of course, provide further reinforcement of your contention that Ava Smith can also experience full recovery from this distressful condition.

Even more convincing, of course, would be if Ava Smith could talk face to face with Gertrude Jones who is a recovered psoriatic (former) client of yours.

Thus, using case histories can be a highly-effective tool which can be used as a means of inspiring clients to change their lifestyles to conform to systemic need. However, when using the case history method to inspire performance, at least two important things should be kept in mind in order to encourage positive follow-up performance:

1. The case histories presented by you to the client should be applicable to him/her in as many particulars as possible, and

2. The case histories should be reasonably verifiable. That is, they should come from a reliable source, from some person whom either you or the client knows, or from some writer in whom both you and the client have explicit faith. Also, the person represented in the case history should be real, visible if possible. Preferably, of course, he should be capable of being contacted by the client either in person or by mail. This, of course, is not always possible.

When case histories are well-presented and answer the above criteria, they usually prove both convincing and inspiring to all but the most skeptical.

91.2.2. Motivation

The majority of sick people who seek out a Hygienist lack deep motivation or much hope. They have usually "been the rounds" before they come to your office. They have listened to and followed the advice of many others who promised "cure" and failed to deliver. They often approach you with many reservations, and even perhaps with tremulous fear. Their motivation to do as you suggest may be feeble.

The feeling of helplessness is widespread. Only a relative few will not accept defeat and come to you already armed with conviction, convinced that they will turn sickness into health!

Dr. Elizabeth McCarter was one of these. Suffering the severe pains of the arthritic, unable to walk without help, she remembered a saying of her mother often repeated in her presence when she was a little girl: "Elizabeth, if you ever have a problem that is seemingly unsolvable, there is usually a book out there somewhere, in some library, that will provide the answer. Your real problem is to find that book!"

Thus, when she was forced with this very real problem, she determined for herself that she could solve her problem, that she would find the way to restore herself to health, that she would overcome this pain, this suffering. It took her well over five years of searching to find the book, five years during which she travelled the world and looked in many libraries, but finally she did find the book. She and I found it right here at home, in the U.S., in a little health food store in Solana Beach, California. What was the name of the book? Why, of course! It was Dr. Shelton's masterpiece, Orthotrophy, Volume II of THE HYGIENIC SYSTEM.

To the scientific mind this book has the impact of a thousand candles upon the darkness of night. It has served to motivate hundreds of thousands of people, both the sick and the well, to desert the herd and seek after the ways of health. Elizabeth is but one of many who were thus motivated and followed through to a successful conclusion, witnessing and participating in a lifestyle change into a high status of health.

Strangers now marvel that, at 82, Elizabeth has the vitality to do all that she does. One reporter even commented quite recently that she has "the grace of a ballet dancer." It is sometimes difficult for us even to remember the "once that was."

Motivation is difficult to define, methods differing as individual clients differ. Some clients have psychosomatic disorders brought about by introspective experiences for which there are few, if any, observable correlates.

For example, the feeling of helplessness that so many clients have may, in part, be rooted in childhood experiences which led to their feeling of having been caught in a trap from which they could not escape. Some develop this feeling because of recent unsettling events or perhaps from continued and exhausting stress which drained their fund of nerve energy.

Sheep that were given tasks to solve but could not soon became neurotic, highly nervous, "unglued," as we say. P.O.W.s, to their credit, often felt trapped and helpless, but maintained some semblance of poise throughout their ordeal. Some became depressed and developed neuroses of one kind or another or various physical disorders. Some actively sought to solve their dilemma and got out of the trap. Jack B. Story, the celebrated Marine hero of the infamous Shanghai prison escape of World War II, is a classic example of motivation followed by action. When properly motivated, people seek after solutions, and when they find a solution adaptable to their peculiar problem, they usually try with all their might to follow through to a successful conclusion; not always, but usually. Sometimes peoples' minds are so cluttered with toxins, they never do find their way.

The Hygienist should understand that, as Dr. Alexis Carrel, M.D., so well stated in Man, The Unknown, "Mind and organism commune in man, like form and marble in a statue." As practitioners we must, understand that with clients whose physical ailments are psychosomatic in origin, the concept of capability, just replace helplessness before meaningful progress can be expected, this whether the immediate trouble is simple or complex and, even, perhaps when the ailments are purely and demonstrably physical, although usually there is a close and often undefinable relationship between diseases of emotional origin and diseases which are more physical. Rarely can they be precisely defined. Regardless of kind, location pr type, they all have a common origin: a toxin-saturated body or toxicosis.

Just this morning a woman, approaching her 50th year, sat in our office recalling the immensity of the restraints placed upon her by her powerfully-built, beer-drinking husband, a man seemingly possessed by an obsession to dominate the very thought processes of his wife.

For over 20 years, during which time she had endured a veritable parade of illnesses, she had meekly submitted to this man, following his every command without question. She became almost a mindless being.

But, one day (and we know not, nor do we care, what caused her to change), her mind suddenly became aware, aware that life had more to offer than this. She determined to improve her health and to get out of her rut before all of life had passed her by.

So it was that four years ago she came to us. She began to learn about Natural Hygiene. She became our private student. She took her physical inheritance and fasted for 14 days on two separate occasions, once at Dr. Shelton's and again with Dr. Vetrano. She made amazing progress physically. The mental changes were slower in coming but they came.

She is taking assertiveness classes now at the local college. She attends Al-Anon.

The metamorphosis, the change, has been wondrous to watch.

This morning we discussed the I CAN concept of living with her. The need is to change an attitude of helplessness to one of "I can," to watch over our own conduct and cease being critical of others, the need to develop a commitment to the improvement of self. This is not the first time we had spoken in this vein to her but one of many. We pointed out to her that it is now time for her to establish a new goal, to select one all-important goal and to direct her thoughts toward it. It is also time perhaps for her to remove herself finally from her restraints, to cast them all aside.

Our client has changed, she has grown. Her husband, unfortunately, has remained just as he was, in a box of his own making. He is sick, but she is now well. She has proved herself because she was willing and even eager to make changes in her lifestyle. He has remained in his box because, stubbornly, he refused to change. His box is made of inferior materials: of beer, steaks, frog legs and wine. She is committed to adventure, determined to explore life and to understand its full meaning.

What did this woman require of us to help her to get out of her box? It took knowledge, it took empathy toward her very real problems, to her pain and suffering; it took repetition time and time again of concepts and principles. It took encouraging words, reminding her of the possibilities. At times, it even took scolding. But, most of all, it required improved health.

The days of whining and wondering are almost over. Our client has set her new goal and we believe she will attain her desire: to be so healthy that no challenge will be too great. Perhaps she will never have it all, but we know she'll give it a good try! And, we think, too, that life will know that this woman passed by and achieved something worthy while she lived.

George S. Weger in his book, The Genesis and Control of Disease, gives us another classic example of how the mind can sometimes control us and even create disease. A young man of 33, happily married, a father, mentally keen, extraverted type, with no vicious habits, and successful in business began to fail in health. He had a nervous breakdown and suffered digestive disturbances, jaundice and became highly emaciated. Like so many others he endured many examinations and much drugging. He became emotionally disturbed.

Dr. Weger also fasted his patient as we did our woman for a period of two weeks and, in the following six months, the man showed remarkable, recovery. Dr. Weger uncovered some amazing psychic aspects which had previously been entirely overlooked by other practitioners.

91.2.3. Health and the Psyche

As quoted from Weger: "The psychic aspects of the case were as follows: During early childhood, an elder brother took particular delight in threatening his younger brothers and sisters with bodily injury, even menacing them with knives and declaring that he would kill them. The patient developed a fear-complex which became more assertive as he grew to maturity. As his health became impaired, he developed an obsession which he tried desperately to repress. He became the victim of an almost unconquerable urge to kill his wife and children. These obsessive inclinations left him in a cold sweat, trembling, weeping, and aghast at the enormity of his weakness. When he learned how this complex had originated in the subconscious and what a momentous effect the repression had on his physical well-being as well as on his mental morale, his complex became sublimated. He was an apt student and soon understood how it was possible for his mental repression to exert a like influence on his physical organism, overstimulating certain endocrines (such as the suprarenal and thyroid) and depressing other glands (such as the pancreas and liver), and how this included also all the functions of digestion and elimination. Understanding in this case was the equivalent of cure."

In the case of our woman client, she was motivated to change by the desire to remove herself from the restraints imposed on her by her thoughtless husband. In Weger's case, understanding that the cause of the psychic aspects of his physical ailments lay in his childhood experiences, motivated him to control his thoughts, to redirect them in more positive channels. In both cases, correction resulted when they became aware that they could be in charge of their own lives. They replaced Helplessness with Capability, the changes in lifestyle then followed, the toxic condition was alleviated by fasting and both moved on to new and more rewarding lives.

Once a client understands that whatever ails him/her is capable of solution and that you, the Hygienic practitioner, have both the understanding of cause and the knowledge of how to solve the client's problem, and that it is possible to change sick ways into health-promoting ways, simply by making certain changes in lifestyle, the client will be more favorably disposed to make whatever 'changes' you propose; at least to take the initial, hesitant first steps.

Sometimes the mere revelation of the source of psychic disturbances, talking them out with a willing listener, will assist the recovery process. It seems that cleaning out the cobwebs that clutter the mind often opens up unknown depths of long-unused thought and makes one more receptive to change.

A case study we have previously written about comes to mind. This woman, as a child, had been subjected to much physical and mental abuse from her father, a prominent politician. Incest had been only one of many frightening experiences. As a teenager, there had been two attempted rapes. When she came to us, she was in her mid-sixties and, up to this time, had never revealed any of these sordid details to another single soul, not even to her husband or children. The story came out in a torrent, the tears poured down her cheeks as she opened wide her soul and revealed how ravaged and unclean she had felt throughout her lifetime.

It was like washing the windows to reveal the day. From then on it was comparatively clear sailing. She was highly motivated to go the distance, to clean out every corner of her physical body just as she had cleaned out the poisons from her mind. She now understood that it had been this mental poison that had gradually taken away her health. Motivation must always precede recovery. The recovery, of course, will necessarily have a dynamic basis and must be conceived in force, desire, goal, or drive. The individuals must devoutly and fervently want health. Indeed, they must be imbued with an inner drive to reach a goal of superior health because it is now a very personal goal.

When the goal becomes a personal thing, even if obstacles arise, as, for example, a temporary healing crisis, they will not be defeated or even diverted from pursuing the goal. The individuals understand that they must cope with any problems confronted because they want to solve them; i.e., they desire to improve health so much that they will do whatever is required, make whatever changes are necessary to attain health, even if it means deserting the herd.

91.2.4. to Change, We Must Desert the Herd

Individual clients must be motivated to desert the herd. As a child we are all biologically dependent on others. As adults we are expected to take command of our own selves. We must remove ourselves from all cultural dependence, from media dependence; otherwise, we devalue Self. Appreciation of Self is important to recovery from sickness. Furthermore, if we don't, we soon lose control of Self.

As Hygienists we equate sickness with the herd mentality. Statistics prove the point for, as a group, the herd is sick. When clients understand this, they become better motivated to withdraw themselves from the herd and adapt more readily to the concept that change is vital.

Sometimes accepting divorcement from the herd and the need to change gives rise to temporary conflict. A conflict, however, which when satisfactorily addressed, serves in the end to motivate a person to remove him or herself even more from the masses, even to the extent that an individual will completely reverse his/her attitude toward life and what is required to achieve the goal of attaining superb health.

But, when sufficient motivation is lacking, failure will surely come. Fortunately for humankind, where sufficient motivation already exists and it is accompanied by an inner urge, desire, force, or drive, success is almost always assured.

It is the happy duty of the Hygienic practitioner to devise ways and means to motivate clients. An emotionally or psychologically healthy person is one who has learned to cope successfully with him or herself and his/her environment. We must motivate our clients to become more poised, to direct them skillfully in such a way that they will attain the superb health which may presently be but a vague dream or hope having no substance.

Motivation is a melding together of want, wish, desire and purpose. Certainly, sick clients want to improve their health, they wish they were healthier than they now are, they have a certain amount of desire to cooperate with you and we should encourage this and, also, we must supply them with knowledge so that they will pursue the purpose which brought them to you.

91.2.5. The Hygienist's Knowledge

The Hygienist who is well-versed in the principles of Natural Hygiene—Life Science— has sufficient knowledge to change the world.

If the world understood and practiced the principles that you are learning in this course and had full understanding of the scientific truth of toxemia being the basis for all diseased states, and lived accordingly, all ailments, diseases, pain, and suffering would be no more. The members of the world population would soon forego their whining, warring, and worrying in favor of enjoying the fruits of healthful living. There would be ample food to feed the world because soil culture would replace what appears to be deliberate sickness culture. Productivity in presently unknown areas of human endeavor would be stimulated as euphoria replaced depression. The hours now spent in laboring would be dramatically reduced and used instead for the full enjoyment of life.

Yes! Natural Hygiene is capable of causing changes which could rock the world. And the Hygienic practitioner who is well informed can be a full participant in the Grand Event. When you have completed this course, if you have been diligent in your studies, you will be fully prepared to do your part.

And you can do your part as you meet every day on a one-to-one basis with the individual clients who seek your help. You can impart to your clients the knowledge of health-promoting practices which, if followed as circumstances permit, will restore them to the vibrant health that is our natural heritage.

At first meeting, however, unless proven otherwise, you must assume that your client has little or no knowledge of Life Science. Obviously, you cannot impart full understanding in one easy lesson.

Clients can often be turned off and become discouraged if we expect too much, too soon. Clients can also be disenchanted by any display of arrogance, the "know-it-all" attitude, on the part of the practitioner.

We will shortly take up some preferred and proven ways to direct clients in their education more effectively so that new practitioners can develop more confidence in their practice, perhaps more patience with their clients, and become leaders in their field.

Perhaps the knowledge learned in this lesson will induce some of our more experienced students to take courage and learn from their failures and in so doing improve their own human-client relationships to the mutual advantage of all.

91.3. Practical Methodology

91.3.1. How to Inspire Your Client

91.3.2. The Practitioner at Work

91.3.3. Motivation

91.3.4. The Hygienist Is a Teacher

91.3.5. Knowledge of What to Do—and How to Do It

In Lesson 90, the student has been presented with some of the psychological aspects of counseling as they may apply in the day-to-day practice of a professional Hygienist. We have in this discussion divided methodology into three main categories and an enlargement on each of these will follow. We should bear in mind, however, that the psychology of counseling can never actually be completely divorced from the more mundane aspects of counseling, from the techniques. The two are inextricably intertwined.

91.3.1. How to Inspire Your Client

We have already put forth our thesis that using specific case-studies may well be the single most effective tool to inspire clients to "go and do likewise."

We have stated that case studies of persons who have successfully recovered from a like ailment will, all other things being equal, have a greater impact on the psyche than will unrelated case studies.

Also, case studies which are given to the client in a printout form and then the information contained therein reinforced by the reading together of the information, combined with an opportunity for the practitioner to point out specific details and/or to clarify others, and for the client to ask questions, will prove a much more effective tool for providing encouragement than using either method alone.

Furthermore, the print-out may be taken home by the client for subsequent re-reading, thus reinforcing the first psychic impact.

91.3.1.1. Me, too!

Inspiration and reinforcement (support) can be augmented by using the "Me, Too!" technique, an easily workable tool. It embodies the "If you can do it, I can, too!" philosophy.

The supporting methodology used here is simple. It is a gathering together of persons with similar affections in a ding, held either at the practitioner's office or home, or the home of a cooperative client.

This group should, ideally, have at least one member who has either made a remarkable recovery applying Hygienic principles in his/her own lifestyle or who, at least, has already witnessed sufficient improvement in his/her condition as to want to share experiences with others.

In the early days of your practice, you may not have worked with a sufficient number of similar conditions to be able to put together this kind of group. In this event, simply set up a support group composed of a few clients having a variety of troubling conditions, perhaps only three or four, just so that they can share their experiences and learn from one another.

Either grouping will work. Indeed, it is difficult to predict in advance which grouping will prove to be the more effective for you. Try them out and see!

91.3.1.2. The Meeting

At the beginning of your meeting, have a round of introductions. At first, just use first names. As time goes on, individuals will seek out and become friends with those persons best suited to them. Repeat these introductions at every meeting so that newcomers will feel at ease within the group and also so that group members will become more closely knit.

The practitioner may pass out case study print-outs—one or two are usually sufficient. These studies may be gleaned from various works by Hygienic writers. They are good to use as an opening wedge to encourage discussion by individual group members. Discussions may range from the negative to the positive. We should not be discouraged by negative stories since such can often provide an excellent base for learning. The practitioner can give explanations of why certain "negatives" (healing crises) occur from time to time and what their portent is.

For example, many clients are disturbed by the initial weight loss so common in the early stages. When the weight loss is explained in terms of tearing down an old structure prior to building a new one, clients, more often than not, accept the rationale of the fact of weight-loss as a prior condition for later health improvement.

We use the blackboard frequently. It can be especially helpful in explaining weight loss. Progress is so often impeded simply by fear when clients do not thoroughly understand why they are losing pound after pound. They begin to question the validity of their whole program! We use the Diagram Method in such situations.

Early Stages: Weight loss begins to accelerate, then slows down somewhat but still goes on, due to catalytic tearing-down and discarding of inferior and diseased parts. All happens under the control of body's intelligence center. Anabolism, the building phase, is submerged to catalysis. Weight is reduced. Swiftly at first, less as time goes on.

At the Mid-Point: Here equilibrium is established. There is no further weight loss because the intelligent control center decides that sufficient inferior tissue has now been removed.

Final Adjustment: As the correct lifestyle is continued, Anabolism begins to accelerate, Catabolism slows down. The individual is well on the road to superior health.

The above is just one illustration of how a practitioner can use group meetings to explain away questions which may trouble many clients. This permits the practitioner to address individual problems in greater depth in private consultations.

At group meetings, all persons should be given an opportunity to speak, to ask questions, to share and to encourage one another. The practitioner should use such meetings to guide, direct, encourage participation and to explain when explanations are in order. As students of this course, you will be well prepared to handle most questions as they may arise from time to time.

Spouses and/or other concerned persons may, with the permission of the client, be invited to these meetings and, indeed, should be encouraged to attend. Hygienic practices are usually totally foreign to their thinking, too, and unless they fully understand and are in accord with what is suggested and taught by you, they may well prove an insurmountable obstruction to your client's future progress.

The key to success in these group meetings may be how well spontaneity is encouraged, and this may well depend on the attitude of the practitioner. Never permit yourself to be bored. Try always to cultivate concern, interest, that deep desire to help. Sick people often suffer much and the spontaneity they feel at your meeting can prove a powerfully positive influence for good.

Spontaneity may be difficult to achieve but if one makes a conscious effort to make these discussions free and open, a time for sharing both successes and failures, more courage seems to develop.

All of us, at times, have to learn to "take it on the chin" when healing crises arise, but often these meetings with other individuals, who have experienced exactly what you are now going through, can enable you to pick up the pieces and begin again, confident that when the crisis is over, you have passed a major milestone on your road to full recovery. If you have to "wing it alone," sometimes you can become discouraged and falter.

Include the quiet ones in the group discussion by addressing them directly as, for example, "Sue, what do you feel about all this?" Note the use of the word FEEL instead of the word THINK.

We all have feelings and most people, even the timid ones, will respond to a FEEL question where they might panic at a "What do you THINK" one!

91.3.1.3. Ending the Group Meeting

Always end your group meetings on a high note! Encourage your clients to hold their head up, to lift up their hearts as well, to turn their thoughts inward to positive channels of "I CAN!" Urge them to unify their energy, to draw down a blind, as it were, on matters of lesser importance and to keep their minds on an inner vision of what they SHALL become. Encourage them to emulate Lillian Russell's way of pushing aside the unlovely, who said that she put a sign on her mental door that read: "Only the serene and the lovely can enter here." She said that a thousand voices might call her away from her resolve, but she trained herself not to hear them. All of us must train ourselves not to hear the negative voices that cry aloud, in favor of keeping our thoughts focused in the direction we wish to go. We cannot let the distracting disruptive outer forces weaken our own resolve. The future can be too beautiful!

Gather your group together in a circle. Let them clasp hands and repeat in unison some simple CREDO, such as:

I AM WHOLE!

I AM PERFECT! I AM STRONG! I AM HAPPY!

BECAUSE I AM IN TUNE WITH MYSELF AND I AM HEALTHY! SO, BE IT!

The saying together of a simple CREDO will help your clients to accept the correctness of their program. It will help them to believe that they can have anything they desire, especially superb health. All that they will be required to do is to approach life's problems constructively, maintaining, all the while, a vision of the possible, and then to work at fulfillment.

Meetings such as we have suggested can challenge those present to continue on, to work for maximum recovery. As conditions of individual clients begin to improve, you will observe that, one by one, they gradually leave the side of the negative newcomers and pass over to become a member of the more positive "Me-too-ers!" Each passover serves to inspire your other newer clients to go forward, not to become discouraged, and, importantly, you, the practitioner, too!

Before closing your meeting, announce a time for gathering together again. Meetings should be held at least once a month. Officers may be elected or appointed to take care of routine announcements.

Usually, a few clients will volunteer to provide certain necessary services such as reminder telephone calls, etc. It is well sometimes to suggest to your clients that they "think" about a certain topic as, for example, "How Important is Exercise in Your Plan for Health?" Then, this subject may be the focus of the group's attention at the upcoming meeting. Be sure to ask those in attendance to sign a registration sheet. After you have been meeting for a while, clients may ask if they can bring a friend. Encourage them to do so. It is within your right to request a minimal fee from clients for your services at these meetings. The money may be used to cover your time and expenses.

Don't forget that you must be a visible example of poise and peace, of successful accomplishment of what the clients themselves desire so fervently. When you are, you have a certain magic about you that you unconsciously impart to those who seek your help, and you will be especially successful in conducting these important group meetings.

91.3.2. The Practitioner at Work

As a practicing Hygienist, you will be pursuing your career at every private and public appearance: when meeting with individual clients, when hosting or conducting a small group for purposes of furthering their education in Hygienic practices, philosophy, and principles; and, certainly, when you begin to hold classes and seminars for the public, which we hope all of you will consider doing, and this as soon as practicable.

You will greatly influence not only the progress of your clients, but also your own, in a number of ways. Intelligent practitioners who wish to become sought out for their expertise will ask themselves many questions, and future success will depend, in great measure, upon what they do to improve in these areas of concern. We especially recommend that you address the following areas:

91.3.2.1. Questions to Ask Ourselves

1. Am I a reasonably good example of what I teach?

2. Do I speak positively, with authority, but not in an arrogant manner? Or am I too hesitant in my pronouncements?

3. Am I able to impart verbally and by my body movements and facial expressions the sense of empathy and concern I feel toward my clients? Do they sense that I really know exactly how they feel; that I understand their anxieties, their concerns? Do I convey to them a confidence in my words?

4. Do I listen more than I talk? Do I use the pronoun "I" too often?

5. Do I appreciate my own value?

Number 1

If the practitioner has recovered from some specific condition, s/he is usually more likely to speak with authority on that subject and perhaps also on the general subject of how best to regain one's health. S/he may even choose to specialize in a particular disorder as, for example, rheumatic or heart disorders.

However, having recovered from a particular malady is not, of course, a prerequisite for practicing as a Hygienist! Even being capable of maintaining a high level of health under the prevailing unhealthful conditions and circumstances, can be, in and of itself, an inspiring challenge to induce lifestyle changes in your clients. In fact, this may well be considered a "plus!"

One's past experiences may well color the tone of the voice, impart a certain glow to one's manner and add conviction to statements, all helpful influences. But a practitioner should not pretend to know what s/he does NOT know nor act a part being something s/ he is not! Deception will always fail. Knowledge imparted honestly will always be more conducive to trust. If a client asks you a question and you do not know the answer, just say that you do not know, but add that you will try to find the correct answer.

If you are still recovering from some condition, say so. Share your progress, even your regressions, with your clients. We recall one time when Elizabeth broke out in a wild rash. It began behind her ears and on to her cheeks. She was a sight to behold and, to make matters worse, the itching was intense. And, to top the whole affair off, we were just about to open an advanced course of study!

We went right ahead with our plans! The class consisted of a mix of old and new students. Elizabeth stood up bravely and announced to those present that the subject of the day was, you guessed right! Healing Crises! We all learned a lot from the experience as the days passed. Students learned about fasting and about what occurs in the body during these days. In fact, those students watched the progress of this entire healing crisis and learned much from it. We are confident that the students who attended that class will not panic when they are confronted with their first healing crises! They will continue on making whatever changes are required in their lifestyle to accomplish their ultimate goal.

The lesson to be learned from this episode is that, if you feel you are lacking in some respect, then you should try as best you can either to remedy the situation or to use it; to cope with it or to accommodate yourself to it. All of us can probably improve our appearance, our attitude, our confidence, in many areas. It is well to take a frank appraisal of one's appearance and assets and to seek actively to improve in those areas where improvement is indicated, or where it might well be to your advantage to do so. Nobody's perfect, but we can all strive for perfection, even if we never achieve it! Remember that you are a living example of all that Natural Hygiene promises. Therefore, why not promise them the best! That will surely influence your clients to make the lifestyle changes you deem appropriate.

Number 2.

Do I speak positively, with authority in my voice, but not in an arrogant manner? Or am I too hesitant in my pronouncements?

What has all this to do with inducing clients to change bad habits into good habits? A great deal! You will be able to induce constructive changes in your clients' lifestyles effectively and consistently, the more talented you become in presenting the changes you deem necessary for a particular client and then follow by explaining the reasons why such changes are vital to your client's well-being. We accomplish this largely through our spoken words, perhaps because they are more personal.

If you are presently hesitant in your manner of speaking or have some other limiting factor, it might be well for you to take a course in public speaking. These are offered from time to time by most schools and colleges and very inexpensively, too, if not altogether at no cost.

Be happily appreciative of your clients. You will reveal this in your manner and in your voice. Your clients have honored you by seeking you out. Leave all arrogance or impatience out of your voice, for such will only serve to turn people away from you.

Everybody likes to hear nice things about themselves. Tell your clients that you appreciate them and especially, remember always to compliment them as they reach a Hygienic milestone. Such appreciation encourages them to go forward and not to either stand still or regress. It inspires them to make the required lifestyle adjustments. Just take a few moments of your consultation time to compliment your client about something. Practice on your friends, the people you meet in the supermarket, wherever you go, and it will soon become natural to you to be more appreciative of others. Remember to compliment those who attend your meetings, the little ones, and the big ones. They have given you a compliment by coming, give them one in return. Inspire your clients by being appreciative of small accomplishments if you sincerely want big changes to follow.

Dale Carnegie admonished his students always to say "WE" instead of "you." Instead of saying, "John, I want you to do such and such," it is better to say, "John, don't you believe we all would be better served health wise, if we would do this and so?" The former gives the impression one is talking down to his client. The latter includes you—the authority—as well as the client—the student. You must make certain lifestyle changes, too!

Avoid the negative in your attitude, your looks and in your words. In fact, having a positive attitude and a positive look about you will often speak louder than words. It may, of course, be necessary to scold a client occasionally, but don't make a practice of it. Avoid it if you can. The shrew soon loses a mate. The scolding or arrogant practitioner soon loses his/her clients, and they lose their opportunity to live their lives healthfully. Talk with your clients, not down at them. Talk in terms they can understand about their concerns, their worries, their problems. Show them how to get rid of their health problems so that their other concerns will either be completely solved, or their impact lessened. We are reminded of a session we had one time with a very obese gentleman, the president of a large corporation. We were obviously concerned about his excess weight, his high blood pressure, and other ailments, about how best to address these issues and how we were to persuade him to make the necessary changes in his lifestyle. We had been consulting with this man for some six months and, of course, had made some progress, but it was limited due to the fact that, like so many obese ones, he had a tendency to revert to his former bad habits from time to time, even to bingeing, all of which retarded his progress. He was psychologically wedded to his old ways and reluctant to change.

However, at one of our consultations he confided that he was extremely concerned about his future. Here was a man in his early fifties. Where he had once been a proud, highly-confident man, he was now a frightened man. It seems he had just been fired from his highly-lucrative position, one he had occupied, and successfully so, for many years, because of certain overseas developments which required worldwide reorganization.

It would have been useless for us to have lectured him about his shortcomings or, indeed, to have talked about anything else. Such a disregard for his feelings and valid concerns would have been inexcusable because his mental state was such as to negate physical reconstruction of the rest of his body anyway. So, during that entire session, we never once directed our attention to his obesity, to his high blood pressure. Instead, we listened and interjected, from time to time, some positive thoughts about how old doors close and new ones open, that we make our own world, our own opportunities; that we can attain whatever we want in life or in this world if we determine what is required of us, what is needed, and then follow through with the doing. We did suggest that becoming healthier, by making positive changes in his eating and living habits, would serve to clear his mind and that this important change would serve to open many doors for him.

When he came back three months later for his next appointment, his blood pressure had dropped dramatically, an examination had showed that over a dozen existing polyps in his colon had either completely disappeared or were greatly diminished in size. He announced with a happy smile that he had a new position which seemed very promising. He had made many of the necessary changes; he had corrected many of his bad habits. Indeed, he was so enthusiastic about his new way of life that he came armed with a whole list of questions for us to answer.

Welcome questions from your clients. Don't be impatient and think that answering them is taking up your valuable time. Your clients are interested, or they would not ask!

Always remember that your clients will be more inclined to change incorrect habits of eating and living when they discuss the rationale with you on a one-to-one basis, when they receive a sympathetic ear to their queries and problems. The questions may seem too simple to devote your valuable time to them, but remember they are important to the one who asks.

Be sincere and open with your clients. Your inner conviction of the rightness of what you have to offer will help to bridge the gap of misinformation which restrains your clients' forward progress and prevents their making necessary changes. Use the spoken word in a confident, but sympathetic way and your clients will usually respond favorably and follow your wise counsel.

Number 3.

Am I able to impart verbally and by my body movements and facial expressions the sense of empathy I feel toward my clients? Do they sense that I really know exactly how they feel; that I understand their anxieties, their concerns? Do I convey to them a confidence in my words?

As students of Life Science, you are preparing for one of the most rewarding careers it is possible for you to pursue. You are preparing for a career of service which, if well done, will fulfill your reason for being—to help others to grow in body, mind, and spirit; as well as rewarding you financially and in many other perhaps intangible ways.

If you naturally feel empathy toward your clients and concern about their needs, you will instinctively impart to them the sense that you understand their needs and are vitally interested in helping them. There will be a "oneness" between you and them and they will respond more positively and be more inclined to follow your directions.

If, however, you do not, by nature, feel this kind of empathy and are planning to enter into Hygienic practice solely for the purpose of making money, then you will surely fail because you will be wrongly motivated and if you are wrongly motivated, you will be unable to convince people to change their ways of eating and living.

However, if you are sincerely interested in helping people to change incorrect habits of eating and living into a more correct lifestyle, then you can develop certain techniques which will assist you even though, at present, you do not naturally feel empathy toward people; and you can do this simply by practicing it!

You may have to pretend at first, to act a part, but all of us do that every day, don't we? By practicing you will soon begin to evidence in word, deeds, facial expressions, body movements, a gesture here and there at the right time, that you really DO care about your clients.

Sincere interest, an encouraging word when needed, a smile instead of a frown, a hand on a shoulder, just touching a troubled person in a friendly and gentle manner at a time of need can change a worried person's whole demeanor and outlook on life, can encourage them to go on when they might otherwise be inclined to give up.

So, enrich your personality by consciously striving to develop a "ONE-NESS" with your clients. It will not only help them over their more difficult crises but will help you in your career.

Sincere interest will cause people to be more confident in their relationship with you and when confident of you and of your understanding of them, they will be less likely to falter and more willing to follow your suggestions.

Consider yourself a rebuilder of men and women, for that is what you are. To rebuild a human structure, unlike beginning to fashion a house of wood and stone, you must have understanding of the mind and soul before you can build a worthy structure.

Work on your personality. If necessary, take personality lessons. Begin with positive attitudes, work at understanding people's concerns, and learn how to support your clients through their most difficult times. Having a sincere empathy toward those who seek your help will not only bring you success in many ways, but it will serve to give many back their lives, to give them another chance to live in health for many years to come. There can be no more worthy calling!

Number 4.

Do I listen more than I talk? Do I use the pronoun "I" too often? There is an old French proverb which, when translated, reads, "Little by little, the bird builds its nest." Just so, clients change bad habits into good habits and learn how to rebuild their bodies.

The ability to listen to other people is a requirement for success in any profession. It is absolutely essential to the successful Hygienic practitioner.

We have to learn how to give up our set notions of how a meeting should proceed and especially of how a consultation should proceed. Of course, we should always have a plan, but sometimes we have to let the wind blow where it will. Crises come and crises go, and current happenings revealed to you as you listen can often direct your immediate course of action.

Always have something in reserve to talk about, of course, some points you wish to express or discuss with your clients but keep the ingredient of spontaneity alive. Let your clients talk. You be a good listener. More often than not, the greatest good will come to your client when s/he has an opportunity to tell another human being about anxieties that lie heavy on the heart and trouble the soul.

Once these have been revealed, they may well influence the changes in lifestyle which you may then suggest as the next desirable course to follow. And, of course, shared concerns and anxieties are already half "cured!" Letting your clients talk can be highly therapeutic.

A part of listening well is learning when to ask the right questions. Sometimes the appropriate question interjected at the right time will lead the interview in the direction you have planned and bring out a consciousness of further need for change on the part of your client.

For example, a woman came to us with many serious health problems. She was so satisfied with her progress by the time her second appointment had come and gone that she failed to keep her third one.

We called to remind her of our appointment, at which time she said how excited she was at her progress and how well-pleased she was that everything was going along so well—so well that she thought she had no further need to consult with us.

We listened as the voice went up and down and when she was apparently finished, we simply suggested that perhaps after some forty years of building disease it might take just a little longer and a little more guidance to rebuild her body the way she would like to, and did she not think perhaps that she might learn something more about herself and about how she functions so that she could have it ALL!

The woman thought a minute and said, "I believe you're right. I guess I really have just made a start. When do you want to see me?"

The appointment was made, and a new study begun. We have been working together on rebuilding her body now for almost a year. Our client has found that there were many more adjustments that were yet to be made and that making them correctly has yielded rich rewards. She now has so much confidence in us that she knows that we will advise her when we think she is ready to "go it alone."

Listening and knowing when and how to ask the right questions is a talent possessed by all successful people. Cultivate it well and you will find your clients much more amenable to change. To be successful we must use every attribute we possess to influence clients to change their lifestyle. Becoming a good listener is one of the best!

Number 5.

Does it appreciate my own value? Inspiring clients' rests on both the tangible and the intangible assets of the practitioner. Hygienists, more than any other practitioners in the whole health sciences arena, should appreciate their own value and, especially the value of their services to their clients.

As a student of this course, you have gleaned true scientific facts of life, you have learned the true science of healing. The Hygienists alone (among the "healers" of the world) understand that people are the "architects of their own miseries" and that it is the Hygienist who can lead people into a harmony of body, mind and spirit which will enable them to reap the wonderful rewards of a life correctly lived.

We Hygienists need to be confident of the Tightness of what we impart to our clients, to appreciate its worth and be able to convey our confidence in that worth to our clients. How else can we expect them to trust us with their most precious possession, their lives?

We Hygienists are valuable and especially so when we have applied and continue to apply Hygienic truths in our own lives; when we ourselves have made the necessary changes in our own lifestyles to demonstrate the worth of what we propound. Once we have conquered ourselves, then we are prepared to become worthy and wise teachers of the healing truths learned in this science of life and living.

It does not matter if you are not handsome or if your face is lined with the ravages of past pain. When you smile at your clients, your value to them shines through. When we are certain of our worth, we can forget self and become genuinely interested in others, and this ability to be un-self-conscious and take interest in other people is actually in a direct relationship to our personal estimate of our own worth!

We should, of course, set our standards high. They should be in keeping on a par with, our value. Only then will we be able to cause clients to appreciate what they themselves can become, to appreciate their own potential and to strive to attain their goal. It is you that can impart to them the reality of organic existence, that life and nature are with them at all times, working on their side, planning and overcoming obstacles and all in their behalf. And it all happens through you, the knowledgeable Hygienist!

In other words, the magic of the sense of your own value will serve to enhance their appraisal of their worth and encourage them to work harder to make the necessary changes called for by their own bodies so that they can become worthy of all that life has to offer to those all too few individuals who are healthy enough to hold it precious. Inspiring clients to make the necessary changes in their lifestyles can be accomplished in many ways. We have named a few. As Hygienists we understand the need for change and are called upon to use every asset legitimately at our command to encourage the sick ones to change sick habits into more health-promoting habits. The practitioner who can, by word, deed, attitude and by his sense of self-worth, inspire others to leave off the old destructive ways and begin a new and healthier lifestyle, will become a leader among peers.

91.3.3. Motivation

In the second edition of Foundations of Health Science by Henkel, Means, Smolensky and Sawrey (Allyn and Bacon, Inc., Poston, 1972. Page 159) we are told that "motivated behavior is behavior that is directed toward the attainment of some goal, object, or purpose. Motives have to do with the wants, wishes, desires, and purposes of the individual and the manner of their attainment."

It would be difficult to find a better way to define motivation as it particularly applies to the relationship between a practicing Hygienist and the client. The successful practitioner should always bear in mind that those persons who seek you out are already motivated to a certain extent to perform. They have a goal and a purpose for being in your presence. They wish to become well again and they hope you have the knowledge either to work some magic or to tell them what magic is needed for them to attain their objective.

The first part of motivation then may be to "disillusion" them, i.e., to help them to reach an understanding that there is no magical road to lead them to a higher status of health. Few understand, of course, that superb health can only be achieved through a process of discarding bad habits followed by a joint effort which involves rebuilding and maintaining. The practitioner must build on the existing foundation of many false ideas and superstitions and then go on to disabuse the client of his original false concepts and change them, to direct clients into new and perhaps unfamiliar and "strange" ways of living and eating.

In Hygienic practice, motivation, in almost every instance, involves "holding out the carrot;" imparting to the clients an enlarged view of what the future CAN hold for them PROVIDED they do "thus and so."

As practicing Hygienists, we learn to judge individual clients' capabilities rather quickly. How well do they respond to large changes? Are they more comfortable, less emotionally disturbed, perhaps, with smaller, less-challenging changes? We adjust our thinking and our suggestions accordingly after full explanation of the fact that an abrupt about-face is always more conducive to a rapid and more complete return to full health than are smaller changes.

However, some clients may be frightened if proposed changes appear too much for them either to understand or to handle, and when this is the case, they do not continue on a Hygienic program for very long. With such clients, we and they are better served when we provide reasonable suggestions which may immediately be met. With these more reluctant clients, a planned program of instructive changes combined with a developing insight into the cause-and-effect relationship in building health can lead to a fuller understanding of the need for certain changes which have been designed by you to bring them into the desired fullness of health.

Group meetings to which family members are invited (a family night, for example) often helps the clients by motivating members of the family to be more cooperative and supportive of their efforts to obtain their goal of better health.

If the suggested changes prove too demanding, then they must be simplified. In other words, they should be adjusted to more realistic expectations. Avoid placing the clients in a position of strong conflict either with themselves, their families, or with you. Some conflict may, at times, be inevitable, but we should strive to minimize it. Remember that individuals differ in their maturity, and we have to be in tune with these differences when we voice our suggested changes.

91.3.4. The Hygienist Is a Teacher

Hygienists are basically teachers of the ways and means whereby the present state of ill health of a client can be changed to one of improved health. In order to bring their efforts to a successful conclusion, they must employ many of the modern tools of education. We will, of course, not be able to suggest all the possible tools of the trade but, hopefully, we can give you some of the ones we have found most useful in our own practice.

1. When to Use Fasting

Fasting represents, in most instances, a giant leap. To fast is always a first priority change when feasible according to the emotional stability and prior "knowledge of a particular client with respect to what is involved in fasting.

We suggest that, from time to time, you hold classes on fasting at which time procedures are given. At these classes case studies may be presented, as well as personal experiences related by clients who have themselves fasted to good advantage. These meetings give a time for learning, for asking questions and for becoming familiar with a hitherto unknown procedure.

2. The "Baby Steps" Technique

Recommended for more timid clients. Both the practitioner and the client should understand that sometimes the recovery period is prolonged and at times even discouraging. Generally, this is a limited technique to use to help less stable clients to make required changes and/or to use with poorly-informed clients. However, the choice between 1 and 2 must be made and all clients will have to be evaluated as to which will prove the more effective and/or acceptable, emotionally, to them.

3. The Historical Review

Sometimes clients become discouraged and think they are making little or no progress even though you know this to be untrue. At such times, it is well to review a client's historical record, noting on a blackboard, when possible, various symptoms shown on first meeting and reminding the client of the positive changes (which you have diligently noted on the client's record at each meeting) which have subsequently occurred, even though these be minor ones.

With some clients it may be advisable to call the client's attention to these improvements at each meeting. This may be especially advisable when a client suffers from a major disorder which is difficult to manage as, for example, muscular dystrophy, which is generally conceded not to be amenable to Hygienic practices especially insofar as expecting a complete "cure" is concerned.

In such cases small improvements can be very significant. We sometimes have to show the carrot frequently, to reassure and reassure, time and time again, in order to encourage the clients to keep their gaze on the light at the end of the tunnel rather than focusing their minds on the troubling symptoms that presently annoy.

4. The Inner Circle Concept

This concept is applicable in more difficult cases and especially with clients who may experience rather frequent healing crises. It helps one to keep clients on course, making the necessary changes in their lifestyles that you feel appropriate at a particular moment in time.

The Inner Circle shows that healing does not occur in a straight line but rather in cycles. We progress from one healing crisis to the next, but these become less frequent and less severe until finally, by our diligent attention to correct living and eating, we reach the Inner Circle, at which time our body, mind and soul are in perfect harmony. Our goal has been reached.

The Inner Circle Concept can be depicted from time to time as need arises to remind clients of the cyclical nature of healing. They often like to estimate how far they have progressed in their healing.

5. The Direct Challenge

Sometimes it becomes necessary to confront a client who is reluctant to make certain changes with a direct challenge. Are you less strong than So and So? So and So can be another client but remember to use a client's name only if you received permission to do so and only then. Otherwise, let the challenge refer to a nameless person, or to a person depicted in one of the printed case studies which you have previously reviewed with the client. Try to incorporate in such clients the "I CAN, do it if So and So can do it" concept. Generally, retaining an inner vision of something we yearn for can sustain us through the rough times and carry us forward to a successful attainment.

6. Family Counselling

When all members of the family are convinced of the need for them to change their lifestyles and to make a mutual effort to do so, success is generally assured. We recently experienced such a happening and have seen how effective the combined motivation can be in achieving a common goal.

The first client was a diabetic married daughter in a certain family. She had been diagnosed as being insulin dependent. Her improvement was dramatic and swift with considerable reduction in her insulin intake. Then a sister who suffered from systemic lupus joined her.

Next came a son, age 7, the child of the first daughter. He was an asthmatic. His improvement was also excellent. Then came the grandparents, the father and mother of the two sisters. They were both in their middle fifties. Finally, the oldest daughter and her husband joined in the program, all with individual problems and goals.

We eventually, by the consent of all, gathered the entire family together in a single series of conferences devoting two hours to each such meeting. At these gatherings, questions and answers were given; each person presented a progress report; there was sharing and planning for the future good of all. Progress was so satisfactory that now we hold these family conferences at three-month intervals, at which time we review, appraise present states, and progress, and provide encouragement. Where changes are required, they are suggested.

All members of the family are very supportive of one another and highly enthusiastic about their new way of eating and living. The grandparents have a pool and the daughters, their husbands, and all the grandchildren often gather for a family party around the pool. They tell us that even those who do not actively attend our conferences are slowly "getting into the act." At any rate, they are all enjoying their "carrots!"

7. Using a Placebo

This technique is sometimes useful when working with elderly, very emotionally distraught clients, who are reluctant to take the first timid "Baby steps."

All of us would probably agree that using a supplement of any kind is unHygienic in principle. However, it can be a useful tool in exceptional circumstances such as when an emotional person needs a rope to hang on to. At such times we have recourse to a pill, one made of vegetables dehydrated in a vacuum at low temperatures. It is relatively harmless, certainly far less so than a sugar pill. We advise our clients that this pill is to be used for a stated limited time to "fill in anything missing" in their diet. This seems to reassure these disturbed individuals. It often calms them down emotionally and gives them the confidence they require to make the first primary changes in their lifestyles. Once this hurdle has been taken, the others seem to follow more easily.

8. Only One Way to Go!

When all medical resources have been exhausted and have failed, as they invariably do, clients are usually more amenable to change. You will all have clients who are in this position. They are, at one and the same time, both easy to work with and difficult.

One of our students was faced with such a situation. She had taken a course in nutrition when she learned that her husband was terminally ill with cancer of the bladder. Armed with her new knowledge about the science of living in health and in disease, she made a complete turnaround in her lifestyle. She refused to place her husband in the hospice, refused to remove him to the hospital as demanded by the consulting oncologist, and said she would care for him by herself and in their own comfortable home. The specialist and a representative from the hospice were permitted to visit whenever they chose to do so. A nurse from the hospice visited several times each week.

The man's diet was changed abruptly to an alkaline diet of fresh uncooked fruits and vegetables. Two items only were served at a meal. On some days only juices were served—fruits and vegetables at suitable intervals. Sunbaths were taken when possible and the man exercised every day to the extent possible. Toward the last, he was gently massaged by his wife and this several times during the day and especially along his spinal cord.

It is interesting to know that this man required no pain killers except an occasional aspirin until the last 24 hours, when he took six aspirin tablets. At his funeral, which we attended, we asked one of the visiting nurses from the hospice if she had ever witnessed such a peaceful conclusion to a terminally-ill cancer patient. She shook her head and then commented that she had never seen anything like this before in her entire practice.

9. Overcoming Compulsive Habits and the "My Doctor Says" Complex

These are perhaps the most difficult of all changes for the client to make, with overeating probably being the most difficult of all bad habits to overcome. In fact, it is said that only about 5% of the obese are successful in reducing their weight to what it should be.

Encouragement and constant prodding are helpful. Consultations should be much more frequent than with other clients. We ask our obese clients to keep a weekly weight record and at each consultation we record any changes. We find it necessary constantly to remind the reluctant ones of their goal, of what obtaining a more normal figure and weight might mean to them in health benefits and of the social and business doors that might well be opened to them.

We also generally ask our obese clients to keep a record of their meals. They usually "confess" to their sneaking and their "bingeing." The old saying states, "Confession is good for the soul!" Perhaps asking for such confession will sometimes be helpful.

Getting over the "my doctor says" complex stubbornly maintained by some clients requires patience on your part. In fact, to overcome it, you have to come up with a better product, so to speak, to be successful with this kind of individual. Of course, we can always remind them, as and when the subject comes up, that they are here—in your office and consulting you—because "my doctor" did NOT have the answers!

In other words, when possible, these clients, if they are to attain their desire to be healthier than they presently are, must be led finally to accept the reality of past failure and replace it with the new opportunity for success now offered to them simply by applying their newly-learned Hygienic ways of living and eating in their own lifestyles.

10. The Bionutritional Blood Test Analysis and Profile

We find this a highly-motivating tool for change, and it is so with most clients, almost without exception. By word and by picture the Analysis and Profile presents to the client the realities of blood condition as revealed by a series of tests made at a standard laboratory which are interpreted and plotted for the client's study. The necessity for change, when such exists, is made clear. We suggest that our clients have these made at six-month intervals. When good changes are observed, as is generally the case when Hygienic changes in lifestyle are adopted, clients are further motivated to improve and make any additional indicated changes.

11. Grouping Clients

The practitioner should take time out to study clients' records, grouping them together by type of disorder being experienced, as follows:

1. Arthritic Clients
2. Diabetic Clients
3. Clients with nervous disorders
4. Clients with heart disorders
5. Clients suffering from respiratory diseases, etc., etc.

Make a critical study of the following as shown in past and present history:

Emotional Lonely Very angry Fears death Jealous etc.

Poisons Coffee, tea Smokes Alcoholic

Cocaine, other drugs etc.

357

Endotoxins

Uric acid

High cholesterol Calcium deposits Purines etc. Deficiencies Poor marriage Eats junk food

Lacks sufficient money etc.

Symptoms

Each client

Make a special listing for excesses, such as: works too hard, eats too much, etc. This will help you to guide individual clients and to suggest appropriate further changes to be made.

When feasible and practical, have group meetings for mutual discussion and analysis of methods used, changes already made, improvements forthcoming, and future planning. Where good results have been slow in coming, these meetings can sometimes be a means of ferreting out hidden causes. They can also provide a meeting of the minds, so to speak, an understanding by all participants of the need for change and for time to accomplish the required healing and, perhaps, even a better understanding of the commonality of cause among participants.

Only those clients who are willing to participate in a frank and open discussion should be included in this type of group discussion because they amount to a "Show and Tell" meeting which sometimes requires disclosure of more intimate details of one's lifestyle. Some clients, of course, are reluctant to participate in frank and open discussion, but with willing clients, the results can often prove highly motivating.

12. "Sell the Rose, Not the Thorn"

Always hold out to your clients the vision of the possible. Do not dwell on the present nor on the past overly long. Clarify all issues involved as they come up, of course, and make clear the possible consequences of incorrect habits, but place emphasis on the salubrious effects of making all appropriate changes in lifestyle. A positive approach is always more effective in selling. Salesmen are advised to sell the benefits accruing to the buyer. The successful practitioner must sell the benefits of living Hygienically and these are legion!

Keep nudging clients along, inch by inch, if necessary. The results can so often be spectacular! A single case study will make our point. Four years ago, a woman came to us seeking help. She had had several massive heart attacks, a mastectomy with lymph nodes extirpated, her shoulders and back were severely curved, and she was fainting seven and eight times a day. Her blood tests revealed an almost impossible state. As we write this today, we have received a letter which reads, in part, as follows: "We have enjoyed our summer and I am glad to report that I haven't had such a feeling of well-being for ages. I really feel good." She is still having some minor problems, a few hemorrhoids, for example. But her improvement demonstrates the magic of Life Science. Sometimes, we and our clients can become discouraged, but motivation and inspiration return once we view results such as this woman has experienced.

91.3.5. Knowledge of What to Do—and How to Do It

This is where Hygienic practitioners come into their own! They have the knowledge of what their clients must accomplish in the way of making specific changes in their lifestyle if they wish to attain a higher level of health, and also, on broad terms at least, of how they must proceed.

The practitioner must, at one and the same time, become the parent who evaluates the situation and determine the proper course of action, the teacher who expounds on methodology, and the overseer who follows procedure to a successful conclusion.

All practitioners have their own personal equipment: ability to lead, respect for the client's needs, sincerity, emotional maturity, sense of humor or lack thereof, appearance, ability to empathize with the client's sufferings. The higher their equipment quotient, the more likely that they will be able to transfer their knowledge of "what, when, how," etc., to clients and thereby maximize results.

The average person's knowledge about him or herself is abysmal though much information is available, indeed an extreme abundance. But, at one and the same time, there is also an extreme confusion about humans and what is required of them to maintain them in a state of excellence.

The modern child has not been taught to read and/or to consult various authors or sources on matters of health, but rather has been taught to follow the advice given in the media, these imparting only the medical view of how to obtain health and to keep it. Early in their lives, people are programmed to consult the medical mentor for guidance as to what to do and how to take care of themselves in sickness and in health and, to the masses, only the medical view is valid.

"Science" divides humans into fragments. Life Science alone treats people as a unitized whole which is governed by immutable laws. Orthodoxy fails to take into account the ethnic, epidemiological and historical nature of man. Hygienists have a conscious realization of cause and effect, and it is this that differentiates the Life Scientist from other more traditional practices and beliefs. It is this difference which must be imparted to clients if they are to fulfill their potential destinies as human beings.

We are required to learn man in his entirety, about the symbiosis of his inner parts and his symbiotic relationship with his environment.

It is impossible, of course, to impart to new clients at first, second or even third meeting, all that we know in this regard. Therefore, our practice becomes a matter of intelligent selection, choosing the more relevant and discarding that which, for the moment at least, is of lesser importance. Evaluation of need, therefore, is a first priority. In our next lesson we will discuss the initial interview. For now, let us merely state that this first meeting is critical but not all-important. We learn a little more about our clients at each consultation, at group meetings, at potlucks, whenever we are in each other's presence. All precise information and all impressions must be considered and evaluated for their importance.

Following evaluation of need we must construct a plan of action based on need as is revealed by past history, impressions, etc. A study of possible causes follows. Here one usually discovers a plenitude of possible causes such as the most common cause of overeating; extremely traumatic events in the past or on-going in the present, such as physical cruelty; overworking; psychological trauma such as worry, fear; perhaps assuming too much responsibility in civic affairs; or exercising beyond one's present capability; eating junk foods; drinking tea, coffee, soft drinks, etc.; alcoholism; prior surgical extirpations of organs and parts; and on and on.

An evaluation of the more important causes should precede the construction of a plan of action. We must always be aware of the fact that most people manifest only an elementary knowledge about themselves and are capable only of revealing things they know to be harmful, and this knowledge is limited. They are usually capable of only tackling easy tasks; this is especially true at the beginning.

We generally find that most people are watchers and followers—not instigators, performers, or doers. They are wary, too, of you and of your advice, unless perhaps they have been referred by someone in whom they have explicit trust. This is especially true when ii concerns their physical selves. Most are deficient and sick. They must, therefore, be led and guided, prodded, and pushed—but gently. As Alexis Carrel wisely said in Man, The Unknown, "Humanity has never gained anything from the efforts of the crowd. It is driven onward by the passion of a few abnormal individuals, by the flame of their intelligence, by their ideal of science, of charity, and of beauty." As Hygienists, our knowledge of what to do and how to do it and when must become our passion, our bright flame, so that our knowledge of life's beauty and its potential as governed by law, can pass over, and become a pan of conscious being of those who, because they suffer, seek our help.

Remember that the mental acceptance of Hygienic principles and practices is a wonderful thing that will come through exercise of the mind. Just as bones and muscles develop through physical exercise, so will the mind enlarge and accept new ideas as it is exercised. As each new principle and practice is expounded by you and practiced by the clients, they will advance another step toward their ultimate goal of better health.

The extent of forward progress will depend on the client's inner discipline which is so often tempered more by peer thinking than by the working of logic. As teachers we must lead clients toward healthier habits of lifestyle by logic, by inspiration and by example, rather than away from bad habits by scolding and lecturing, by imparting to them the wondrous vision of what is possible for them to achieve and to enjoy. We must not express that which must be taken away, but instead tell about that which will be given. Few clients will learn the right way to live and eat solely by lecturing. The desire to know the beauty of life lived in its fullness is that which can attract, guide, and hold.

The greatest desire of humankind is for health and youth. Men and women alike spend their lives and their gold most often in a fruitless search of illusions. It is well known that we wear ourselves out more often than not by our excesses, our lack of moral discipline, our overdoing in so many ways. The science of life is Truth-gold. It is based on the known facts of physiology and anatomy, not on illusions or ideas; on natural and universal law not on mere concepts. It shows us up for what we have been but also opens up the door to what we can become.

Once we have imparted to our clients the secrets of life, we will have taught them how to keep their bodies whole; we will have returned to them their control and have placed them at the steering wheel of life. They will have received knowledge of many of life's secrets so that for all of life they will be able to keep intact the vigor of their body, its beauty, and the capacity to enlarge their mental sphere.

To accomplish all that we might like to accomplish requires a well-thought-out plan of action. The practitioner should have a general plan which can be modified to fit individual clients' needs. The plan must address all of the biodynamic requisites of organic existence: how much exercise, precisely what changes are required in feeding, what bad habits must be eliminated immediately, etc. All must be considered and addressed as individual need dictates and as progress is reported from time to time.

Mice kept overlong in cages in close confinement and subject to manifold stresses soon wear out, but when given freedom in larger pens where they can burrow and explore, and when they are fed and fasted appropriately, their life spans are extended in health. So, it is with people. When simple Hygienic habits of organic existence become a part of our clients' thinking and doing, they receive the gift of a knowledge which will favorably influence them for the rest of their extended life spans.

Clients will, of course, experience adjustment difficulties. Some will fall by the wayside and then we must learn to "let go." We must not waste our energies in futile pursuit but rather expend it in more useful ways and with more receptive people so that greater success will be assured.

Basically then, we must ascertain the facts to the best of our ability, exploring our clients' knowledge about both the past and the present. Then, we are called upon to formulate a plan of action realizing full well that a plan is just that. It is not a rigid edifice which cannot be changed as need arises. The Hygienist who meets need as it arises with a correct solution will be successful, not only financially, but in having satisfaction in work well done.

It is wise to cultivate both in oneself and in one's clients positive attitudes which will yield positive results. Every forward step, every replacement of a bad habit by a positive change in lifestyle is conducive to improvement in the quality of life. We need to impart to our clients the idea that they have the greatest health-building machine ever built and that when they work with it and answer its simple needs, it will provide them with a fulfillment of riches beyond all their fondest dreams.

91.4. Questions & Answers

It seems to me that holding group meetings and giving lectures would take up a lot of time. Do you think the time spent in such activities is worth all the effort and expense?

Definitely! I say so for several reasons. Practitioners who keep to themselves will soon have no clients, for one thing. For another, they will become stale. They will not be in tune, as we say, with clients' needs as well as when they meet frequently with clients in group meetings and also when they have contact with the public. Group and other public meetings provide a time for the exchange of ideas, to hear other points of view, to learn what is going on in the community, to keep abreast of developments. Additionally, it is interesting how often your words spoken perhaps a year or more ago will remain in the minds of those who heard you speak and cause some persons to seek you out when need arises.

I have a client who is quite elderly, in her late sixties; she is frightened of fasting. What would you suggest as a possible procedure for me to use in handling her case?

Each client is different, of course. However, with such timid and uninformed clients, I would not insist on fasting unless the condition is so far advanced as to require it. But, even then, I think it advisable to take some time, if at all possible, to teach the client about fasting, to provide study materials about fasting, and lay the groundwork which might cause greater willingness to fast.

Sometimes, too, we are called upon to use alternative methods, such as a 24-hour or a 36-hour fast followed by mono or duo meals which place limited stress on the digestive organs and conserve energy resources.

I think we have to remember Alexis Carrel's statement that the mind and body are inextricably one. I believe he said, as if etched in marble, so intertwined are they. A client beset by fear will not progress very well. Sometimes it is necessary to back off before we can go forward. So, my advice would be to take it easy and make small but important changes before taking a giant leap.

You make it all sound so easy. Is it really as easy as this lesson makes it out to be to influence clients to change?

I'm glad you asked that question. The answer is a resounding "No!" Of course not. Theories and methodology are always comparatively easy to recite but can be extremely difficult to put into practice unless one is very skilled in handling people. However, these are workable tools to use. Using them day after day, month after month makes us grow in our ability to work with people. Remember that practice makes perfect! We become more skilled as a practitioner the more we practice. It takes time to build a house. It takes time to build disease. It takes time to build health. It also takes times to build one's skill in helping people.

Article #1: Faith

Obviously, if we are to be successful in our endeavors, we are called upon to have faith in the fact that what we do is correct. If we are not convinced that our program has merit, that it will bring health; indeed, that it is the only possible way to achieve a better life for ourselves, then we will never reach our goal. Even a poor regimen will often produce astounding results, if the patient believes with all his/her heart that it will make him/her better. And how much more spectacular the results can be when the regimen adopted is one in perfect harmony with our body's needs.

Once upon a time, or so the story goes, there was a Sultan who, for some time now, had been very, very ill. He was much beloved by his people, and they begged his learned physicians to make him well. The exalted men of science had given him numerous remedies and drugs, they had bled him and given him snuff, this being the medical custom of that day. But it had all been to no avail. The Sultan continued to grow ever weaker.

At length, one of his physicians, wise among men, instructed the Sultan's craftsmen to fashion a hammer of wood. He told them to make a hollow hammer, both the ball and handle were to be hollow inside. When they had finished the hammer, they were instructed to bring it to the sage together with a block of wood fashioned in a hollow cube. And so, it was done, according to the wise man's instructions.

When the hollow hammer and the hollow cube were brought to the exalted one, he filled them, each in turn, with many different drugs, remedies selected by the most learned men in the kingdom. They came from far and wide with offerings of their art. When all the hollow parts were filled, he instructed the craftsmen to seal up the hammer and the block so that none of the powerful and exotic drugs could escape. Then, the wise one went to the Sultan, there on his bed so close to death, and directed that the bed and the Sultan be lifted up and carried out of doors into the open courtyard. And it was so done.

The great man told the king that, early in the morning before "breaking fast," he was to strike the hollow cube with the hollow hammer, now filled with the potent drugs, until such time as the Sultan should sweat profusely. He told the poor sick king that the aroma wafting from the drugs encased within the wood would, in this manner, be gently wafted about his royal person and, at the proper time, the Sultan would be cured. Day after day, the king followed instructions. And, it came to pass as it had been predicted.

The Sultan grew strong and vigorous, the people rejoiced and waxed eloquent in their praise of the wise physician. He was given much gold and silver and robes of purple and gold.

While this is only an allegory from the Arabian Nights, it imparts to those who see and understand, much wisdom. It tells us the futility of using drugs in any program for health. By inference, we know that it was not the drugs that brought the gift of life, but rather exercise, rest, fresh air, pure water, time, and FAITH. Faith plus the doing can make health happen!

Article #2: Desire Plus the Doing

Desire is not enough! We must also have the doing! Sir Francis Bacon (1561-1626) wrote as follows: "We denounce unto men that they will give over trifling, and not imagine that so great a work as stopping and turning back the powerful course of nature can be brought to pass by some morning draught, or the taking of some precious drug; but that they would be assured that it must needs be that this is a work of labor, and consisted of many remedies, and a fit connection of them amongst themselves."

We can have all the desire in the world and yet never achieve our goal of being healthier than we now are. As Sir Francis indicated, we must gather together all the known attributes of health, the Biodynamic Principles of Health applied according to the Vital Laws of Life, and with these we must work at building health. There will, of course, be times when all will not appear to be going well but, like Robert the Bruce, we must continue to do those things which we know to be required if we ever expect to be better than we now are.

Many long years ago, Cicero said, "The only difficulty, if any there be, consists in making a beginning." So, here we are. We have travelled a lifetime together; we have learned many new and wonderful things about living. We know that this earth might well become a place of joy, if man would but follow natural law. The sages of all time have taught us that the simple ways of life bring health to body, mind, and soul. It is the simple ways that cause the blood to move gently within the arteries and to course merrily through the veins. Obedience to Law causes movement to quicken and the spirit to soar, the memory to clear and wisdom to come. We know that sickness shortens our years, even as health prolongs and gladdens them. We must now make a beginning, for each one of us is required to travel this magic road to health alone; it must be our desire and it must also be of our doing.

In this century, a young woman spent her body's energies caring for an invalid mother. She, too, lay sick and dying. So ill, in fact, was she that a new young doctor in the village where she lived, was afraid to be seen treating her. He feared that, if he offered his services to this dying girl, that he might lose the few patients he had just obtained. There was no other doctor to whom she could turn.

Her family, knowing no other way, closed her up tight in her room thinking to keep her warm and snug. They fed her freshly boiled broths and did their best. However, this giving, loving girl continued to weaken, and her pain became almost unbearable. She finally concluded that death would be a welcome release from an existence such as this. She begged her troubled father to carry her out to the lawn and there to place her on a mattress. She told him to bring her no food and no drink for she was determined to die, but she was also determined to die under God's heavenly blue sky. She asked him to bring her a stick and then to leave her there.

The father, himself weary with life, did as his daughter quested. He carried her out of the comfortable warm house and placed her on a mattress there on the lawn. No one brought her food or drink, only some pure fresh water. The girl amused herself with her stick, feebly digging from time to time in the earth, first on one side, then on the other.

She looked up at the blue sky and watched the birds on the wing. She talked upon occasion with the passersby. And so, the day passed by, but still she lived.

The next day she continued to dig, but she ate no food and had no drink; only, pure, cool water. The days passed, days turned into weeks and weeks into a month and still she did not die. This feeble woman, no more than a child in years, began to dig deeper and deeper. A strange and unexpected thing began to happen; she grew stronger and stronger. Suddenly, one day she decided she wanted to LIVE!

In fact, she knew that the reality of life could be hers and it was revealed to her how she could bring it all to pass.

How excited she was. She cried out for food, and they brought her the foods she requested: only God's sun-ripe fruits would she have, and these in abundance. Soon, she was able to sit up and they then placed her on a couch, still under the blue sky. She continued to dig, rolling first on one side and then on the other, reaching down to the round. In time, she arose from her couch, and her joy was complete. Like the birds she had watched for so long, she, too, was now on the wing. Health had returned, a gift of nature. It had been there to receive all along, but it had taken a deep desire to live and then the knowledge of how to achieve life plus living according to the demands of the human structure and function.

Sometimes we, like the young girl in our story, require no food. Perhaps we can use only the sun, the air, the fresh cooling breezes. Perhaps all we need to do is to forget that we are sick and look around us at this beautiful world and enjoy the free gifts that can bring health. Perhaps all we need is cool, pure water until that time comes when we, too, can reach out and touch a life that is beginning to blossom again. Knowledge, Desire, followed by the Doing! Could these be the magic keys to health?

Article #3: A House Divided

We Must Get Involved

"A house divided cannot stand!" We are all familiar with this saying. It applies to families, to countries, and to professions. The voices are loud in extolling the advances of mankind, yet does it not seem paradoxical at this time in our history, when so much progress is reported in so many diverse fields, that we are witnessing so much confusion in the field of health science?

We walk on the moon and communicate to the far reaches of space. We explore the innermost depths of land and of sea with equipment and instruments from a never-never land of make-believe. More money, time and effort are probably being spent in research into the realm of disease than ever before in the long history of mankind. The amount of dollars expended in this country alone troubles the mind.

Astronomical sums are gathered each year for the investigation of our modern-day scourges: arthritis, diabetes, cancer, multiple sclerosis, and heart trouble. Name the disease and there is probably a fund being collected somewhere. Each year, with a regularity that provokes admiration, come the appeals for money, offering ever anew the hope of meaningful progress around some illusive corner. The hunters are on the loose, or so we are told, ready to search out and destroy all the deadly robbers of health—if they can only find them. But it takes money! and MORE money! and still MORE!

Scientists, nutritionists, dieticians, physicians of all persuasions—all offer "cures," "treatments," and opinions, these latter being almost as diverse as the grains of sand on the shore of the sea! There are divisions within divisions. Preventive medicine is also a "Big Thing" but even here there is disagreement as to how to prevent disease in the first instance.

Where are the teachers of health? We do not find them among these. All seem to be concerned with the sick, with disease, and a few with health! How can we know anything about health when we concentrate solely on disease? Where are those who teach the laws of the body—laws which have always determined our state of being, whether we are healthy or whether we suffer from some degree of diminished health? Where are those who can show people how to build a health bank account and can point out and demonstrate forcefully by their own doing, the exciting and as yet unexplored realms of discovery that may lie ahead for the person whose health account is in good order?

Instead, depending on whom we consult, we may be told that our sickness is just a sign of the times. We probably suffer from acidosis or anemia, either a high or a low blood pressure. Perhaps we take too few calories, or could it be, too many? We no doubt eat "too little" protein. Everybody does, you know! Our metabolism is, without a doubt, sadly disarranged and our body chemistry is surely a mess. We need iron, or iodine, or folic acid, perhaps; and of course, Vitamins C, X, Y, and Z!

In all likelihood, too, we could use a little magnesium, potassium, zinc, or some other mineral right off the chemist's shelf. And then, it's easy to see that we must, of necessity, shed that pot-belly, or could it be that we could use just a wee bit more padding to balance us off? To top it all off, of course, our endocrine system is worn to a frazzle giving us severe emotional problems and we definitely need a few shots and a psychiatrist. And, of course, there's always the possibility, too, that there's absolutely nothing wrong with us. Of course, that's it! It's all in our mind and we'd better get with it, or else! And so, humankind sickens and dies, often prematurely and in great pain.

...Sickness is everywhere about us, but no one sees the message to be found in sickness. Sickness and death give way only to more of the same. The hope of humankind lies in understanding the ways of health—THE HYGIENIC WAY!

We Must Get Involved

A house which is so divided causes confusion and many problems. It gets nowhere. Therefore, we feel it is important for all of us, whether we are actually engaged in this business of teaching health or whether we are just ordinary persons who want to live out our days in joyful health—all of us must become more open-minded, more informed, so that we can get some new ideas. We must trade the consensus of sickness for the consensus of health. We must learn the Vital Laws of Life which are circumscribed for all living creatures, even Man, and we must understand that unless we live in accordance with these laws, that we have no choice but to become a part of the herd; a part of all the sick, the suffering and the diseased, all those who cry out in pain among our midst.

Man is so easily misled. He tends to place his trust in man instead of in Nature, which provides a grand design for man, a design planned to the last detail: the food he should eat and the environment in which he must live. Man has always tried to improve on Nature or to make Nature accommodate herself to his own ideas of the way things should be and the way they should be run.

It might, of course, be very nice indeed if all of our parts and systems would adapt themselves to our wishes and whims but, unfortunately, they just won't! We are unable to change our physical equipment in any real way; it works in its own sequence and patterns to sustain life. So, it appears, that at least for the present, we must learn to accommodate ourselves and our habits of living to our physical self because, if we refuse, the parts will wear out in far too short a time and we simply won't have a chance to back up and try again for, you see, we will be very, very dead.

Excerpted from "Superior life Management"—5 study lessons—by Robert and Elizabeth McCarter.

Article #4: The Several Doors to Your Personality

Put This Bright Finish on Your House

How Fine You Look!

Unlimited Choice of Furnishings

Do This Today for a Guaranteed Future

A Strong Ally for a Bright Future

Your voice is the "front door" to your personality, and like the front door on a real house, much of the impression that folks get of what YOU are like "inside" depends upon the atmosphere about that "front door" of yours. If it is warm, friendly, sincere, and readily opened, folks will get the impression that they are going to LIKE what they find inside.

When you open that door to let your personality COME OUT, the kind of person people see and hear leaving that "house" of yours will depend upon what you say, and HOW you say it. So, your "personality house" will need several doors.

It will need the door of good conversation, through which you enter into cooperative relationship with others, by the exchange of ideas and thoughts, by intelligent listening to others, and by asking complimentary questions.

It will need the door through which you can step and make effective presentations of your good ideas to groups of people, guided by thoughtful, prepared speech, delivered in an interesting, attention-claiming manner.

It will need the door through which you use your voice and words, to inform others— to instruct—to guide—to influence. Those you meet as you step through this door will be your family, the people with whom you work or have social relationships. (And, of course, your clients!—The Authors.)

The best "hardware" with which to hang these important "personality doors" is a broad vocabulary, an ever-expanding vocabulary, acquired by listening and reading, and choosing new words and phrases as your own.

Put This Bright Finish on Your House

Now with your "house" structure completed, we can add some of the finishing touches, starting with the color scheme. One basic material is yours to work with here, and with it you can put the most attractive finish on your house. This material is OPTIMISM. (Remember that when the principles of Life Science are applied by a person filled with sufficient residual energy to initiate and sustain the recovery process, you will approach a success rate of 100%!—The Authors.)

Take a good look at this world of ours, and what is happening every day, and at just how we are getting along. Take a GOOD look, and you'll see that this old place is basically going along in an OPTIMISTIC manner! Things aren't perfect—but there's a lot more on the POSITIVE side than on the negative. And if you CONCENTRATE on this fact, you will ALWAYS find that there are two sides to every condition—no matter how "dark" something may seem at any one moment.

You can add the perfect decor—the perfect "color scheme" to your personality, by DEMONSTRATING that you can and do find the "bright side" of this world—OFTEN—very often!

Optimism—and all the congenial, happy attitudes it infers—will make YOUR "house" an outstandingly attractive one in the eyes of everyone.

How Fine You Look!

Then, of course, you will want to add the distinctiveness of a good landscape job, so you accomplish this through DRESS and GROOMING.

You know, if we went around in practically nothing but our skins, as do some of our brothers and sisters in other parts of the world, (totally in keeping, of course, with Hygienic principles!—The Authors), we might say that we could greatly simplify this whole matter of wardrobes, and taking care of our clothes, and being concerned about how we "look." But just suppose that we did make a fantastic switch in our culture and decided to try it the "South Sea Island" way, with loin cloths, and beads and grass skirts the "fashionable" dress. It doesn't take any imagination to picture what would happen to the personalities of all of us, does it? I don't think I would want to argue the merits of such a "fashion" for myself.

I am sure that when you consider the ramifications of the two extremes of culture, the "grass-skirt" motif as compared to the fully-clothed motif, you will see the great responsibility and dependence we place upon clothes and grooming in the kind of society in which we live.

Others don't see the real skin-clad you. They see the clothes you wear, and the condition of the exposed portions of your body, such as hands, arms, face, hair. Therefore, they are constantly appraising and evaluating you, upon the basis of the quality, cleanliness and good taste of your clothes and grooming.

Harmonious color combinations, good choice of accessories, well-cared-for hair, all add up to the way to "landscape" yourself, so that people will have a continuously agreeable reaction to the kind of person you are. For this reason, your wardrobe should be considered an INVESTMENT—and your grooming a careful preparation for your appearance as an actor or actress on the "Stage" that is your everyday world.

Unlimited Choice of Furnishings

And finally, of course, you will want to furnish your house. Here you have unlimited choice of materials because you furnish your "personality house" with KNOWLEDGE. Learning, the seeking of knowledge, the ACQUIRING of knowledge makes your personality grow and prosper. Through an expanding pattern of knowledge in your life, and its expansive effect on your personality, the adding of days and months and years to your life, ACTS IN YOUR FAVOR. Each day that brings you NEW knowledge adds to the power of your personality, and if each changing day brings this knowledge from a DIFFERENT source, adding variety to your inner resources, your personality IM-

PROVES with age! A most desirable circumstance, isn't it?

In your "personality house," there are many rooms to furnish, and so there are many opportunities for using a variety of knowledge. Seek to furnish each room distinctively, through positive, progressive knowledge concerning your vocation, your avocation, your interests, world affairs, community affairs, and the people with whom you associate. Good knowledge of all people and things that concern your everyday living will make your "personality house" one that is COMFORTABLE for you and for others.

Now you know what it takes to make an ideal "personality house." You know the materials that are required to build one, or to "remodel" your present one. You know HOW to do it. Most important is the fact that you can have a "personality house" that is distinctive for YOU, and which will be seen by others as being most ATTRACTIVE.

You can create the attitude within yourself that will ENABLE you to have this house by doing two PROGRESSIVE things, TODAY!

Do This Today for a Guaranteed Future

First, make an honest inventory of your personality assets and liabilities, by comparing your present habits and attitudes (and the results as they affect your life), with the STANDARDS' set out for you, as we build that IDEAL "personality house." Persons who have objectively made such an inventory, under this plan, have had good experiences, because they ALWAYS found that the "remodeling job" suggested to them was easily within their ability to accomplish. The important thing was the they

MADE the inventory, so they knew exactly what to do. This is equally important to you, and the results will be equally valuable. (Could this be an appropriate tool, also, in helping clients the better to understand areas of concern in their lifestyle habits?)

Second, based upon your inventory, make a plan to do that "remodeling job"—beginning TODAY! The very act of making this plan, and of taking your first step to ACT according to the plan, will result in a favorable change concerning your future.

From then on, each step that you take to improve your "personality house" will be a forecast of a favorable future.

A Strong Ally for a Bright Future

You have an intimate ally which will go to work WITH you, as you take this inventory, and make this plan. Perhaps I should say that this is an intimate ASSOCIATE, since it can conceivably NOT be an ally.

I am referring to your subconscious mind, that inner part of your mental resources that records all you do, and in turn, influences you to act the way you do. It has always been working this way, and it influences negatively or positively, depending upon what you caused to be recorded there. Record an abundance of negative reactions from the things that you do, and your subconscious mind will be impressed accordingly, and will tend to cause you to continue to act this way. But if you record an abundance of positive ideas and thoughts, your subconscious mind will be impressed by THESE, and will try to get you to continue along the same path. In that case, it will be your ally. Right?

If you apply yourself wholeheartedly to your inventory and your plan, your subconscious mind will be greatly impressed, and it will HELP you go into action on your plan. I know that this is what you are going to do, so I know it will be your ally.

... For every moment of the future that is controllable by you, your attitudes and habits as reflected in this IMPROVED personality, will work POSITIVELY to effect a FAVORABLE control.

Your "personality house" is you. Make it comfortable, pleasant, and secure for yourself, and distinctive in the eyes of others, and the future for YOU is predictable. It cannot help but be a fortunate future!

From Personality and Your Future by Charles M. Simmons

Article #5: Excerpt from Man, the Unknown by Alexis Carrel, M.D., Nobel Prize Recipient.

Young and old people, although in the same region of space, live in different temporal worlds. We are inexorably separated by age from one another. A mother isn't usually a sister to her daughter. It is difficult for children to understand their parents, and still less their grandparents. Obviously, the individuals belonging to four successive generations are profoundly heterochronic. An old man and his great-grandson can be complete strangers. The shorter the temporal distance separating two generations, the stronger may be the moral influence of the older over the younger.

From the concept of physiological time derive certain rules of our action on human beings. Organic and mental developments are not inexorable. They can be modified, in some measure, according to our will, because we are a movement, a succession of superposed patterns in the frame of our identity. Although a human being is a closed world, his/her outside and inside frontiers are open to many physical, chemical, and psychological agents. And those agents are capable of modifying our tissues and our mind. The moment, the mode, and the rhythm of our interventions depend on the structure of physiological time. Our temporal dimension extends chiefly during childhood when functional processes are most active. Then, organs and mind are plastic. Their formation can effectively be aided. As organic events happen each day in great numbers, their glowing mass can receive such shape as it seems proper to impress permanently upon the individual. The molding of the organism according to a selected pattern must take into account the nature of duration, the constitution of our temporal dimension. Our interventions have to be made in the cadence of inner time. (Emphasis by the Authors.) People are like a viscous liquid flowing into the physical continuum. They cannot instantaneously change their direction. We should not endeavor to modify a person's mental and structural form by rough procedures, as one shapes a statue of marble by blows of the hammer. Surgical operations alone produce in tissues sudden alterations which are "beneficial," but recovery from the quick work of the knife is slow. No profound changes of the body as a whole can be obtained rapidly. Our action must blend with the physiological processes, substratum of inner time, by following their own rhythm ... Our interventions in the building up of body and consciousness have their full effects only when they conform to the laws of our duration.

A child may be compared to a brook, which follows any change in its bed. The brook persists in its identity, in spite of the diversity of its forms. It may become a lake or a torrent. Under the influence of environment, personality may spread and become very thin, or concentrate and acquire great strength. The growth of personality involves a constant trimming of our self. At the beginning of life, a person is endowed with vast potentialities. People are limited in development only by the extensible frontiers of ancestral predispositions. But at each instant a choice must be made. And each choice throws into nothingness one of their potentialities. They have, of necessity, to select one of the several roads open to the wanderings of existence, to the exclusion of all others. Thus, they deprive themselves of seeing the countries wherein they could have traveled along the other roads. In our infancy we carry within ourselves numerous potential beings, who die one by one. In our old age, we are surrounded by an escort of those we could have been, of all our aborted potentialities.

Every human being is like a fluid that becomes solid, or a history in the making, or a personality that is being created. And our progress, or our disintegration, depends on physical, chemical, and physiological factors, on viruses and bacteria, on psychological influences, and, finally, on our own will. We are constantly being made by our environment and by our self. And duration is the very material of organic and mental life, as it means "invention, creation of forms, continual elaboration of the absolutely new." (Quoted from Creative Evolution by Henri Bergson, Henry Holt and Co., Inc.)

Article #6: Excerpt from "In Tune with the Infinite" by Ralph Waldo Trine

Fear and lack of faith go hand in hand. The one is born of the other. Tell me how much one is given to fear, and I will tell you how much s/he lacks in faith. Fear is a most expensive guest to entertain, the same as worry is so expensive are they that no one can afford to entertain them. We invite what we fear, the same as, by a different attitude of mind, we invite and attract the influences and conditions we desire. The mind dominated by fear opens the door to the entrance of the very things, for the actualization of the very conditions, it fears.

"Where are you going?" asked an Eastern pilgrim on meeting the plague one day. "I am going to Bagdad to kill five thousand people," was the reply. A few days later the same pilgrim met the plague returning. "You told me you were going to Bagdad to kill five thousand people," said he, "but instead, you killed fifty thousand." "No," said the plague. "I killed only five thousand, as I told you I would, the others died of fright."

Fear can paralyze every muscle in the body. Fear affects the flow of the blood, likewise the normal and healthy action of all the life forces. Fear can make the body rigid, motionless and powerless to move.

Not only do we attract to ourselves the things we fear, but we also aid in attracting to others the conditions we in our own minds hold them in fear of. This we do in proportion to the strength of our own thoughts, and in the degree that they are sensitively organized and so influenced by our thought, although it be unconscious both on their part and on ours.

Children, especially when very young, are, generally speaking, more sensitive to their surrounding influences than grown people are. Some are veritable little sensitive plates, registering the influences about them and embodying them as they grow. Those who have them in charge should be very careful in their prevailing mental states, and a mother should be especially careful during the time she is carrying the child, since mental and emotional aim on her part will so greatly assist her approach to labor and to the care of her newborn infant. Let parents be careful how they hold a child, either younger or older, in the thought of fear. This is many times done, unwittingly on their part, through anxiety, and at times through what might well be termed over care, which is fully as bad as under care.

I know of a number of cases where a child has been so continually held in the thought of fear lest this or that condition occur, that the very things that were feared have been drawn to the child, which probably otherwise never would have come at all. Many times, there has been no adequate basis for the fear. In case there is a basis, then it is far wiser to take exactly the opposite attitude, so as to neutralize the force at work, and then to hold the child in the thought of wisdom and strength that it may be able to meet the condition and master it, instead of being mastered by it.

But a day or two ago a friend was telling me of an experience of his own life in this connection. At a period when he was having a terrific struggle with a certain habit, he was so continually held in the thought of fear by his mother and the young lady to whom he was engaged—the engagement to be consummated at the end of a certain period, the time depending on his proving his mastery—that he, very sensitively organized, continually felt the depressing and weakening effects of their negative noughts. He could always tell exactly how they felt toward him; he was continually influenced and weakened by their fear, by their questionings, by their suspicions, all of which had the effect of lessening the sense of his own power, all of which had an endeavor-paralyzing influence on him. And so instead of their begetting courage and strength in him, they brought him to a still greater realization of his own weakness and the almost worthless use of struggle.

Here were two who loved him dearly, and who would have done anything and everything to help him gain the mastery, but who, ignorant of the silent, subtle, ever-working, and all-telling power of the thought forces, instead of imparting to him courage, instead of adding to his strength, disarmed him of this, and then added an additional weakness from without. In this way the battle for him was made harder in a threefold degree.

Fear, worry and all kindred mental states are too expensive for any person—man, woman, or child—to entertain or indulge in. Fear paralyzes healthy action; worry corrodes and pulls down the organism and will finally tear it to pieces. Nothing is to be gained by it, and everything to be lost. Long-continued grief at any loss will do the same. Each brings its own peculiar type of ailment. An inordinate love of gain, a close-fisted, hoarding disposition will have kindred effects. Anger, jealousy, malice, continual fault finding, lust—each has its own peculiar corroding, weakening, tearing-down effects.

We shall find that not only are happiness and prosperity concomitants of righteousness—living in harmony with the higher laws—but bodily health as well. The great Hebrew seer enunciated a wonderful chemistry of life when he said, "As righteousness tendeth to life, so he that pursueth evil, pursueth it to his own death." On the other hand, "In the way of righteousness is life; and in the pathway thereof there is no death." The time will come when it will be seen that this means far more than most people dare even to think as yet. "It rests with ever-growing splendor and beauty, or in a hovel of his own building—a hovel at last ruined and abandoned to decay."

The bodies of almost untold numbers, living their one-sided, unbalanced lives, are every year, through these influences, weakening and falling by the wayside long before their time. Poor, poor houses! Intended to be beautiful temples, brought to desolation by their ignorant, reckless, deluded tenants. Poor houses!

A close observer, a careful student of the power of the thought forces, will soon be able to read in the voice, in the movements, in the features, the effects registered by the prevailing mental states and conditions. Or, if he is told the prevailing mental states and conditions, he can describe the voice, the movements, the features, as well as describe, in a general way, the peculiar physical ailments their possessor is heir to.

We are told by good authority that a study of the human body, its structure, and the length of time it takes it to come to maturity, in comparison with the time it takes the bodies, of various animals and their corresponding longevity, reveals the fact that our natural age should be nearer a hundred and twenty years than what we commonly find it today. But think of the multitudes all about us whose bodies are aging, weakening, breaking, so that they have to abandon them long before they reach what ought to be a long period of strong, vigorous middle life.

Then, the natural length of life being thus shortened, it comes to be what we might term a race belief that this shortened period is the natural period. And as a consequence, many, when they approach a certain age, seeing that as a rule people at this period of life begin to show signs of age, to break and go downhill as we say, they, thinking it a matter of course and that it must be the same with them, by taking this attitude of mind, many times bring upon themselves these very conditions long before it is necessary. Subtle and powerful are the influences of the mind in the building and rebuilding of the body. As we understand them better it may become the custom for people to look forward with pleasure to the teens of their second century.

There comes to mind at this moment a friend, a lady well on to eighty years of age. An old lady, some, most people in fact, would call her, especially those who measure age by the number of the seasons that have come and gone since one's birth. But to call our friend old would be to call black, white. She is no older than a girl of twenty-five, and indeed younger, I am glad to say—or I am sorry to say, depending upon the point of view—than many a girl of this age. Seeking for the good in all people and in all things, she has found the good everywhere. The brightness of disposition and of voice that is hers today, that attracts all people to her and that makes her so beautifully attractive to all people, has characterized her all through life. It has in turn carried brightness and hope and courage and strength to hundreds and thousands of people through all these years, and will continue to do so, apparently, for many years yet to come.

No fears, no worrying's, no hatreds, no jealousies, no sorrowing's, no grieving's, no sordid grasping's after inordinate gain, have found entrance into her realm of thought. As a consequence, her mind, free from these abnormal states and conditions, has not externalized in her body the various physical ailments that the great majority of people are lugging about with them, thinking in their ignorance that they are natural, and that it is all in accordance with the "eternal order of things" that they should have them. Her life has been one of varied experiences, so that all these things would have found ready entrance into the realm of her mind and so into her life were she ignorant enough to allow them entrance. On the contrary she has been wise enough to recognize the fact that in one kingdom at least she is ruler—the kingdom of her mind, and that it is hers to dictate as to what shall and what shall not enter there. She knows, moreover, that in determining this she is determining all the conditions of her life. It is indeed a pleasure as well as an inspiration to see her as she goes here and there, to see her sunny disposition, her youthful step, to hear her joyous laughter. Indeed, and in truth, Shakespeare knew whereof he spoke when he said, "It is the mind that makes the body rich."

... Would you remain always young, and would you carry all the joyousness and buoyancy of youth into your maturer years? They have care concerning but one thing—how you live in your thought world. This will determine all. It was the inspired one, Gautama, the Buddha, who said, "The mind is everything; what you think you become." And Ruskin had the same thing in mind when he said, "Make yourself nests of pleasant thoughts. None of us as yet know, for none of us have been taught in early youth, what fairy palaces we may build of beautiful thought—proof against all adversity." And would you have in your body all the elasticity, all the strength, all the beauty of your younger years? Then live these in your mind, making no room for unclean thought, and you will externalize them in your body.

In the degree that you keep young in thought you will remain young in body. And you will find that your body will in turn aid your mind, for body helps build the mind the same as mind builds the body.

... Full, rich, and abounding health is the normal and the natural condition of life. Anything else is an abnormal condition, and abnormal conditions as a rule come through perversions. God never created sickness, suffering and disease; they are man's own creations. They come though his violating the laws under which he lives. So used are we to seeing them that we come gradually, if not to think of them as natural, then to look on them as a matter of course.

... Give the body the nourishment, the exercise, the fresh air, the sunlight it requires, keep it clean, and then think of it as little as possible. In your thoughts and in your conversation never dwell on the negative side. Don't talk of sickness and disease. By talking of these you do yourself harm and you do harm to those who listen to you. Talk of those things that will make people the better for listening to you. Thus, you will infect them with health and strength and not with weakness and disease.

To dwell on the negative side is always destructive. This is true of the body the same as it is true of all other things ... "We can never gain health by contemplating disease, any more than we can reach perfection by dwelling upon imperfection, or harmony through discord. We should keep a high ideal of health and harmony constantly before the mind... "Never affirm or repeat about your health what you do not wish to be true. Do not dwell upon your ailments, nor study your symptoms. Never allow yourself to be convinced that you are not complete master of yourself. Stoutly affirm your superiority over bodily ills, and do not acknowledge yourself the slave of any inferior power ... I would teach children early to build a strong barrier between themselves and disease, by healthy habits of thought, high thinking, and purity of life. I would teach them to expel all thoughts of death, all images of disease, all discordant emotions, like hatred, malice, revenge, envy, as they would banish a temptation to do evil. I would teach them that bad food, bad drink, or bad air makes bad blood; that bad blood makes bad tissue, and bad flesh bad morals. I would teach them that healthy thoughts are as essential to healthy bodies as a strong willpower, and to brace themselves against life's enemies in every possible way.

I would teach the sick to have hope, confidence, possibilities. No person's success or health will ever reach beyond his/her own confidence; as a rule, we erect our own barriers.

"Like produces like the universe through. Hatred, envy, malice, jealousy, and revenge all have children. Every bad thought breeds others, and each of these goes on and on, ever reproducing itself, until our world is peopled with their offspring. The true physician and parent of the future will not medicate the body with drugs so much as the mind with principles. The coming mother will teach her child to assuage the fever of anger, hatred, malice, with the great panacea of the world—Love. The coming physician will teach the people to cultivate cheerfulness, good-will, and noble deeds for a health tonic as well as a heart tonic; and that a merry heart doeth good like a medicine."

Lesson 92:

Planning a Transition to Better Living

92.1. The Typical Client

92.1.1. Fred—Case Study

The typical client who consults with a Hygienic practitioner will most likely have had recourse to various "therapies" and will have plied him or herself well with a variety of chemicals which may well have ranged from all manner of prescribed drugs to over the-counter concoctions; to vitamins, herbs, and a variety of assorted supplements. Many will also have sought a magic release from their many ailments from practitioners of diverse disciplines. Almost without exception, they will be lacking in hope and seek out the Hygienist as a last recourse, lacking any real faith that this time they will be successful in their quest, the finding of a "cure" for whatever ails them.

It will be rare, indeed, to find clients who will appreciate the fact that, so long as sufficient vital force exists to power the effort, the erstwhile dream of attaining a higher level of health can become an accomplished reality and this through something they had all along: the healing power within. And, too, they will fail to realize that the magic solution they have sought for so long will require effort on their part; that the attainment of better health requires a planned transition, a gradual organized rebuilding which will, when adhered to in all particulars, take them from their present here of sickness and suffering to the thereof dreams fulfilled and euphoric joy in living.

92.1.1. Fred—Case Study

Fred was typical. In his late 70s, Fred came to us suffering from digestive trouble and a prostate enlargement which caused him to urinate frequently, especially at night, and was the source of much discomfort. For several days prior to his first visit, he had been unable to retain any food, vomiting, as he said, "even a poached egg."

A widower for some ten years, Fred was lonely. He recounted a sad tale of how he and his wife had travelled many miles and counseled with many "specialists" in search of a cure for his wife's cancer, but to no avail.

Sadly, he told us that it has "cost me well over $70,000.00 to bury my angel."

It was obvious that Fred was still grieving and living in the past. Like so many others, following his wife's death he, too, had begun to fail and, like so many others, too, he had begun yet another, so far unsuccessful, search for a better life. He recounted how he had consulted with several medical men, including a specialist in internal medicine how, almost in desperation, he had finally gone to see naturopath and a nutripathist; all without, of course, a noticeable improvement.

Fred told how he had taken the pills, the enemas (low and high), the various drugs, herbs, and vitamins. In fact, he said that he had a whole box of vitamin bottles and with a gesture, indicated a box large enough to house a food processor! Fred sadly shook his head. He knew that he had foolishly spent a fortune on yet another fruitless pursuit. And now, said he, "I am here to see what you have to offer."

Fred's predicament is not at all unusual or rare. Unfortunately, his case, while not wholly typical in all particulars, does demonstrate the emotional valley it which so many of our new clients find themselves. The practitioner must be ready to respond in a constructive way to this kind of negativity. Perhaps the most valuable service the Hygienist can offer in the initial stages of transition is to supply the missing ingredient of hope.

92.1.1.1. Our First Move

To instill an element of Positivity into Fred's thinking we invited him to one of our potluck parties. At that particular meeting, we had 13 guests besides him. He was surrounded by people in various way stations along the transition road. All had achieved some measure of success some amazingly so. Fred had to take notice!

We watched and listened as Fred asked questions received positive input and encouragement. One couple, in particular, cornered him and we heard the give and take One little child, age eight, a recovered asthmatic, climbed up on his knee and asked, "Do you like fruit, too?"

The table was spread with all manner of salad makings. The washed fruit filled a number of plates. There were steamed potatoes for Fred and some steamed green beans, and he wisely ate very little. But his eyes darted hither and wonder watching what other guests chose for their meal.

Fred asked for his second appointment before the evening was over. We asked him to keep a record of his food intake and set a time for our next meeting. Fred was ready to begin his own transition into better living. The meeting together with friends had successfully supplied the missing elements in Fred's life: faith and hope.

92.2. Superb Health the Norm

Almost every person who consults with a practicing Hygienist will be experiencing some degree of diminished health, sometimes even serious.

Few clients will comprehend that superb health should be the norm. Few, if any, will understand that (aside from that which may come as a result of accidental injury), all disease, all suffering, all sickness and, in fact, all the accompanying and/or subsequent pain and travail that so often comes with impairment of health, are signs that the body is in an abnormal (or toxic) state, and is trying to cleanse itself.

This may well be the first important concept that must become a part of a client's thinking. This is the first "Baby Step" most are required to take as they begin their hesitant transitional steps to better living. And yet, for some, this will be a giant leap into a strange new world, a world of new thoughts, new ideas, new concepts.

The client must learn that each person creates his own suffering, his own pain, by a series of multiple errors in eating and living and that the amount of diminished health, which is presently being experienced can, in all instances, be traced back to and accounted for by some rather simple principles.

Each of us represent the sum total of countless generations of people and, for this very reason, we enter the world with our very own personal collection of strengths and weaknesses. We all have strong parts, but we also have a few weak ones. The sum total, of course, represents our constitution. All of us, too, make mistakes. Our present condition represents a lifetime of multiple errors in eating and living, errors which no doubt began on the day of our birth.

Most clients willingly accept this concept but there is also another concept which they must learn and it is even more important, and that is that the converse of the preceding negative aspect of life is also true: namely, that it is possible to manage our lifestyle, beginning now, at this moment, in such a manner as to cause us to progress from the present HERE of pain and suffering forward to a THERE of euphoric joy, at which time full health becomes our constant companion, replacing the former dour shadows of sickness.

Additionally, the practitioner should make clear to his client that this transition can be accomplished by faithfully following a planned sequence of biologically-acceptable, scientifically-sound, steps and procedures designed to change a health-damaging lifestyle into one more in tune with all hidden systemic needs.

In other words, the client can become somewhat inspired if s/he comes to appreciate the fact that it is entirely possible within the framework of sound scientific principles to change frustration and despair, always the unwanted fruits of a diseased state, into a wonderful joy-filled experience. Developing a more positive attitude about life and living will, in and of itself, help one and all to take new forward steps less timidly.

And, finally, in the context of this present discussion, clients who become actively involved in the planning and execution of a pattern of behavior will, all other things being equal, be more willing to further actively their own cause: THEIR transition into better living.

Perhaps the hardest concept for new clients to accept is the knowledge that there is nothing outside of the body that has any power whatsoever to heal body hurts and, even more vital, that there are no outside wisdom, guidelines, or intelligence which can fully assess, define, determine the complete nature or the extent of the client's own peculiar needs; that there are no gadgets or machines which can accurately determine the cause or possible multiple causes of the particular sickness or ailment. The client must gently be urged to an understanding that there are no outside forces or substances or combination of forces or substances which can fabricate blood, lymph, and other body fluids, or direct them to where they are most needed. As practitioners most of us once stood, figuratively speaking, where the clients now are, and we must be aware of the existing deep medically-oriented programming that has up-to-now dominated their thinking. It will be difficult, on first hearing, for them fully to comprehend the truism that there is no outside force(s) or substance(s) which can correctly evaluate the situation and decide which cells are to be replaced or retained, or just where the precise place is where they may be needed to enhance systemic functioning or meet structural needs. Should some be discarded, or perhaps recycled? Most of us don't have sufficient wisdom to make this determination consciously, but, wondrously so, it is inherent in our subconscious being.

To most clients the exposure to this life knowledge will represent a new dimension in their thinking, one that requires them to discard the "magic bullet" concept, the belief in a health fairyland, in favor of mind and self-control, certainly not an easy transition to make. This kind of reorientation requires considerable change in the clients' thought processes and it may take time for them to fully grasp the entire significance of the idea that all healing power lies solely within the body itself and that making it fully operational will depend upon how well individuals meet their own very personal needs and that the extent of wellness it is possible for them to achieve will depend on how well they meet those needs and upon the amount of vitality they yet possess to power the transition to a successful conclusion, to the better living they so fondly envision.

In other words, at the outset, the client should be helped to reach this understanding. Briefly stated k means that all healing, by the very nature of the life process, must be and is a biological evolution. Old and sick cells must first be torn down and usable parts salvaged before new and healthier cells can be formulated by a commingling of recycled materials with the incoming tide of higher quality nutrients.

The client must be brought to an understanding that the first new cells represent only a beginning, a start on a transitional process that will witness a parade of generations of cells, each being just a little healthier than the preceding generation.

This fascinating journey towards better living represents an amazing series and variety of transitional implementations, a biological rebuilding which proceeds cell by cell. In no way, can this transition be brought about by a single giant leap over mountains of hidden systemic obstacles accumulated perhaps over a period of many years; impedimenta composed of the residues of pills, potions, procedures—the multitudinous errors of the past.

Healing is a very human happening, one made operational the moment the inner self receives the tools of life: good food, fresh air, pure water, friendships, warmth and sunshine—the essences upon which life depends. In other words, if we would walk in health, we must walk in the ways of health!

92.3. Introducing The Toxemia Connection

92.3.1. Early Introduction Advisable

92.3.2. Orienting the Client as to How S/he Relates to the Seven Steps to Pathology

92.3.3. Building Reasonable Expectations

92.3.4. Zeroing In

92.3.1. Early Introduction Advisable

In working with our own clients, we feel it is advisable, at an early opportunity, to introduce the Toxemia Connection. This concept, like that of self-generated healing, will generally be completely foreign to clients' thinking and accepting it as a totally valid premise may also require some major adjustments on their part.

Most clients have followed the herd all their lives. Almost without exception, they will have been nurtured on the germ theory of disease. Almost all will have willingly accepted the prevailing idea that their pain and suffering are the direct consequence of the foul work of some outside agent, be it germ or virus. They also have dutifully been well-programmed to believe that healing will require some powerful force to "do away with" whatever is at fault. Certainly, of course, and in their view, their illness is hardly of their own doing.

To discard these popular notions requires some mental handsprings, as it were, by the clients. The toxemia theory of disease which they must now learn represents the firm foundation upon which all Hygienic practice is based. Therefore, the connection between toxicosis and disease must be set forth in plain terms for the clients' enlightenment. It is vital for each client to develop a deep understanding of all that is involved in the toxemia connection and what can reasonably be predicted to evolve, and therefore reasonably be expected to happen in their own selves, once the theory has been well examined, cerebrally accepted, and then intelligently acted upon.

Briefly, as Life Science students have already learned, the Toxemia Connection is based on the fact that all diseases, barring those of accidental origin, have their beginnings in a deranged state of the fluids of the body, in a departure from the norm brought about by an abnormal accumulation of metabolic acid debris which has more less exhausted vital power.

The nature of the disease itself will depend on the kind of poisons present, upon the amount of waste present and, to some extent, upon the peculiar inherited weaknesses of the affected individual. The extensiveness and intensive-ness of the ailment will likewise be similarly influenced; the possibility for full recovery, upon the vital power.

Multitudes now live in pain. More multitudes have died writhing in agony because they did not have this knowledge, or, being informed, refused to walk in the ways of health.

92.3.2. Orienting the Client as to How S/he Relates to the Seven Steps to Pathology

The client's next mental adjustment concerns the fact that any departure from the normal condition of the body fluids will always result in a biological evolution, but this time it will be a reverse evolution from the norm to the abnormal. This departure will always proceed in a more-or-less predictable fashion from simple cellular fatigue (enervation caused by cellular constipation), in its earliest manifestation, to a more-or-less complete saturation of cells, fluids and tissues with acid metabolic waste debris, this last in its later stages. Such accumulation and the ensuing defensive measures instigated and kept operational by the nervous system in an effort to retain the life of individual eventually exhausts the vital force, at point death ensues.

Concisely put, the Toxemia Connection simply means that most people become ill and subsequently die prematurely, not from a particular disease, per se, but rather from organ failure; usually the failure of the liver, or kidneys, or heart, or some combination of poorly-functioning organs which can no longer meet the systemic needs of the life process due to a derangement brought about by the accumulating poisons.

Thus, the body cells that make up the faltering organs and the total society of cells, overcome as they are with acid wastes, simply are forced to cease their functional duties, causing the life process to come to an end: the electrical power that sustains life is no more.

Throughout the entire reverse biological evolution many cries for help are constantly being given off by body cells in the form of pain and suffering. The disease itself, however manifested, represents the body's attempt to reestablish normalcy and it is only when the vital force becomes exhausted that the pains of protest and the systemic attempts to normalize the situation, the symptoms formerly expressed, now cease because the healing vital power has been wasted. None remains to fuel the effort.

92.3.3. Building Reasonable Expectations

Here is where the blackboard becomes almost indispensable. As our practice is strictly educational in all respects we use this tool frequently. We write down the seven step; in the evolution of pathology which have previously been delineated in this course; to review, they are briefly Toxicosis, Enervation, Irritation, Inflammation, Ulceration, Induration and, finally, Fungation.

Next, we note the various symptoms characteristic of each stage and encourage the clients to share with us any symptoms they may recall from their own past. Clients are then amazed at how closely their own medical history will correlate with what they now see on the blackboard before them. By this kind of active participation, they begin to develop an understanding of the nature and origin of, disease and, what is even more important, just how their own past lives, their errors and omissions, may have contributed to their own reverse biological evolution.

Additionally, the practitioner can perhaps, at a later time, when the clients may become discouraged by their seemingly slow progress, remind the clients of this evolutionary transgression and to what stage they may have progressed before beginning their own transition to better living. The building of reasonable expectations often depends on the client being exposed early in the transition to this knowledge.

Of course, full acceptance of such a radical change in thinking may require some time. However, we do not hesitate to suggest, even at this early stage, that it is possible now to set the stage for a more or less complete turn-around; to put the brakes on, to make a new beginning, this time in the opposite direction, toward health. In other words, we have an opportunity to encourage the clients to begin their own transition towards better living.

Often we find that gaining this new understanding of the nature of healing and coming to realize that it may be entirely possible for them to reverse the biological evolution, to turn it in a more positive direction, is often sufficient to supply the missing element in their thinking: the Hope mentioned earlier.

Hope often supplants their former fear because they can now see both where they have been and the positive direction they can now begin to take, provided that they learn what they themselves must do to enjoy this totally new experience, this transitional journey from HERE to THERE, to the time and place when superb health will be their constant companion.

Using the blackboard to define and illustrate the transition that must be made in every instance helps the client also to an understanding of the fact that the more severe their symptoms (that is, in whatever stage they place themselves, either correctly or incorrectly, in one or perhaps even in several), the longer it will probably require for them to achieve full recovery if that, indeed, be yet within the realm of probability, considering their present condition. In other words, the foundation for reasonable expectations can thus be laid even this early in the transition, possibly alleviating future disappointments.

Enthusiasm for this new way of living coupled with Desire, Hope, the Will to Act and having Reasonable Expectations may well prove to be an unbeatable combination!

92.3.4. Zeroing In

Clients usually have some difficulty in grasping this new concept of the nature of disease and, since this understanding is essential to future progress and peace of mind, the true nature of the disease process should necessarily be introduced early in the transitional reeducation period.

Certainly, if this theory is correct—and it is becoming increasingly accepted among modern cellular scientists if not among the orthodox hanger-on, and if symptoms were not forthcoming, the individual would soon die. Thus, the diagrams can help the new client to understand the WHY and the IMPORTANCE of Symptoms.

Using the blackboard and/or the diagrams to illustrate the role of toxicosis in disease making provides a graphic representation, to the clients of their own past, the present and future possibilities. Intelligent clients soon realize, perhaps for the first time, that an opportunity is being presented to them to begin a totally new life, one filled with attainable promises of a better life and this, too, for ALL life!

Blackboard and diagrams help the client to realize that if the body did NOT unload its excess acidic waste, the cells must soon be adversely affected, both in functioning ability and in their structural integrity; in other words, that these acids will damage. Also, a natural conclusion follows that organs composed of these deranged, confused, and damaged cells would then, in due course, likewise deteriorate in the same manner. Once this understanding is reached, it is only a simple and direct conclusion for most students to make that if they desire a better life, they must reduce their own systemic toxicity, that they must begin a program to normalize their own body fluids.

92.4. A Practical Demonstration of Procedure

92.4.1. Symptomizing

92.4.2. Levels of Tolerance

92.4.3. The Evolution of Pathology

Let us go back and see how we worked with our client Fred whom we met at the beginning of this discussion. At age 77, a widower, very lonely, without relatives, he was in a very depressed state of mind. At 5 feet, 7 inches, he weighed 169 pounds. A review of his medical history showed the following:

1. Pyloric end of his stomach excised some years ago, time uncertain.

2. Part of vagus nerve removed.

3. Diagnosis of prostatitis made.

4. Desert fever.

5. Nodule in lung.

6. Unable to retain food for the last three days with frequent vomiting prior to that time.

7. Constipated. Necessary to take frequent enemas.

8. By prescription of naturopath, he was presently taking 26 vitamins and other supplements daily.

9. Feeling terrible.

Recommendation: Fred was to brew a day's supply of vegetable broth made from carrots, potatoes, green beans celery and zucchini. For a total of four days, he was to make a fresh supply of this broth. Also, he was told to remain in bed, having access to fresh air at all times. The broth was to be taken in quantities of 6 to 8 ounces every two hours, or as needed, from 6 a.m. until 6 p.m., after which only distilled water could be had, as and when required only.

Following the four days bed rest with broth, Fred was to rest for two hours during the day and then to be up for two hours. At two-hour intervals he was to have freshly made vegetable juices (Fred owned a juicer), extraction them from carrots and celery, these to be alternated with freshly-extracted fruit juices (orange or grape). These juices could be sipped slowly every two hours, if needed. For his evening "meal," Fred was told that he might enjoy a single variety of fresh fruit. We call this our "Two-Two Transition Program."

Following the four days bed rest, Fred was encouraged to do some elevated leg exercises, just a few at first. These exercises are done lying flat on the floor and raising the legs to a vertical position. The legs are then "pumped," bending the knees and then extending the legs again to the vertical position.

Fred was advised to reduce his vitamin intake but was cautioned about the possibility of a crisis should he attempt to eliminate them completely at this time. Obviously, Fred had become accustomed to false stimulation.

Fred was provided with our study book on the colon.

Three Days Later

Fred telephoned. It seems that, in the intervening few days, he had experienced rather annoying pains in the abdomen (perhaps a mild crisis?). However, he reported that he was now feeling much better and would renew the Two-Two Program. We suggested that he might find a hot bath useful should he again experience any pain, this to be followed by bed rest using a hot water bottle.

One Week Later

Our second consultation: Fred had lost 14 pounds. Said he felt MUCH better and was definitely more relaxed. The chief difficulty during the previous week had been the expelling of gas. A discussion on fermentation and putrefaction followed and Fred was advised of the pressures caused by such gas production on various organs including the prostate gland, the heart, etc. He was advising that poor posture can add to this discomfort. The study book on the colon was gone over with the client. A chart of "Good Things to Eat" was reviewed, as well as informative charts about the colon, the digestive system; list of flexibility exercises was provided with several being pointed out as being advisable in Fred's case. Face and neck exercises were demonstrated. A new dietary program was suggested, as follows:

1. Meal One—Fruit—A single variety.
2. Meal Two—Salad plus vegetable soup.
3. Meal Three—Salad plus:
4. Lamb or chicken, OR
5. Ricotta cheese, OR
6. Baked or steamed potato

Fred was now to eliminate salt, pepper, and all beverages except distilled water. Since he had never used any of these to any great extent, we all felt he could make this part of his transition rapidly.

Once his future course of action was agreed upon, we have a brief discussion on the Seven Steps in the Evolution of Pathology and Fred left with his next study book which uses the condition of arthritis as a means of illustrating this biological evolutionary process.

Second Week

Fred returned for his third consultation the following week. The student will observe that only one week was given between consultations with this client. This was felt best since, being alone, he required encouragement to keep him on course.

He was asked how he had managed. Response: Fred was well pleased and felt much improved. On his new diet, he had experienced much less gas and very little discomfort. Additionally, he was now sleeping well, being required to get up only once each night. (Previously, he had gotten up to urinate as often as five or six times every night.) He was delighted with his progress. Fred had eliminated most of his vitamins and other supplements on his own.

The origin of pathology was reviewed and the seven steps in its development. This time, the various symptoms indicative of each stage in this evolutionary process were depicted using the blackboard. We suggested that our PLAN was to reverse this process of toxemia buildup and thus prevent further damage. We pointed out to Fred that his present condition was the result of 77 years of systemic mismanagement and that it would take time to have the level of health he desired. In the first study book Fred learned what errors may have led to the development of the colitis condition which had been diagnosed some years previously. He actually was able to cite many of his former errors. These same errors, as time went on, had perhaps led to benign growths that had also been diagnosed and to the proctatitis condition.

In the second book and through our discussions, he saw revealed, for the first time, the evolutionary nature of body damaging and recalled many of the symptoms experienced in his own life that had been characteristic of the seven stages. Now, he was ready for his third study book, this one to present the four categories of causes of toxicosis. By this time, Fred could hardly wait to get on with his studies because he was naturally of an inquisitive mind. We contrasted for Fred the high cost of using apheresis to cleanse the blood with the Hygienic way, the former costing as much as and perhaps even more than

$32,000.00 for a series of "treatments;" the latter, the Hygienic way, simply adherence to principles and practices ordained by human design. We pointed out to Fred that the Hygienic way is self-help, working with biologically-sound principles, while the other represents a purely mechanical cleansing which is hit-or-miss at best, and one that carries no guarantee. We emphasized that the Hygienic self-help plan not only cleanses the body fluids but also removes the cause(s) of impairment while apheresis is, at best, only a temporary expediency, a refined type of bloodletting, a technique long ago discarded as debilitating and useless, since cause remains behind to make future trouble.

Over fifty years ago animal experimentation showed that the blood of animals could be removed, cleansed, and then be replaced. This was all well and good, of course, but it was soon learned that, in a very short time, the blood returned to the exact same condition it had been in before the cleansing procedure!

Why did this reversal occur? Simply because the tissues had not been changed, the organs remained as they were, and functioning efficiency of cells remained unchanged. Cause, you see, had not been removed—It seems obvious, does it not, that apheresis will be similarly ineffective long-term as a means of restoring health and for the very same reason: cause remains. Only natural methods have any chance to restore.

The Fourth Consultation

Another week had passed. Fred was immediately asked what he had done to assist his body's cleansing efforts. He said that he had been gaining considerable insight into what had brought about his present condition. He had reviewed all his studies and now, having read this newest lesson, he understood many of the things he himself had done, and had failed to do, which had led to his being so uncomfortable. He felt that overnutrition; overstimulation through the use of coffee, salt, sugar and meat; the emotional stresses of his wife's long illness and her subsequent death; the financial worries during this long period; and, finally, his self-imposed social isolation and subsequent loneliness—all had contributed to his "downfall."

He reported that, being a good religious man and at our suggestion, he had attended church during the last week, something he had not done for some time. We encouraged him to continue to do so and also to attend weekly meetings at church and to go to some of the community's programs for older citizens. In other words, we encouraged him to socialize. We also invited him to another of our "parties."

On examination, we say that Fred's tongue was a nice pink. He said his stomach felt like a new stomach. He thought he could begin his exercise program in earnest now, so we provided him with a series of exercises we thought suitable for his present capacity and encouraged him to walk every day. He promised to do so.

We then reviewed all past lessons and told him that, since he had done well, he was ready now to learn about proper food combining. For the next two weeks he was to read and study about how to formulate his meals correctly and to practice doing so. We requested him to keep a record of his own meals and to bring this to his next appointment, at which time we would all go over them together to see how well he had done. We supplied him with a copy of The Tree of Life, and a Food Combining Chart, this last to hang in his kitchen as a guide to meal-planning.

What Was Accomplished in These Four Weeks?

1. Fred became convinced that his former visits to various other practitioners, and there were many, had all been in vain.

2. Fred learned that healing was residual within the body and could not be put into the body from some outside source or by "treatments."

3. He learned that health comes only as the fruit of healthful living.

4. Fred resolved to learn how to live so that he could enjoy a higher level of health.

5. Fred learned about the colon and its purpose in the body.

6. He learned about how toxemia affects all cells of the body, and eventually damages organs and tissues. He has stopped taking pills.

7. He learned the seven steps in the evolution of pathology and characteristic symptoms of each.

8. He learned about the four categories of toxemia and related them to his own life experience.

9. He found that his body responded favorably as he put his new knowledge to work in the marketplace—in his own body—and he was pleased with the results.

10. He became imbued with enthusiasm to continue his studies, to learn more, so that he could become even better physically, mentally, and spiritually.

11. Fred made the initial transition quite successfully.

12. He is looking forward to his next consultation because we have told him that, at that time, he will learn how well he has done with his own food combining and then will learn about the six steps he must take to perfection.

13. Finally, his blood pressure, which was, on first visit, hovering around the 200 mark, is now reading 120 over 78. Fred is ecstatic.

92.4.1. Symptomizing

Symptomizing, of course, often causes new Hygienists to "snap back." Consequently, they fail to find themselves. It is vital, therefore, for new clients to understand that the continuance of life actually depends on this gift of life: the body's ability to channel a toxic overload to various accessory exit points whenever a toxic overload presents an emergency situation, one that is life threatening.

The symptoms that arise, whatever they may turn out to be (and each individual will respond with his own peculiar symptoms which may be either severe or light, or even somewhere in between, depending on many variables; and may even be nonexistent in some cases) can reveal much about the client. The greater the amount of residual vital force, the more violent the symptoms are likely to be. As the individual grows older and his vital force has been wasted to a considerable extent, the healing symptoms may be quite mild, if at all. This is, of course, why chronicity becomes established. As the individual lives his years wasting his vital force needlessly because of a destructive manner of living, the horrendous specter of chronicity makes its entrance when the power has been so reduced that health-saving symptoms are no longer possible. Thus, diseases of late years tend to become progressively more intensive and extensive, symptomizing more emotionally trying.

However, when clients adopt a more Hygienic way of living, they have the opportunity, with the help of the practitioner, to establish in their minds that, from this point on, health-building will become their business. If they can do this, they will develop a belief in themselves, in their ability to create their own lives and to create them in the very best image of themselves. Belief in oneself can be equated with success. Clients who believe in their bodies' inner power to heal will be more inclined to begin the business of health-building and will recognize each symptom experienced as a success story, a confirmation of their own creative abilities. It will help them to give consistency of effort and bring their efforts to a successful conclusion. Confidence in self, in the Hygienic program, in the practitioner, will all help to keep hesitant clients on course and make the transition a successful one.

Developing an understanding of the possibilities involved in the transitional process can often rapidly metamorphose students' thinking and cause them to become very enthusiastic about their own possibilities. How far can they go? Could it be that they could become like "him or her, or them"? Even practitioners sometimes have to remind themselves that, with full acceptance of responsibility for oneself, an amazing amount of recovery awaits their clients' best efforts. We must remember, too, and tell our clients that symptomizing means that the business of health-building is being successfully pursued.

92.4.2. Levels of Tolerance

Clients will, of course, have developed their own levels of tolerance. They should, in our view, learn something about this concept early in the transition. It will help them better to understand this matter of symptomizing. We provide study materials about how the constant introduction of poisons into the body from external sources or by the generation of excessive amounts of metabolic poisons within the system itself through life's errors, can not only damage cells, tissues, and organs, but can actually lead to an increase in the systemic toleration to 1. individual specific poisons and/or 2. to poisons in general.

Of course, the client should be led to an understanding that there is an unfortunate result of such increased toleration: the body constantly functions under a handicap and thus wastes the vital force. The higher the level of toxic toleration, the greater the wasting effect.

Rapid wasting naturally leads to such disorders as, for 'example, Alzheimer's disease, organic brain syndrome, and many others generally, but incorrectly, associated with the aging process.

92.4.3. The Evolution of Pathology

I. TOXICOSIS	Cellular constipation starts to build.
II. ENERVATION	General Feeling of malaise, of not being "up to par." Cellular functioning ability decreases.
	Person may feel irritable, nervous, anxious, depressed without sufficient cause, etc.

III. IRRITATION	Sensation of pain. May come and go in predisposed areas, of varying intensity.
	Previous symptoms, if evidenced, tend to worsen. Constipation
	Occasional diarrhea Headache
	Dry cough
	Itching, pimples, mild rashes, etc.
IV. INFLAMMATION	Fever, redness. Runny, red nose.
	Some swelling and mucus formation. Previous symptoms tend to worsen.
	All "itis" diseases, named according to location.
V. ULCERATION	Hardening of tissues, stiffening of movement. Walling off of lesions; benign tumors form. Scar tissue.
	Sclerosis.
	Advanced degeneration of organs, especially of liver and kidneys.
	Onset of senility, abnormal behavior patterns.
VII. FUNGATION	Cellular replication out of control: true cancer.
	In early stages: organ failure, especially of the heart, kidneys, liver. Tuberculosis
	Gland malfunctioning—breakdown of hormonal system, especially the hypothalamus and pituitary.

92.5. Decision-Making Time

92.5.1. The Power of the Past

92.5.2. What's Wrong with Medical Science

92.5.1. The Power of the Past

Certainly, the client's present condition should have made him fully aware of the power of the past. His past errors have produced his present. The life script of the past is gone, it cannot be relived. He has an opportunity now to create a new life script. He must not permit himself to resist becoming the best he can be in favor of the past. Unfortunately, it would appear that far too many humans feel they don't deserve being the best they can be. They tend to hold back, to retain the past, until they simply get "fed up" with the present.

However, it is decision-making time for the clients. The diagrams hopefully will make them appreciate the fact that, as human beings, they can change. The knowledgeable practitioner can help make clients fully aware of the fact that, as human beings, they can put an end to their former destructive manner of living which produced negative degeneration and a poor quality of life, and create, instead, positive regeneration of mind, body, and soul: the "I CAN" philosophy.

Clients must ask themselves these questions: Why am I here? What am I doing to change? Where do I want to go? How would I like to look and feel? Is health REALLY important to me? How important? Can I make the required changes? WILL I? Will I desert the herd, the past, in favor of a more promising future? In their answers lie the success of both the clients and the practitioner.

92.5.2. What's Wrong with Medical Science

But there may remain one question that may arise in a practitioner's initial dealings with clients, and it must sometimes be addressed, that question being, "What's wrong with medical science?" The answer, of course, to this question, which is so puzzling to many clients, has been given by many writers and can best be summarized, we feel, as follows: Namely, that medical science is wrong because it is always changing!

Truth never has cause to change because truth is always truth, in any age and in all circumstances. We can never depart from truth and remain truly scientific.

The ability of the human body to heal is always there so long as life remains. That doesn't change! The replication of cells goes on and on and on, generation after generation, so long as life power exists. That doesn't change! It may become a more feeble effort, but it is there. The body secretes the same secretions, in the same way, and for the same purposes, each possessing its own specificity. That doesn't change! All things, forces, actions which are characteristic of life remain. The only changes which take place are in the wasting of body power through erroneous behavior and the subsequent wasting of cellular functioning capability, and thus, too, of organs and systems.

It is never pleasant for any person to hear that he has been worshipping at the feet of a false god. We had a consultation at one time with a man whom we'll call Albert. We had just covered much of the information discussed thus far in this lesson. Albert listened attentively as he learned how it is often possible to retrace the downward path and restore a higher level of health. His face soon began to reveal deep frustration and anger. He commented, "What a fool I've been! I have wasted not only my health but also my wealth in pursuit of a mirage. Just a month ago, I attended a lecture, and the lecturer offered a panacea for all my ills. I fell for his line, and it cost me well over a hundred dollars. I have done this countless times, and for what? For a lie! Now I can see that I have played a leading role in a total farce!"

To cite another case. Morrie weighed over 300 pounds and suffered from arthritic pains. He recounted how he had consulted a total of 26 medical doctors over the past years and had found no relief. To the contrary, he has seen his pains worsen, the swellings grow larger and become harder, his muscles stiffen. His last physician had referred him to a specialist in rheumatic troubles. This consultation had been "the last straw" for Morrie. It had lasted a total of 15 minutes. His bill had been $60.00. His advice? "Take aspirin whenever you feel the pain."

Morrie had been taking aspirin for years! Completely baffled and disillusioned, confused, and desperate, Morrie was a prime target for some medical "quack" to take him on. Fortunately, he came to us. It was now our immediate task, as it will be for all practicing Hygienists, to make real the body's ways: of the healing inner power, of the body's awesome wisdom to manage the healing effort, to bring it to a successful conclusion. If this is not done, the transition road may well prove to be difficult because a mind clouded by its past shadows will remain filled with doubts, even fear. It behooves all practitioners to "set the stage" as near perfectly as possible. In so doing, they help their clients to make a successful transition from the past into better living.

To be successful, we have to motivate if we expect clients to change. Otherwise, they tend to invest their energies (vital force) in staying where they are rather than making those changes all humans must make if they desire success. An established faith must be cultivated before hope of progress can become a realized fact. Clients must be encouraged to invest their vital force now in building a better life rather than in staying as they now are; if not indeed, becoming increasingly worse. Life is such that each one of us has this choice: to remain a prisoner of our past errors or to get on with the business of living into a better life, perhaps one that will be even better than we might ever hope to enjoy. Thus, during the first phase of client's transitional journey, we must set the stage. We introduce to our clients some new thoughts, new ideas new concepts, a new faith, and new hopes. In other words, we introduce Natural Hygiene!

92.6. The Six Steps to Perfection

92.1. The Problem

92.2. The Plan the Client Reports the Story of Bess

92.3. Priority

92.4. Performance Rubber-Banding

92.5. Patience

92.6. Perseverance

92.1. The Problem

The client must now begin his personal transition to better living. The first step entails a clear recognition by him and the practitioner of the PROBLEM, its extent, and its intensiveness. Various tools are pertinent here: the medical history, the diet profile, conversational give and take.

The client must realize that acknowledging the problem and/or the vulnerability to a particular condition is the first step to solving it and that, whatever this may be, it is capable of solution through the systematic application of proven Hygienic (truthful) practices and principles, all the concepts gained in this Life Science course. We must reach the subconscious mind and establish a BELIEF, perhaps not complete at this early stage, but beginning to emerge, the belief that, "YES! I CAN DO IT! I can make this transition!" The Master Plan Chart which follows can be used to good advantage as an explanatory tool.

92.2. The Plan

The second "P" toward Perfection is the formulation of the client's personal PLAN OF ACTION. In order to formulate such a plan, the practitioner working with the client's cooperation must first examine the four categories of possible causes of illness (Poison Habits, Deficiencies in eating and living, Excesses in eating and living, and Emotional Causes) and then ferret out those considered most responsible for the client's present impairment. The Master Plan can prove useful here.

For example, clients will see that exercise is an organic requisite, part of the MASTER PLAN OF LIFE. If clients have heretofore lived rather sedentary lives, they will more readily accept the fact that now, if they desire to live better, in the full meaning of that term, then they MUST exercise. As part of their plan, a suitable exercise program should be included, this being one of their first "baby steps" to Perfection.

The Diet Profile must be studied and changes in the dietary regimen made as may be indicated. Each organic requisite in the Master Plan can be considered in turn until the client's own PLAN is complete.

As we were writing this section, the gentleman whom we met early in this lesson, Fred, telephoned. He is eating and enjoying his meals and, what is more, he is sleeping throughout the entire night now, something he has not been able to do since his wife's death. Additionally, the terrible gas pains that seemed to grab at his heart are completely gone. He confessed that he had been gripped by a fear that he, too, would die of cancer and, remembering his wife's years of torture, he had, at one time, even contemplated suicide. He called because he wanted his next appointment to be scheduled earlier, if possible. Fred is now in a hurry. He sees perfection now as a real possibility! And for him, too!

Clients must be brought to realize that they can no longer live in the "World of If." IF I had only eaten correctly! IF I had kept up with my tennis. IF I had only rested more and partied less! IF only I had accepted the responsibilities of being human. IF only I had not eaten all those horrible foodless junk foods! The World of IF must be laid aside. It is time to weed out all the causes of ill health, one by one, perhaps; or even all at once if that is so indicated.

Specific errors in lifestyle will be revealed by the client from time to time as confidence in the practitioner, and in Hygienic practices and philosophy, grows. Each should be addressed at the time.

The most difficult of all poison habits to identify are, without a doubt, those of emotional origin. The importance of the psyche upon physical wellness is also one of the most difficult to bring to the conscious attention of the client. Clients hesitate generally to advance to public view their private fears and to weigh the deadly effects of such imprinting.

Joan provides us an excellent example of how one client coped with a devastating emotional web of fears and sorrow. In her late 60s, Joan was a widow. She had recently buried her husband, a victim of cancer. She went through some of the early steps of transition hesitatingly because she had mental reservations. We had been working with her for well over a year before we found out that she harbored deep fears about her future. Alone, without close family ties, she wondered about her economic well-being, her health future, about her ending up her days in a nursing home like so many of her peers, or even perhaps in the agony of terror she had witnessed in her husband's last days. Fears and sorrow pervaded her very soul and limited her progress.

We encouraged this woman to join a bereavement group. There she found companionship. As she grew in health, she began to make plans. She sold her home, the upkeep of which cost her heavily, and subsequently moved into an apartment complex where she was constantly with people of all age groups, particularly at the little recreation center maintained by the owners. She began slowly to put her fears aside and the first thing we knew Joan was laughing again. And, as her joy in living increased, so did her wellness. Joan now looks for solutions, instead of suffering defeats.

Most of us have been brainwashed in the past and by current medical teachings to separate the cerebral centers from the rest of the body. In reality, however, this cannot be done, for our cerebral centers consist not only of isolated nervous matter but also of fluids which bathe the cells. By virtue of human design, these fluids have their composition regulated by the blood serum which, in turn, contains all the secretion emanating from all the cells of all the glands and tissues, these permeating and diffusing throughout the entire body.

Every organ contributes to the chemistry of the brain, as does every cell; and the brain imprinted thusly sends out its constant messages. There is not a square centimeter within the entire community of body cells that will not be imprinted by the distress of cerebral cells exhausted by emotional upheavals or by toxins contained in the fluids which sustain them.

An ever-present fear of what the future may bring can cause that future to materialize and become the present. Worry can impair and even paralyze the digestive organs. So it is, that hidden fears must be found and the client led into a deeper understanding of the importance of mind control. Positive action must replace the "If s" and concerns of the past.

The client and the practitioner both must comprehend that there is no such thing as suspended forward motion. For health to happen, we must change into health. This is why formulating a workable PLAN—one deemed so by clients themselves—is essential to future progress. If clients are ever to break the toxemia connection and begin a transition into better living, they must identify and recognize their problems, develop an understanding of possible causes of their problems, and then, with the practitioner's help and guidance, develop a sound, workable plan to solve the problems.

The practitioner must further impart to the client the concept that NOW is the time for him/her to take control of his/her own life, to learn intelligent self-management, this to be based on sound physiologically-, biologically-, and anatomically-proven facts; that s/he can no longer afford to base wellness on demographic ally-controlled news releases, or on medical therapeutics which have failed in the past. S/he must now learn to manage the body and mind intelligently according to the capabilities and limitations established by personal design.

All the familiar patterns of self-abuse must be penetrated, identified, and corrected. This is why the PLAN can never be static. It must be subject to on-going change and modified from time to time to meet all specific needs as best they can be determined. It should be made quite clear that if the clients manage themselves well and supply adequately the needs of life (the Master Plan) they will begin to enjoy an ever-higher level of health. I they do not, of a certainty, the converse will rear its ugly head.

The Client Reports

Upon introduction of the initial changes, we ask the client to report back in seven days or, at least, within two weeks. S/he is encouraged to respond to such questions as: How did the stomach react to the dietary changes? Was the client able to sleep better?

How many pounds were lost, if any? We encourage and note all positive responses. These serve to inspire both the client and the practitioner!

The holidays are always difficult times for newcomers to Natural Hygiene. Last Christmas we hosted a Christmas day party. We all enjoyed a Hygienic meal and the fellowship. No one missed the health-destroying practices so prevalent at this time of the year and it is interesting to report that few of our guests suffered from spring cold and not a one "enjoyed" having the flu. We will repeat this kind of party from time to time.

Unfortunately, some clients may meet with resistance from family members or from their peers, and so may begin to falter. It is essential for such as these to "psych" themselves into following their plan exactly. They must learn not to feel guilty about not eating or acting exactly as the other members of the family do, or as the masses. They can be helped over these difficult times by teaching them to reaffirm, over and over again, if need be, both silently and aloud, "I NEED to become healthier than I am. I NEED to eat this way. I MUST eat this way. I WANT to live better and the ONLY way I can enjoy life is to DO WHAT I MUST DO. Therefore, I WILL DO IT! PERIOD!"

Clients must reach, early on, an understanding that everything they may now hope to become depends on how well they meet their basic nutritive needs now. Students of this course have much knowledge to impart to those who seek their counsel. They know how to set up eating formats, about food quality, where to go to purchase organically-grown foods. They know which foods are best adapted to humans by virtue of their structural design and biological requirements. This must be imparted to the clients, else they will forever be dependent on other; Included in the PLAN must always be specific instruction on the subjects of air and water quality, the amount of food to be eaten at any one meal or throughout the day, as well as information on how and when to eat. There is much for clients to learn and so little time to share all the knowledge.

The time of transition is a learning experience. It is period that requires much change, both in thought and practice. Clients must learn the practices, the foods, the substances, and forces that are anti-vital, destructive of body cells, of the life force. They must also learn how best to manage themselves into a new and better dimension of life. Ideally, it will progress from the simple initial physiological, physical, and sensory, almost resting, phase to the first strange ways of assembling and eating foods; and then the coupling together of a host of helpful changes in the total lifestyle. At the conclusion of the transition, ideally, there should be full acceptance by the client of the Hygienic manner of eating and living, this having been encouraged by the positive results obtained.

The Story of Bess

The PROBLEM possessed by any one individual can be present in actuality, it can be of the here and now; as, for example, a painful arthritic condition; or it can exist in a VULNERABILITY, a predisposition by virtue of an inherited systemic weakness to some condition, either known or unknown. Erroneous cultural habits often lie at the root of such problems of "vulnerability." We inherit the cultural errors of our childhood teachers; not, in actuality, the tendency to a disease!

Bess, age 34, presents a classic example of the latter. When she first consulted us, she was beginning to experience some shaking in her hands which, under stress, became quite annoying. She recalled that her mother, toward the end of her days, had suffered from Parkinson's disease, the "shaking" sickness. Bess was terrified.

We worked out a plan for Bess which was new and strange to her, but she followed it successfully for about six months. The shakiness disappeared, even when she found herself under stress. So, Bess became somewhat careless about working her plan and being single, she began to go out with the girls now and then for a pizza, and then more and more frequently. She failed to keep an appointment, so we dismissed her from our client list.

After about a year, a penitent Bess was back in the fold, this time perhaps even more frightened than before. The shakiness had returned, so much so that she was no longer able to meet adequately the demands of her very responsible position. Her "vulnerability" had finally penetrated Bess' conscious mind. She knew now, with a far deeper understanding, that she was vulnerable in that her nervous system could not withstand the careless assaults she had been making upon it. All doubt about the need for her to live Hygienically was removed. She knew with a certainty that, from now on, she would have to invest in herself. She decided that she wanted to "let all of life in" and would invest her all in making this new life. This time she decided to take the important THIRD STEP toward Perfection.

92.3. Priority

Yes! Bess decided to make the attainment of superb health her FIRST PRIORITY. This is what psychologists refer to as "GETTING TO THE YES POINT." After reaping a sick harvest from following the ways of the masses, Bess found herself haunted by the sick shadows that walked beside her, ghosts of the past. Thus, it was that reality brought her to the YES point. The attainment of superb health, by necessity, became her FIRST PRIORITY.

Previous to this point, of course, Bess had passed through a series of emotional storms wherein she resented the demands of her own Self. Thus, for a time, as many clients try to do, she attempted to fantasize herself into a higher state of wellness and so took the detour which led to many emotional, physical, and mental skirmishes which put her back in touch with the realities of organic existence. She found that, like all humans, she was subject to organic laws. She had become submerged and actually enmeshed by FEELINGS instead of in touch with her real self. The results of her fantasizing feelings, instead of keeping in touch with her real self, and her completely unrealistic expectations, finally caused her to become aware, probably for the first time in her 34 years, of the systemic needs of self. This period of storm and uncertainty is often called the period of "Low Think." Bess survived it and has since adapted fairly well to her new way of life.

Clients can be helped to pass through the period of "Low Think," and then on to the establishment of superior health as their personal FIRST PRIORITY once they begin to see their own small successes as they follow a series of planned sequences. Printed, well-chosen study materials often can help a client to reach the extremely important understanding that the Hygienist has a larger view of nutrition than the simplistic views espoused by most dietitians and medicos. To the Hygienist, nutrition is not only a mechanical-chemical process vital to life, but also one that is intimately personal, involving, as is always true, emotional, cultural, and psychological factors, mores, etc. To the Hygienist, nutrition includes everything that happens to food once it is introduced into the mouth: mastication, digestion, absorption, transportation, assimilation and, finally, elimination; and all the factors, influences and substances that can affect each or the whole. The Hygienist and the client must comprehend all these manifold aspects of the nutrition scene and also that all must be made as nearly perfect as possible, if full health is ever to be achieved.

If the clients decide that they now wish to break the toxemia connection and remove their burdensome toxic overloads, they must give active consideration to this most important aspect of self-management and follow through with intelligent implementation.

The transition period is, first and foremost, a learning experience of major proportions, one contrary, in most instances, to all previous training. It includes necessarily the development of an understanding that the client's previous heterogeneous manner of eating, drinking, and living created systemic frenzy and failed to meet systemic needs. The client must learn that food is used by his/her body solely for replacement purposes. Additionally, s/he must acquire the knowledge that certain common practices, foods, substances, and forces are anti-vital, and actually destructive of body cells and the life force. It must also include discovering how best to manage himself, often against considerable societal and personal odds, into a new and better dimension of life. Ideally, it will progress from the initial physiological, physical, and sensory simple changes to the full acceptance of the Hygienic way of life. The practitioner should not forget that this is no mean feat!

But it is this experience which can finally put clients back in touch with themselves. They begin to love themselves so much that they no longer have any doubt that the attainment and maintenance of full health must become and remain their FIRST PRIORITY because upon their doing so, all else depends. This is when the client begins to reach an understanding of the practical value of expectations based on organic reality instead of on myths which lack life substance. This is when clients begin to take hold of conviction, and establish as their main purpose in life, the need to build as high a standard of wellness for themselves as it is possible for them to achieve. They will do this not only for themselves but also for the benefit of those they may happen to love and for society at large. Once the windows of the mind have been opened up, the clients can then enter into a new and hitherto untraveled dimension of their lives, one filled with undreamed of opportunities.

92.4. Performance

The clients have their problems. With the practitioner's help, they have devised a plan. After a certain amount of accommodation and soul-searching, they have decided that they love themselves enough to make health-building the First Priority. Now they must work the plan, they must PERFORM.

As practicing Hygienists, we cannot accompany our clients home and supervise their performance. THEY must work their own plan.

Once the plan is instigated and in force, with the needs of the body now being adequately met, the cerebral powers begin to take a new direction according to the following organic law:

"When the quality of the food coming into the body is of higher quality than the tissues of which the body is made, the body immediately begins to discard all lower grade cells and tissues which are then recycled. All usable materials are incorporated along with the incoming top-grade nutrients and used to formulate and construct new and healthier tissues, this being accomplished in an ongoing, biological evolutionary process with each generation of cells being healthier than the preceding generation."

The client, for this reason and according to this law, must expect certain salubrious changes to become operational because his/her own body intelligence will, by due process, recognize immediately that certain improvements, both in lifestyle and in eating, are now forthcoming. Curative, health-building changes will begin, which may prove disconcerting at times. It is at such times that the client necessarily becomes acquainted with the power of the only healing ability s/he has, a healing force resident wholly within. S/he has it ALL! And it is a powerful force that will always guide in the direction of perfection so long the Plan is followed. Having a workable plan and working the plan—PERSONAL PERFORMANCE—will inspire the required constructive INNER PERFORMANCE. Personal performance brings positive inner performance and its twin, Positive progress, not only physically, but also mentally and spiritually.

The client soon realizes that nature's efforts, unlike the drug response, are not due to simple chemical actions and reactions, but are, rather, vital changes, changes which have been designed with exactitude by the body's own intelligence to correct that which was incorrect, and that all such will be brought to a successful conclusion, in due course and as may be required, by cell destruction (catabolism) followed by cell multiplication (replication and cell formulation (anabolism). The quality of the performance will, as a certainty, determine the quality of the correcting vital work—and all will be under direction of the sympathetic nervous system.

To state our thesis simply, the client must discover to best to manage self (the Plan), reach the grand decision the First Priority; and then perform in order to realize this potential that lies sleeping within. Perfection awaits the willing performer and, in the performing, lies a world filled with creative processes intended to write a new life script one which increasingly witnesses the fulfillment of potential. All that is required of the client is that s/he bear faithful witness to organic authority.

Rubber-Banding

But being a faithful witness to organic authority is sometimes difficult for some clients. Often newcomers to Natural Hygiene have a tendency to revert, to go back to the old, palate-pleasing foods and their tantalizing former lifestyles, even though they may comprehend, at least at the surface of their minds, that these incorrect foods and habits are the very same ones that damaged them.

This very common tendency of people to revert to the more familiar past is called by some psychologists "RUBBER-BANDING," a snapping back into old habits that please instead of following new directions that challenge and even, at times, become painful. Adaptation and accommodation are required, both mentally and physically, if such snapping back is to be simply a momentary happening.

The practitioner should help clients to recognize the cause of this rubber-banding: receiving false instruction, which come either from a damaged body and mind OR from habitual happenings of the past, many of which were written in childhood memories and are illustrative of the child mind. As health-seekers, clients must now enter into their own new worlds, in which they will constantly receive new instructions of a much higher value instructions programmed by an awesome inner wisdom each designed to transport them into an ever-growing wellness of being.

Clients will make an easier transition if they accept the fact that they are not being deprived of something desirable but, rather, are being offered a splendid opportunity for ENRICHMENT! Once this awareness takes over, they are usually ready to adopt the new pattern for living and begin, too, to set forth their own goals, small reachable goals at first. The wise practitioner permits these easily attainable goals and then goes on to encourage clients to take the necessary baby steps to reach Goal Number One. At that point, rubber-banding can often be avoided, if a period of adjustment taking a varying amount of time according to individual differences if allowed. This permits a time for body balancing.

When full accommodation has been reached, then Goal Number Two becomes a new challenge. This procedure is then followed until the desired level of wellness the achieved reality; the challenge has been met.

Such helpful guidance encourages clients because the) experience a rewarding pattern rather than feeling they are being deprived of something of value. In this way, the client is helped to assume the: "I AM IN CONTROL!" position instead of being locked in the "Low Think" jail of past imperfection and failure.

92.5. Patience

In working his/her plan, the client may not always progress in a straight line; indeed, few will. Many clients become beset with societal concerns that can have severe emotional impact. For example, clients may become worried that other people won't like them, that they may consider them "odd," or "different" from themselves.

Let us share a part of a letter we received just this morning from a young man who is beset with just this kind of emotional concern. A salesman, handsome, talented, witty, a man of many talents, had the early signs of rheumatoid arthritis. He was in considerable pain.

This young man, let's call him Kurt, began his program in a suicidal frame of mind. Because of his youth and willingness to perform, he made rapid progress and soon forgot about his former aches and pains. In their place, however, came a new worry, "I am getting too thin! I look like a skeleton," he complained. So, he reverted, at least partially, to his past. He became a rubber-band.

In his letter he dismisses us saying, "You have been a great help and inspiration in my life. I am not a true vegetarian. It didn't agree with me or my hectic lifestyle. (He has failed to understand that it may well have been his hectic lifestyle that led to his rheumatic ailment.) I just became too thin, felt weak and started feeling upset. Therefore, I have compromised. No hamburgers, steak, chops, etc. I just eat lots of chicken, fruit, vegetables, but still love mashed potatoes, etc. God bless you." and he signs his name.

This young man will return to Natural Hygiene. How do we know? Because his symptoms will return! As Dr. Shelton so well said, "We cannot disobey the laws of life with impunity."

We must encourage our clients to have the PATIENCE to let their bodies fully accomplish the necessary work. Otherwise, they fail and perhaps we ourselves fail to some extent. But, if we do our best, then, of course, we must learn to "let go." New

Hygienists have a choice: to endure a hurting body, or to be content to let other people "do their own thing," to go their own way while they live into a new and higher level of health such that these others will never be privileged to experience.

Novices in the science of life must develop conviction of the correctness of their plan. This, of course, will come only as the fruit of knowledge, knowledge about themselves and how they fit in with the life process. They must get into life and realize just how important life really is, that it is worth their very best efforts. To make this adjustment can be difficult because all of us are so bombarded by herd mania, but patience will make it happen.

Knowledge can help to build a kind of security system around clients, one that will serve to protect them from outside negative comments, thoughts, and forces. A security system based on knowledge coupled with a sense of the worthiness of self will often survive throughout the transition to perfection. Clients must not close the door of their mind to truth but rather they should learn to open it to organic reality.

Kurt, unfortunately perhaps, made too much progress and made it too rapidly, within a very few weeks. His pains left too quickly! He is now thinking, not about his future, but rather about all the pretty young girls he would like to date. We must expect this behavior, from time to time. Those who lack intelligence or who, like Kurt, possess false standards, may not complete their on-going journey toward perfection. They lack patience.

But the vast majority will! They will come into a full realization that the body will do its own metabolic balancing, that it will somehow and in some manner discard all that needs to be discarded: all the putrid, messy, decaying filth that accumulated in the days before self-became important. Kurt mistakenly believes he now has Perfection! Instead, he has been inspired by FIRST IMPROVEMENT to become a rubber-band. His lack of patience will prevent his reaching, at least for now, the ultimate goal of euphoric wellness.

Elderly persons can better appreciate the fact that they must get control of their mind and of themselves. They must have a full measure of patience, sufficient to get on with the involved work of health building.

We must do our best to teach clients to flow with the certainty of the life process, with conviction that there is no other way to have their desire, that perfectly functioning and peaceful body. We must exert our best efforts to develop the understanding that every mistake, every error, will leave a lasting imprint, that it will damage the body. Our clients must be led to appreciate the fact that, upon the patience they now manifest, will depend the quality of all their future life.

Learning about Natural Hygiene means learning about cooperation: all persons with themselves, and themselves and all others. We must do our best to teach our clients to look at life, to anticipate life, knowing that a full, enriched life will surely come to them, if they but have the necessary patience and will to let it happen.

92.6. Perseverance

The twin of patience is, of course, PERSEVERANCE. We humans can't put ourselves on "hold." We can't say "maybe" or "perhaps," or "next week." The body never remains in a static position. It will move either forward or backwards depending on whether or not we answer systemic needs, these varying from individual to individual.

As the energy level rises, or falls, this movement, whatever the direction, will begin to accelerate. So, once we embark on this transition to better living, we must persevere in the doing, knowing that our plan, our performance, our patience, and our perseverance will reward us with gifts, enormous dividends, if you will; to name but a few, in the form of:

1. Improved health and peace of body and mind.

2. Economic dividends of immeasurable value.

3. Internal cleansing to set free formerly wasted reserves of vitality, these providing an enlarged capacity to live always in health.

4. Reduction or total elimination of internal handicaps that restrain and limit functional excellence.

5. Provide new spiritual insight into life's meaning and one's purpose for living; a statement of "Why was I born? Why was I chosen to receive this precious gift of life?"

6. Remove our former dependence on manmade pseudo foods, drugs, potions, and all false stimulants.

7. Provide us with a new beginning, a new dimension of life that can be exciting, provocative, promising and immensely rewarding both to ourselves and to others.

8. Establish a permanent euphoric joy in living.

9. Provide a worthy example to others of what living Hygienically might possibly accomplish in the lives of those we meet as we travel our own life course.

10. A rare opportunity, known to but few, to write our own challenging life script and this, too, regardless of our chronological or physiological age.

92.7. The Call and the Challenge

This then is both the call and the challenge of a transition into better living. Someone once said, "We do not 'ooze' into health, we choose it!" Each client must love him or herself so much that s/he chooses to follow the Six Ps to Perfection. S/he must come, by whatever means, to realize the authority of organic law and, being desirous of the whole of life, then choose to give far more than lip service to this authority and, instead, choose to live in accordance with it, and, even more important, to persevere no matter how long it may take to reach his/her own ultimate goal.

In other words, the client who will be successful makes the grand decision to desert the sickened herd and chooses, instead, the good rich life, the better life, of perfect health. Once this has been done, all that remains is for the client to focus seriously and deeply on this goal, always motivated by the good results that follow in the wake of intelligent performance.

Harry is a case in point. He had watched himself become a 50-year-old "baby," completely dependent upon others, a burden to his family and to himself. At our first meeting, his eyes were filled with terror.

Harry has been a Hygienist now for the better part of a year and has reached that point where he is fully confident that one day, he will no longer be dependent on others for his total care.

Harry has yet to fast a whole day but, undaunted, he says, "Don't worry, I'll make it. I'll do it!" And we are sure he will. This is the confidence required to reap the rewards of a successful transition. Harry is already looking forward to the day when he can, in person, attend one of our potlucks or other meetings and there tell his own wonderful story so that others may develop his deep sense of the rightness of the Hygienic way. Harry usually replies, "Do you think I can do that?" Our reply comes, "Why, Harry, of course you can do it!" And then a smiling Harry usually replies, "You know, I believe I really can!" The challenge has been accepted.

Someone once said, "Minds grow by reaching, not by resting." Our clients will surely make a successful transition when we help their minds to reach into the wonder that is life's scientific truth; when we impart to them the knowledge that life is never static, but rather always a dynamic play of forces; and that, by adhering to nature's gentle ways, they can participate in a positive dynamism that will, with certainty, fulfill all their dreams. Client and practitioner alike must honor the call and accept life's wondrous challenge. After all, we are all in the process of BECOMING, and what we will to become, that we will BECOME!

92.8. Questions & Answers

I know Natural Hygiene works. Remember how my blood pressure dropped from near 200 down to normal? Well, now it's back up there again. And I'm back on my medication again. I have it under control again and with the lowest dosage I've taken in many a year, but I just can't seem to stay on course. I'm all right until the evening hours. Then, what do you know, I'm at that popcorn and beer again. And, as you can see, I've gained over ten pounds since I was here last. What can I do?

Many beginning clients revert. We call this "rubber-banding." I would like to point out to you one very important fact that you have apparently overlooked. In spite of your momentary slipping back into a past bad habit, you tell me your medication level is now at its lowest point. That should tell you something. You have been successful! You have accomplished something you had been unable to do for years. You don't have to poison yourself. Your Hygienic program is working! Now, you must resolve to take the next step and develop mind control. When the popcorn calls, don't buy it! Take the dog out for a walk, or drink a glass of hot water, or start working on that crossword puzzle. Direct your mind forcibly into some other activity. Resolve, no matter what, to stay on course. Get to the point where you will no longer require that crutch, the popcorn, or any other crutch. You can do it. Don't permit yourself to snap back. You know, we usually get what we want out of life. If you want superb health and all that THAT can mean to you, then you will do whatever is required of you to obtain it, even giving up popcorn!

At one time in this lesson, you said something about the body doing its own metabolic balancing. What do you mean by that?

I am glad you asked that question. You see, there are practitioners at large who charge fantastic prices for their counseling. They claim to be able to balance the metabolic activity of their clients by juggling various kinds of mineral and other supplements. One woman we knew had just been released from the hospital after having suffered with pneumonia. Naturally, she felt weak and tired. She was lacking in strength. She got taken in tow by one of these juggling artists. She purchased (from him, of course) dozens of bottles of hormones and enzymes, of vitamins, various kinds of potassium and selenium pills; she took zinc and calcium tablets. In fact, she owned a veritable "health" food store! She was being metabolically "balanced."

After a time, she was filled with minerals, hormones, vitamins, and with a whole host of supplements. She became even weaker and totally confused. You see, in full health, our, body is never confused. In full health, we are metabolically balanced. We have within us suitable amounts of all nutrients, our cells take in the nutrients they require and give off their wastes which are dutifully rounded up, transported to the proper destination, and then promptly eliminated. In full health, a state of equilibrium—homeostasis—pertains. This is what the Hygienists mean by metabolic balancing. And, to set the record straight, there is no exact way to determine the precise needs of any human system at a particular moment in time. Our needs change with each nuance of life, with each nerve message transmission. No human mind can possibly prescribe human-formulated doses to meet this changing kaleidoscope of systemic needs. Only your body can do that. Once we begin our own transition into better living, that is exactly what begins to happen. The body begins to balance itself. And without outside interference, it will do a grand job.

My hangup is milk. I manage the fruit meals, but I've drunk milk for as long as I can remember. My father was a Physician and he used to bring home a whole gallon of milk for us two kids. Will it hurt me if this is my worst habit?

The childhood script can often prove to be the most demanding of all our life experiences. You see, your experiences and habits in childhood were reinforced by parental authority in which you had complete trust. However, you and I are now adults. We are each writing our current life script, travelling our own life course. We must excuse parental error. We now know that all milk, except breast milk in infancy, is a nonhuman food; that using it can lead to clogged arteries and damaged hearts, to arteriosclerosis and all manner of degenerative conditions. We must also accept the known fact that milk is an indigestible menace. To the extent that you drink it, you will be damaged. If you are willing to accept that damage, and you, of course, at this time have no knowledge of exactly what it might be, then you can go on drinking your milk, you can go on being a child again. You will have only yourself to blame for whatever the damage may prove to be. We sometimes call this kind of reverting, "killing softly!"

I recently went to a clinic and the medical staff there put me through the Cytotoxic Testing. It cost me almost $300.00 but they determined I had some 58 different food allergies. What on earth can I eat? They took me off wheat, office cream, off all meat except lamb. Golly! they've taken away just about everything good to eat. What is your advice?

My advice to you is to consult with an experienced Hygienic practitioner and begin your own transition to better living. In other words, it's time for you to place your body house in order! I guarantee you that if you follow the Life Science Road, you can soon forget all about your 58 allergies and, furthermore, you will begin to enjoy every

411

mouthful of food you bite into. What is more, you can forget about medical clinics and their personnel and—even more importantly—about their advice! Your allergies are evidence that your body is fighting desperately to protect you from all these so-called "good foods" you have been eating. My friend, I'm afraid you have been living in a fool's paradise. Remember what we said, "Life is never static." You are at a crossroads now. I hope you'll choose the Hygienic transition road to better living. It is a road that can be filled with accomplishments, with promises fulfilled.

My daughter is so obese that she was recently discharged from her job because she was so slow in her movements that she just couldn't keep up with her co-workers. She was watching her diet rather well, we thought, but when this happened, she defrosted a huge pizza, poured some canned hot sauce on it and now she is on a pizza and hot sauce binge and vomiting all the time. What can we do with this girl?

In the first place, it's time you stopped your parenting! Your daughter is approaching middle age, as it is commonly measured. It is high time for you to stop watching over your baby and enter into a new life, to take care of your Self. As for your daughter, the proper thing for her to do would be immediately to stop eating anything until her system settles down. In short, she should fast until the condition rights itself. I would advise her to go to a Hygienic retreat for an extended rest and fast. She would then look better, feel better, would have greater speed and flexibility; in short, she would be better prepared to manage her own life and to leave you free to do the things you need to do at the here and now in your own life course. In any event, permit your daughter to manage her own life and you get on with the business of managing yours.

Article #1: Supplementary Text Material by Guylaine R. Aragona

Recently we received an Answer Sheet, a final examination paper, from a student in New Hampshire, the wife of a chiropractic physician, who is also one of our students. Her comments are well worth our consideration at this juncture. Therefore, we have included them as supplementary reading.

Most individuals play and use their bodies carelessly, believing that the body is made to function on overuse and abuse. The people of this gender will be your McDonald's hamburger joint people; candy and potato chip, canned and ready-made, quick-to-prepare-food eaters, laced with every chemical under the sun. They are the ones that feel great, but cannot perform certain tasks, nor do they possess a normal range of motions with their bodies, only because they are not 16 anymore. Poor excuse! My grandmother was in her 80s and could possibly have still turned cartwheels. Of course, she had her own vegetable garden, which she diligently worked in, and she also prepared all of her meals with most of what her garden produced for her. To bed at 9 p.m. and up at 6 a.m., energetically ready to begin her day, with a family, home and all that entailed a day's work. Now, why is it that in her 80s, she was as fit as a fiddle? Because she was in tune with her body, what went into her body, and with life itself.

These days, people are into trying to make a "fast buck," overstressing their bodies, and putting into their bodies anything that will satisfy "hunger" or just anything at all that tastes "good," such as junk foods (candies, chips etc.). When they don't feel well, they blame it on age, or "the bug that's going around," but never on their own self-abuse. Gradually, when arthritis hits them, they search for relief with a drug or drugs, still without realizing that they have to change their gross habits of eating and living believing that they will miraculously be healed. Why do for yourself what a few pills will do for you? And, if an organ or some bones can be removed or fused, and one can still continue to function, even yet in gross ways. Obviously, most people are brainwashed to believe that they can continue to abuse the body and that drugs and chemicals can cure one's self-inflicted sickness and disease. For shame, that so many people's lives are regulated by "take this pill for your ulcer at 4 p.m.; take this pill for your gallbladder at 4:30 p.m., and be sure you take your mineral pills at 8 a.m. and, before bedtime, at 9 p.m., etc. etc." The money spent on chemicals that your body was never intended to absorb to begin with, causes one's body to work overtime to fight them. This takes away from the body its ability to help itself, its own healing ability. The secret is to teach people how to take charge of their body by proper natural nutrition and proper exercise for their bodies. It will take much to teach them, especially those who do not yet have arthritis, joint degenerative diseases, the fusing of the osseous structures, etc.

All the factors of self-help must be used, and this includes feeding one's body fresh raw vegetables, raw vegetable juices as well as fresh fruit juices and fresh fruits. Also included must be rest and sleep, sunshine and warmth, fresh air; cleanliness, internally and externally; eating at regular intervals. I understand that this may be difficult for an individual, at first, but we can start a bit at a time. In my opinion, any vegetable, whether cooked or raw, is better than none, and most especially, better than meats of any kind and a host of junk foods. To break one of such gross habits takes patience and also, most importantly, understanding, and, always, great positive direction. (Ms. Aragona has presented the task quite well. Such is the familiar pattern of self-abuse that must be penetrated and corrected. And this is why the Plan cannot be static. It must be subject to on-going change and modified from time to time to meet each client's specific needs as best they can be determined.)

Article #2: The No-Breakfast Plan

Note: Sometimes clients cannot accept the No-Breakfast Plan as originally espoused by Dr. Edward Hooker Dewey, M.D., an early Hygienist who lived in Meadville, Pennsylvania. To help them overcome is difficulty, the following true story as related by Prof. Hereward Carrington, Ph.D., in his fine book, Vitality, Fasting and Nutrition, may prove helpful. The story as told related to a Mr. Van R. Wilcox who fasted for 60 days and used no solid food for a total of 70 days.

The result of this fast was that Mr. Wilcox was completely cured of every one of his many infirmities (we counted 10 such depicted in the text!). In so fine a physical condition was he, indeed, such a high state of health had he attained—that he set about walking across the American continent—from New York to San Francisco—a distance of some three thousand six hundred miles, as walked—which remarkable feat Mr. Wilcox performed in 167 days—an average (taking into account the fact that Mr. Wilcox could not walk as the "crow flies") of slightly more than twenty-two miles per diem—he carrying, throughout, from twenty to thirty pounds of baggage! During this period, Mr. Wilcox was exposed to dangers and hardships galore; the temperature being at times 125° F. in the sun; at others 13° F. below zero. During all this time, though the physical exertion was as great as it was, not once did he eat a breakfast.

... Surely this should explode once and for all the fallacy that a hearty breakfast is required by those doing hard muscular labor—since there is no exercise more taxing than walking, or one that arouses more keenly the appetite.

Note: If Mr. Wilcox had walked at a consistent pace of 4 miles an hour, he would have had to walk for almost eight hours every single day! Apparently, he did just that!

Article #3: Holistic Approach: Relying on the Doctor Within by John M. Barry, N.D., D.Sc. & Dawn Lyman

You have within you a tremendous capability both to defend yourself against becoming ill and to heal yourself when you do become ill. Medical practitioners have long referred to this capability as your defense mechanisms. These defense mechanisms include your mind and emotions as well as your body.

They include all your physiological and psychological functions as well as all your glands, organs, and inner systems. All these functions, glands, organs, and systems interact in whatever way is needed for your well-being according to some inner wisdom which is obvious to researchers and practitioners alike, but which is poorly understood.

Dr. Albert Schweitzer called these defense mechanisms your "doctor within" when he advised physicians they would be at their best if they gave the doctor who resides within each patient a chance to work. Your "doctor within" is inborn and functions involuntarily throughout your life to repair injuries and keep you well; or return you to health after an illness. If you give this "doctor" a chance to work, s/he can even "cure" the common cold. S/he can compensate for the loss of a large part of many of your organs, including three-fourths of your liver, an entire lung or kidney or adrenal gland, restoring your functions to nearly normal. S/he restores normal functioning, not because you only needed one lung or one kidney or one-fourth of your liver to begin with and, by some happy chance, just happened to have extra; but because s/he is able to improvise with whatever is left of the injured system to compensate for what has been lost.

Whether you call it "the doctor within," "innate intelligence," the body's immune and defense mechanisms, or whatever, this is the only force capable of healing you of any disease. Only this inborn healing capability knows exactly what is really fundamentally wrong, and how corrections should be made. There is more information stored in the billions upon billions of cells which comprise you than is stored in all the libraries on earth. This information is used for continuous improvisations of your peculiar and specific mental and physical systems. No scientist knows how this works. And no battery of instruments can indicate how it works. In addition, how it works in your case is entirely different from how it works in others.

You may wonder why you get sick in the first place, if your "doctor within" is so marvelous. Well, even if you weren't exposed to such debilitating factors as pollution, stress and poor judgment as well as circumstances beyond your control (the new baby has colic and you have to go to work after getting 87 minutes sleep), you would still have to deal with entropy, the process by which all things break down into the elements of which they are composed. Because you are subject to all these deteriorating influences, you need to take some action to assist your "doctor within" in order for him/her to maintain your health.

Most health practitioners try to assist your "doctor within" in one way or another. Of the available methods, the orthodox medical approach is the most popular and most widely accepted. Drugs, radiation, surgery, and dangerous invasive procedures have become part of the orthodox medical approach and supposedly are used to assist your "doctor within." And, in many cases the need to assist the "doctor within" is secondary to malpractice liability which usually dictates that doctors provide the "correct" (acceptable to the medical establishment) treatment regardless of expected outcomes. The orthodox approach relies on drugs which in most cases are used simply as symptom-relievers. When a symptom poses an immediate threat to your life, it must be dealt with directly and at once, and drugs are used in such cases as a last resort.

However, trying to outwit the myriad of complex and still mysterious chemical, hydraulic, mechanical, and electrical systems which comprise your "doctor within" by repressing symptoms with chemicals is a lost cause, like spraying flies around a pile of manure. As long as the manure is not removed, you will always have more flies to spray, no matter how many you kill. No amount of observing of symptoms or performing of tests will show the entire, united, sub molecular workings of the human system. Therefore, swatting symptoms with chemical drugs does not remove the manure pile of ill health causing the observed symptoms. In fact, some symptoms can be caused by the healing process itself and are just reactions from the improvising used by your "doctor within" in his battle for maintaining health and should not be interfered with.

In addition, both the safety and effectiveness of any drug is open to question. Each drug is tested by its own manufacturer," not by the Food and Drug Administration (FDA) as many assume. Each manufacturer selects the persons used as subjects, selects control groups, designs the experiments, and selects which data it will submit to the FDA. The FDA makes drug decisions based on what the drug company presents as findings about a product from which it hopes to derive a profit; long-term adverse reactions to the drug are never considered.

The orthodox medical viewpoint has emphasis on germs, viruses, and specific aberrations rather than on the knowledge that poor health is usually caused by the elements of your lifestyle and environment which contribute to eroding the strength of your "doctor within." Factors contributing to disease are infinitely varied. A partial list might include contaminated water, food, or air; improper nutrition; unnatural chemical interference (including prescription and/or over-the-counter drugs); psychological or physical stress; lack of exercise; lack of fresh air; lack of sleep; and allergies including specific food allergies. These disease-causing factors are brought under some control, not by drugs or the technology associated with medical science, but by the actions of farmers, plumbers, legislators, garbage collectors, pest exterminators, food inspectors, and many others. Diseases such as beriberi, pellagra, pernicious anemia, rickets, scurvy, tuberculosis, as well as many of the contagious diseases and parasitic infestations have not retreated in modern industrialized nations because of drug therapy of medical science. They have retreated from improved sanitation, better nutrition, refrigeration, food and drug laws, meat and dairy inspection, rapid transportation of fruits and vegetables, inside plumbing, clean water standards, sewers, proper garbage disposal, more bathtubs, heater-ventilation codes, the forty-hour week, elimination of "sweat shops" in industry, labor laws, etc., etc.

As the methods used by the "doctor within" become better understood, more and more orthodox medical practitioners are turning to a more holistic approach to health. The holistic method acknowledges, in effect, that you can't repair a broken sidewalk without cement, aggregate and water. To repair a sidewalk, you need to use those elements of which the sidewalk was made in the first place. You also can't repair a sidewalk under adverse conditions (while people are walking on it, for instance, when the temperature is too low). Likewise, the "doctor within" needs favorable conditions in which to make repairs and the elements of which human tissue is made.

The holistic approach is one that assists the body's defense mechanisms by supplying the proper items and conditions needed for good health. This approach, because it involves your entire lifestyle, requires your knowledgeable participation, since only you are privy to all aspects of your life on a running day-to-day basis. The responsibility for your health belongs to you. A condition of total wellness can be attained only by learning health-building principles and applying them in your life. It is up to you to supervise your own nutrition, sleep, exercise, stress reduction, and mental attitude. You are the one to avoid pollutants and self-destructive habits. You are one that should examine the social and economic factors your life which may be contributing to ill-health. If give your "doctor within" the proper tools and conditions, s/he will provide a state of happiness and harmony within yourself, with others and with the environment.

Reprinted from the Herald of Holistic Health

Article #4: Pleasures, Instinctive and Acquired

Remember the meanings of joys or pleasures are elative. The inveterate cigarette smoker may insist that he gets pleasure from smoking. But this same man will have to agree that this feeling of pleasure primarily had to be acquired. The first cigarette was everything but pleasant, but in spite of it, by conformity the habit is started. Later, the inevitable effects of drug addiction take hold and the smokers find "pleasure" in smoking the smoke containing the alkaloids.

In a similar fashion, sensations of pleasure can be cultivated from the eating of harmful foods. Think about the candy, doughnut, cake, and soft drink habit, all giving relative "pleasures."?

Surprisingly, animal flesh belongs in the same category of providing "pleasure." In this case it is obtained from the meat containing alkaloids, with their stimulating action. It may be shocking to some of us to learn that we are imbibing narcotics when partaking in the eating of meat.

We have digressed somewhat to establish the meaning of pleasure. The point is knowing that there are several types. Some pleasures are deeply inherent, instinctive and satisfy constructively. Other pleasures are of relative significance. They later had to be learned in the overcoming of inborn natural protective instincts. This explains the sickening feeling after the first cigarette or the belching or burning signals uttered by protesting digestive organs. We could also include the resulting disgust most of us experience when passing a butcher shop. The "enjoyment" of meat is definitely a relative and learned pleasure.

What is amazing is to discover our own immense capacities for adjustment. Once the mind has appropriated the truth, an unrelenting change in our feelings surges ahead. Natural instincts again take over, with a reshuffling of pleasure concepts.

Not all of us can benefit from such a reform, directed by our own free will. When I returned from Argentina with the evidence and pictures of Dr. Roffo's cancer experiments, showing the horrible and gory results of smoking in my professional classes, I could always expect a certain percentage of my students to quit the habit.

I mentioned a "certain percentage," why not all of them? Simply the message did not go through, their minds refused to accept it. Remember, only some of us, not all of us, do recognize the truth, when it is presented. When the pupil is ready, the master will appear.

An excerpt from the book, The Health Secrets of a Naturopathic Doctor by M. O. Garten

Lesson 93:

Teaching your Clients About Fasting

Article #1: Health Secrets of a Naturopathic Doctor by M.O. Garten

93.1. Introduction

Instinctively, every person knows that the living body is maintained by nourishing it. We are all aware of the fact that little children will not grow unless they receive proper food. We observe little ones being stuffed beyond capacity all around us. As a result, many are bloated beyond belief, their small bodies already foul cesspools of rapidly-accumulating poisonous debris.

We are also aware of the fact that unless the human body, child, or adult, receives its full quota of nourishment, it will, in time, cease to be; the life spirit will depart, returning to the source from whence it came.

For centuries the custom has been to ply invalids with what is termed, "good, nourishing food," and this often to their undoing for, instead of contributing to an increase in wellness, the food wasted the vitality of the sick to the extent that it proved instrumental in either prolonging the recovery or causing the demise of the person so abused.

Humans, unlike other animals, do NOT instinctively know or understand that abstaining from food can be an effective means for the body to cleanse its stagnant fluids, one wholly compatible to nature; a natural happening which will permit the restoration of a degree of health as predetermined by the potential for recovery that lies dormant within.

In this lesson, therefore, we will examine some aspects of fasting that may have been previously touched upon to some degree but which, in our view, warrant further attention and then, by means of various case studies, we will show how certain individuals became convinced that fasting was worthy of their consideration and eventually became a part of their pattern for transition into a higher level of health.

93.2. Energy Flow, Fasting and Mind Control

Vital force is essential to recovery. When a person is tired, s/he will eventually be compelled to lie down and go to sleep and, normally, such a one will sleep until such time as the cerebral centers recognize that the body has regained sufficient electrical (vital) force to fuel life's usual activities. In health, s/he will awake in due time. We cannot sleep too much but, obviously, we can sleep too little.

In the last century Russell Thacker Trail, M.D. pointed out that nothing is remedial—that is, conducive to the healing process—except those conditions which economize the expenditure of the forces of the sick organism.

Most people agree that the only real curative agencies are those decreed by nature. Hereward Carrington, Ph.D. reminded us that this is so, then we should look to nature: to the animals in the wild, to observe what they do. How do animals live, what do they do when injured or when sick? He further pointed out that, in every instance, we find that when animals live in a congenial environment, they eat their own food; they abhor and refuse all "foreign" food and, in sickness, they, more often than not, refuse food, often for days and, in severe cases, for weeks. Eventually, weakened but recovered from their ailment, they begin to forage for food. Instinctively, animals know when it is time to eat and when they should refrain from eating and thus begin to conserve their bodily energy through the process of sleep. Instinctively, and prompted no doubt by the sensation of thirst, they also drink a far greater quantity of water than they usually do. In other words, in sickness or injury, they resort to fasting. There has never been a time in all of recorded history when man did not fast, for one reason or another: to attain spiritual, mental or physical excellence and, at times, to achieve a worldly objective. Obviously, mankind would not have consistently fasted unless he derived considerable benefit therefrom. We find the rationale for such benefit from what Trail said: namely, that if healing is to take place, then the available vital resources must be permitted to be focused on that effort and not directed elsewhere in all manner of extraneous pursuits.

It is well known that the digestion of food requires a vigorous mechanical effort which can exhaust not only the overworked muscles which comprise the alimentary canal, but also the vital resources in supplying the means of digestion. The process requires a well-stocked larder of secretions and enzymes for the efficient completion of the highly-complex chemical resolutions required to change the larger food molecules into organic molecules of a size suitable for transport across and through the cellular barriers of the mucous membranes and thence into the bloodstream of life.

These secretions are not just there. They have to be manufactured, stored and transported, processes which expend vital force. Dr. Robert Beaumont, M.D., in working with the wounded French trapper, Alexis St. Martin, found that whenever the man was ill, any food eaten would simply lie in the stomach for periods as long as 40 hours, during which time it was not digested but rather subjected to fermentative and putrefactive agents. This remains a vivid demonstration of the fact that the control center in the brain knows full well when food should not be taken into the body and sends out the dictum by urgent means (via the autonomic nervous network) to cease the digestive effort because there is a greater need in illness: that of physiological rest during which time the resources of the body can be conserved with the energy redirected into more appropriate channels, to the healing of wounded and/or ailing parts.

Dewey, Densmore, Trall, Jennings, Upton Sinclair and others all recognized that, during abstention from food, minimal bodily activity goes on and, consequently, there is little "wear and tear" on the organism in general, a fact which, as a direct consequence, would, under cerebral guidance, permit the fasting individual to subsist on his/her own resources even for a few months, while, at the same time, the necessary energy, supplied through appropriately chosen channels, is directed to the areas where a need exists.

Herbert M. Shelton, in his book Natural Hygiene, Man's Pristine Way of Life, quotes Dr. Isaac Jennings discussing a fast being taken by an acutely-ill child, as follows:

"There is now little action of the system generally, and consequently, there is but little wear and tear of machinery; and like the dormouse, it might subsist for months on its own internal resources, if that were necessary, and everything else favored. The bowels too have been quiet for a number of days, and they might remain as they are for weeks and months to come without danger, if this were essential to the prolongation of life. The muscles of voluntary motion are at rest and cost nothing for their maintenance, save a slight expenditure of safekeeping forces to hold them in readiness for action at any future time if their services are needed. So, of all the other parts and departments; the most perfect economy is everywhere exercised in the appropriation and use of the vital energies."

It is this ability of the living organism, and man is no exception, to self-direct the digestion of its own tissues during periods of abstinence from food from outside sources, combined with the inescapable fact that, when ill, animals, including man, tend to lose their appetite and are thus forced into abstinence that leads us to conclude that fasting is a method decreed by nature to conserve body energy by reducing normal activity for the purposes of redirecting available energy to more essential purposes. It would appear that this is a concept and fact of sufficient importance to be brought to the attention of our ailing clients. It is one of those things that makes sense. The fact that fasting is a sensible procedure when illness or injury exist is further supported by another clearly observable phenomenon—namely that, unless the brain cells have been so damaged that they cannot function any longer automatically, up until the point of cessation of cellular activity, death—the mind remains in control of all bodily activity, the autolysis being carried out in a precisely-defined order or urgency: first, the elimination of excess toxic materials which are either already in solution or capable of being made ready for elimination; then, the fatty tissues, wherever located, these to be followed in due course by the disintegration and elimination of wens, tumors, diseased parts in general; healing; all long before vital muscular supports and/or organs are broken down.

The last point which serves to give credibility to fasting as a naturally-given means of healing is that before vital organs even begin to disintegrate, the fasting individual, usually experiences the sensation of hunger which is frequently extremely intense; sometimes, less so. Additionally, the tongue assumes the pink color indicative of a cleansed blood and the secretions begin their more normal free flow.

Often by this time, the individual has been reduced to a skeletal condition. However, it is the amazing ability of this skeletonized structure to commence and sustain the rebuilding of its own tissues while, at the same time, the energy grows, that can really captivate the mind.

All these factors combined should put the coup de grace to all illogical objections to fasting, which by being voiced at all, demonstrate fully the lack of all logic. The final product, with normal weight established, reveals the extent of the body to restore itself to an amazing degree of wellness. And, amazingly too, is the fact that the exercise of normal bodily functions will actually hasten the process of rebuilding. The entire process, from start to finish, is under exact mind control.

Knowledge of these fundamental organic truths can often assist a doubting client to give over his/her childish misconceptions in favor of adult conclusions, these to be followed, in due course, by adult behavior in that the client makes his/her first initial mind acceptance of the rationale of fasting. Mind control of the total self, more often than not, will open the way for bold new experiences; perhaps even acceptance by reluctant clients of fasting as something for them to consider as they evaluate the options specifically open to them.

93.3. The Hygienic Experience

93.3.1. How Long Should We Fast?

93.3.2. Why Clients May Need to Fast

93.3.3. Nerve Channels Must be Free

93.3.4. The Role Played by Water in Fasting

93.3.5. Fasting "Cures" Nothing

93.3.6. Dr. Buchinger's List

93.3.7. Other Possible Reasons for Fasting

93.3.8. Fear of Fasting

As the students of Life Science well know, fasting is not well-accepted by "traditional" medicine, especially in this country; this in spite of the fact that, generally, it is well accepted abroad and this by many otherwise fully orthodox practitioners. Much of this acceptance in other lands is due to the persistence of Dr. Otto Buchinger, formerly fleet surgeon in the German navy, who had been elevated in 1917 to this high command, one equivalent to that of rear admiral in the U.S. navy.

Upon receiving his appointment, however, Dr. Buchinger was too ill to carry on with the manifold duties which the appointment necessarily entailed. It is said that he was totally incapacitated by arthritis as well as severe gallbladder and liver disorders. Fortunately, for all students of Natural Hygiene, he was referred to a Dr. Gustav Riedlin, one of the earliest of European pioneer fasting specialists.

Under Dr. Riedlin's guidance, Buchinger fasted for some 19 days and found that the arthritic condition had been greatly improved. After a suitable interval, he then fasted again, this time for thirty days, with the astounding result that all his organic troubles had been completely done away with.

424

Needless to say, Dr. Buchinger became an enthusiastic advocate of fasting and eventually operated two large sanitariums in Germany where records of literally thousands of patients were admirably kept and completely documented. It is said that more than 70,000 people fasted at the Buchinger retreats. Orthodox practitioners confronted by such well-documented case studies began to open their own fasting clinics and spas.

We well remember visiting with a medical professor in Madrid who reported that he had come to a well-known medical college in America to study but left in short order. He said that he was dismayed to learn that medical doctors in this country seemed to know nothing about fasting. All they were concerned with was "gadgets and drugs!" He further stated they seemed to have no knowledge of "the healing hand" that soothes away all hurts.

In this country, Dr. Herbert M. Shelton has been the leader. Others have followed in his wake: Dr. Vivian Vetrano, Dr. Robert Gross, Dr. Scott. Probably together they have supervised well over 100,000 fasts. Other fasting retreats around this country have supervised tens of thousands more, while innumerable individuals have successfully fasted on their own.

Not all fasters are successful in achieving total recovery, of course, but those who possess sufficient vitality to commence a fast and then to sustain the period of recovery for a sufficiently long period of time, have achieved what has often amounted to almost unbelievably salubrious results.

Even short fasts, from three to five days, add up in benefits. Last Christmas, for example, we received a card from Rod. If you recall, Rod suffered from arthritis so badly that he could no longer hold a pen or pencil and so was forced to give up his career as an accountant. We first learned about Rod from a client who told us that he had sought relief from pain first in Arizona, then in Nevada; but all in vain. His lack of muscular coordination and the pain just went on and on, even worsening.

Then he was referred to us and began a Hygienic program which, even without resorting to prolonged fasts, just shorter ones, enabled him to go back to work again.

Rod is now home again and, on his Christmas, note he reported to us that he is doing so well that he was fully able to cope with the extreme cold which buffeted all this last winter. He reminded us of the fact that prior to beginning his fasting the cold weather had caused him great suffering.

This young man began to fast one day a week and then three days every month. What has this fasting done for Rod? Just a few years ago, Rod cried out with pain in our office and asked us if we could help him. Today he is back home again, working and his last message to us read, "I'm doing just fine!"

93.3.1. How Long Should We Fast?

Experience shows that the fasting period varies from individual to individual. Few persons fast, however, to completion. On an average, fasting clients abstain from all food for from 10 days to two weeks. In some drastic, cases, persons fast as long as 30 or more days before the signs indicate that the internal cleansing and healing has been completed.

In very severe chronic cases, Dr. Shelton found, it sometimes necessary for patients to fast three and four times before experiencing a complete cleansing and healing.

Many Hygienists have found a yearly 10to 14-day fast highly beneficial. Others fast one day each week and two to three days every month and find this method quite satisfactory. When the fluids of the body are kept reasonably clean and pure by adhering to strict Hygienic practices and principles both in eating and living, then even in today's stressed and polluted frenzied environment, one can maintain a high level of wellness and have amazing vitality compared to the rest of our diseased population with only an occasional cleansing fast of comparatively short duration.

Fasting, it seems to us, has no further need to be proved as a body-accepted and, therefore, correct healing modality. The mechanisms for conducting a fast "come with the design," so to speak, just as the method of cleaning a piece of equipment is dictated by its structure. An engineer must know his/her equipment to be a successful engineer. Unfortunately, most humans neither understand nor appreciate their "equipment," their own bodies! In the exact same manner, the proper method of cleansing the human body is ordained by its structure and, therefore, more proper to it than other artificially-conceived modalities as, for example, the blood-letting of former years and the "marvel" of today's technology, apheresis.

93.3.2. Why Clients May Need to Fast

Since all diseases (excepting of course those due to traumatic causes, injury and the like) are the direct result of abnormal metabolism (which, being ongoing, results in certain chemical changes which, by the very nature of things, cause a gradual decline in cellular efficiency and organ degeneration due to the infusion and precipitation of toxic waste by-products, known to German physicians as ZELLENSCHLACKEN, or cell cinders), it follows that such debris should be removed with dispatch and with unerring accuracy and in the order of urgency as best determined by the cerebral powers of the body and not by unproven and questionable powers of man-conceived substance or gadget.

Obviously, if such waste debris were allowed to remain, the entire systemic transportation system would be interfered with, starting first at the more-or-less porous cell membranes where the infusion of debris rapidly begins to set up membrane blockages which reduce the infusion of nutritive materials into the cell and interfere with free flow of arterial blood and its venous return for oxygenation in the lungs. In truth, the whole cleansing of the body is reduced, the endocrine regulation of body chemistry is strangulated and, subsequently, as a natural sequence, every single chemical and/or other cellular work becomes somewhat other than normal.

93.3.3. Nerve Channels Must be Free

It is not only the free flow of fluids and the possibility of blockages occurring in the arterial and venous channels that are of importance. Still another concern arises, namely, that all bodily activity depends on the free conduit of nerve messages via the nervous mechanisms of the body. Situational problems must be relayed to the central control centers. There they must be evaluated, conclusions reached, and proper solutions determined. Suitable directions to be involved and/or troubled areas must then be transported with precise areas or sites being predetermined. Subsequent follow-up instructions for cells must be carried to wherever a need or problem exists.

Should the sympathetic nervous system be interfered with by any unusual build-up of wastes, the possibility, even the probability, of error exists. The entire body mechanisms could conceivably falter and be subject to error, certainly a matter of grave concern.

To the rational mind, it seems quite obvious that probably every disease to which man is heir can be traced back to this one simple circumstance: that any degree of metabolic abnormality produces an abnormal amount of toxic debris which can build up and interfere not only with the free transport of nutrients to the cells and the subsequent removal of cellular waste but also with nerve message transmission, always with the possibility of single and/or multiple errors occurring either occasionally or constantly, and these being either limited in scope or totally systemic.

If all this be true, and we can see no sound physiological basis for concluding otherwise, then fasting to accelerate the removal both of the waste and its autolysis by proper organic built-in methods which are always under cerebral guidance would appear to be the only proper method to cleanse the system so that free transport through all channels would once again become a reality.

93.3.4. The Role Played by Water in Fasting

Water is, of course, the greatest of all solvents. Having access to pure distilled water is necessary to a successful fast. All the diseased parts, already "burned up" by a most carefully-controlled autolysis, all the systemic poisons can thus be dissolved in the water and flushed out of the body, no longer a threat to life.

93.3.5. Fasting "Cures" Nothing

It is important for students to understand that fasting "cures" nothing. Its sole purpose appears to be to permit the system, through physiological rest, to lessen its expenditure of energy, to reduce any buildup of metabolic waste by-products to a minimum, and then to divert all conserved energy resources to certain tasks which have been selected through cerebral evaluation as being needful of a more concentrated effort just at this time. In this manner, autolysis of inferior parts and the elimination of collected waste debris can be accelerated and systemic equilibrium, the recognized hallmark of good health, can be more quickly established.

It is at this precise point, when systemic balance has been achieved, that disease ceases to be a problem and a condition of wellness takes over. As Dr. Allan Cott, psychiatrist, says in his book, Fasting: The Ultimate Diet: "Fasting is certainly not a panacea for all ills, but it may be effective in treating many more varieties of sickness than orthodox medicine is ever likely to concede."

Dr. Buchinger found the following illnesses either improved or were totally eliminated by fasting and insisted that the merit of fasting should be considered in all such conditions.

93.3.6. Dr. Buchinger's List

1. Obesity, chronic underweight, diabetes in initial stages

2. Rheumatic disorders of joints and muscles; sciatica

3. Heart conditions

4. All circulatory problems involving blood vessels such as high or low blood pressure, hot flashes, many symptoms of aging

5. Stress and nervous exhaustion

6. Skin diseases of all kinds

7. Diseases of the digestive organs

8. Diseases of the respiratory organs

9. Kidney and bladder diseases

10. Female disorders of many kinds

11. Allergic conditions including hay fever

12. Eye diseases such as chronic iritis, retinitis, etc.

13. Conditions which follow venereal diseases or the condition itself

14. The many forms of glandular disturbances: ovarian, thyroid, etc.

15. Periodontal diseases

16. Fasting in readiness for operations and for better and easier recovery afterwards

17. As a preventative measure (to prevent cancer, etc.)

18. Diseases which have their origin in under-nutrition and malnutrition

19. General fatigue, spring-fever.

There are probably many other reasons for fasting. We present the following for the consideration of our students:

93.3.7. Other Possible Reasons for Fasting

1. To attain spiritual insight, mental acuity, sensual acuity, increased perceptual awareness, etc.

2. To lower the cholesterol level.

3. General body clean-out.

4. To give the digestive system a rest.

5. In the case of wounds, to give the body time to heal.

6. To relieve tension.

7. To sleep better.

8. To regulate the bowels and provide better elimination through this channel.

9. To slow the aging process.

10. To save money in many, many areas of life.

11. To feel and look better, younger.

12. To improve one's sex life.

13. To help a person eliminate smoking, drinking, and/or other addictive habits.

14. To reduce or totally eliminate pain.

15. To provide rest for all organs, muscles, and systems; to restore vitality and full energy flow.

16. Just to save time (the average person spends three hours a day and more in preparing, serving, and eating his/her food!)

Dr. Shelton pointed out that with disorders of the alimentary canal, fasting removes three sources of local irritation, namely:

1. The mechanical irritation brought on by particles of food that come in contact with the raw inflamed mucosal linings;

2. The mechanical irritation which results from the vigorous contraction and expansion of the walls of the stomach and the wrinkling of the surfaces as they receive and handle foods; and

3. The chemical irritation caused by the secretion of strong acid gastric juice.

Dr. Shelton maintained that in such disorders the fast should be continued until systemic renovation has been completed. It seems logical that these same conditions should pertain with all disorders affecting the entire canal including, for example, the miserable condition of colitis which can cause individuals to become extremely nervous, irritable and, at times, almost hysterical due to headaches and other discomforting symptoms that often accompany this ailment.

93.3.8. Fear of Fasting

The fear of fasting is widespread due (in great part it seems to us) to what amounts to medical hysteria whenever the subject comes up. Few clients, in fact, will have ever even heard of fasting as a valid means of restoring health. We ourselves had never heard of it in this connection until many years after we had begun our own worldwide search for improved health.

Out of many, many thousands of medical treatises, and books on all manner of diseases, methods, opinions, statements, and whatnot written and disseminated in this country, fewer than one percent probably even mention fasting as a means of recovery from illness. If the subject comes up at all, it is referred to as "starvation," which is enough to "make the hair stand up on end," as the saying goes. It is only in recent years that some physicians have found merit in treating obese patients in this manner.

The reasons for this unwarranted fear are, of course, obvious: negative pre-programming, the prior conditioning about fasting as being something "far out;" a total lack of education about fasting. What people do not understand, they fear. Therefore, persons who are ill and desirous of once again experiencing the euphoria engendered by complete wellness, need to become more knowledgeable about the subject and especially about how a series of shorter fasts but, importantly, a more prolonged fast, might benefit them.

Dr. Ragnar Berg, the celebrated nutritionist, and Nobel Prize Winner stated that he knew of fasts that lasted over 100 days and that he also had supervised or controlled fasts up to as long as 40 and more days, while he himself often fasted as long as 21 days while continuing to work 11 hours daily either in his laboratory, actively engaged, or at desk work. Innumerable stories, both documented and undocumented (in this case from reliable sources) witness to the fact that we need have no fear of either dying from hunger or from not knowing just when to terminate a fast. However, newcomers to Natural Hygiene, for the most part, have to go through a developmental process before they can cognitively accept fasting as a rational experience for them to consider, a healing measure of nature which can accomplish only good.

The mental condition of the fasting patient is of utmost importance to success. All negative thoughts, all fear that worries and depresses the mind, should be eliminated. It is of crucial importance that, before undertaking a fast, the client be well-schooled. If not, should s/he experience any unpleasant and unanticipated symptoms, s/he is likely to magnify the seriousness of what is happening and even to become panicked into terminating the fast too quickly, thus possibly undoing much of all of any benefit accruing to the fast.

This is particularly true of the new fasters. Even though they may be somewhat knowledgeable about the subject, mentally they will perhaps unconsciously anticipate trouble, this because that which they are presently experiencing is so entirely foreign to all that they have yet known. They can become anxious, uncertain, even perturbed, and especially so if not well-schooled.

In all cases, therefore, it is our view that clients should be well-educated in the fast before undertaking one—except, perhaps, in rare circumstances when, at the discretion of an experienced practitioner, an immediate fast may be indicated. The question arises then as to how best to impart this information to the client.

Sometimes we must do so abruptly. For example, just last evening we received a call from out of state from a friend of many years. He wanted to bring his wife to Tucson so that we might devise a suitable diet for her. On inquiry, however, we learned that about a year ago she had received a diagnosis of lymphoma of the parotid gland on one side of her throat and that she had been subjected to radiation and chemotherapy and was presently in, the hospital to have biopsies made of new swellings which had appeared in her throat and right breast. She had-been advised by the supervising oncologist that he feared that the lymphoma had already begun to spread throughout her body.

It was our sad duty to inform this gentleman that, at this late time, just improving the diet would have minimal effect. Because of the seriousness of her condition and the unfortunate "treatments" she had received, probably the only chance his wife had to recover any degree of improved health would lie in her resorting to a prolonged fast.

And, knowing the complete confidence this woman has in medical procedures and in her physician, we very much doubt if she will accept our recommendation. However; there was, in this case, no time for delay.

93.4. What We Have Learned Thus Far

Thus far, we have brought forth the following points for our students to consider:

1. People do not know instinctively, as animals do, that abstaining from food can be helpful in acquiring a higher level of wellness.

2. The rationale of fasting lies in a controlled diversion of energy flow from ordinary duties by keeping these to a minimum through enforced physiological rest, and then directing of all thusly spared energy resources by the autonomic nervous system to the area(s) where healing is most needed.

3. The only real curative agencies are those decreed by nature. Fasting is such an agency, this fact being witnessed and confirmed by design and results achieved following its application!

4. A fast is self-directed.

5. All vital parts, including the brain, are spared in fasting, with the mind remaining clear, until cessation of all systemic activity.

6. Following a prolonged fast during which the individual may be reduced to the skeletal structure, the body has the ability to reconstruct, and this in a more perfect manner than prior to the fasting experience.

7. The salubrious results of fasting have been well-documented. Of this, clients need have no doubt.

8. Not all fasters receive total recovery.

9. While fasting can be a useful means of recovery in a wide variety of illnesses, it is not to be a panacea for all. We have, therefore, listed those conditions which are known to have been greatly improved when fasting was resorted to.

10. Fasting is a means of removing cellular debris which when allowed to accumulate can produce certain adverse chemical and obstructive changes which can be destructive of a high degree of health.

11. Pure water is essential to a successful fast.

12. Fasting should not be considered as a "cure."

13. Fear of fasting is widespread and, therefore, it is encumbent upon the practitioner to teach his clients about fasting because all anxiety, all worry, and ungrounded fear can negate any benefit which might accrue to the faster. The mental condition of the faster must be positive for the fast to be successful.

93.5. The Learning Process Can Vary from Person to Person

After we have had several consultations with a client and arrive at the conclusion that a fast would be beneficial to him or her, we introduce the subject as quickly as possible. Probably every practicing Hygienist has his/her own way of acquainting new clients with the manifold possible benefits that may accrue to an individual who fasts.

We go over the various points and information which we have practiced. We encourage our clients to ask questions. At first, of course, few know just what kinds of questions to ask, but we observe that as we go along, clients begin to ask intelligent questions. We present them with copies of articles about successful fasts, especially of persons who have been restored to a higher level of health who previously suffered from the same identical condition as the client; or, if we do not have such, of related cases.

For example, suppose a client suffers from a stubborn rash. S/he will be greatly cheered if s/he reads about the successful healing of another person similarly afflicted after taking a fast of 10 days. This client may even be inclined to begin his/her own fast.

We suggest books for the client to read, easily read books such as the following, many of which are available inexpensively in paperbacks:

1. Dr. Cott's book, Fasting, The Ultimate Diet previously cited.

2. Fasting Can Save Your Life! by Dr. Herbert M. Shelton.

3.   About Fasting by Dr. Buchinger, previously cited.

4.   Dick Gregory's Natural Diet For Folks Who Eat: Cookin' With Mother Nature, Harper and Row, Publ. Inc.

5.   Natural Hygiene: Man's Pristine Way of Life by Dr. Shelton

6.   Vitality, Fasting and Nutrition by Hereward Carrington, Ph.D. available in a reprint from health research, Mokelumne Hill, California

7.   Others by Densmore, Sinclair, and other Hygienists.

Life Science in Austin, Texas, can suggest other books and supply the same to interested students. The Carrington work is for the more serious student.

Some students respond quickly to their new knowledge, others less so. A few will even begin short fasts on their own. With reluctant fasters, patience is required. A very few will not accept fasting as a valid and effective means of restoring a higher level of health until forced by circumstances to do so. To illustrate just how a number of clients were able to surmount the barrier of fear and come to accept the concept of fasting and, eventually, to fast, we follow with some actual case studies. As always, these studies represent true examples but, for obvious reasons, we have changed the names and some of the exact circumstances. The first case represents a very reluctant faster.

93.6. Case Studies

93.6.1. Case Study—Alex M.

93.6.2. Case Study—Gladys G.

93.6.3. Case Study—Dr. J., a Ph.D.

93.6.4. Case Study—Susie and Bill

93.6.5. Case Study—Ethel

93.6.6. Ethel's Diary

93.6.7. Case Study—Rachel—Her Story

93.6.1. Case Study—Alex M.

When he first came to our attention, Alex M. had just celebrated his 51st birthday. His immediate problem was obesity coupled with a sense of more-or-less constant fatigue.

He was also disturbed about the rather sudden appearance of a circular band of very visible capillaries which underscored the rib cage in the abdominal area.

Alex was a difficult patient to work with. A professional man, highly intelligent, comfortably placed financially, he was confident of his own expertise in certain scientific disciplines, including biology and chemistry. Reluctantly, therefore, he conceded that perhaps there were some areas of healing of which he had less knowledge than he had previously thought. But he was, at least, willing to listen and to learn.

As time went on Alex gradually adapted well to a Hygienic diet. He began to exercise and even occasionally worked out at a spa. He was able to reduce his weight from about 225 pounds down to a slim, trim 173 pounds and admitted to having the vitality of a man at least 20 years his junior.

Alex was very proud of his accomplishments, and with good reason, because adapting to Hygienic living had meant a complete turnaround both in his thinking and in his habits. The gourmet eating of his past had to be replaced by an abstemious well-chosen and-combined 80% raw food intake. Sheer willpower enabled him to give up salt, meat, and bread. Giving up sweets proved to be a major obstacle, but we overcame it by permitting him one very unhygienic indulgence once a week, namely, a huge hot fudge sundae complete with real whipped cream! How Alex looked forward to Fridays. This was HIS day!

But, you know, this strange technique worked! It wasn't too long before Alex confided that those hot fudge sundaes didn't seem to taste too good anymore; in fact, they kept him awake all night with his stomach and bowels growling and churning. So, on his own, Alex decided not to give in to his pathogenic desire for hot fudge sundaes and other processed health-destroying sweets.

However, fasting was another matter. In spite of reading the literature on the subject and also in spite of his acceptance of the fact that natural methods had already worked what amounted to a miracle of healing in his case, he still refused to consider fasting as something he should do. The capillary ring, so noticeable on his skin under the rib cage, and other symptoms which seemed to indicate the probable existence of a deranged liver, continued to concern him but not to the extent that he would consent to a fast as a possible means of restoring better living function and perhaps even doing away with his disfiguring ring.

Alex's refusal to fast lasted for almost six years. We saw him from time to time. He kept on his program. In fact, he told us that he had finally converted to eating just two meals a day, one of these being a fruit meal and the other a vegetable salad. When we saw him, we could scarcely reconcile his appearance with that of the obese "problem child" we had first encountered. Alex had become quite a Hygienist, but he had still not fasted, not even for a single day in all those years.

Then it happened! Alex began to lose weight. The pounds began to roll off him like water off a duck's back. He couldn't stop losing weight. He came to us almost in a panic. We backtracked. We again explained to Alex about housebuilding; about how nature will first tear down the old before building the new and better house. We once again reminded him that nature will have its way, all in due time.

We reminded him of some of the previously-learned facts about fasting and postulated the thought that if he had fasted originally, this might all have been over long ago in short order and that he would have long ago had his brand-new house.

This concept made good sense to Alex, but would he fast now? Again, the answer was a negative one. Alex would still not fast. He decided to eat nuts and sweet fruits in abundance, to begin weight-lifting in earnest now. That would do it. Of that he was confident.

About three months later, Alex was back. His body had refused to give in to his desires, his wishes, his dictates. Nature would have none of the nuts or sweet fruits, it seemed. He hadn't gained a pound! Instead, there had been a new and highly-disconcerting development: Alex's back, sides and rib cage had burst forth in blossoms! He was literally covered with hive-like lesions, some the size of a small saucer. They itched and itched, unbearably so. At times, he could neither sit nor stand still in comfort.

He was able to sleep but fitfully. Alex had reached the end of his resistance. Alex consented to fast, but he would do it his way.

He first fasted for 24 hours. He waited a month and then fasted for 36 hours. The blossoms continued to annoy. So, Alex decided to try a three-day fast and found that the itching had lessened considerably, and the lesions had grown smaller. There seemed to be some healed areas in the midst of the larger lesions. Our client was pleased with himself. So, a week later, he began another fast, one of five days duration. At the end of this longer fast, the lesions had completely healed. Even the capillary ring appeared much less noticeable.

Then it was that Alex confided to us that actually fasting wasn't too bad after all. He thought he might even try it again sometime!

Alex's case study demonstrates that some clients will be most reluctant, due to their previous negative programming, even to consider undergoing a fast. We never know at the outset what we may encounter when we begin to talk about this subject of fasting.

Many clients will not fast until compelled, like Alex, by unexpected developments, to do so. However, let us point out that, in spite of his reluctance to fast, during the intervening years, Alex had become much more knowledgeable about the subject of fasting and about what to expect during the fasting experience. In other words, he finally had become so knowledgeable about fasting that when he began to fast he was mentally prepared for whatever uncomfortable symptoms might appear and fully confident of the fact that fasting would bring to him only salubrious results. It was his knowledge that cast the dice, so to speak, in favor of performance.

His former fears, although unfounded, yet real, had long since evaporated to be replaced by willingness, albeit reluctant, to follow nature's way of dealing with physical, mental, and even spiritual problems and concerns.

The lesson for Hygienists to learn from this case is that of the need to have patience, not to give up, even though, at first, a client may refuse absolutely even to consider the fast as a probable methodology in his own very special case. Every change for the better will produce curative changes within a sick body, even though they be small and, for the time at least, unnoticed. In the end, small changes all add up and eventually produce major health benefits. Just so, the constant repetition of a thought, an idea, a concept, even about fasting, will leave its imprint and may eventually do away with surface acceptance and change it to cognitive acceptance. Cognitive acceptance is usually followed, in time, by correct and positive performance. In the final analysis, therefore, through knowledge, even the reluctant client may conclude that his or her own return to health may be hastened if s/he does undertake to fast. S/he may then even follow through and take action.

93.6.2. Case Study—Gladys G.

Gladys G. provides another example of delayed fasting, but for a different reason. Gladys became a private student about two years ago after having been referred to us by another client. At first, she took our course in applied nutrition and then decided that she could benefit from private consultations.

Gladys was fully aware of the fact that she was seriously ill, suffering as she was from a weakened heart; at 5' 4" she weighed only 85 pounds. She had also almost reached the point of complete exhaustion. Her general appearance showed a woman whose whole constitution was gravely debilitated. Full recovery seemed very problematical, so much so that we even hesitated to undertake her reeducation in the ways of natural healing.

However, we agreed to do what we could. Obviously, our client was too debilitated to go on a prolonged fast at this time. There were also other family considerations which made fasting impossible, at least for the time being.

Gladys was inclined to be a "symptom-searcher," a trait characteristic it seems of many highly-debilitated people and especially if they are inclined to be somewhat neurotic. At each consultation, Gladys would come armed with a long-written list of day by-day minor aches and pains. Not one would be missed! For example, if her left eyelid happened to be somewhat itchy, or puffy, that fact would go down on Gladys' report.

However, there was one thing that worked for us as we began to teach Gladys about Natural Hygiene.

Since she had originally come to our attention upon the recommendation of a fellow church member in whom she had complete trust (in fact, her minister), she was inclined to take everything we said as "gospel," no matter how strange, at times, our words must have sounded to her. Thus, it was that she followed instructions religiously.

Gladys faithfully took her mid-day rests, performed all suggested beginning exercises, attended to her regular sunbathing and was especially careful in formulating all her meals according to our instructions. Additionally, she studied her assigned lessons every day.

This client's progress was slow, but steady. Even her friends began to compliment her upon how well she was beginning to look even though she remained quite thin.

But still Gladys was reluctant to fast, her immediate family being extremely hostile to this idea because they thought her too thin, although in all other ways they were extremely loving and supportive. However, we continued to talk about the possible benefits accruing to fasting. From time to time, during our consultations, we would bring up the subject and hand our client a case study to take home with her to read and think about.

A whole year and a half went by. One day she came all smiles and revealed that for the entire preceding week, she had been able to manage very well on just two meals a day. Gladys was very proud of this accomplishment, so we began to write on our blackboard, for her to visualize all the several "successes" she had achieved since we first met. They included:

1. Eating well-combined foods.

2. Eating better-quality food, much of it organically grown and up to 80% of this eaten raw.

3. Exercising more now than formerly.

4. Foregoing all snacking, all "junk" foods.

5. Adopting—and adapting to—a frugivorian diet, eschewing all animal flesh and all animal-derived products.

6. Rarely eating bread or any other type of cereal.

7. Avoiding all legumes, except those she sprouted.

8. Rarely, if ever, eating anything grown underground.

9. Socializing more than she had been doing.

10. And now, adopting the Two-Meal-per-Day Plan.

Gladys beamed as we examined the list, a fact which inspired us to make her even more aware of how her newly-acquired lifestyle had been instrumental in bringing her many major health benefits as well as important personal health-promoting changes which would bear fruit in future years. With her active cooperation, we began to list them on her blackboard:

1. For six months now she had not taken a single dose of medication.

2. She was now able to sleep all night long, something she had not been able to do for many a year.

3. She was no longer symptom-searching because she understood that symptoms were the evidence of on-going healing within.

4. Her nervousness had been considerably reduced. Even her family, loving as they were, found her easier to get along with.

5. All signs of edema were gone.

6. She rarely coughed up mucus now, except for some slight amount when she got up in the morning.

7. She was now involved in many church projects and making a full contribution in that work where once she had been compelled to sit on the sidelines and watch.

8. She had developed a natural-looking nice pink color, this replacing her former wan and pale look.

9. She no longer had recourse to such "crutches" as vitamins, minerals, and other supplements.

10. She no longer drank tea, coffee, or soft drinks of any kind; just pure distilled water.

11. Obviously, Gladys had recovered a considerable measure of her lost health.

The time was ripe. We suggested to our client that having made such wonderful progress through her initial timid steps into Natural Hygiene that now perhaps was the ideal time to take a bold new step: why not fast for just 24 hours one day every week?

We wrote on the blackboard: "A beginning fast—24 Hours—from one evening meal to the next evening meal. I CAN DO IT!"

Buoyed up by her successes, Gladys agreed to try. And try she did, for when she came back after a six-week interval, she reported that "it wasn't as bad as I thought it was going to be!"

Probably the biggest surprise of all to this client and to her family was the fact that she had gained two more pounds, and this one but two meals a day with one day each week lived without her eating any food whatsoever.

Our client's family was at a loss as how to explain this miracle. Our client herself was so enthusiastic at this point that we knew it was time for her to set a new goal: for the next month, she was to fast now for 36 hours once every week. Gladys eagerly complied and fully met the challenge. For the next six months our client followed this fasting schedule, fasting for 36 hours each and every week. As a result of her total fasting experience, she achieved some remarkable health improvements:

1. All heart palpitations and spasms were done away with. She reported that she no longer was able even to feel her heart beating when she lay on her left side at night.

2. No digestive disturbances of major import. In fact, she reported that her stomach felt "at peace."

3. There are no visible signs of edema where on first visit, her legs had resembled the so called "piano legs" we so often observe in obese people (and remember that Gladys was emaciated at that time with the edema embarrassingly noticeable).

4. She rarely even has to clear her throat now. When she first began her timid way into Natural Hygiene, she had a severe bronchial condition.

5. She now weighs about 94 pounds and feels confident that she will now continue to gain until her weight becomes normalized. But even this small weight gain represented a 10% improvement.

6. She is full of smiles now. Her former distressed and worried look has entirely disappeared. She knows that, at long last, she has brought herself in tune with nature's ways and that they will not let her down.

7. Her vitality continues to astound not only herself but all those who knew her "back when."

However, in spite of all the above remarkable improvements, this client has agreed to continue on her present regimen until such time as her family agrees that she would benefit from a longer fast. Because she has made such splendid progress, all of us anticipate that the presently ongoing family opposition will soon melt away and it will not be too long before this lovely woman will be on her way to an even longer fast.

This is a determined woman in many ways, and a highly intelligent one, too. Remember that she accomplished all of these short fasts while surrounded by the anxious, worried countenances of her devoted, but unschooled, husband, children, brothers and sisters. We are fully confident that one of these days, in the not-too-distant future, Gladys will call to tell us that she has done it: she will have, at that point, taken her first three-day fast!

In this case study, we see vividly illustrated how family opposition can retard a client's adapting to a fast. However, this did not stop the learning process. It did not stop our client from moving forward because the knowledge spurred her on to performing in small, hesitant, but fruitful ways. The initial forays into the fasting experience were taken without apprehension on her part. She knew fully what to expect and so was prepared. The results were as anticipated.

93.6.3. Case Study—Dr. J., a Ph.D.

Doctor Joe weighed some 295 pounds on first visit. He was a graduate of many colleges and universities, a man of diverse talents. He had been directed to us, as is usual with most clients, by a former student. He said he had been looking for someone with whom "he could feel compatible." He felt we might satisfy his requirements!

Because of his intellectual bent, we immediately started Joe on a study program. We made no specific recommendations as to either his eating habits or his lifestyle, just assigned him a certain number of pages to be covered within a certain time frame. When he had completed each assignment, we discussed and analyzed what Joe had read. Being skilled in speed reading, our client turned out to be a voracious student, gobbling up the information as fast as he received the materials. Therefore, it was necessary to reassign, from time to time, certain studies whenever we felt he had skimmed over them too rapidly for full cerebral acceptance of concepts.

While Joe had started out basically as a skeptic, he began to see that the principles and practices espoused by Hygienists were both intellectually acceptable and scientifically sound. He began to study the physiology of the digestive system and to pore over anatomy books. But even though several months had passed, during which time we had made helpful suggestions as to the ways and means whereby our student might change his lifestyle and reap certain benefits thereby, he had not, as yet made his personal commitment.

Finally, however, he did. He decided to shift into a more sensible health program, made an appointment with us and requested that we set up a regimen precisely tailored according to his specifications! Since this was, of course, a very unusual procedure, we delved a little deeper.

It seems that Joe had decided that for him to make an immediate changeover into a strictly Hygienic regimen would be too trying. He would, therefore, take 1 1\2 years to achieve his goal, at which time he would weigh in at 210 pounds, be muscularly fit and superbly healthy!

We cautioned Joe that, because of his obesity and several previously diagnosed conditions, including a slight hypertension, digestive troubles, and some liver impairment, that he might not fully achieve his goal in such a short time without having recourse to a fasting program. Joe, however, was convinced that, for him, all things were, indeed, possible.

Joe was a gourmand, delighting in exotic foods. But, in spite of his obesity, his grossly inadequate eating habits and his health impairments, our client was an extremely vital man. He possessed many good habits. He was happily married with a wife who was so supportive of his efforts that she immediately agreed to join in the adventure. Since he was semi-retired, age 62, and she was also a woman of leisure, they decided to devote all their efforts to accomplishing the goals Joe had set out for himself.

Therefore, at the outset, we designed a tentative regimen for both to follow. Initially, they were to give up all processed, canned, and frozen foods. All sugared goodies were immediately taken off Joe's favorite foods list. Instead of having meat of some animal derived product three and more times a day, as had been their custom, their intake of this kind of "food" was to be limited to one serving daily.

A walking schedule of 30 minutes per day was set up, plus stretching and flexibility exercises for morning "wake-up." Neither Joe nor Julia, his wife, had previously followed any particular exercise program; in fact, both had lived extremely sedentary existences.

Because of his obesity, Joe was to take two rinse-downs daily under the shower and this without fail. (We remind our students that most obese people have a pronounced body odor due to the fact that fat so often serves as a storage vault for toxins.) Both of these students were encouraged to forego their intense studying now in favor of more exposure to fresh air and the great outdoors. They talked things over and agreed that one month would be the correct interval to overcome their first hurdle; that this would be acceptable risk-taking. No further changes in their routines were put forth by us at this time.

In 30 days, Joe and Julia made their report in person. Every suggestion had been followed precisely, except for one. They had decided to review all their studies thus far and had set aside 15 minutes each. morning for this purpose. (We have several couples who have since adopted this same routine and have found it amazingly helpful.) Joe reported that he had lost only about three or four pounds, but both said they felt much improved and were sleeping better.

Our couple decided that Phase Two should now begin and that this, too, would be adhered to for one month. It was agreed that they would now reduce their coffee intake to one cup per meal from their customary two or three, and to drink it now without sugar. They would consume no other beverages except distilled water. Salt would be restricted also and used now only on their meat allowance which was to be reduced at this time to only four times a week. We mutually agreed that these steps as outlined would prove helpful. Additionally, they were to extend their walking now from 30 minutes to one hour daily. On leaving they were given an assignment: they were to read Dr. Shelton's book, Fasting Can Save Your Life! They promised to do so.

Before the month was up, Joe and Julia telephoned to make an earlier appointment. They were excited about fasting. Joe had lost a full ten pounds, the first time he had really been able to accomplish such a weight loss without "starving" himself, as he put it. While not yet mentally prepared to fast, they both wanted to get on with their program. A fast? Well, that was another matter. That would require considerably more study and personal evaluation.

So, we made some new assignments. They were to study all about food combining and to plan their daily food intake according to a three-meals-per-day format and to keep a daily record of their food intake for purposes of review by us.

The formats suggested were:

1. First Meal A variety of like fruits (up to three different, but compatible, kinds); plus, celery.

2. Second Meal A large salad with either a baked or steamed potato or baked brown rice.

3. Third Meal Medium Salad, Steamed green vegetable(s), Protein

For the protein meal, they were to restrict their flesh intake now to but two servings a week approximately three ounces of either lean lamb or poultry. One day per week, they could have either coddled or poached eggs or cottage cheese. The remaining four days of the week they were to serve their choice of any of the following: one whole medium avocado, four ounces of their choice of pecans, walnuts, almonds, or Brazil nuts; or two tablespoonsful of sunflower or pumpkin seeds.

As a learning experience for them, we requested that they keep a food diary which we could review together. They agreed that this might prove helpful.

It is not necessary at this point to tell how Joe and Julia progressed each month and precisely what changes were made other than to say that within eight months, they were eating only two meals per day, Joe had reduced to about 250 pounds and both he and his wife were well pleased with their progress. Neither had experienced any undue healing crises although Julia had suffered from an uncomfortable itching sensation for a period of a few weeks.

Thus, it was that Joe and Julia agreed it was now time for them to begin to fast, but they would do it on their own and would not go to a fasting institution, this in spite of our recommendation that they would be better served by doing so.

Shortly they successfully accomplished their first three-day fast. Julia reported that on the third day she had fainted and had immediately taken some fruit juice and thus did not quite complete her fast. Once this was accomplished and behind them, they agreed that they were ready to proceed on their own and advised us that they would report into us every three months.

And so, they did, most faithfully. They progressed from three to five days and then to seven. Julia fasted for seven days first. Then they took turns. As one fasted, the other stood by, ready to step in should the need arise. However, all went exceedingly well. Joe amazed us all with how well he stood up during these weeks. He had so much vitality, as a matter of fact, that while fasting five days he was able to work in his garden for hours on end, even though he had been advised it would be far better for him to conserve his valuable energy reserves for the healing effort.

At the end of 18 months, Joe weighed 205 pounds. He had reached his pre-set goal, but he now realized that his original ideas about himself and how nature works had been somewhat in error and that it would now just be a matter of time until his own self dictated what his normal weight should be. Both he and Julia looked at least 10 years younger than when they first began this new adventure into the fasting experience. They were now confirmed Hygienists and were fasting 36 hours every week.

We have presented this case study to illustrate that sometimes we will have clients who are determined, for one reason or another, to "go their own way," to some extent. While they may lean on the practitioner in some matters since they do respect, to a certain degree his/her judgment, background, and experience, they still have such explicit confidence in their own intelligence always to make correct choices, that they become somewhat difficult to work with. As practitioners, we must recognize that highly-intelligent individuals are somewhat locked in their egos; they are often difficult to work with. We have a choice to make: 1. To dismiss them as beyond our ability to cope, or 2. To help them as best we can through education and thus minimize their errors.

If we choose the latter course, one we personally prefer since such persons represent a real challenge, then we must guide carefully and have patience and understanding. Generally speaking, their innate intelligence and willingness to learn will lead them to make more correct choices than otherwise. And making incorrect choices, as any experienced Hygienist can testify, can be a great learning experience!

93.6.4. Case Study—Susie and Bill

In relating clients' case studies, we rarely use correct names. All matters discussed between the client and the practitioner should remain private. However, the people are real even though their identity remains their own private space. Their problems were their own as were their solutions and results—all were very real. We can all learn from their experiences, from their triumphs and from their rare defeats.

Susie and Bill are to be commended. They have diligently worked, and their bodies have accomplished an amazing return from severe long-established chronic conditions to a superb state of health. They have accomplished this, too, without the continued guidance of a Hygienist except for an occasional consultation plus periodic telephone counseling sessions.

Susie, like so many other women in their middle sixties, suffered from a painful arthritic condition which had caused her to retire early from her work as a dress designer. Bill had a rather severe skin ailment which had bothered him from time to time for many years: a type of granuloma. Susie and her husband had been on medications of various kind for many years.

With this couple, the wife was the leader. She insisted that Dr. Robert do a bio nutritional blood test analysis and profile for each of them. She next began to take a class in Applied Nutrition and was soon followed in this effort by her husband. It was not long before Bill became just as devoted to health-building as Susie.

Their first initial changes were made in meal planning. Bill began to garden. When possible, they drove to ranches in and around the Tucson area to pick fruit and obtain fresh vegetables which they did not grow themselves.

Susie bravely took the first 24-hour fast. Bill held back; a bit reluctant to take this "drastic" step. Next came the 36-hour fast, then a series of three-day fasts. Susie took them all in her stride and began to notice small improvements. Inspired by Susie's example and her improvement, Bill finally began his own fasting schedule. He really was brave: he began by skipping breakfast! But it wasn't too long before they were both taking turns, fasting from three to five days. They carefully monitored one another while fasting, recording temperature, respiratory rate, and pulse according to a rigid schedule:

1. On arising
2. At noon
3. At bedtime

The first five-day fast was taken by Susie and she found it more trying than her previous shorter fasts in that, on the fifth day, she experienced so much pain that she broke the fast abruptly and while still in pain. As a consequence of this error, she found it extremely difficult to regain the weight she had lost both during and subsequent to the fast. She reported that she also felt very tired at times, much more so than she had felt before. About six months ago Bill fasted for five days and just recently reported that he was, at that moment, on the third day of his second five-day fast.

This couple have been on a Hygienic program now for over four years. Needless to say, both have accrued much benefit from their learning experience. Susie has made a complete recovery from her arthritis. Her vitality is simply amazing, the admiration of all her friends and relatives. Bill's skin ailment is well under control now, but he is not completely free of lesions. He weighs a trim 135 pounds. Both look extremely well and happy.

They are both well-pleased with what following a sound Hygienic program coupled with periodic short fasts has accomplished for them and are only too happy to share their experiences with others whenever we schedule a lecture or have a potluck. They are very caring people and demonstrate it in their smiles and willingness to give the gift of health to others. They are unstinting in their praise, too, for the ones who, from time to time, guided them during their transition. Recently we were their guests for dinner.

While at the restaurant, we chanced to meet another non-Hygienic couple whom we know. With a beaming smile, following introductions, Bill said, "These people have given me 20 more years to live and enjoy my life!"

It is results like these that we practitioners can impart to hesitant clients. In and of themselves they can be a learning experience with great value. Additionally, the method, the steps taken by Bill and Susie may prove useful to other individuals and/or couples from time to time. With Bill, remember he started by missing his first breakfast!

93.6.5. Case Study—Ethel

Ethel, like so many of our students, began her Hygienic debut as a student in one of our public courses. Rather quickly, realizing her need, she became a private student.

Ethel was afflicted with many ailments, including extreme nervousness (she was almost hysterical), rheumatic involvements, skin problems, constipation, adrenal insufficiency, digestive troubles including passage of enormous quantities of gas; additionally, she was extremely depressed and enervated. There were also family troubles which were emotionally quite trying and no doubt these had contributed in a major way to her rather neurotic state. At times Ethel just didn't appear to be a participant in the real world but lived instead in a closed society of her own making.

In her middle 40s, Ethel had been on a medical merry-go-round for over 20 years. She had had it all! However, fortunately, she had escaped surgical intervention, possibly because for the last 12 years she had been under the care of an elderly chiropractic physician who dutifully kept her "propped up" with hormones and vitamins and other supplements and did not insist on her seeing a medical doctor. While debilitated to the extreme and somewhat confused, we felt she had sufficient vitality on which to build and, in the end, this conclusion was verified by the happy results which, in due course, followed.

This particular woman began her fast in the late summer. For the better part of a year, she had been under our care. She had gradually been introduced to a program which included improved nutrition, exercise and all the other Biodynamics of Life as and when they could be utilized, including having been, from time to time, schooled in the art of fasting.

Our client first began with a series of 24-hour fasts. She then went on the Transition Diet for a period of two weeks. Our students will recall that this regimen combines juices with two fruit meals per day. She rapidly advanced to three-day fasts, all of which were extremely well-tolerated by her.

During this time Ethel's condition had steadily improved until the time came when we felt she was in a condition to warrant a longer fast at an institution under expert guidance. Ethel, fully realizing the fact that she had improved steadily under some simple Hygienic care after a fruitless search for improved health for over 20 years, was eager for this new adventure. Arrangements were made for her to fast at Dr. Shelton's Health School and off she went.

We had asked this particular client to keep a diary. We were especially eager for her to do so because of her long history of being on various medications, including cortisone, various antibiotics, and hormones. She had also taken much aspirin and other pain killers and had been on megavitamin "therapy" for the last 12 years. No medication or supplements of any kind had been taken during the previous six months.

We recount her experience in her own words because they give us a rather vivid account of what can happen during a longer fast and especially when drugs have been taken for many years, but it also demonstrates how this one woman, well-fortified with knowledge about fasting, was able to go on in spite of all that happened during and subsequent to her initial longer fast.

93.6.6. Ethel's Diary

First Day Ate my last meal at noon.

Day Two My case history was taken.

Day Three The second day of my total fast. I am starting to feel very weak. My chest feels very heavy. I can hardly breathe. The lymphatic glands under and down my arm ache terribly and my left knee has been aching all night. In fact, I had to apply heat to it all night. I'm awfully hungry.

Day Four Unable to sleep. Too much pain. Pain in my knees, my chest, my hips, and lower back. I crawled out of bed, got a blanket, and wrapped it around me and huddled under a pile of other covers. I also had a heating pad and hot water bottles all around me. Chills, pain, and more chills. I'm really hungry now but don't much fancy eating anything. Just too much pain.

Day Five I ached all over, all day. No sleep. Same program as last night. Hurt too much to write any more.

Day Six Ached all night again. Only got an hour of sleep. Don't feel hunger at all today. Sat up most of today. My legs don't ache quite so much when I sit up. In bed, I can hardly stand them.

Day Seven Went to lobby. Slept really well last night. Awoke about 4 a.m. Legs at it again, ached. Sat outside a while today and then took a steam bath for about 30 minutes. That made me feel very weak. Went to bed and stayed there all afternoon. When I woke up, I found my stomach all covered with spots. Surprisingly enough, I felt real good this morning.

Day Eight Golly am I weak! Still have rash. I had a nosebleed this morning, too. Only got up twice today. Knees and hips real painful. Heating pad helps some, but not much.

Day Nine Feel pretty good, but awfully weak. Sat outside some in the sun. For the past three days, these pimples have been itching and I have had nose bleeds off and on, too.

Day Ten Feel fine. Sat in the sun for almost a half hour. And then in shade for several hours. Good day!

Day Eleven Woke up with sore gums. They got little bumps all over them. Sore throat, too, and a fever sore on my lip. Can't control the gas. It seems to come out through the vagina and rectum both. Sometimes it just piles up in me and it's hard to expel it. Pimples on ray stomach again and now on my legs. My lips are very sore.

Day Twelve The eleventh day of my fast. I feel very weary, very tired. Pimples are all over my stomach and now in the vaginal area. Some of them are forming pus heads, but we haven't seen any pus. Received a thorough examination today, which really relieved my mind.

Day Thirteen Had my first bowel movement and it was very odoriferous. More breaking out on my legs. I am so awfully weak. I could hardly make it back to the bed after that trip to the bathroom. And then I kept turning and tossing. My stomach is aching just awful. Did manage to crawl out of bed to fix a hot water bottle. No one else around. After that I fell asleep. I slept until after 4 and then I sat up a while but had to go back to bed again. So terribly, terribly weak.

Day Fourteen I have been fasting now for thirteen days. I am so tired. My chest still hurts bad.

Day Fifteen Day 14 of my fast. Very weak and tired. Haven't had to use any blankets now for the last two or three days. No real pain today. Just very, very weak.

Day Sixteen Broke my fast.

As the student can see, this fast was concluded before the return of hunger and even before her tongue had cleared or she had experienced any return of vitality. She remained for another week at the school. She knew she should have remained longer to permit a fuller recovery but, for financial reasons, she had to return home.

However, she immediately called us, and, under our guidance, she carefully followed a prescribed regimen which emphasized rest. She adopted a greatly restricted all-raw food diet which consisted of two mono fruit meals plus one salad meal composed of four vegetables, two of which were lettuce and sprouts. Every two months, she fasted for seven days and after six months, she undertook to fast for ten days and this on her own.

It might prove of interest to our students to observe what happened in the days immediately following her return from Shelton's School.

Day 1. Before I got through with my lunch, I had a bowel movement that filled the commode. I was sick at the stomach for the rest of the day. Dr. McCarter told me to stay in bed and rest.

Day 20. Swollen feet. Bad sinus trouble.

Day 21. Feet still swollen. Nauseous. Had watermelon for supper. Still have those pimples on my stomach. Dr. McCarter tells me to be patient, that they'll soon heal.

Day 22. Swollen feet yet. Pimples on stomach and legs again. My eyes just feel sick, and I have diarrhea.

Day 23. Feel pretty good today. Day 24. Feel pretty well.

Day 27. Didn't feel at all well tonight. Ate a lot of melon. Too much, I guess.

Day 28. Been feeling well, at least better, up until today. Felt "icky" after my noon meal of lettuce and nuts. Had BM three or four times during the last four days. Feel terrible tonight. Had some more watermelon.

Day 29. Slept outside for almost 3 hours. My arm hurt. Stomach ached. Had to use the hot water bottle again.

Day 30. Didn't feel well all day.

Day 31. Fasted. Didn't know what else to do. Dr. McCarter said it was okay. Slept two hours. Weak. Finally had BM. Felt better.

Day 32. Stomach hurt all day.

Day 33. Stomach feels better. Didn't eat this morning. Had avocado, alfalfa sprouts and tomato for lunch. For dinner, the same. Did eat a few nuts later on.

Day 34. Stomach feels better. Light lunch. Just nuts this evening. Felt quite well today.

Six Days Later. Fasted for three days. Stayed in bed. Not too bad. First day after the 3-day fast. Felt good.

Second day after the 3-day fast. Felt great! Better than I have felt for the last 20 years. Just absolutely GREAT!

Ethel continued to make so much progress that even her friends began to comment on how well she was looking. Her complexion became radiantly "alive." Her voice, which had been high pitched, developed more quality and depth to it. She had a sparkle about her that was entirely missing before she began to fast.

Much of the follow-up discomfort this woman experienced might well have been avoided if she had been able to continue her original fast at least until all her pain had disappeared and, better yet, of course until the return of hunger. As it was, only a partial cleansing of a highly toxic body took place and this, too, while the poisons were still in flux, but, as we have seen, in spite of all her pain and discomfort, this woman had been so well-prepared for her fast, that she persisted and continued her Hygienic transition. Within the year, she was back at Shelton's and fasted for another 14 days, this time with little or no discomfort.

How does this client feel about fasting? She has continued to fast one day every week, three days once a month and, every two months, she fasts for five days. In fact, we have to put the reins on her to keep her from fasting too frequently. She "checks in" every three months at which time we evaluate her experiences and her progress. Instead of sled riding downhill as she had been doing all those previous years, she is now confident that she is on the right path, using nature's own methods and tools. She has become radiantly beautiful and, if it were not for her still existing family disorientation, she would be at peace, not only physically, but also mentally and spiritually. Under great odds this woman has accomplished a small miracle. She has successfully confronted herself, has weeded out all the worms of doubt and, with deep conviction, has removed herself not only from the bondage of the current mass hysteria but also from her previous addiction to her own pet beliefs. She knows with a certainty that is unshakeable that she is one with nature and thus fears nothing that nature has to offer. She has learned the laws of life and they are serving her well.

93.6.7. Case Study—Rachel—Her Story

We will let Rachel tell her own experience with fasting. She tells it so much better than we could ever do because she tells it from her heart. When this was written, Rachel was in her late sixties. In her own words, this is Rachel's story:

"My name is Rachel. I have been asked to speak about my experience with fasting and its benefits on the body. And I'll tell you how I learned about the Shelton School of Health where health is built, not bought."

"I'll start by telling you how it all began. In early January of 1979, I started bleeding from the uterus, and hoping that it would go away. After it stopped for a while, I did nothing. In February, a friend asked me if I'd like to attend some nutrition classes given by Dr. Elizabeth McCarter, and after finding out the fee, I said, 'I can't possibly afford it!' My friend, however, told me that the first class was free, and said, 'Why don't you go?' So, I agreed.

"At this class I was convinced of all the things I was doing wrong for my body and, after attending all the sessions, I was convinced that this was money well spent.

"While Dr. McCarter spoke she also told us about Dr. Shelton's book which she carries with her in these sessions, and how she recovered her own health some fifteen years ago by following the rules outlined in his book. She had learned about the importance of fasting and its help in building the body back to health. (Editor's note: It was actually considerably later that we learned about Dr. Shelton and about fasting, but it was about this time that we began our search for healing.)

"At one of the classes my bleeding had again started, and I asked Dr. McCarter what I should do, and she said, 'Fast and rest.' I went home, missed one meal and my husband, Al, wouldn't hear of any more of that. My bleeding stopped again, until the first of May, when it started again. I knew I had to find out if something was the matter, so after three doctors from May 11th to the 14th, I was to have a DNC on Thursday, May 17.

"On the 19th, the doctor called to tell me, 'You have cancer! We'll set a date for an hysterectomy as soon as you have an IVP, lower GI, and X rays of the bladder, chest, etc.' 'The works,' as he put it.

"Again, I called Dr. McCarter and told her I didn't want to go through all of this as I had had two major surgeries in the past and problems with both. Since her talk in class, I had been wanting to cleanse my body by fasting, but never thought I'd ever have to do it, but I could see now was the time to consider it. So, I sought the Lord's guidance in prayers. These are the very words that flashed in my mind:

'Abide in Me.' 'Greater is He that is in you than he that is in the world.' And 'I will purify you; I will cleanse you; I will make you white as snow.' I was so thrilled and surprised as I had wanted my body cleansed and felt this was my answer from God.

"On Tuesday night I finally told Al about my condition. He was shocked and wanted me to have the surgery. Instead, I presented him with three alternatives since I felt this was my body; that I, too, should have a choice. I told him about Tijuana and the laetrile therapy, and about Dr. Shelton's School of Health in San Antonio, Texas. The third choice was simply to continue to lie around and rot.

"Al said, 'Not Tijuana!' And thus, it was, our choice was to lead me to Texas. "I called Dr. Vetrano at the school to see if they could accept me and, when she heard about my problem, she advised me not to have the X rays and all the rest but to 'come as soon as you can.' We set the date for the third day after that. So, I cashed in all my stocks so as not to worry my husband with anything. I had enough to buy my plane ticket, a few travelers' checks and to cover my stay at the school.

"On my arrival I felt strange. Here I was alone, in a strange town, and down in spirit because of all the opposition from so many people including most of my family, something which hurt me more than my condition. Besides never having fasted in my whole life, I can truthfully say that I was really frightened.

"... Feeling the way I did, I told one of the doctors there that I wasn't sure this is what I wanted, and, in fact, I called some friends who lived in San Antonio to come for me. While I waited, however, two ladies who had finished fasting talked to me about it and said, 'Since you have come so far and it will do you so much good, you ought to stay.' My worried friends arrived, and I asked them to sit down with me to talk about it. They listened quietly and when I had finished, I told them I felt much better about it all and would stay. It frightens me now to think that, in a split second, I could have thrown down the drain all I had set out to do for my body, and this experience alone was a worthwhile lesson for me. I thank the Lord again for helping me and keeping me there.

"I was not to begin fasting for two more days, so I decided .until then to interview the patients and get some information I wanted. When you fast, you are to remain quiet, talk little, walk slowly, etc. Let me tell you about some of the people I interviewed that day.

"One lady, only 25 years of age, showed me a small lump on her hand which she said had been as big as an English walnut, and after fasting 27 days, this was all the remained. She stayed two weeks longer and all of it had vanished. She left one week before me and returned the following Friday night to bring me a bouquet of flowers from the florist.

"Another lady, I'd say in her forties, who was in a wheelchair with muscular dystrophy, the wife of an M.D., who came against her husband's will to fast and had finished seven days of fasting. Soon after I came she had discarded her braces and was walking. She was so excited, as all of us were, when she told us she hadn't walked in years. She called her husband, and he didn't believe her. She was so thrilled with the results of the fasting that she was on her second seven-day fast when I left.

"One man and his wife had just finished a 30-day fast. Five years ago, they had been there. He is an M.D. They found cancer in his lungs and had scheduled surgery. He heard about the school and decided to try it. They also fasted 30 days and rested 30 days, went back home for more X rays and his lungs had cleared.

"An older man from Puerto Rico has been coming to the school since 1954. As I talked to him, I could see the small print in the book he was reading—and without glasses, too.

"A lady in her seventies, her son an M.D. in Texas. She lives in New York but also has a home in Germany. She came against her son's wishes because she had doctored with five physicians for years with fungus in her ears, under her nails, and her heart bothered her. She wasn't worried too much about her nails, just so she could get some relief for her ears. Well, in seven days of fasting, her ears and nails both cleared up. And she also had had hemorrhoids ever since her son had been born. She sunned these daily in the Solarium and she said that they, too, had dried up. She will go home a happy person.

"One of my roommates was a young girl, very stout who had fasted 27 days. She lost fifty pounds, and she had also had a yeast infection—whatever that is—and it had also left her. When she returned home, she called to see how I was. Everyone at the School was so nice, just like a big happy family, all there for one purpose, to get their health back.

A man in his late 60s drove all the way from Indiana. One day I was sitting in the lobby while fasting and he came up the steps two at a time. I commented, 'You can tell you are not fasting.' He said, 'Oh, yes! I still have another week to go for my 30th day!' He stayed until the day I left.

"I could go on and on. About 100 people from all over the world were here. My fast was fourteen days and I felt that I should have gone on to at least 21 for nature had not told me to quit: my tongue was still coated and my throat in back didn't tell me I was hungry but the lump in my breast the doctor wanted to take out when I had the DNC had disappeared.

"We had so many young people there fasting, which made me happy that they are learning so early in life how important your health is. In the lectures we learned what to expect during fasting, which made it easier for us. I had no problems since I gave up coffee after Dr. Elizabeth's classes and I took no drugs. Your body will smell, your mouth will fill with a salty, bitter saliva; your legs and parts of your body will ache, a backlash from those drugs in your past; the urine will darken, and many other things might happen. But it will all be for good. You will have to shower more often and brush your teeth. You will not be given drugs, enemas, pills, coffee, liquor, cigarettes, cooked food, milk—nothing except pure water, pure fruits, vegetables, and nuts—raw—the last three only after you have finished fasting. You are to remain the same time longer as the time taken to fast, in order for you to recover properly. This is important, I found out.

"Wouldn't it be nice if all the surgeons who have patients ready for an operation would say to them, 'Go home and fast for fourteen days and if you still need surgery, then we will operate.' Just think of how many would not need that surgery! For, by fasting, you rid your body of the toxins that are causing your problem in the first place, and when surgery takes place, your organs are removed, but you still have the poisons to cause more problems, for still more organs to be removed. Besides all that, you will be given more drugs and shots and pills and hard telling what else which also adds to your problem.

Some of the churches, not mine, are building their own hospitals. Wouldn't it be nice if these were used as Schools of Health, like Dr. Shelton's, where we might go and cleanse our bodies, and keep our organs? I purchased Dr. Shelton's tapes. I'd like all of you to hear them. He tells it like it is. (Wonderful to use at group meetings—the Authors.) "This is the way I feel about sickness:

1. Seek God's guidance first.

2. Fast. This is mentioned so much in the Bible.

453

3.   Eat the fruits, vegetables and nuts just as He gave them to us—raw. If only we will do this, we will live a healthy life.

We have let Rachel tell her own story because it demonstrates so well some of the points we have made in this lesson and in our lesson on the elderly. Not all, of course, but most of our clients are at least of middle-age, most are older. They bear the imprinting of all their past days, months, and years. They all, even the very young, come to the practitioner with their private hidden fears. Prior to their seeking Hygienic counseling, many have been engaged for years in a life-and-death balancing act, trying this, that and the other "cure." Many, if not all, have had significant psychological problems, chief among which have been depression and varying mood swings. Many of their friends and relatives to whom they look for support respond negatively, even to the point where they judge them to be crazy. It becomes the job of the practitioner to show them they are not. Few practicing healers, regardless of in what discipline they may work, comprehend that long-term illness of itself has a devastating effect on the emotional well-being. Multiple stresses arise and they certainly do not go away when first the client enters a Hygienist's office. In fact, they may well multiply. Suddenly, they are offered hope to replace despair; action to replace inaction. All this can be stressful, too.

All this can be especially true when it comes to fasting. Just as Rachel indicated, thinking about the possibility of not eating is a totally new experience. Such a thought can actually terrify timid individuals. But, have our students taken note of how Rachel's fears were quieted by hearing other people talk about their experiences with fasting? What she heard broke through the psychological barrier and prepared her mentally and emotionally. In fact, she went so far as to anticipate the benefits accruing to her by fasting. She began to build up positive mental images of future wellness, these in and of themselves, being conducive to good results.

Clients must be prepared by the practitioner to accept fasting as something which will specifically help them. Rachel was prepared before she went to Shelton's School, but she retained hidden fears. Clients can be helped across inner barriers by individual testimonies like Rachel's (it was given by her at one of our group meetings), by classes such as the ones Rachel attended, these being offered to the public for a fee. We hope our students noticed that the first class was offered FREE! Case studies such as we have cited often prove very helpful in acquainting clients with what fasting has to offer and, of course, Hygienic literature offers a wide range of these.

And did our students observe how varied the fasters were in Rachel's account? How different were their problems but, in every instance, through fasting, they obtained favorable results. Did our students also note that many, like Rachel, encountered family resistance which they had to overcome? And did our students observe that the fasters received emotional support and guidance from other fasters? These are among the many valuable lessons we can learn from Rachel's account.

We kept in touch with Rachel for a year or so but have now lost contact with her. We know that she periodically continued to fast on her own and became an enthusiastic supporter of the Natural Hygiene way of life.

Rachel was prepared to accept fasting as an opportunity for her to recover her own higher level of health, rather than a means of depriving her and placing her life at risk. Our society wants instant "cures," of which there are none. They are fascinated by the magic of a heart transplant, for example, and fail to look beyond the implant to the years of worry, concern, and always-present fear of sudden death from rejection by Self. It takes someone very special to take the steps that Rachel took to overcome the psychological buzz-sawing to which our people are constantly subjected on all sides. It also takes someone very special to guide troubled clients into and through a successful fast. This is what Rachel did and this is how she did it:

1. Being frightened by a personal physical problem, she took a course in Natural Hygiene; others seek solutions elsewhere.

2. During her class sessions, she learned how to eat, and how to live so that the precise needs of her body would be met.

3. She learned about the Toxemia Theory and about the seven steps in the evolution of pathology.

4. She learned about fasting and decided she loved herself enough to try this method of body cleansing.

5. She decided to make a change, to desert orthodoxy: the proposed surgery, the X rays, the drugs, in favor of Nature's own way of cleansing—self-autolysis; she decided to fast.

6. She began to plan. Step by step she made the necessary arrangements, prepared her family, got her finances, together, etc.

7. She began to work her plan.

8. She persevered and was successful. Her life, like so many others who have preceded her, is no longer being lived in the shadows of fear. That can be the priceless reward of teaching our clients all about fasting.

93.7. Useful Assignments for Reluctant Fasters

Reluctant fasters are child personalities in adult bodies. They are prisoners of prior imprinting. With such it may be useful to make the following assignment:

1. Write down how much you like yourself and tell why. Be specific.

2. Are you scared of the future? If so, tell what is bothering you.

3. Would you like to change? If so, why?

4. Tell how you would like to change. For example, if you suffer from disfiguring skin lesions, you might like to get rid of these. Put this down. Would you like to be more mentally alert? If so, that should go on your list, too.

5. Do you have any method or plan at the present to bring about the changes you would like to make? Tell us about it.

6. How do you think you can accomplish all this?

7. Have you given any thought to fasting as a means of helping you to change? If not, why not? Can we assist you to make a decision?

These are just sample questions to assign from time to time as you work with clients. Getting private thoughts, desires, ambitions down in writing can often open the door to

Action so that the bridge between the desire for something and the accomplishment of same can be successfully travelled.

In working with your clients remember, too, that short-term pay-offs are pleasurable and very important to your clients. They need to be made aware of them from time to time. Also, they should be aware of the fact that while small successes do add up in time, the ultimate health benefits will accrue only to those fully adult persons who desert their media-inspired, culturally-fostered and lifelong patterns of living and choose, intelligently and with dedication, the life-long rewards which the fasting experience will certainly bring.

93.8. The Elderly Client and Fasting

93.8.1. Transition into Fasting by the Elderly

In a previous lesson we have commented that those few persons who survive to an advanced age in today's polluted and frenzied environment, are the "tough ones." In order to survive, they have demonstrated not only physical stamina, but also mental stamina, this being witnessed by the very fact that they have, if mentally sound, successfully overcome all the many and varied kinds of emotional assaults that can arise to trouble all of us as we travel on that train that seems to gallop us all through life.

Each problem situation as it arose had to be evaluated by these people, and then dealt with as they saw fit.

The elderly clients who seek the advice of a Hygienic practitioner will, in most instances, listen carefully to what they hear, they will read the printed materials carefully, will listen to the stories by others in group meetings and in lectures, but then they will reach their own conclusions, whatever these may be: they will either find merit in their new knowledge or will discount it as not worthy of their trust.

If, in their view and according to their past indoctrination, they find their newly-acquired knowledge sound, they will be more inclined to follow the Hygienist's recommendations; if not, they will be reluctant, hesitant to do so. With emotional reservations, they may adopt whatever regimen is set forth.

Many times, clients will come to the practitioner exhausted, both physically and mentally but, nevertheless, they will have in reserve sufficient strength to resist change, especially if it is too abrupt. Therefore, we have found it advisable to advance rather slowly with our elderly clients. This is especially so when we believe that eventually a fast may be needed to bring about a successful resolution of a particular condition, say a chronic ailment of long duration.

In such cases we suggest the advisability of a prolonged fast immediately but then we "back away," offering an alternative regimen which begins with simple dietary and other suggestions. We then proceed on a planned program of detoxification that is even more prolonged than the one detailed in the lesson on hair. However, we do proceed as circumstances seem to indicate the time is at hand to move forward.

93.8.1. Transition into Fasting by the Elderly

Step One

An all-fruit day once each week, each meal to consist of one, two or three compatible fruits. Examples supplied to each client as, for example:

Oranges

Oranges and strawberries Grapes Bananas

Bananas and dates, etc.

To be continued for two weeks.

Step Two

An all-fruit day once each week with no more than two fruits to be served at all three meals.

To be continued for two weeks.

Step Three

TWO all fruit days per week, one of which is now a mono fruit day, the other permitting a variety of two fruits per meal.

To be continued for two weeks.

Step Four

One mono fruit day per week.

One partial fast day—only two fruit meals permitted on this day.

Thus, two days per week are now divided between a mono and a two-fruit-meals per-day regimen.

To be continued for one month.

Step Five

One mono fruit day per week. One 24-hour fast day per week. To be continued for one month.

Step Six

One mono fruit day per week.

One 36-hour fast day every other week. To be continued for one month.

Many elderly people will progress this far but will not progress any further. With a few, the practitioner may find them prepared emotionally to advance as follows:

Step Seven

One mono fruit day.

One 48-hour fast every other week.

Step seven should be followed for several months after which it would be appropriate to suggest that the client now fast one day each week and perhaps even a three-day fast once a month.

Using this step-by-step progression, the student will observe how easy it would be, should it prove necessary, to put a client on "hold," until such time as s/he would feel comfortable; or even to back track a step, should that prove necessary. Using this method demonstrates to the client that you are working with him/her and in his/her best interests. Few elderly clients appreciate being "pushed" into strange and unfamiliar territory, which fasting undoubtedly is, to fast. We must always strive to work within their levels of acceptance.

Few experienced Hygienists will permit an elderly client to fast at home, on his own, for longer than three days or longer than ten days even at a fasting institution under close supervision. The reasons should be obvious:

1. Their bodies bear the imprinting of many years of incorrect living. It is impossible to predict what biological storm might erupt to throw an unknowledgeable and uneasy client into a panic state, always a dangerous situation, which could even prove fatal.

2. The reserves of the elderly are generally limited, and it is often exceedingly difficult for an older person to regain the weight lost during the fasting period.

Thus, it is that we should be extremely thorough in our instructions and careful in working with clients as we teach them about fasting. In fact, it is far better to be cautious to the extreme than to risk negative responses, either emotional or physical. This is true with all clients but especially important when working with the elderly persons who seek our help.

93.9. The Learning Experience

93.9.1. Be Prepared

This lesson on teaching fasting to clients is intended as a learning experience for practitioners, a growing. Its intent is to open up avenues of thinking which can then be translated into methods to be used in the instruction of newcomers to fasting.

As our students have no doubt observed, we have not tried to hide the fact that, at times and with seriously-ill and/or highly-medicated or neurotic individuals, the fasting experience can be quite trying. This you should know.

It is our belief that everything we teach should be firmly rooted and have its bases in physiological, biological, and anatomical truths and that the more the practitioner knows about the mysteries of and the many possible experiences and/or problems possible while fasting, the better prepared s/he will be to teach clients about this important healing aid.

There are several aspects to be considered in teaching our clients about fasting. In order, these are:

First orientation

1. Personal needs of each client

2. Personal adjustments that may be required as the client considers the possibility of his/ her resorting to a fast

Overcoming fear

1. Overcoming anxiety and the loneliness of the fast itself

2. Making necessary economic adjustments

The obtaining of comfort while fasting

1. Physical

2. Emotional

Due consideration of past indiscretions and the extent of the existing physical decay as they may influence:

1. Length of fast—the determining factors

2. Intensity, extensiveness, and possible frequency of healing crises while fasting, as well as kind of symptoms

Each of these subjects has been addressed in some degree, many in an oblique manner as revealed in the several case studies of fasting clients.

93.9.1. Be Prepared

In teaching clients about fasting, it is well to be prepared. It is our feeling that our students are better prepared in this respect than students in any other healing discipline. However, we follow with some basic guidelines for students to consider as they work with their clients.

1. Be prepared. Know your subject and have some very definite points you wish your clients to consider at this time in learning about Natural Hygiene's principles and practices.

2. Cultivate a listening ear. Hear what your client's specific concerns are, not what you may think they are. Identify them as emotional? Economic? Real? Or fancied?

3. Be explicit in explanations. Don't hem and haw about or evade answering questions. Be open and direct, not evasive. If you don't know, say so but be sure you attempt to find the answer and then communicate your answer to your client.

4. Encourage your clients to ask questions about fasting and related subjects. They may reveal hidden fears and anxieties which can be cleared up at the onset of the learning session. Questions may also provide a grand opportunity for the practitioner to suggest certain reading materials to the client. His interest in a particular subject can then be enlarged and addressed.

5. Don't cover too much at any one session. Decide on specific aspects of fasting you wish to cover and then try to "remain on target."

For example, a series of discussions might well address the following topics «and in the order given:

1. What is fasting? How does it differ from starvation? Historical background and some of the reasons why people have fasted in the past, and also in the present.

2. Why should a person fast? What is meant when we say that the mind is in control?

3. Who should fast? Dr. Buchinger's list and our own list of other reasons for fasting may be a good place to start.

4. A follow-up of "c" with various case studies to be considered at the session and then taken home by the client for re-reading.

5. Where are suitable fasting facilities to be found? How much does it cost? Type of facilities, what to expect, etc. All information given should be as specific as possible.

6. Healing crises while fasting. What happens within the body?

93.10. Questions & Answers

I fully understand that fasting would help me with my sinus trouble. I also suffer from constipation and digestive troubles although both of these are responding to my improved diet. However, my family, and especially my husband, are totally against my missing a single meal, never mind going on a prolonged fast that may last two or three weeks. How can one resolve a problem like that?

Family opposition such as you describe may not be capable of full solution. From time to time we have family group meetings. If your husband would come to some of these, he might learn something about fasting and eventually give his consent for you to embark on a prolonged fast. If not, then continue on your present Hygienic path, being sure to meet all your body needs adequately. Miss a meal occasionally, several if and when you can. Healthful practices add up, in time, to major health benefits. It will just take you longer.

Will fasting help a person with a mental condition?

It all depends upon the underlying cause of the mental condition. If, for example, it is due to some kind of mechanical misconstruction, then it is doubtful that a fast would be of much, if any, benefit. However, if the sickness has come about through unhealthful eating and living practices which have in turn produced an inner toxic state, then the fast might be conducive to healing. It would all depend, of course, upon how much irreparable brain damage had occurred. However, in any case, a fast is worth trying before other, perhaps more dangerous, practices (such as surgery, hypnotism, and the like) be resorted to.

Isn't the fear of fasting an irrational fear?

It may well be, but it can be very real to the person thus afflicted, so real, in fact, that it can prevent his ever beginning a perhaps badly needed fast or it could actually produce great harm should the person who is overcome with fear nevertheless attempt to fast. This is why we emphasize the need not only to acquaint clients with the fasting concept but also to school them thoroughly before they undergo even a rather short fast. We should remember that best results are always obtained when a client has explicit faith in the fasting procedure and, also, in the practitioner.

Why is it that fasting is beneficial in some conditions, but less so with others?

That is a good question and one that perhaps needs to be addressed more in our studies. People are different. Diseases, with a few exceptions, all have a common cause, namely a toxic state of the body brought about by multiple errors in living and eating, these sustained over a varying amount of time by each individual and in differing ways and intensities. The greater the number of assaults, the intensity of the assaults, the kind of morbidity developed—all such will determine the nature of the condition and the extent of wasting of vital force which has subsequently ensued. Now if nerve tissue has been completely destroyed, it will be irreparable. Once brain damaged, always brain-damaged. If bones have been grossly abused, then full recovery may be impossible. Just as individuals differ in their respective backgrounds and life experiences, so will the forthcoming results of a fast differ. Additionally, the attitude of the fasting person will influence, either for good or bad, the results of a fast.

However, let us emphasize that, regardless of the nature of the illness, if the individual embarks on a fast by first becoming well informed about the fast, what to expect from the fast, etc., s/he will receive benefit from it in many ways, chief among which will be a greater systemic peacefulness. Even in terminal cases, the patient's last days can be made more comfortable when the fluids of the body have once been cleansed.

I am still at a loss to know just how we can tell when a fast should be broken.

Can you perhaps clarify that for me?

Most Hygienists will agree that it is impossible to tell, in advance, just when to break a fast. It is important to make this point clear to your students. Ideally no time limit should be set forth at the onset of the fasting experience. The fast should, and again let us say, ideally, continue until certain definite signs appear. The return of natural and usually quite acute hunger is probably the most important sign that the need to continue the fast has ended and that the person should now begin to take in food. This is a sure sign that the digestive system is ready to receive, process, and absorb nourishment and, further, that the system is ready to assimilate the nutrients as received at their final destinations, the cells. There are also other signs, such as the clearing of the mucus overlay from the tongue, the return perhaps of a more normal pulse, etc. The individual body should be the sole determiner of the precise time to break the fast simply because it will give forth with these reliable signs, signs which should not then be ignored.

Whenever a fast is broken before nature's clear signs have indicated the need for termination, then we should understand that while nature has cooperated with us thus far, a complete cleansing has not, as yet, taken place and that more remedial work will have to be undertaken at a later time. I think that much of the post-fast discomfort that Ethel, for example, experienced and the fact that she had to undergo a whole series of fasts for a period of some years before she experienced the resurgence of health for which she was looking, was due, in large measure, to the fact that she broke her fast far too early, not because she wouldn't have been willing to go on, but purely because of her economic limitations.

What do you consider to be the most important role of the practitioner when it comes to the fast?

That question bears right down to the subject of this lesson. Our role should and must be to acquaint our clients with fasting, to tell them about the possible benefits that might accrue to them through fasting, to inform them about the possible symptoms that might arise during the experience, and WHY they may occur, and how such can be helpful rather than harmful; etc. In other words, we should help our clients to understand how fasting might help THEM to recover from whatever ails them.

Article #1: Health Secrets of a Naturopathic Doctor by M.O. Garten

"Cell Cinders" as Causes of Diseases The

"Towel—Salt Water" Experiment

Secondary Changes that Happen

The Process of Autolysis

Action of the Stomach During the Fast

The Gallbladder

The Pancreas

The Small and Large Intestine

Heart and Blood Vessels

The Pulse

The Blood

The Lungs

The Skin

The Kidneys and Bladder

"Cell Cinders" as Causes of Diseases

The European terminology of "cell cinders" as cause of disease most accurately drives home the point. It is generally agreed that civilized eating practices make all of us prone to overeat. It is said that up to the age of twenty, a man can eat as much as he can—up to forty as much as desired and after that he should eat as little as possible. Hippocrates made the statement that "if a sick person is fed—one feeds the disease. On the other hand, if the sufferer is withheld from food the disease is fasted out." How true, as I have observed in thousands of cases.

The disease process begins most gradually, but insidiously. In metabolism we find two stages, one of building up—the other of tearing down. The latter stage is the guilty one. Foods are not completely torn down and eliminated as formerly mentioned. Uric and carbonic acid remnants may undergo crystallization, obstructing metabolism. Cholesterol may clog lining of vessels and capillaries, where in some cases it may create

464

starvation in the midst of plenty. Calcium carbonate may infuse joints, muscles, or vessel structure, bringing on arthritis, rheumatism or hardening of vessels.

The "Towel—Salt Water" Experiment

For best illustration, let us take a small towel. Let us dip this fabric into a solution of salt water. The towel is permitted to dry after which we will find a drastic change in the appearance and "feel" of the material. No longer does the towel feel soft and pliable— it is now rigid like a board and feels hard and brittle. In the immersion, the salt water saturated through the fabric as a liquid but in the drying process changed into crystals. On closer examination we would find the crystals over, under and around every fiber.

Such is the case as so pointedly termed "cinder infusion" by the European experts as bringing on a ravages of disease.

Secondary Changes that Happen

It is axiomatic that Secondary changes usually occur as the result of this cell strangulation. Tissues, organs, or glands become diseased and undergo degeneration. Necrosis, (tissue destruction) is frequently observed in post-mortems. This, incidentally, may explain the disagreeable stench given off by some chronic cases during the fast. Putrefactive changes can also be noticed which explains the body odor. The entire disease origin problem gravitates into the symptoms of blockage. Remove the obstruction and the channels and fibers of life throb into renewal activity and good health.

The living organism must maintain its oxidizing mechanism in order to keep from dying. During the fast, the food now must come from within. The body economy now can accomplish chemical changes so perfectly as being unmatched by any other laboratory process. Uric acid can actually be transformed into protein, from whence it came. Cholesterol is reconverted to fat—carbonic acid changed to starch or sugar. It is the great transformation or operation without the knife which takes its course with the greatest of precision.

The Process of Autolysis

The process of autolysis (self-consumed) is inaugurated. All tissue components, not essential, are oxidized or burned in order to maintain life. This is the incredible manifestation of higher intelligence taking over command.

Many alterations can now be observed in the entrance to the digestive organs. Most noticeable is the coated tongue and disagreeable mouth odor. This unpleasant emanation does not come from the newly displayed phlegm but mostly from the lungs. Here we find body chemistry in a noble effort to bring about elimination of hardened infusion, liquified by the fast. This cleansing is carried out predominantly by the blood and lymph stream, using kidneys, bowels, and skin as an exit for the dissolved waste products.

The sometimes-obnoxious odor could also come from partially degenerated organs undergoing dissolution. Last, but not least, the odor generally also originates in the colon, the great "sewer pipe" of the body. Sluggish bowel action and impacted fecal material could contribute by the production of noxious gases which in turn reach the lungs through osmosis to be removed to the outside through the breath. While fasting, it is advisable to stay away from people as much as possible. The coating from the tongue should be removed twice daily with a stiff toothbrush.

Action of the Stomach During the Fast

Under a complete fast, where only water is consumed, hydrochloric acid production is greatly reduced. This is the one significant improvement to the juice diet in which stomach acidity is not always retarded. Consequently, hunger sensations may become prolonged, making the juice diet more difficult to withstand.

The first two or three days of the fast are the most trying to go through. After that, most hunger pangs disappear after which the individual seems to "float," strangely feeling free of many disagreeable sensations in the abdominal region. Buchinger reached this stage only after the fourth day when he stated that "everything became quiet on the Western front." Rumblings from fermentations lessen; all organs appear to greatly appreciate the new well-deserved rest.

An important change in the stomach is its shrinkage during the fast. The normal healthy stomach in an adult is supposed to equal the size of two fists, holding a little more than one pint. That this is not the case in us "civilized" beings can be attested by all surgeons or morticians. I have seen stomachs in post-mortems measuring several times the normal size. Such distended stomachs have exceedingly thin walls resulting in defective function. In the prolonged fast, the shrinking process of the stomach goes on and stops, whenever the normal size has been regained.

The Gallbladder

Here we may find drastic reactions to the sudden withdrawal of food. Secretions of gall continue to accumulate in this reservoir, in some cases in an increased tempo. The solution may often regurgitate into the stomach, giving rise to temporary spells of nausea or vomiting.

The Pancreas

In the fast, the pancreas reduces in size. The functional integrity of the digestive portion of the gland is greatly enhanced. The endocrine part (Islands of Langerhans) often becomes so reactivated as to reduce implications of diabetes.

The production of hormones or digestive ferments is somewhat sluggish immediately after the fast. It may take several days to bring about normal secretion, explaining the importance of breaking the fast correctly.

The Small and Large Intestine

The small intestine also shrinks in both length and diameter. The colon, besides shrinking, undergoes a decided reorganization.

About 75%, or three quarters, in the amount of stool is made out of bacteria, dead or alive. It is interesting to learn that the colon may become completely sterile in a ten day fast. Still more significant is the problem of impacted feces. A British surgeon once made the statement that the average man carries with him such hardened bowel wastes to the extent of between several ounces to as much as fifty pounds. I have seen colons on the marble slab practically being rigidified with unelimin ated retained stool. Only a small opening in the center permitted passage of some bowel content.

During the fast, the impactions clinging to the colon wall loosen, and copious stools are passed. This is one of the most perplexing experiences to a faster, when no food has been ingested.

Heart and Blood Vessels

The heart again assumes normal shape in the fast; vessels become freed of their clogging infusions (cholesterol). The average size of a well-fed "civilized" heart is enlarged, which is now being corrected.

The vessels and capillaries of the heart (coronary) receive a most thorough cleansing, restoring normal fluid circulation. It is also possible that the fast could absorb scar tissue formations in cases of rheumatic heart conditions. How else could one explain the amazing improvements achieved by the fast in such cases?

As to abnormal blood pressure, it is amazing how quickly and efficiently the fast comes to the rescue. High pressure ratings lower from day to day—most likely due to the absorption of cholesterol. In the case of abnormal low pressure, the explanation is more difficult. Undoubtedly, the adrenal glands are involved, where functional integrity is brought about by the fast.

The Pulse

The pulse is usually increased at the start, then falls below normal as the fast continues. Rates may vary from forty to one-hundred-twenty beats per minute, which may become erratic from time to time.

Should the pulse remain irregular for longer periods, or when extremely low or high pulse rate prevail, the fast should be broken.

The Blood

While the quantity of the blood volume is reduced in proportion to loss of body weight, the quality of the blood is greatly improved during the fast. It is amazing to observe the gradual increase in red cells in the blood picture.

Dr. Weger and Dr. Tilden reported cases of pernicious anemia where the red count doubled in periods from one week to twelve days. The abnormal high white count had also been reduced two-and-one-half times during these observations.

The primary reason for anemia accordingly is not nutritional deficiency, but cellular obstruction in organs and glands preventing utilization of the food. The blood-building mechanism in bone marrow, liver, spleen, etc., is put into a higher degree of perfection by the cleansing action of the fast. This does not mean that nutrition is of no consequence to the relative state of the blood. This, however, is always secondary—improper body chemistry coming first. This is why many top European sanatoriums inaugurate dietary reforms with temporary food withholding.

The Lungs

The gradual absorption of mucus from the miles of hair-like tubes in the lungs make deep and effortless breathing a most pleasant experience to the faster. The voice becomes clear and resonant.

The fast does provide an excellent opportunity to practice deep breathing. In some of such experiments it was established that the volume of breath intake (air) doubled. In connection with skin brushing with dry brush, great improvements in the general oxidizing mechanism of the body can be attained.

The Skin

The skin as well as the teeth are the parts that reveal a true indication of body condition.

With the lowering of metabolic efficiency, the skin becomes pale, then and dry with development of many folds. Secretions of perspiration lessen with an increasing difficulty of keeping warm.

During the fast, the skin resumes more effectively its role of body cleanser. Perspiration may become odoriferous as it may carry dissolved particles of uric acid, decomposed cells, etc.

One of the most gratifying effects of the fast is the observance of changes of the skin. The once shiny cigarette paper appearance, particularly on extremities, changes over to a more velvety texture, the skin loses its shine and many folds, and becomes thicker.

The Kidneys and Bladder

Constituting the great filter apparatus of the body, it can be seen that the kidneys participate greatly in this new effort of body reorientation. At the start of the fast, the urine is invariably dark in color, strongly acid in reaction, and of high specific gravity. Dissolved uric acid, phosphates and bile pigment are making up the ingredients responsible for the relative "thickness" of the urine. The odor may become offensive.

As the fast progresses, the color of the urine becomes lighter, being less odoriferous. This improvement in urinary characteristics is in direct proportion to the amount of cellular waste being "melted" out of the body structures. It must be remembered that next to the colon, the kidneys carry the largest load in the removal of metabolic waste from the body.

To fully appreciate the benefits bestowed by a fast to the urinary system, one should follow a typical case. A male patient came to me, complaining of constant burning sensation in region of bladder. The patient submitted to a twelve-day fast, after which all burning sensations disappeared and the man slept through the entire night.

Buchinger made a thorough study of this kidney-bladder phenomenon and broadly speaks of specific antibodies produced by the body during the fast. Accordingly, the fasting organism in its concentration on worn put or diseased tissues, manufactures certain "medicinal" agents from the diseased organs to be used in the healing or repair of such organs. This protective mechanism partially explains seemingly impossible correction of long-existing disease processes. Other investigators have corroborated Buchinger's assertions and claim the faster's urine to be virtually a healing concoction.

Incidentally, Buchinger's first patient, a woman physician, aborted a handful of kidney stones after an eleven-day fast.

From the book, Health Secrets of a Naturopathic Doctor by M.O. Garten

Lesson 94:

Exercise and Children

94.1. Introduction

94.2. Exercise from Birth to Adolescence

94.3. Conclusion

94.4. Questions & Answers

Article #1: Exercise for Baby by Dr. Herbert M. Shelton

94.1. Introduction

With today's current trend of "sit-down" activities, America's facing a grim reality—our youth population is not as physically fit as we thought it was. In tests done to determine strength, endurance and physical ability today's youth scored very poorly. It is not uncommon to read about a teenager succumbing to a heart attack while performing intense physical training. Passivity has a strong foothold on the youth of today. With the availability of video games, television, computers and all the other leisure devices, our children are gradually becoming less and less capable of sustaining any substantial physical activity.

Many children who dwell in the large, industrialized cities throughout the U.S.A. (and elsewhere) are being deprived of experiencing the "real" outdoors. They have no working knowledge of nature—no connection whatsoever with wildlife and many could not even tell you where the food they consume came from.

It is very disturbing to think that the vast majority of our youth are daily ingesting pseudo-foods and would rather die before they sample some wholesome foods. The parents in today's fast-paced, make-a-quick-buck society are relinquishing their obligation of protecting and taking care of their children and are oftentimes leaving their children's dietary needs to the whims of the junk food manufacturers and physicians who are less informed about nutrition than even they are. It is no big surprise when our children are constantly placed on the treadmill of visiting doctors to having no stamina at all in accomplishing the simplest physical task.

Parents, your children are being victimized and so are you. It is time you grab the reins and take control! Don't allow the manufacturers of trash foods to pollute your children's bodies, nor their minds.

You need to pay close attention to the types of foods you buy, the types of influences that your children receive and last but not least you the parents should be setting the prime examples for your young ones. This includes a rigorous exercise program that you can include your children in.

Natural Hygiene recognizes the value of physical fitness and advocates it as one of the main essentials in life along with a diet of fresh, raw fruits, vegetables, nuts, and seeds; fresh air; sunshine; pure water; etc. Natural Hygienists teach that your child needs to spend most of his/her time in an environment that promotes healthful habits and is conducive to building strength and stamina and endurance. This environment would be one where the child derives pleasure in using his/her body to its maximum potential. The sooner you start providing this environment, the better.

94.2. Exercise from Birth to Adolescence

94.2.1. Different Stages of Development

94.2.2. Other Factors Exercise and Females

94.2.1. Different Stages of Development

94.2.1.1. Infancy: Birth to First Birthday

To a lot of people, the mere suggestion of exercise for an infant brings all sorts of reactions. But a factor that has been long ignored is that behavior patterns established early in life tend to be self-perpetrating. The child is much more likely to be receptive to physical activity if exposed at an early age than a child who is not exposed at all or much later. As parents then, the job of insuring your child's total well-being is entirely yours, and it is crucial that only the best quality of input is directed at your child.

Today children are being shortchanged. In this increasingly demanding society where both parents are forced into the workforce just to "make ends meet" children are viewed as mere appendages—as tax write-offs of extra expenses. They are not viewed as replacements for the previous generations to carry on the work of tomorrow. If they were, they would be treated with more dignity and be allowed to grow and learn in a natural environment.

Most children nowadays are sentenced to spending the day inside artificial environments called day care centers. On the way to and from there they spend strapped into car seats. When they go out, instead of being allowed to walk they are strapped into strollers and rolled down the street. At home when mother and dad have no time for baby, he or she is placed in a mechanical swing set, a jolly jumper, or a playpen to keep out of mother or dad's way. This allows the parents to catch up on all they were unable to do all day because they had to be away at work. In this type of situation, a child can scarcely grow to be supple and strong as when I was a child. I (and most people in my generation) grew up able to run and play all day to my heart's content. I got plenty of fresh air and my heart got a good workout. Most of the mechanical contrivances to imprison children were not yet invented. Also, parents did not have to work so hard to earn a living as the cost of living was not so high as today—generally the mother remained at home with the children to teach them how to grow.

In many cases now the only muscles that are developed in infants are those in their jaws and mouths. They're constantly being fed as a pacifier as it takes less effort to feed them than to indulge in physical activity with them. Parents, the key word is active. A child needs to be allowed to stretch and move him/herself without binding. Encourage him/her to crawl and make other physical motions.

The First Six Months: This time is spent getting acquainted with your newborn, giving love and warmth. It is also a good idea to move the infant about while holding him/ her to get s/he familiarized with motion. Even though the child might seem floppy at first, don't be alarmed. With practice certain exercises will stimulate the muscles and strengthen them.

Besides merely moving the infant about in your arms, use gravity to produce physical activity in your baby. Hold your infant in the air horizontally, face downward. S/he will instinctively use the muscles of the neck and trunk to support the head and body against the pull of gravity. You can begin this activity as early as four weeks and as the weeks progress you will notice a remarkable difference in your child. S/he will be able to raise the head, arms, and legs on his/her own.

Remember that at birth the strongest muscles are in the back of the neck. The child is better able to support its head when face down than face up.

By ten weeks you can start pulling the child up by both arms slowly. At first his/ her head may bob about a little, and that due to a lack of control in that area, but with continued effort more strength is gained, and more control of the neck and trunk will be noticeable.

Another activity is holding the child in a standing position so that s/he supports his/ her own weight. The infant pushes with its feet against whatever surface (your lap, the floor) it is stood on. This activity can be started early for maximum benefit—by the time your child reaches around 26 to 28 weeks. Such maneuvers will be rewarded by your child being able to make bouncing and dance-like movements which will lead to the child cultivating the habit of carrying his/her own body weight. Your child will sit earlier, crawl earlier and walk earlier than most children whose parents haven't taken the time to properly exercise the child. S/he will also have much better control in these activities.

At the end of the first six months when the infant gains the strength and ability to sit, be sure that s/he is well propped up at all times. Also, the use of the arms and hands shouldn't be restricted to allow the muscles in those areas to be developed.

Most parents today with all the demands placed on them by society are finding less and less time to spend with their children and are often inclined to purchase "timesaving devices" that are pawned off as aids to mom and dad and junior. Contraptions such as mechanical swing sets, jolly jumpers, walkers, and mechanical rocking chairs to name a few. These devices encourage passivity in children and should be discouraged. They give the child a sense of movement coming from some force other than him or herself. As a parent it is imperative that you make time to see that your child receives all the physical activity possible. That is the key—allow your infant to fully experience freedom, freedom from diapers and other binding clothing whenever possible, freedom to explore the environment, freedom from all mechanical contrivances and restraints. Again, as a parent it is your responsibility to inspire active exercise in your children and with the practice you gain in the first six months of your child's life, your next six months will be even more fun as the effort you had put forth is now being rewarded.

As your child begins to show signs of more physical development such as crawling and creeping, you can add to his/her exercise by providing pillows and large cushions to his/her path. This will teach your child to crawl over obstacles and further develop the muscles. When s/he begins to stand and walk (which varies from child to child—usually within the range of 8 to 13 months), s/he will find other uses for the pillows and cushions. A child might use pillows for carrying toys around or any number of uses s/he might conceive. This process helps the child to develop muscular strength and a feeling of accomplishment.

As your child's ability increases, you will need to use your imagination more to maintain his/her interest. Here are a few suggestions: Pile larger stacks of pillows to form a tower, provide a large cardboard box that could be used as a tunnel or a house, etc.

At this age you can also try the wheelbarrow. This exercise is quite simple. Place the infant on a comfortable surface face down. Lift the bottom half of his/her body holding the child by the waist or legs around the ankles. On the onset the child might not respond, but soon will try to support his/her own weight with the arms.

Now as your child develops you must consider the matter of child-proofing your home. Some parents attempt to restrict their child's movements around the house as a means of insuring noninjury to child and damage to their valued possessions. This usually ends up in frustration for both parents and child.

It has been my experience that the sanest thing to do is to child-proof your home or apartment. What does child-proofing mean? It simply means that your house will not be a smorgasbord of temptation to the now mobile child. Everything you don't want your child into or that may pose a danger to him/her must be placed out of sight and out of reach plus a few other safeguards. Example: Place a gate near the stairways as the child has no concept of danger of heights at first. Remove all floor lamps, floor plants, covering electrical outlets, etc. My experience is that all the things you cherish when placed out of sight and reach can make for a more relaxed environment for the child and the parent. The child will be able to explore at his own pace without restriction of physical activity. Another important piece of advice—each year children are poisoned by household chemicals, paint removers, insecticides, and other harmful health hazards. If you do use these, keep them in a well-secured area preferably where they're locked up. If living

Hygienically, however, very few chemicals will be around the house (exceptions may be those used for hobbies and crafts).

Parents, exercise caution when it comes to the well-being of your youngster. Don't settle for cliches from so-called "experts." Be conscious of all phases of your child's growth and development. At this stage of development mother's milk is the optimum food. In discussing physical health, it is imperative that the subject of diet be brought into play. Besides lack of physical activity, the conventional diet of high fat, high protein and high calories is a main contributing factor of juvenile obesity and other maladies. During the Vietnam War autopsies performed on the U.S. soldiers showed that the vast majority had the beginnings of heart disease. The majority of these soldiers were no older than twenty-two years of age. Disease does not always appear immediately. It tends to be cumulative. The common notion that if it doesn't harm me right away all is well, is deceptive. Remember all things take time to develop, even disease. The sooner we adapt a healthful lifestyle, the better the chances are of continuously enjoying our lives.

94.2.1.2. Toddlerhood: One to Three Years

This is the time which your child is fully experiencing his/her strength and skills. The entire world is at his or her command. S/he is constantly doing things that meet with parental disapproval. It might seem like the child is totally oblivious to anyone else's needs but his/her own. But the truth of the matter is that the child is exercising his/her independence, which can be very annoying at first. Your usual pace is slowed down by your child's insistence in taking care of him/herself. It will eventually soak in that this will be the way things are going to be, and it is the parent who will need to adapt in order for the child to grow. Let your youngster run, climb, hike, ride a tricycle—anything that will promote physically-motivated activity. At this point, the best you can do as a parent is to encourage the child and to create a sense of enjoyment in what s/he is doing. Playing to exhaustion is a natural state for a child. However, we are programmed from our youth to feel that it is harmful to be exhausted—to sweat and get sore or experience any kind of pain from activity. Strenuous activity (play) that causes perspiration has been suppressed vigorously in this society. There are even campaigns by large deodorant manufacturers denouncing sweating as something abnormal and they've invested millions of dollars to promote such misinformation.

So, parents, the ball is in your hands, and your goal now is to continue to provide inspiration for your youngster. Some children need less attention in this area than others. My sons need little inspiration to exercise. They are three and six years of age and have the energy of two cyclones which keeps my wife and I on our toes and in shape.

Remember to play hard whenever you play. The benefits are countless. Not only will you get yourself in shape, but you will instill an attitude of positivity toward physical activity in your child. The example parents set for their children now will determine his/ her outlook on life in the future. So now is the time to start the exercise program for you and your children that you have been putting off for so long.

I also recommend that when you engage in physical activities that they be done outdoors as much as possible. It doesn't matter what the activity, when done in the fresh air it provides a great exchange of carbon monoxide and I oxygen and strengthens the lungs. But not every day will the weather be perfect and for those days when you might be forced to be indoors, you can pass the time and continue developing your child's wellbeing with some of these exercises:

The Back Lift: This is an excellent exercise for your toddler as it develops strength and flexibility in the back and shoulders, and it is easy to learn. To execute this exercise your child should sit on the floor with legs out in front. The legs should be flexed moderately at the knees so that only the feet and buttocks are touching the floor. He/she then should lean backward placing the arms behind the back with fingers pointing backward and away from the body. From this position the child lifts the trunk off the ground supporting his/her entire weight with the feet and arms. This posture as stated before will strengthen the back and shoulders, ankles, and arms. Incidentally, this exercise can also be done outside, weather permitting.

Your youngster will need your enthusiasm and guidance in doing exercises. Keep the exercises varied and short to enhance the period spent doing physical activity. As your youngster matures, more of his or her time will be spent outdoors at least part of the year, depending on the region you're living in.

It is common practice for parents to restrict outdoor activities during the winter months. This is not very wise because the child should be enjoying the cool fresh air that the winter brings. Another practice that is common is for the parent to overdress the child believing the child will "catch cold" if not bundled up. This bundling renders the child totally immobile—the child resembles a blimp ambling around the playground not being able to fully experience the outdoors. I've observed that children after a few minutes of hard play begin to shed layers of clothing naturally. From this I have come to the conclusion that if the child is dressed for movement and is allowed to remove clothing as needed, the body will generate its own heat on the strength of the physical activity the child is engaged in. When the weather is cold, it is wise to treat the situation as a normal occurrence. Let your child experience it and save yourself some aggravation by dressing your child so warm, that s/he is unable to move and comes indoors not knowing what to do with him/herself.

94.2.1.3. The Preschooler: Three to Six Years

This phase of your youngster's life is when s/he begins to demonstrate skills such as talking, limited reasoning abilities and more concern for others. S/he is capable of executing oral instructions but still likes to have a guide handy to take him/her through the paces. Your youngster is now developing a personality. Your child will let you know his/her dislikes and likes. S/he is forming attitudes and character that will serve him/her throughout the rest of his/her life. It is very important to recognize this and to instill only positive attributes.

Your youngster's motor skills are now well defined and activities like swimming, skating, and running are more to his/her liking. S/he is now ready for vigorous activities and delights with being offered challenges. This phase of your child's life is important as are all phases of growth and any wrong programming will have to be deprogrammed in the future to accomplish any progress. Parents, be aware that girls are also entitled to develop strength and endurance, courage and all the benefits that go along with physical activity (more on this further on in the lesson).

Your youngster's body is now capable and functional and should be exposed to activities that will promote strength, endurance, coordination, and conditioning. If you are like many parents, you will be entertaining visions of a star athlete in the family, but it will do you well to put such thoughts in the background for a while. Let your youngster enjoy the pleasures of being active without great expectations. Running is a very good way to introduce your youngster to sports/fun activities.

Swimming is another excellent activity. At this point in your child's life, it is important to be conscious of his/her limitations and you should not try to push the child beyond his/her capabilities. It is a good idea upon engaging your youngster in any sports activity that he or she be provided the proper clothing to begin with. Loose-fitting cotton clothing is necessary to allow for movement and the skin to breathe. Also, an ill-fitting shoe could cause much discomfort and contribute to the child not being able to sustain any prolonged activity.

Remember also that your youngster enjoys the outdoors and that every effort should be made to see to it that s/he gets an opportunity to experience rain or snow, to touch, feel and be a part of the natural weather processes. At this time skills that your child has already developed should be built upon. To add to his/her basic abilities keep in mind at all times that childhood should be fun. So whatever activity your youngster is engaged in should be approached with an attitude of fun. This will minimize the chance of him/ her becoming bored and disinterested and eliminate the need for parental pressuring to excel. Also don't stand by and criticize how your child is doing. This can cause your child to lose interest.

Your main function as a parent/coach is to monitor which phase of your child's daily exercises needs more attention. This can be determined by the following: How does s/he use the body to jump, run, drag heavy objects, or do chin-ups, sit-ups, push-ups, etc. These exercises promote strength and are within your child's range of capabilities and should be encouraged. Watch your child progress in these and make suggestions to the child as to what exercises need to be improved, whether the back should be straightened, which ones should be done more, etc.

The above-mentioned exercises can be classified into two groups: resistance and nonresistance. Resistance exercises are when the muscles are made to contract against an applied load, such as in weight training. Nonresistance exercises, on the other hand, are natural and involve the body to work against gravity with no outside items necessary. Within these two groups are subgroups: isometric and isotonic. Isometric exercises involve the muscles shortened by the tension of the exercise but does not contract. Isotonic exercises cause the muscles to contract under constant tension.

Nonresistance exercises are safer than resistance exercises but are not as effective when it comes to building strength since the pull of gravity is the only load against the child's body. This type of exercise is limited by the size of the child and child's potential ability. Another plus for nonresistance exercises though is that it can be started at any age including infancy.

Resistance exercise training should not be introduced until age nine or ten and only after your child has been involved in nonresistance training to firm up the muscles and tendons for stress that is involved in a resistance exercise program. Remember nonresistance exercises are performed without the use of added load or resistance. Gravity and the child's weight are the only load on which the muscles work and requires minimal supervision. These, of course, can be performed by boys or girls.

Push-ups are one of the many nonresistance exercises. To execute the child lies face down and flat on the floor, hands next to the shoulders and palms down. Legs should be straight back with the heels together and the toes on the floor supported only on the hands and toes. The child should then push the body straight up until the arms are fully extended and the elbows are straight. The youngster then dips down by bending at the elbows until the chin and chest barely touch the floor, then straighten up again. It is important to keep the spine straight while performing push-ups—don't allow the tummy to sag to the ground. For a variation of this exercise place hands about two hands widths to the side of the shoulders.

Sit-ups are another excellent nonresistance exercise. The child lies flat on the back, hands clasped behind the head, legs bent so that the thighs and legs form a right angle with each other. The soles of the feet should be flat on the floor. Next s/he lifts up the trunk, curling the neck, shoulders and back completely off the floor. S/he then leans forward, touching the elbows to the knees. For added stress, the exercise can be performed on a slant board with head on down end. It is necessary to use a strap or a bar if your slant board is not equipped with one. This will prevent the body from slipping down the board. Also, the slant board should be used only after some degree of strength has been obtained by the child in doing sit-ups from the floor.

Knee bends are good as well. The youngster stands straight, feet about shoulder width apart. Hands are to be clasped behind the head or neck. S/he then squats down to an almost sitting position or below, keeping in mind not to drop the buttocks all the way down. This will flex the knee joints and create stress on the cartilage and ligaments in the legs. The child then returns to the original standing position straightening the legs at the knee. Placing a box or chair behind the child will aid the child from squatting too low. Caution should be exercised with this maneuver. Attempting to increase stress by squatting to a full deep knee bend position can be injurious to your child's knee joints.

Performing this exercise to maximum capacity can be boring and difficult for a child. To avoid these pitfalls, on this particular exercise you could determine the quantity of repetitions by the child's age times three.

Back to resistance exercises. The muscles work on a specific load while shortening. The muscles contract against an immovable object and develop tension but do not shorten. Programs that are classified as isotonic include weights, rubber bars, springs, etc. In this program the youngster performs the absolute maximum number of repetitions possible beginning slowly and gradually working up to eight and then to twenty repetitions. As the weight increases, the repetitions decrease. It is important to note that many repetitions with moderate weight increases muscle size more so than it adds strength. Performing with heavier weights increases the strength but you need to decrease the number of repetitions. So, selecting a weight load that would permit a large number of repetitions is the way to go for large muscular appearance. Caution though: these exercises should not be introduced until your child starts showing physical signs of adolescent development.

94.2.1.4. School-Age: Six to Twelve

Ah, time for the youngster to be out in the world experiencing as an independent individual. Physically, the school-age child begins at the onset to lose the first baby did tooth and culminates with an appearance of a pre-adolescent growth spurt. The body is now taller and trimmer, height is increased by 30% and weight increases by as much as 100%. During this period, the body proportion becomes more adult-like. The legs are not as short, and the head is not as large as before. Along with physical growth comes proportionate strength increase.

Also noticeable is the six-year-old's improved coordination, balance, and motor skills. The child at six tends to be restless and is better at starting a task than finishing it. This should be taken into consideration when you contemplate your child's exercise regimen. When the child is nine or ten, his/her capacity to follow through is a lot more developed. This will make it easier to introduce a routine and have it fulfilled. The youngster is now more prone to think in terms of long-term goals and what is involved in attaining them. This is the time to begin serious athletic training if you are so inclined.

The six or seven-year-old is still introspective and shows an interest in imaginative play, which soon dwindles. The five or six-year-old is usually cooperative and eager to please his/her parents but by ten or eleven the influences of persons outside the household tend to diminish the authority of the parent, i.e., teachers, coaches, peers, etc. The ten-year-old child might suddenly seem resentful toward the parent's control but might take advice from a total stranger better than his/her parents. This is a process that although it may be disturbing to the parents is all a part of the growth process. In some children it occurs at ten and in some it occurs during adolescence. Another thing that oftentimes occurs at this age is your youngster may develop a hero worship stage (normally not the parent) which can be a positive stage providing the hero is of good moral character and possesses positive attributes.

You may wish to involve your school-age youngster in some physical activity outside the household. Example: Enroll him/her in a karate class or a dance class, etc. A word of caution is in order here. A child's attitude at this phase is shaped by his/her friends, coaches, relatives, teachers, etc., and this leaves the child open to all sorts of inputs. He or she is at the mercy of others who are not the parents.

I can remember my childhood sport experience quite well. I played baseball, basketball, soccer, did relay running and broad jumping. Because what I did, I was good at, I was constantly sought after to play on some team or the other. Now all this was exciting until I grew older and realized that everyone always expected the best from me. One of my teammates went on to become a professional baseball player for the Minnesota Twins, but when I got older, I lost interest. I can still remember the disappointment everyone displayed when I decided against pursuing a career in baseball. I learned real young that when you are good at something you are never allowed to be a mere human anymore. As long as you're able to bring in a home run or stop a run from being scored, you're fine. But once you fail at an attempt, everyone forgets, and you stand alone. That's a terrible feeling—especially for a youngster. I have added this bit of history because I have seen perfectly rational parents get very excited over a simple baseball game which their child is involved in—this places a lot of stress on a child.

Another factor to consider when involving your youngster in sports is injury. This is one of the many causes of deformity in youngsters today. Children are forced in little league to perform tasks that they are not ready for, i.e., pitching for long innings can cause permanent damage to the arm of the child who has not yet fully developed his/her arm. Mistakes like this one are committed oftentimes for the entertainment and pride or ego boost of the parents.

94.2.1.5. Adolescence: Twelve to Eighteen

This is the age of rapid change. Your youngster is now experiencing a remarkable increase in strength and body shape. It is time for primary and secondary sexual characteristics to form. In boys a deeper voice is developed, facial and pubic hair as well, etc. With girls' pubic axillary hair, enlarged breasts, broader hips, etc., develop. Along with outward physical signs there is also the onset of menstrual flow at about the age of thirteen to fifteen (younger in the less healthy, older, or not at all in very athletic, healthy girls) and in the male the production of sperm occurs at this time.

Adolescence is a time for self-examination and concern for worldly affairs. Great concern is placed on the adolescent's role in society. How s/he fits into peer relations is now more in the foreground than ever. It is not uncommon for your youngster to perform crazy and sometimes dangerous stunts to gain overall approval from peers or to impress a member of the opposite sex. At this point all that energy should be channeled into more constructive endeavors, namely physical fitness programs and other health promoting activities. Example: swimming, skating, tennis, etc. Experiencing physical fitness brings excitement and joy to the youngster as well as respect for the body and health. With the adolescent who strives for fitness, engaging in the health-deteriorating practices of tobacco, liquor, drugs, etc., that are so common among our youth of today, are of less appeal than to someone who is less health oriented.

Again, this time proves to be difficult for the parent. The youngster continues to disregard his/her parents well-intended advice. Like in the earlier stages of the child's development, this is an expression of independence from parental influence and is quite normal. As a parent, your only solution is to offer guidance when requested.

If your child is involved in sports, the instructor will assume the role of surrogate parent in regard to career choices, advice, etc., and you should work closely with him/ her to insure your child's total well-being. In adolescence the parent once again will notice the youngster's weight change rapidly. Infancy and adolescence are the only times in life that one produces fat cells and once these cells are produced, they remain forever. Dieting shrinks the cells but doesn't eliminate them. An overweight teenager is a sad sight as this will continue throughout life without the individual constantly monitoring his/her weight. Current statistics indicate that the average American is more overweight than ever in the past when people did more physical jobs for a living. The reason for this national weight problem, of course, is lack of exercise and the overeating of high-fat, high-protein, highly processed foods.

It is recommended that as your youngster gets older s/he be introduced to fasting. Fasting is a natural and time-honored means of providing the mind and body with rest and recuperation. As the body rests while not having to digest, absorb or metabolize food, it is freed to go about its business of self-cleansing. The blood, the kidneys and the entire intestinal system rids itself of accumulated waste. The brain and nervous system refresh and retune themselves also. Hints on fasting you should start with a very short and slow fast, say twelve to eighteen hours and gradually build to forty-eight hours. That is the safest and sanest approach to take when dealing with a teenager. Fasting means absence of food or drink, except pure water which should be consumed as needed. Avoid prolonged physical exertion (brief exercise is okay). Avoid long exposure to the sun or heat. Rest. The fast should be broken slowly, starting with fresh-squeezed fruit juices followed by solid foods a few hours later. The meal should be complimentary to the fast, i.e., long fasts should be followed by a small meal and vice versa.

One final note: In adolescence your child might be more prone to find solutions to problems in his/her own way. If you will recall, you probably did the same thing. I know I did. Some problems are less urgent than others but to your teenager all are urgent. And today's make-a-buck philosophy makes the teenager a prime target for all the fads that are currently swamping the market. Parents, everything that your child will ever be starts with you!

94.2.2. Other Factors Exercise and Females

Women in the U.S. have been handicapped by the old misconception that women are not supposed to do physical activity. This misinformation has served the U.S. males well in keeping their women in the background. I have lived in other societies where the women were allowed to take more control of their lives and they had fewer problems when they arrived at child-bearing age. The American female generally arrives at child-bearing age not being physically or mentally fit which explains the high incidence of congenital deformity that occurs daily in the hospitals throughout the United States. Most American women have difficult pregnancies and childbirth largely due to a lack of physical conditioning.

It has been standard practice to allocate less dollars for female physical education and athletic scholarships than for males (if any at all). It is finally dawning on the North American society that both girls and boys have the same physiological needs, and the only difference is that girls have been excluded from any type of physical training programs.

94.2.2.1. Sleep

Sleep is an individualized process and can only be determined by the way the child functions throughout the day. If during the day the child appears irritable or sleepy, that child should nap. In studies done in the U.S., it was found that children who are active need less sleep than say a child who is passive and lacking in mental stimulation. So, sleep then is determined primarily by the degree of, activity, diet and mental condition of the child. Most youngsters dislike bedtime as they're afraid they might miss something. It is often a battle of wills to get them to bed. The best thing to do is to establish a nightly routine of showers, dental hygiene, and bedtime stories. This works quite well with my sons. Of course, a different routine is necessary with older children. You need to work out a program of sleep patterns that works for you and your family.

94.3. Conclusion

It is important to encourage your child to indulge an opportunity to be physically active. Help your child become involved in a sport of his/her choice. Develop interest in sports as a family. Do specific exercises with your child to help him/her supplement normal physical activity. Run or jog at least three times a week as a family.

Discourage the use of junk foods. Try not to keep foods you don't wish your child to consume in your house (rather than prohibit it). Read all labels carefully and educate your children to do likewise (not necessary if eating only raw fruits and vegetables—no labels). Follow a Hygienic regime of proper diet and lifestyle—consumption of fresh, raw fruits, vegetables, nuts, and seeds; take plenty of fresh air and sunshine; and exercise.

Here's to a future of continued good health to you and your family.

94.4. Questions & Answers

How does a family of four with both parents at work all day manage to follow an exercise program?

Ask yourself this question: am I going to allow my family's health to deteriorate which will be more costly in the long run or am I going to grab every opportunity I can get to engage in physical activity? It should be quite clear what the answer to this question is. Here are a few suggestions: Instead of watching TV in the evening, spend an hour or so going for a walk in a park or forest nearby your home. Take time on the weekend to go bicycling with your family. Enroll at a fitness center. These are just a few things you can do-to safeguard the health of your entire family. I'm sure you could think of others. Just eliminate a passive activity from your daily routine and replace it with an active one. Your family will love you for it and you'll all feel great!

My son shows no interest whatsoever in physical activity. He just wants to watch TV all the time. What can I do?

As far as the TV is concerned make rules as to how much television he can watch each day. When the amount of television has been watched, he is to do something else. Your child's lack of interest could be for many reasons. Find the reason. He might be the type of person who needs to be inspired or motivated. Or perhaps he had an injury which you are unaware of and has pain. The type of diet your child consumes also plays a key role. On tests done with athletes, those who were placed on a diet of natural and wholesome foods performed better and had more of a desire to do so than those on the conventional diet of processed, adulterated foods.

My son seems to sleep less now that he is enrolled in a karate class. Is this, okay?

You have absolutely nothing to be concerned with, it is perfectly normal. You see the more physical activity the body gets, the less sleep it requires. This is great for your child. He will now have more time to indulge in the activities of his choice.

Article #1: Exercise for Baby by Dr. Herbert M. Shelton

It is unfortunate that we have so long depended upon physicians with their drugs, their condoning and encouraging of bad habits, their fear of exercise and their anti-natural approach to all the problems of life and have not given more heed to the physical educator with his more natural approach to life. We are paying a terrible toll in suffering and premature death for our faith in the destructive agencies of physicians and our rejection of the constructive things of nature.

The physicians have established, for our guidance, a whole series of false (and low) standards based on averages of abnormals and then, they have resisted everything that will assure true (and higher) standards.

To the everlasting credit of Sylvester Graham, Drs. R. T. Trall, Geo. Taylor, Chas.

E. Page, and others who were the real pioneers in the Hygienic movement, they made a study of physical education and employed its principles in their care of both the well and the sick.

Beginning at birth with a program of physical education for the baby, Dr. Page insisted that babies should be placed face-down upon their beds and not upon their backs, as was, and is, the rule. He insisted that they developed better and faster in this position. When an infant moves its arms and legs in this position it does so against resistance. Merely kicking the air with its legs and waving its arms while lying on the back offers no resistance. I have watched an infant push its way across the bed lying face down, at only one week of age. Here is real exercise; exercise that calls for vigorous use of the muscles, especially those of the legs and thighs. The infant will raise its head, shoulder, hips, and thighs backward, thus giving vigorous exercise to its spinal muscles. The beauty of the cords of muscles on each side of its spinal column is matched only by those of the strongman.

Suppose from birth, kittens, puppies, calves, colts, and chickens were placed on their backs and never permitted to use their legs for anything more vigorous than merely waving or kicking them; would these animals ever walk? If young monkeys and apes were placed on their backs and not called upon to use their legs and arms, if they were not also forced to swing by their arms, what slow development we would logically expect! Why must we continue to hamper the development of our own young by placing them on their backs and keeping them there?

Dr. Tilden, after years of employing this plan, wrote in his Care of Children (1916): "Place the baby on its belly (Dr. C. E. Page's method), and allow it to stay on the belly rather than on the back. The Page method works out well. Children walk and run much earlier.

The fetal spine is a flexed spine. To bring it into a position of extension and hold it there requires the development of the spinal muscles. The wiggling and squirming of the infant, while lying face-down, develops the spinal muscles as they cannot be developed if it is placed on its back.

When the baby with well-developed spinal muscles comes to sit up, and it will do so at a much earlier date, it will sit erect, because its muscles will be strong enough to hold it erect.

I have emphasized the development of the spinal, arm and leg muscles that takes place in the prone position. It is necessary that I mention that the side muscles and the muscles of the abdomen are also called into vigorous action by the movements of this position. The strength of these muscles also helps to hold the baby erect when it sits up.

Does this mean that the child should never be placed on its back; or, on its side? By no means. It needs the vigorous, spasmodic kicking of its legs and flinging of its arms to develop these. All of its muscles need and must have exercise in various ways.

Crawling, or creeping, calls for a certain amount of strength in the muscles of the arms, chest, and shoulders. This strength is developed faster if the baby is placed on its face and allowed to use its arms against resistance. The baby will learn early to lift the upper part of its trunk with its arms. Also, it will early learn to draw its legs and thighs up and assume the knee-chest position. All of this strength and use of the muscles must be acquired before it can begin to crawl.

There is more involved in the exercise of the baby's body than that of muscular development. There is also mental development. The baby learns to do things. It becomes conscious of its muscles and of its powers. Muscular consciousness is gained faster if the muscles are employed against resistance than if the limbs are merely flung wildly about. Neuromuscular coordination also is gained more rapidly if resistance is offered to the movements of the parts of the body than when no resistance is offered.

The period in which the infant crawls is one during which the trunk muscles and those of the arms and legs and thighs are strengthened. Especially the muscles of the abdominal wall, lower back and shoulder girdle are strengthened by the act of crawling.

Play pens, now popular with ignorant and lazy mothers, are an evil influence in the lives of babies. Babies confined within the narrow railings of these abdominal prisons have no incentive to crawl far, thus they miss this much needed exercise.

Dr. Page contrasts our methods of caring for babies with those employed in nature in caring for puppies, kittens and the young of other animals. We hold the babies, carry them, put them in baby carriages, coddle them and make of them little tyrants that are constantly demanding attention.

"The young of some species," says Page, "are, upon occasion carried by their parents from one point to another; but beyond this they furnish their own transportation. Their parents roll and tumble them about, more or less, for mutual pleasure; but in the main they are from the beginning forced to rely upon themselves. Everywhere among animals we observe the same thing: the young are never over tended. They have no baby carts in which to spend a great part of their time, to their physical disadvantage; like our pampered baby aristocrats. They are not taught to sit down with a box of playthings in front of them to prevent them from being tempted to make their way to distant objects. If they chance to see anything they want, it never comes to them. It is Mohamet and the mountain every time; the creature and the thing never come together, except through the exertion of the creature! Hence, they grow lusty and strong and healthy. They earn their diet, and therefore it is digested and assimilated. Their frames are covered with well-knit muscles—not a continuous fatty tumor, with scarcely any sound muscles beneath. In short, they are from the very outset, kept in 'condition'."

This emphasis upon exercise for infants needs to be re-stressed. They need to be rolled and tumbled about as do the other little animals, and they and their parents derive as much sheer joy from this as do the lower creatures.

In The Hygienic Care of Children, I have emphasized the evils of toys. Babies do not need and should not have these playthings. They need opportunity for activity—for exertion.

The normal baby is able, at birth, to grasp a pencil or other appropriate object in one hand and hang from this, holding up the weight of its body with but one hand. In "authoritative" works on babies we are told that they soon lose this ability. This is true, however, only if they are not permitted to use their hands in this manner.

Physical educators are agreed that hanging by the arms affords the best type of activity for the development of the chest, shoulder girdle and arms of the child. I can see no reason why this activity needs to be delayed until the child is three or four years old. It may be started at once—at birth. A good strong grip developed early in this way, will save the child many falls and injuries a little later. The infant of two months will delight in holding on to your fingers and by the use of both arms and legs, doing deep knee bends and squats.

We have an unfounded fear of permitting a baby to stand on its legs before these are "strong enough to support its body." There is no better way of strengthening the legs than that of permitting the baby to use the legs against resistance in this way.

By the third month, the normal baby, will hold on to your fingers, stand up and raise up on its toes. Babies are not ' the frail little animals we seem to think, and they are as fond of activity as puppies and kittens.

It is perfectly true that babies are more helpless at birth than most young animals and this period of helplessness lasts longer than it does in animals, but the principles of proper care for both groups are the same. Babies need exercise and they need to be permitted to do things for themselves. How are they to learn to do things for themselves if these are always done for them? I know a nineteen-year-old girl who does not know how to tie her own shoes, because, and only because, her mother or others have always done this for her.

Lesson 95:

Exercise in Sickness and Recuperation

95.1. Introduction

While only too often neglected and even rejected in the past by many orthodox practitioners as being correct procedures to be employed in the treatment of the sick or as valuable tools capable of hastening restoration of health during periods of recuperation, the many possible forms of exercise are now receiving increasing popular and professional acceptance.

Where once patients recovering from surgery were often kept confined to their beds and permitted only limited movement, they are now often encouraged to leave their beds and to walk up and down the hallways or about their rooms. Physical therapists are frequently called into service when the physician in charge deems it advisable as in cases where paralysis constrains movement.

We understand that both the arthritis and muscular dystrophy foundations now pay for hydro exercises for persons suffering from these ailments. Groups of patients, under the guidance of a therapist, perform certain movements while immersed in a swimming pool. They report feeling much improved following these planned exercise sessions. Hydrotherapy was much employed during the last century by hydro therapists, most of whom were devoted practitioners of Natural Hygiene. Modern orthodoxy was reluctant to adopt it but is now utilizing hydrotherapy to a limited extent.

However, even now for the most part, invalids, and the elderly, especially those confined in nursing homes, languish in their beds. Individuals and practitioners alike have not as yet learned to appreciate fully the value of exercise and activity in sickness and in the restoration of health to those persons who are no longer, suffering deeply from some ailment but who, as yet, have not made a full recovery.

Hygienists have long recognized that exercise is essential both in sickness and in recuperation. In fact, George S. Weger, M.D., believed that positive exercise was contraindicated only in profound states of enervation or in cases of inflammatory fever, or cardiac depression." Dr. Weger had his fasting patients do tensing movements for periods of from ten to thirty minutes, depending upon the vitality and muscular vigor of the person.

Hygienists contend that rest and exercise are twin requirements of a healthy life, one being dependent upon the other and of equal importance. In sickness they are often far more important than food. This latter concept is the exact opposite of the prevailing notion that weakness requires feeding and that both the quality and the quantity of food should be increased. As a result, patients are fed much and often while activity is neglected.

Strangely, orthodoxy does not seem to learn from the fact that, more often than not, those patients that are fed the most, if they progress at all, recover more slowly than those who either are fed abstemiously or fast altogether, assuming, of course, similar circumstances and conditions.

Orthodoxy fails to realize that just because a certain quantity of food is eaten does not necessarily mean that the same amount has been assimilated and utilized by the body for reparative and healing functional activities. While the sick can perhaps digest a certain amount of food and absorb it into the system and then even transport it through its many channels, there is no guarantee that it will be assimilated by the cells and put to constructive use.

95.2. Activity Is Required

95.2.1. Exercise and the Arteries

95.2.2. Muscular Activity Creates an Appropriate Response

95.2.3. Specific Benefits of Exercise

95.2.4. Need for Balance

95.2.5. as the Strength Improves

95.2.6. Slow is Best

95.2.7. Exercise, a Natural Tonic

For food to be beneficial to the sick, the conditions which encourage assimilative powers must prevail; that is, there must be activity commensurate to the nutritive intake. Otherwise, the food will promote further toxemia, and thus the intensity of the illness. It does so by encouraging further enervation and thus weakening cellular functioning capabilities. All wasting of vital force in this manner is anti-vital.

Exercise, carefully planned and judiciously employed, serves to direct the nutrients to those areas where they may be needed most. When a demand for nourishment is issued by a certain part, area, muscle or group of muscles, the appropriate response will be forthcoming, and the need will be filled. Healing and repair will be facilitated.

However, when no demand is put out, the cells do not receive the nutrients required for the more extended efforts of healing and repair, or even for simple upkeep, and can make but feeble efforts toward this end. Thus, the period of recovery can be not only prolonged but also less thorough, leaving the patient vulnerable to relapses should he be subjected to unusual stress demands.

Dr. Herbert M. Shelton has stated that "many invalids fail to recover their health, even though all other factors are favorable, simply because they could not be induced to take 'sufficient or appropriate exercise.'"

Shelton goes on to say that while numerous other methods are utilized to increase nutritive acceptance by various parts, none of them are as effective and devoid of harmful consequences as muscular activity. "None of them are so prompt, none so localized, none so economical of vitality."

He further contends that "artificial agents and measures employed for this purpose occasion other actions and induce irrelevant changes and needless vital expenditure. These methods involve a harmful and uncompensated expenditure of the patient's power."

Exercise, to the contrary, represents a compensated expenditure of vitality in that the important tools required for healing and repair are delivered right to the premises where they are most urgently needed, and this takes place in exchange for a minimal loss.

Without such proper and regular delivery of supplies, cellular function will remain half-hearted and even faulty with the whole process of recuperation prolonged and, as previously noted, perhaps not as solidly constituted.

Where artificial stimulation, rather than exercise, is employed, it does not take much imagination to decide whether or not the effect on the body will be enervating or conducive to healing. Whipping organs and parts by using medications, for example, has the effect of expecting plants to grow without providing the proper soil.

But, when the individual is sick and his functional abilities reduced and these are stimulated by means that do NOT result in enervation, then better function can be expected. As function improves in certain weakened areas, the effects are felt throughout the entire body, including the mind, and these effects are good effects.

Exercise and activity are stimulative in kind, but they are proper stimulants. The Law of Dual Effect, in a positive way, is in effect. The exercise requires energy, true, but it stimulates the kind of activity that is conducive to the restoration of health. The use of medicines and other types of enervating modalities does not bring any compensatory values to the individual but, to the contrary, either introduces or causes to be formed certain toxins which add further encumbrance to an already enervated body.

95.2.1. Exercise and the Arteries

The arterial vessels, large, small, and microscopically tiny, are extremely numerous and capable. As is well-known they carry necessary supplies to and from the cells, wherever located, and then collect and eliminate the discarded metabolic wastes via nearby, strategically located, venous channels.

Not so well-known is that there are two areas within the human body where these vessels are especially numerous and capable, namely in the brain and in and around the organs where there is much vital action, those parts where important vital action is constantly taking place, where changes important to recovery occur. For example, in the liver.

In sickness many of these vessels are either constricted by calcareous deposits or by malformations of one sort or another, such as twisting or bulging in spots. Important to this discussion is the fact that these same arteries are capable both of being enlarged, if too small, and diminished in size, if overly large.

If an arm in which the muscles have become wasted through disease is habitually and vigorously exercised, the arteries slowly begin to expand, and the muscles soon become more fully developed. This is a natural happening. Exercise creates the demand for nourishment. The clear signal of need is relayed to the cerebral centers which correctly interpret the signal received, decide on an appropriate response, and give forth with certain directives which are relayed to various organs and systems concerned with supply. The necessary nutritive response takes place with lightning speed.

Sick and hurting cells receive glucose for fuel, to maintain body heat; necessary fatty acids and amino acids for rebuilding and repairing purposes; vitamins, auxones, enzymes, hormones, minerals—all the supplies required both to maintain organic function and to improve it and, above all perhaps, to revitalize the nerve force, so necessary for full recovery. All are received on demand.

The twin companions of the arteries are the veins which are even more numerous and entwined than the arterial divisions. By incorrect habits of living and eating, the veins become clogged and deformed. In such a state, the venous web cannot adequately remove toxic wastes and thus the toxemia continues to mount and the deterioration of the body to accelerate. Exercise can intervene and hasten the elimination of the health destroying toxins. As the blood becomes less sticky and viscous, as the veins themselves become enlarged and less malformed, the channels open and transportation of wastes begins to improve, as does general wellness.

95.2.2. Muscular Activity Creates an Appropriate Response

The human body is constructed and designed in such a way that muscular activity in any particular part will immediately call forth a response by the autonomic nervous system directing energy and supplies appropriately enough to those organs, tissues and cells being moved, there to be used for constructive functional purposes. Blood and nerve power are directed to those areas where a demand exists.

In other words, if the invalid is encouraged to move the fingers of his right hand, the cells comprising the muscles and other parts in that area will receive an appropriate response: they will be fed, and toxins will be gathered up and removed. All such appropriately fed and cleansed parts will increase both in substance and in wellness.

Illustrative of this phenomenal organic wisdom is the fact that scientists have long recognized that the physical capabilities of a mature individual may be very much dwarfed if his vigorous play life as a child was limited and almost in an exact proportion, all other things being more or less equal. Sick and weakened adults must deliberately choose to exercise if they would enjoy its health-promoting benefits.

Their previous usually sedentary lifestyles have undoubtedly contributed greatly to their present state of diminished health and vigor.

95.2.3. Specific Benefits of Exercise

As humans age and vitality is lessened and when they are ill, exercise is very much needed, even though this idea may be contrary to popular thinking. Exercise is essential to keep the heart and lungs in good condition, to keep the blood and other fluids replenished and their movements active. Exercise is needed to improve the digestion and to encourage elimination of the toxins which have brought the patient to his present unfortunate state, to create the demand for nutrients to be directed to specific areas where the most need may exist.

95.2.4. Need for Balance

The chances for recovery are enhanced when a careful balance is maintained between feeding of a diet well adapted to the patient's present impaired state, if feeding be indicated at all; rest in an amount and a kind, including physiological rest, as to increase energy flow for healing and reparative purposes; and, finally, exercise and activity geared to the present capacity of the patient to accept and as specific needs may require as, for example, a stiffened knee or elbow, or other damaged or weakened part.

When given a well-chosen, easily-digested diet with the foods properly combined in simple combinations or served in mono fare, if permitted to rest when the body signals its need for sleep, and when certain parts of the body totality are exercised regularly and in accordance with capacity to accept, then the patient can expect full recovery so long as sufficient vitality yet remains to initiate the recovery process and then to sustain it for a long enough time to accomplish the objective.

If insufficient vital power remains and the patient is greatly debilitated, his vital force nearing exhaustion, recovery may be initiated but perhaps not be sustained sufficiently long to achieve the desired results. In that event, of course, exercise would be contraindicated since it would serve only to deplete the systemic resources even further and thus it would be more in keeping with organic reality to postpone forcing the activity until such time as the improved vitality gives a different and more positive signal. In such a case physiological rest might well be a more immediate need.

95.2.5. as the Strength Improves

As clients become stronger, the exercises should become more vigorous and more complex—involving more muscles over a wider area and to a greater depth—and the activity extended for a more prolonged period.

Various types of exercise should be incorporated gradually into the daily program and should be utilized in the mornings and evenings as well.

95.2.6. Slow is Best

However, exercise should not push development too far or at too rapid a rate. The goal should be not to harden the muscles and create extraordinary mass but rather to keep them well shaped, supple, and flexible. All excess, even in bulk, is anti-health. Moderate, intelligently-used exercise will provide the greatest efficiency to accomplish the desired health benefits while excessive exercise can only serve to waste the vital force for no good purpose.

In sickness moderation is extremely important, especially when the patient is greatly debilitated. We shall presently see how exercise may be utilized in a gradually more complex series of movements with greatly debilitated patients as the energy flow increases and capacity improves.

But we should bear in mind the admonition of J. H. Tilden, M.D. that the muscular system and the liver are allies, that exercise, even though it be limited, will use up energy (sugar) and this the liver furnishes. Tilden points out, and validly so, that if the muscular system, even in sickness, is not intelligently worked, the liver will become engorged with glucose, or the glucose will be fed into the circulation for excretion by the kidneys, a definite waste of nutritive material as well as vital force, a loss the patient can ill afford without receiving compensatory value in nutritive "gold."

We are all reminded by the admonitions of the Doctors Robert Walker, Sylvester Graham, Russell Thacker Trall, Shelton and others that in caring for the ill and incapacitated, we must always bear in mind the needs and capacities of the patient. Just as with food, exercise should be geared to these three considerations: 1. Constitution, 2. Present condition, and 3. Ability to perform or work. To do otherwise would be contrary to the best interests of the patient and would, in all likelihood, retard his progress, and perhaps even bring it to a halt.

We should remember, too, that nerve depletion precedes the illness, it does not follow it. Therefore, the primary requisite for recovery is rest. Only when the body is well rested should activity be introduced. Otherwise, exhaustion will follow and make full recovery unlikely. When a person attempts to do anything to fast, he inevitably experiences a negative nervous system impact. Therefore, in working with persons suffering from any degree of diminished health, and especially with highly debilitated patients, we must avoid all temptation to push too much activity upon them or to make the exercises too complex or to extend the exercise periods overly long. In such cases, slow is always best!

Graham states our thesis this way, "A certain amount of exercise or labor is ... as essential to the highest welfare of man, as food or air. By a rigidly abstemious diet he may live on, with an exemption from actual disease, and perhaps attain to what we call old age, with very little active exercise. But in such a life he can never know that vigor of body and mind, that perfectness of health, that vivacity and buoyancy of spirit, that habitual serenity and cheerfulness and high enjoyment of which his nature is capable. But we have seen that every vital action is attended with an expenditure of vital power and waste of organized substance, and that every vital function necessarily draws something from the ultimate and unreplenishable fund of life. Hence, so far as voluntary exercise or labor is necessary to the most healthy condition and perfect functions of the human system, it is a blessing; and beyond that, it is in some measure an evil; for in proportion to the excess, life is always shortened, and the body predisposed to disease."

95.2.7. Exercise, a Natural Tonic

Modern therapeutics employ tonics of one kind or another to stimulate the body. They fail to realize that all such stimulation is accomplished by raiding the vital resources of the body and especially its vital force. The ultimate result of such foolishness is, of course, the inevitable wasting of the body even though a temporary feeling of wellbeing may be experienced. This is only the top of a sine curve. The deep valley will be sure to follow!

Exercise, on the other hand, is a natural tonic, one unfortunately that is generally overlooked. The same salubrious effects can be achieved and more healthfully so, by the employment of proper exercise and pure air. In keeping with organic reality, there just is no other way conducive to a resurgence of health. All other agencies and means employed in an attempt to restore health, while they may temporarily relieve the symptoms, will, in the long run, actually aggravate the condition and shorten the lifespan.

95.3. Positive Versus Negative Thinking

95.3.1. Words Alone May Not be Sufficient

95.3.2. Getting Out of the Self-Destructive Phase—the Mental Rollover

95.3.3. How to Plan for More Positive Mental Activity

95.3.4. How to Encourage a More Positive Mental Attitude

Thus far we have been addressing the issue of physical activity, the moving of muscles. However, there is another form of activity which is perhaps equally important, if not more so. We refer to mental activity. This can be both health-enhancing and health destroying.

The sick are often depressed. They have a negative attitude toward life and living. They tend to find fault overly much with almost every aspect of their life. This negative imprinting has a profound effect on wellness. As J. H. Tilden, Weger and others have said, discontent and general lack of poise can be instrumental in poisoning the entire system. Understandably so, a lack of poise is a direct result of years of piling up poisons through erroneous living. A vicious cycle is initiated which gnaws away at wellness, since all such negativity spawns even more poison.

Sometimes the measures employed by the client to relieve his own inner anxieties wear on the people around him. In turn, they react negatively which further impinges on his emotional well-being. In such an event the client turns his mind inward and concentrates his efforts in such a manner that he begins to conjure up and magnify all kinds of symptom complexes.

We worked with one client a few years ago who was a master at turning inward and discovering all manner of supposed negative happenings, all a result, of course, of her improved lifestyle and diet. In fact, this habit became so intense with her that she began to keep hourly and daily records of passing variations in her condition even down to such minute happenings as a tingling in a certain fingertip or a passing itchiness behind an ear, the correct ear and area being again precisely identified. In the beginning she filled page after page of notebook paper with this kind of detailed information. Rejected outwardly by her peers, she had turned inward to make Self-important.

However, this kind of attitude can kill. In this case we had to direct the woman's attention to more positive things in order to promote more positive responses. It is important always to raise the clients' own self-esteem first, by making positive things happen insofar as their general feeling of health is concerned and second, by imparting to them the concept that they are in charge, that they can bring about whatever degree of health they wish to achieve and that it all can be accomplished by learning the requisites of organic existence, how to impart them to the body and how-to live-in accordance with them, and then actually doing it! This is mental activity at its best.

Elsworth F. DuTeau, in an article in New Age, entitled "Positive Thinking," shows how important the acceptance of personal responsibility can be when he states, "There are those who during their income years have a good life. Then, after those years ended, they find a gradual erosion of their savings and security through inflation and misfortune, even having to sell their home to obtain capital to sustain them and provide the necessities of life. For them, self-pity and bitter, passive, resignation only deepens their gloom. It is then that they need positive thinking and action more than ever. They must know what to salvage, where to go, what to do to reconstruct their lives. They can't just stop doing. They, through positive thinking and action, must persevere. They should remember that there is no failure except in no longer trying, no defeat except from within."

If we, as practitioners working with the sick and ailing, can impart this concept of positive thinking PLUS action—the doing—the working effort to build health—performing by Self—to our clients, the results will be salubrious beyond our fondest expectations.

Small successes are very important in this connection. Every small improvement intelligently conveyed to the clients will become incorporated into their thinking and help to initiate a more positive attitude. A series of such small successes will, by directing the thought processes from their former depressed and defeated pathways into more constructive channels, actually give birth to a resurgence of vital force which can then be directed computer-like by the individual's own cerebral centers to those areas where need is urgent.

Supplied with the necessary nerve energy and as nutritive transport is powered and nutrients arrive, the cells respond with revitalized effort, healing and repair proceed at an accelerated rate, the state of health rapidly surges.

Without the proper mental attitude, unless the mind is re-directed into positive channels, unless it actively foresees the future well-being, unless the positive vision of euphoric joy and happiness are written on the subconscious, the ill will proceed thus far—perhaps even enjoy some measure of improved health—but they will never enter into that rare condition of perfect health as described by Graham and previously quoted in our discussion.

The mind can be active both in a negative way which produces negative results, and especially where one's health is concerned; or, it can be active in a positive way, not only anticipating but actually producing favorable results.

Thus, it becomes the happy duty of the practitioner to plan a program to bring about this necessary change—a more positive thinking on the part of the sick and to encourage a like mental metamorphosis among those persons who may have made thus far only a limited recovery, for one reason or another, and now need not only instructions as to what and how to do and behave, but also that essence of superior health, Inspiration, an inner rebirth of accomplishment already achieved or easily capable of achievement. Such is a primary principle of vital improvement, the importance of which cannot be overlooked.

Unfortunately, in the care of the sick orthodoxy attempts vainly to disassociate the rest of the body from the mind. This cannot be done because they are by the very nature of design, one, a single entity, symbionts which can favorably or adversely affect each other.

Both the body and the brain are subject to precisely the same laws of organic existence. Obedience to these universal laws governs the vital powers of the body and the manifestations of that vital force, whether they be perfect or something less than perfect. This is a principle which cannot be denied and one that should be primary in Hygienic thinking. Orthodoxy is wrong when it does not actively encourage positive thinking on the part of the sick. Enter into any hospital ward and view what is transpiring there. Bells ring sounds of all kinds intrude and confuse. Nowhere is there any careful addressing of this primary need of the human soul. And yet, a constructive attitude, an active acceptance by the mind of the POSSIBLE, the fact that full health can be attained by adherence to organic law, this is of primary importance in recovery, probably as much so as the will to live.

We listened to a woman today who revealed how, for three months prior to her annual physical, she became engulfed by terror, so much so that she became unable to deal with her customary obligations and duties. Instead of anticipating a healthful life for ALL of life, she "knew" that sooner or later at this yearly ritual, she would hear that she had "caught" some horrendous disease! This engulfing fear made her nauseous, irritable, headachy and, as she put it, she became "completely unglued." Fear not only gripped and strangled her mind, but it also grasped in its tentacles her physical body and soul.

When the mind has been rendered enervated and distraught by an incorrect manner of living, the physical body will be equally and just as deeply etched. If the thoughts be wrong, the entire organic domain will suffer and to the same extent regardless of how well we may do in other areas. Instead of neglecting this "soul power," as is common among orthodox practitioners, we Hygienists should become better informed. We need to study and understand more and more about human behavior and learn how to encourage greater depth and breadth of understanding of principles on the part of those who seek our aid as to the amazing possibilities that await, the fact that a lifetime of great joy, happiness, achievement, personal satisfaction and perfection of health are there to be had. But they must be earned! The mind plainly controls exercise and health, but equally activity and health influence the mind. All are symbiotically intertwined.

95.3.1. Words Alone May Not be Sufficient

Admonishing any person, and especially one who is ill, to think more positively may not accomplish a changeover from negativity to a more hopeful, forward-looking life script. Most sick people have a tendency to look inwardly, not outwardly; to today, this moment, rather than to the future except in negative ways. Many ill persons are filled with a doomsday attitude and develop the "Poor Little Me!" syndrome.

It is time for such people to shift into health. They must be taught that they are not helpless and hopeless, that health can be destroyed, to be sure. They have already proved that. But it can also be built! But to accomplish this, they must accept the reality of organic living, namely that all their troubles, whatever they may be and however intensive and extensive, have their origin in toxemia which itself came about through enervation and that enervation was the inevitable result of disobeying organic law, either through ignorance or deliberately.

Due to their enervated state, sick people are often child personalities and must be led. Since most are also novices at Natural Hygiene and do not think as we do, nor have our knowledge, their minds must be fed. They must be taught that all behavior has pay-offs. Bad behavior in the life script means illness and suffering. Good behavior, as evidenced by adherence to the immutable laws of our organic existence, carries its own immense rewards: the keys of life that open the doors to all of life!

Sick people often need to grasp a new concept, too; that the attainment of a higher level of health represents a long-term pay-off and cannot be compared to the short-term "relief" that so soon fades away. This latter is a transitory thing which only compounds error while the planned, long-term building contract that we make with ourselves is an on-going growing step-by-step series of small successes which, in the end, add up to full attainment of our goal.

We can impart to the sick and ailing that they have an opportunity now, at this moment, to make a choice: to continue their present downward path that all their medicines and treatments had failed to stop, or to reshape their lives. They can be made to realize that sick as they may well be, they still have certain strengths and that these can become stronger, that positive choices expand the mind and facilitate construction (the healing and repair); that they can "get around" this sickness that binds them in their chains by activating their minds and thus enter into a new and much more enjoyable dimension of living, one in which they will begin once again to feel together and solid.

As this feeling grows in depth they will experience a growing sense of inner peace. Once they come to realize that all of life awaits, that the world can benefit by their presence and by what they have to contribute—at that moment, they will be well!

The knowledgeable Hygienist realizes that successful recovery can often depend on the establishment in the mind by the client of the importance of certain long-range health goals; that temporary inconveniences and/or hurts must often be abandoned or laid aside to accommodate more worthwhile long-range objectives. Often such a motivated person will say, "I can bear it!" When the sick persons can do this and refrain from settling for "relief" in favor of real health, they make their strengths stronger and lessen the importance of their present symptoms. These then no longer cloud their mind to the actual healing that is taking place.

Persons who are able to make this transition learn to speak to parts of them that are in need and with a positive voice. They develop a higher perception and appreciation of their own body's capabilities. They know that they possess a power to focus in on themselves in such a manner that healing begins to accelerate.

Learning that we can get around our bodies with our mind can be a powerful vital force. It can help us to break down long-standing habit walls and make a place both in our minds and in our physical bodies for new and healthier patterns of living that will make our future journey into health shorter, easier, and, above all, rewarding beyond our fondest expectations.

95.3.2. Getting Out of the Self-Destructive Phase—the Mental Rollover

For recovery to be assured, clients must move their minds out of and away from the self-destructive phase of their past that may have thus far restricted their progress. For example, persons who have believed all their lives that germs and viruses are primary causes of disease actually have child minds and exaggerated egos. Egos so powerful as to believe that "they" can do nothing wrong will be reluctant to accept cerebrally the fact that their present debilitated conditions are direct results of errors, errors that they themselves perpetrated and this over a long period of time and in every aspect of living.

This is a monumental admission for some ego-centered persons to make. Those who are able to move out of this self-destructive phase will be successful in recovering wellness; those who do not, will fail.

Then there are those individuals who live in the past. Such as these must do some mental gymnastics. Their minds presently are constrained by regrets: If only I had done thus and so, or if only I had not done that. Or they may even say, "As soon as I do this, that or the other, I will be well!" But they constantly fail to move their minds out of this nonactive mental vise which constrains all progress into a more active stance: from going to make the required changes and adjustments because they lack an active, forward looking mind into motivated performance, the actual doing of what is required of them if they are to achieve their objective, that peace of body and mind which can be experienced only in total wellness.

In order to move the mind into a state of willingness to write a higher and better life script, the student of Natural Hygiene must actively decide WHAT s/he wants to do. S/he must first establish the objective. The. mind must move out of the past and begin to create mentally an entirely new life. This kind of mental gymnastics, known as the Mental Rollover, requires graduated changes:

1. The DECISION that the past was lacking in some respects and, specifically in this discussion, that health was less than perfect.

2. The change in ATTITUDE, moving from egocentrism to a less-dominating role— that of a penitent, of course, but a forward-looking penitent, one who can participate in change.

3. A change in THINKING and here we refer to the development of the mind to such an extent that the client begins to open hidden recesses and exercise cerebral capabilities, these having been long neglected insofar as addressing the physiological and biological needs of the body were concerned.

Establishing in the mind that the client is no longer grasped by the "Poor Little Me!" syndrome because s/he is now and always was someone deserving of a far better life, can actually do it and, not only that, but can do it on his/her own, all by him or herself.

This is the final change, UNDERSTANDING that life is not a dress rehearsal, but the here and now, a reality in the making. There is no magic about living the healthy life; it simply requires knowledge about what to do and then the follow-through, the doing. Understanding that you ARE, that there is a hidden potential that lies deeply within all of us and also that there, within us, rests the person we can be, is perhaps the ultimate mental activity that can cause an actual birthing and future development of that presently sleeping, but potentially healthy, being to awaken.

The changed activated mind can create, cause, and control the becoming of the soul. In understanding lies the key, the cerebral acceptance of the fact that our future is actually our present, that what we do and accomplish this day will bear fruit tomorrow. If what we do today is health-promoting, then we will, on the morrow, become healthier.

This then is what is required for patients to move into health, to move out of the Self-Destructive Phase. Before meaningful progress can be hoped for, they must first of all make this Mental Rollover. They must stop playing the popular game of Victim, they must establish firmly in their subconscious their own self-worth. They must shift their minds into high gear, begin to think through their problems, figure out realistically what they need and must do to change their present state of diminished health into a higher degree of wellness and then begin to appreciate the fact that to achieve their objective it is reasonable and truly scientific for them to start by meeting their known physiological and biological needs, and that while certainly they will be called upon to initiate continued and vigorous movement of muscles and bones, they will also find it necessary to activate their mental processes. They must develop the willingness to learn new things, entertain new ideas, and develop new concepts.

Someone has said that most people would rather do anything else than think. To achieve whatever goal has now been established, the novice Hygienist, the one who desires above all else to achieve a high degree of health because s/he knows that everything else s/he may enjoy and experience of goodness in this world will be of his/her own making, the one who wishes above all to leave the Self-Destructive Phase as represented by the past, into a new and more promising dimension of life, must now fully activate the mind and learn to think in an expanded way and a higher plane.

95.3.3. How to Plan for More Positive Mental Activity

There are probably as many ways to stimulate positive mental activity in clients as there are individuals. Rarely will we be able to actually intrude into the herd to obtain our clients. Those persons who do seek our help can usually be divided into three classes:

1. Those who seek our aid in desperation, having exhausted all known traditional sources.

2. Those who wish to keep their feet firmly planted within the herd but have a faint recognition of the fact that in Natural Hygiene there is something of value that they may

possibly put to good use in their own lives, although they remain, at this moment, uncertain of what that may be or how it may be applied by them; and

3. Those persons who, perhaps by chance, become exposed to Hygienic principles and practices and become convinced of their soundness and resolve to learn more and perhaps even to apply it in their own lives.

The practitioner will soon learn that there will usually be but limited success in activating the minds of the first group. Members of this group may progress to a limited extent but, at the first health crisis, even though it be minor, they tend to seek "relief" for whatever ails them. They thus revert back to their former ways even though they may feel that the practitioner has their best interests at heart. Their minds have been too well programmed in orthodoxy to make the giant leap required to become true Hygienists.

With members of our second group, the ones who are reluctant to renounce totally the ways of the masses, the practitioner can often achieve a fair degree of mental activity. There will be acceptance of concepts and principles, but limited application with the health benefits being commensurately curtailed.

The third class will become the achievers, the performers. With open active minds, they will challenge concepts, analyze them, reject some and accept the best. These they will incorporate into their personal plan for living, their plan for the future. In these persons, the Hygienic practitioner will find his/her rewards, soon learning to classify clients and be able to arrive at a fair approximation of just how much a prospective client will be able to achieve in new mental activity in the days that lie ahead. It then comes down to "how best to achieve results?"

95.3.4. How to Encourage a More Positive Mental Attitude

Since in this limited discussion we do not have time to develop ideas and minds," we will simply list some of the ways and means of mind activation that we have used and found applicable in many instances. They may then be weighed, evaluated, rejected, or utilized in practice as they may or may not prove useful with individual clients.

1. At each consultation it may prove stimulating to present a pre-planned orientation which deals with a topic, idea, problem, concept, etc., which, in the opinion of the practitioner, best pertains to a particular client. For example, with almost all clients, it will prove highly motivating to introduce them to the concept that chronic disease represents a long and traceable biological evolution. Another thought-provoking (activating force) idea to consider is that disease is self-caused. This gives the practitioner and the client the opportunity to explore the four categories of causes of disease: Poison Habits, Emotional Causes, Excesses in Lifestyle and Diet and Deficiencies in Lifestyle and Diet and to see how these may relate to a client.

2. Relate all topics, ideas, problems, etc., which are discussed specifically to a particular client. In this manner, the client begins to think about how s/he may have arrived at his/her present sorry state. S/he often actively begins to sort out life errors, a prerequisite for making correct decisions in the future.

3. Group discussions should be sponsored as time and opportunity permit. Here new clients can come face to face with more experienced students and in sharing with them enlarge the learning experience.

4. Tape recordings. These can be listened to either at group meetings or in the privacy of the client's home. The practitioner may either keep a lending library of these tapes for individuals use or make them available for group meetings. Clients may also be encouraged to purchase certain tapes which the practitioner considers worthy of a particular client's attention. Tapes can reinforce concepts learned elsewhere.

5. Reading. Clients should be given printed matter in the form of short discussions deemed of particular value to a client. A practitioner may operate a lending library for a fee, or s/ he may simply recommend certain articles and/or books to clients.

6. Seminars that clients may be encouraged to attend.

7. Conventions where the client may have an opportunity to become acquainted with the widespread interest in Natural Hygiene, with persons whom s/he may only have read about but whose opinions s/he values and meet and talk with individuals who may be in various stages of recovery from a similar ailment.

Clients who participate in as many of the above kinds of activity as possible will find their minds expanding. Their acceptance of new ideas will also grow and, in due time, the salubrious effects of this kind of positive imprinting will be experienced throughout the entire body, in every organ and system and, importantly, in the mind as well.

A stagnant mind will soon atrophy and become little more than diseased tissue. But, a mind that remains active, constantly challenged by new ideas, thoughts and concepts will grow and expand in health. Learning about the true science of life and healing (Natural Hygiene) can fill this basic systemic need.

95.4. Physical Exercises Suitable for the Bedfast

95.4.1. Aerobic Exercises

Health is impossible without exercise. This pertains to all persons but especially so to bed-fast persons who, if not exercised, will grow weaker with each passing day.

All bedfast individuals should either exercise every day on their own following a well-planned sequence of movements as presented to them by a skilled practitioner or, if incapable of voluntary movement, have their muscles and bones moved by an attendant as need suggests and capacity to accept permits.

The best way for bedfast patients to begin an exercise program is to use tension exercises. These should be followed faithfully and methodically in a planned sequence. Proceeding in this fashion accomplishes more than just muscle participation. George M. Weger, M.D. points out in his book, The Genesis, and Control of Disease, that exercise assists in "the development of self-control and self-discipline, which are so necessary to those who wish to acquire poise and to become master of self." As J. H. Tilden and others have pointed out, superior health is impossible without first developing poise.

Tension exercises are simple to perform. They can be performed in depth or shallowly, in a prone position or sitting up, either in or at the side of the bed. The arms, legs, abdomen, and neck can be used.

Each person should exercise in this fashion at least twice each day, every day, in the morning and evening. The time devoted to tensing will depend on several factors: the willingness of the person to participate, the client's age, vitality, muscular ability, and willpower. Unless the client is in an extremely weakened condition, s/he should start with from five to ten minutes devoted to tensing of muscles.

Weger reminds his readers that to obtain the maximum good, the muscular contraction should be positive, and the mind should be concentrated on every movement. It should be willing participation. Otherwise, the exercise will prove of little value. The time spent in this voluntary activity may be increased as progress indicates with fifteen minutes per session being advisable but with thirty minutes being the maximum.

Other Movements. Progressive movement of muscles in the following recommended sequence:

1. Flex fingers (bend at joints) of both hands simultaneously starting with a count of five and building up gradually to a count of twenty-five.

2. Clenching fists and proceeding as above starting again with five reps.

3. Making a circle with full hand in motion. Increase reps to 25.

4. Reverse circle and repeat.

5. Holding arms straight out in front of body, with hands parallel to the bed or floor, move to right and then to left keeping arms still.

6. Assuming same position, bend at wrist and move hands vertically upward then follow with a downward thrust so that tips of fingers point at the bed or floor.

7. Bend arms at elbow and bring into side of body. Thrust forearm forward while simultaneously flinging wide the fingers. Repeat.

8. Repeat forearm thrust outwardly and to the side. 5 to 10 reps.

9. Bend arms at elbows and raise shoulder high. Now thrust vertically to the ceiling flinging wide the fingers. 5 to 10 reps.

10. Lie prone in bed. Pull shoulders up to ears several times.

11. While lying prone, flex toes forward, then backwards. Do hot bend the entire foot, just the toes. 5 to 10 reps.

12. While lying prone, bend the entire foot forward pointing the toes. Return to position and then pull the toes back toward the legs. Repeat with 5 to 10 reps, or more.

13. Keeping knee of right leg straight, raise to vertical position. 5 to 10 reps.

14. Repeat with left leg.

15. Move right leg parallel to bed and out toward the right. Repeat using the left leg and moving it to the left. Increase distance and number of reps from 5 to 10.

16. Simple rotation exercises first with the arms while in an upright position, then with the legs in prone position. Be sure to keep elbows and knees straight. 5 to 10 reps. These can then be followed by rotating the shoulders.

17. Face exercises may be included, such as grinning, yawning, blinking, and screwing the mouth from one side to the other.

18. Neck exercises should be done two and three times a day: turn headfirst to right, then to left; pull head forward to chest and then as the strength and vitality improve, resistance may be given to these movements by exerting an equal and opposite pressure by holding the palms of the hands against the head. The head may also be moved first down to the right shoulder and then to the left.

19. Place a blanket or pillow under the shoulders thus allowing the head to fall back. In this position a number of movements may be carried out as, for example, raising and lowering the head; moving the head in various ways as in rotating; tensing and relaxing of the abdominal muscles; kneading of the muscles of the abdomen using the fingers or the knuckles.

20. In a reverse position with blanket or pillow under chest and the client on bended knees, move body to full upward hump and then downward again.

21. Sway body first to right and then to left while in the same position.

22. If the client can sit on the side of the bed, s/he should attempt as many of the following movements as possible and as vitality allows leg lifts, leg rotation, bending torso forwards and backwards and from side to side. The spine should be twisted first to right and to the left. If the room is large enough, while doing this right-left twist, the eyes should be focused on three successive points each located directly in front of the client: first, on floor, next to a point directly ahead and lastly to a point on the ceiling. In this manner the eyes will not be neglected but will also be exercised and thus strengthened.

These same exercises will prove useful to clients who are not bedfast but can walk and move in an upright position. In either case, the client should be given a printed chart explaining the different exercises and the number of reps to be made.

It is always helpful, too, to furnish each client with his/her personal chart. On the chart s/he can note the day of the week, the number of the exercise(s) performed, and the number of repetitions of each, plus the total time exercised.

Other exercises which can be exceedingly beneficial in recovery when the client possesses good movement and sufficient vitality is obtained through free-form dancing. Here the client simply sways and moves to music. If the client is in a comparatively debilitated condition, the music selected should be kept subdued and it should have a rather slow beat. Sliding of the feet along the floor, raising legs by bending at the knee, turning, twisting, dipping, and many other movements are possible in slow free-form dancing. Older clients who have led sedentary lives enjoy these kinds of sessions and especially when they can join a group in the activity.

As the health, vigor and endurance increase, the beat can be speeded up with the movements therefore being made at a faster pace and even becoming more extensive and of a greater variety.

Free-form dancing imparts a good feeling to the participant. It provides emotional release which is always beneficial.

Tennis, badminton, perhaps even skiing and weightlifting being careful at all times not to expend too much vital force without compensatory nutritive reward.

95.4.1. Aerobic Exercises

Rarely are aerobic exercises recommended for persons in a highly-debilitated state. They divert too much energy away from the healing and reparative efforts so essential to recovery. We observe far too many unfit persons actually doing themselves more harm than good as they jog along the roads here in Tucson, even in the hottest weather. Their efforts would be better utilized and produce greater good if restricted to the type of activity outlined in this lesson and we refer to both aspects of activity, both mental and physical.

Recovery from illness demands much energy. In illness, we should conserve our energy and permit it to be directed where it will do the most good rather than expending it in exercising overly much without receiving compensatory value in return.

In recovery simple movements will encourage the circulatory powers sufficiently to transport the required nutrient tools to those areas where the need exists. When the recovery so indicates, walking may prove to be the most beneficial of all exercises. As the health continues to improve, sprinting for short distances can be introduced. Alternate walking and running, increasing the tempo of the walk are useful additions to the exercise regimen. Only the fit should jog and even then, the time and distance should not be such as to create undue fatigue.

Swimming for short periods in water with the temperature not exceeding 85° Fahrenheit, can be beneficial during recuperation. As the health, endurance and strength continue to improve, the client may choose from a wide variety of possible sport activities, such as tennis, badminton, perhaps even skiing and weight-lifting being careful at all times not to expend too much vital force without compensatory nutritive reward.

95.5. The Role of Feelings

One important adjunct to recovery from illness that needs to be addressed when planning mental and physical activity for a client is that of Feelings. Seldom do sick people express their feelings in a positive way. They are usually revealed in negative attitudes, words, and actions.

The client who slumps in his chair reveals perhaps that he is listless, tired, or simply not interested in the present activity. He also reveals that his body is highly toxic.

The facial expression may be tense, the expression worried. The spoken words may be sad words, not happy ones. The eyes are often dull, lacking the sparkle of interest in life. The whole attitude can be one of removal from the real world, of extreme depression. When the mind is depressed, the organs and systems are in a like state.

When exercise is first proposed to such clients, they often, on first venture, tend to withdraw, even to express verbally a reluctance to participate. This is where group activity can prove enormously helpful. If our depressed and discouraged clients can be stimulated to perform even a few simple exercises they soon find their former depressed feelings being replaced first by the satisfaction of accomplishment, however limited, and, as time goes on and they become more skillful and begin to acquire increased endurance and strength, they often become imbued with a sense of happiness, of joy, which is in and of itself highly conducive to a resurgence of health.

Replacing negative depressed feelings with a series of Positive Belief Systems causes a realignment of the thought processes which project into the consciousness creating a climate in which problems are capable of solution. Once Belief engages the consciousness, it is sometimes amazing to watch the physical responses that begin to take place. For example, skin disorders that may have troubled for years often clear up with surprising speed.

When the system is engulfed by such feelings as jealousy, worry, anxiety, anger, superior health is impossible. When the system is engulfed by the feeling of Fear, this can be the ultimate confusion which can destroy life.

Whenever a person is ill, any feelings that are held in tend to distort the whole person. They can soon undermine the health of the mentally tormented person. We find that women and men alike, as they begin their middle years, the so-called middle-crisis years, are often actually terrified at the prospect of the future. They fear the horrible diseases they feel are sure to come. Are they not all around them?

Are not all older people decrepit and senile, a burden on society? Do not the young desert the old ones and leave them totally alone? Is THIS not the only possibility the future can hold for ME.

We must change all that! This kind of negativity will give way when confronted by knowledge. We must convince clients that this kind of unfounded fear is a cover-up, pure and simple, a cover-up for not acting intelligently and for not actively pursuing the kind of lifestyle that is known to be more conducive to health than that pursued in the past. We must show our clients that when one harbors a vision of a future filled with diverse diseases, then the body is not only already well filled with toxins but is continuing to gather more.

Only when fear is driven out of the body can the individual be free again to activate both mind and body in such a way that forward movement toward improved mental and physical health becomes a matter of fact and not an impossible dream.

When the fluids of the body once again course through the arteries and veins in a cleansed and purified state, then disease becomes impossible. The tormenting visions leave, never to return.

Healing begins the instant that tenseness, depression, fear, and other feelings depart.

At that moment positive things begin to happen.

As the minds of clients are activated to believe that the future lies almost entirely in their own hands and that their destiny can be of their own making, they rapidly begin to show improvement.

Goodness always feeds upon itself and draws to itself even greater good. The pains of life are revealed in feelings, to be sure, but these psychic pains can be used to motivate. Activity, mental and physical both, can help a client to let go, to fight for the health rewards that are sure to come when the lifestyle habits become normalized; that is, in tune with organic laws.

Certainly, if the future is to be at all normal—lived in health—then clients must begin now to incorporate into their lifestyle all of the known requisites of human existence, including a full quota of correct physical and mental activity. Often just knowing that they can do it can motivate a client to make the necessary changes.

Bernard Jensen in his book, You Can Master Disease, says it quite well: "More important than the cleansing of the bowel, more important than correcting a mechanical maladjustment in the body, is teaching the patient how to remove fear, how to control his emotions, and how to get ease of mind."

And, to quote Shelton, "Joy and happiness are essential to health. There are few Hygienic influences that are equally as conducive to health and long life as a cheerful, equitable state of mind." (From Living Life to Live It Longer.)

Free-form dancing or performing tensing exercises to a happy lively tune cannot help but cheer and activate the mind, sending it spiraling in a new and healthier direction. Encouraging such activity, which combines both the physical and the mental, can greatly assist the sick, the mentally weary, the depressed to enter a totally new dimension of life, one rooted in feelings of joy and happiness and destined to grow in health.

95.6. Four Case Studies

95.6.1. Case Study No. I

95.6.2. Case Study No. II

95.6.3. Case Study No. III

95.6.4. Case Study No. IV

95.6.1. Case Study No. I

Irene was 42 years of age. Her husband was an alcoholic. Her days of parenting were completed, the children on their own. For the past five years she had suffered from an assortment of "allergies" which made her life miserable. She had been injected with various drugs, so many she couldn't even remember their names. She constantly had to sniff antihistamines in order to breathe. Her whole attitude was one of depression. She could find nothing good about this life and confessed that she had often thought of suicide.

Upon review of Irene's past life and of her present lifestyle, it was obvious that changes needed to be made. A dietary regimen geared to the Extended Detoxification Plan was advised and begun. Our client was encouraged to take daily walks, to sunbathe as often as she could, and to begin a program of study in Natural Hygiene to learn the why and how of her new regimen.

This was, of course, all good. If followed carefully, there was no doubt in our minds that Irene's health would improve but, because of her greatly troubled and depressed attitude toward life, her improvement would, in all likelihood, be quite slow. She needed more. She needed to be lifted out of her depression, to be helped to realize that life really is worth the effort, that it can be happy, and joy filled.

To accomplish this objective we proposed certain steps for our client to take: 1. To look around for some hobby or interest to replace her former parenting, the absence of which now left a vacuum in her life which required filling; 2. To go to an Al-anon meeting and there to listen and learn how she might better cope with the demands put upon her and the frustrations she now was experiencing in her life because of her husband's alcoholism, and 3. To attend such group meetings as we might present in the coming weeks and months.

Irene agreed to cooperate in all these suggestions. She took a course in Reflexology as well as all of the courses that we have written over the years. She became a faithful attendant at Al-anon meetings and at our group's study and social get-togethers. In addition, she reported her progress to us every three months.

Not too long ago, Irene telephoned to share a success story with us. It seems that her family had always "put her down," perhaps because she had always been rather "sickly," as she described it. But the evening before, she had received a long-distance telephone call from a sister who had developed a severe bronchial condition which, according to her physician, required surgery. So impressed was the whole family at the improvement in Irene's health, what Irene had accomplished, that they had advised this sister to call upon her for advice! Irene was "on cloud nine!" That had never happened to her before in her whole life! Mental and physical activity combined with appropriate changes in her eating and lifestyle had accomplished what we had set out to do: to so improve her health that she would be an inspiration to other sick and depressed souls.

95.6.2. Case Study No. II

"Sam," actually short for Samantha, was in her middle fifties. She was at least 75 pounds overweight, outwardly happy as a lark, but inwardly disturbed about life and her precise role in it. She had reached a point in her life which many people reach who live from day to day without purpose or direction. She had just drifted through life.

She had been a willing follower of the masses, enjoying their destructive lifestyle, with no thought of the future.

Suddenly, and totally without warning, or so she said, she was confronted by a major health problem. She had just been diagnosed as having hypoglycemia. She was angry now at the whole world, albeit still wearing her habitual light-hearted expression which, during our initial consultation, proved to be but a mask to hide her inner confusion and anger.

A review of her eating habits revealed the customary diet of persons who suffer from hypoglycemia and diabetes, one overloaded with all kinds of processed carbohydrate foods such as sugar and white flour; all the many kinds of foods concocted from these substances, plus considerable emphasis on processed convenience-type packaged foods, many of which contain large amounts of fats and pure cane sugar. Foodless foods such as these overwork the pancreas and other endocrine glands until the body is simply not able to utilize its inherent balancing mechanisms with the result, of course, that a metabolic disaster scene results with the blood glucose levels fluctuating abnormally.

Sam told us that she had become very forgetful and had difficulty in concentrating. In fact, her mind often went blank. She had lost her temper at work on several occasions, a new trait for her. She said she was usually quite easy to get along with. She had times when she felt faint and suffered from headaches, also a rather recent symptom. She had always felt so well! And as for fatigue, it seemed that now she was always tired, never rested.

Obviously, Sam needed help. We prescribed for her an immediate fast for three days, the entire time being spent in bed. She was to remain as quiet as possible. Following the three-day fast, Sam was introduced to Hygienic living. Because of her excess weight, vigorous exercise was not to be recommended at this time. Therefore, a twice-a-day walking schedule was decided on. Sam, like all of our clients, began a basic course of instruction with the purpose of directing her mind into more positive channels, to help her to realize that her present apparently hopeless situation was really not so devoid of hope after all. Later Sam joined a class in exercising designed for older persons. She was thus being reprogrammed in three different directions: A new diet, daily exercise geared to her present capacity, plus a planned educational program designed to present her with a new perspective on life's rules.

Sam lost weight slowly as planned, but consistently. Her listlessness and fatigue, her forgetfulness, the headaches, and other symptoms have all either completely disappeared or been much alleviated. Her mental outlook is again one of genuine cheerfulness. Sam knows exactly where she is headed and fully confident that she will achieve her new goal: perfect health.

95.6.3. Case Study No. III

95.6.3.1. Encouraging Activity in Sickness

Mrs. M. arrived here at the Institute extremely debilitated, so much so that it was deemed advisable to put her immediately to bed. Her blood tests revealed that her entire system was operating in low gear and that she would have to be handled with extreme care. Her medical history confirmed our appraisal since it revealed that for many years this woman had been a willing subject of medical mismanagement on a grand scale.

Through the years she had suffered one extirpation after another including the removal of tonsils and adenoids at an early age, this followed at age 28 by a cauterization of her womb after having partially recovered from typhoid fever. At age 37 a complete hysterectomy was performed because of profuse bleeding during menstruation, this proving to be a most trying time.

At about 54 the gallbladder was removed and, just "as a precaution," the surgeon thought it best also to remove the appendix, this decision apparently having been made during the operation and without the patient's consent or knowledge.

Several heart attacks followed in rapid succession and for the three years preceding her seeking Hygienic care, Mrs. M. had lived the life of an invalid unable to carry on even simple household tasks. As with so many, she had exhausted all orthodox avenues as well as her financial resources before seeking the only method of health care based on physiological and biological truth. She did so at the request of a relative newly introduced to Hygienic care.

Following two days of complete bed rest combined with physiological rest, Mrs. M. brightened. It was thought advisable to encourage some activity on her part even though it was obvious that vigorous exercise was, at this time, completely out of the question. However, we knew that it was vital that the blood flow be encouraged. Because of her weakened heart and a generally-debilitated condition, it was agreed that this client could not go on a prolonged fast which might have rested the heart and encouraged reparative processes. Therefore, it was decided to place her on a juice diet for a few days, both vegetable and fruit juices being used alternately during the day in two-hour intervals. As an adjunct to this light feeding program, we decided to begin a scaled-down activity program, one which would require both physical and mental responses.

Only too often, it is not realized just how important both mental and physical activity can be in illness. When the mental processes become dull, a similar reaction can be observed in the physical body. Thus, mind cooperation and mind control are both helpful and necessary to full recovery. Mood swings, especially when the valleys of depression are deep and the peaks are overly high, can undo other measures being used in a constructive manner and even though these may be based on sound physiological and biological bases of fact. Therefore, it was decided to introduce both kinds of activity this early in the program but to do so only to a very limited extent.

95.6.3.2. Mental Activity

In her debilitated condition, Mrs. M. had little awareness of events or things. She was too concerned about her condition to display interest in external happenings. The anxiety so evident in her facial expression was being mirrored internally in lessened systemic efficiency as well.

It has long been known that superb health is impossible when the mind is disturbed, depressed and anxious. It was important, therefore, to direct Mrs. M.'s attention away from herself toward other things of a happier nature. Therefore, we placed1 Mrs. M's bed in such a manner that she could watch the bird feeding every morning and evening. At feeding time, we would visit with her and identify the various birds and tell something about their habits. We recounted how one Arizona roadrunner became crippled in one leg, but did that stop him? No, indeed! Every day, in fact twice every day, he came to the feeding ground hopping around on one leg. We told her that, at first, this valiant bird barely made it but, as time went on, he became stronger and stronger until, finally, he was hopping with the best of them.

We told her that this is the way with all living things; that so long as they obey nature's laws, feeding and living in accordance with the body's needs, then repair and healing will take place. No doubt, this great strong bird had been severely injured but rest, suitable food plus determination had produced the healing required for him to live a reasonably good life. We reminded her that she was no different, that her body had the same wondrous capacity to heal itself, too, and that now, at long last, she was embarked on a journey into health. There was much to learn and do but, like the valiant and brave roadrunner, she could make of this a highly-successful journey.

Thus, Mrs. M's mind was focused in a new and more positive direction. It was activated to believe that by following after the principles and practices espoused by Natural Hygiene, she just might be able to enjoy life again instead of having to endure the mental hurt of being totally dependent on others for her care and nurture and this, too, for the rest of her life. At age 62, this thought had become a nightmare that ate away at what little wellness she had left. Now, for the first time, she had hope. Her mind that had turned now became imbued with and activated by an inspiring song of hope.

Some comparable tactic can often be used with similarly anxious clients. Some may have a latent interest in knitting, others in listening to good music, still others like to listen to stories about what other people in similar circumstances have done to improve their health. Whatever sparks attentive interest should be explored.

95.6.4. Case Study No. IV

At age 27 Mark was schizophrenic. He lived in his own private world and had done so for well over a year when we were brought into the picture. At first he would not even meet with us, even when we went to the home. Therefore, our initial steps had to consist

517

of improving the food intake. Both parents cooperated fully and within a few months Mark began to make tentative steps out of his mental prison.

Our first glimpse of the young man came when, on a house visit, he peeked around a corner and quickly withdrew. We seemingly ignored his behavior and Dr. Robert began to talk about weight-lifting and suggested that perhaps Mark might enjoy this kind of activity. Mark's parents thought this might be a good idea, so they agreed to purchase two five-pound dumbbells for a trial run, so to speak.

The experiment worked. Mark "took" to the dumbbells and, before long, he had acquired some skills. His mother said that this was the first time since the mental curtain had descended on Mark's mind, that he had shown any sign of interest in anything or anyone.

On our next home visit, three months later, we were delighted to find Mark sitting in the living room, a big smile on his face. He could hardly wait to show us his new dumbbells. They were ten-pounders! To our delight, he willingly demonstrated his newly-acquired skill.

Mark still has a long way to go on his journey into health, but he is on his way. The next step? We have suggested that his parents now join a fitness club so that Mark can see and be with other young people and thus further activate his mind, as well as his physical body. His parents have agreed to take this important step. Mark has expressed his willingness to join them in this new adventure.

95.7. Conditions Where an Exercise Program Would Be Contraindicated

1. Moderate to severe coronary heart disease that causes chest pain even with minimal activity.

2. A recent heart attack. Usual recommendation is to-wait for three months and then begin a light program under supervision.

3. Any severe disease of the heart valves. Slow walking may be tried.

4. Certain types of congenital heart disease.

5. Greatly enlarged heart.

6. Severe heartbeat irregularities.

7. Uncontrolled sugar diabetes with high fluctuations in blood glucose levels.

8. Hypertension with blood pressure readings, for example, of 180/110.

9. Extreme obesity. Walking permitted.

10. During acute diseased states, especially where there is fever.

The above restrictions pertain, of course, to vigorous and sustained exercise. Exercises which are performed slowly and for a limited time or if done with assistance can prove beneficial in most cases, even in patients suffering from one or more of the above ailments.

The patient requires careful observation during exercise periods and the exercises should be immediately stopped if the patient shows signs of weariness, of if the skin turns either blue or excessively pale, or if the patient begins to breathe overly hard.

The rule of thumb is to start with simple movements. Observe the response and the reactions given by the patient. And, to build slowly!

95.8. Questions & Answers

When a person is very weak from a long history of erroneous living, I fail to see how exercise could possibly benefit that person. Can you clarify this for me?

I will do my best. That's a good question. In extremely weak persons, exercise might properly be contra-indicated. A fast with complete bed rest might be in order for a time. However, remember that most ill persons have lived a sedentary life. Healing and repair will not be possible until their wounded sick cells have their toxic load removed and they then receive the nutritive materials they require for reparative and healing purposes. By exercising specific areas that is exactly what we encourage: the directing of the lymph and blood to the area's most in need of cleansing and feeding by free-flowing fluids.

How do you know when it is time to introduce exercise?

That's an easy question. You try out a few passive exercises and observe the response. If the patient soon exhibits fatigue, you stop, wait for a suitable resting phase and then you try again.

Why is the lymph so difficult to activate?

The lymph flows first into the lymph nodes and has to be squeezed out by the contraction and relaxation of the musculature in that section of the body where the lymph nodes are located. By this squeezing action, the lymph is sent forth into the lymphatic channels and thence into the bloodstream. As you see, therefore, without exercise, this lymphatic flow is minimal.

Why are feelings so important in healing?

The mind gives a clear picture actually of the body. When the mind is sad, the whole body is sad, also.

All the metabolic activities throughout the entire body are similarly depressed. When fear grips us in the thought body, it also grips body action via the autonomic nervous system. It can even stop digestion entirely. We have all degrees of feelings. As they fluctuate from happy to sad, so does our body activity. Illness traps our feelings in depression, sometimes quite deep. A healthy state imparts a happy state, not only to the mind but actually throughout the entire body, a state revealed by systemic harmony. George S. Weger, M.D. was the first person, I believe, to note the importance of mental poise to health. His views were supported by J. H. Tilden and, in later years, by much research.

I like the tension exercises. Why do you especially recommend them for ill people. Would they not be good for everyone?

Certainly. As you perform them, you will probably notice that you will use muscles you have not used for some time. You will note that, if you perform each exercise in sequence, that you will have exercised just about every part of your body. And all this without needlessly wasting your vital force as so many people do without understanding the purpose of exercise, which is to encourage circulatory flow of fluids to accomplish two purposes: 1. to remove toxins and 2. to bring food to the cells. Do we need hours of exercise to accomplish that purpose? Let's use our heads!

As for the first part of your question. They are especially good for ill people just because they do not call for any undue expenditure of vital force. Also, the number of reps can be adjusted to individual strengths as well as the depth of the exercises being used.

Article #1: Fitness Guide

Nothing is either good or bad but thinking makes it so! Your brain can make you ... or break you! It takes in, and interprets, each situation you face. It sparks your every thought, emotion, action ... conscious or unconscious. Hippocrates sensed this over two thousand years ago as the cause of "our joys, delights, laughter ... the fears and terrors that assail us, some by night and some by day."

Emotional stress cannot be measured. It has no meaning except in the way you react to your own life problems! ... Nothing is either good or bad but thinking makes it so!

Don't get the wrong idea about stress! Like fear, stress is no new thing. It has been with man since man began.

The tensions, anxieties, fears ... the stress of our atomic age ... are no worse than those our forefathers faced ... only different! Man dies as surely by axe or arrow, by sword or spear, as he does by bullet or bomb!

Life is a perilous adventure. It always has been ... and a perilous adventure it seems sure to remain. Only the problems change with the changing generations ... the pressures never do.

How your mind and body react: Above your kidneys lie your adrenal glands that secrete the hormone adrenalin. Sudden anger, sudden fear, trigger these glands. Into your bloodstream shoots adrenalin.

Your blood pressure jumps. Your heart pounds. Blood from your stomach and intestines is shunted to your heart and muscles. Your breath comes fast. You tense to act ... but you can't!

Why? Because your problem differs vastly (though your body does not) from the one your ancestors faced a hundred thousand years ago. How to save their skin (yet eat) was their problem. To live they must have food. To get food (and keep it) often meant to kill or be killed ... to fight or to flee! At such moments, their anger, their fear, triggered adrenalin into their blood ... for sudden extra power to their blows ... or sudden extra speed to their legs, if they had to take to their heels to save their skin!

Not so with you, an executive faced with the kind of opposition you cannot batter down with your fists! Only a slight tremor of your hand as you hold a paper may betray the anger you smother! What irony! That swift dose of adrenalin nature intended to help you, hurts you ... if time after time after time, over the months and the years, you smother your anger or fear!

What combat studies show: In combat, every so often, a soldier, will succeed in an astounding feat, utterly impossible to a man not triggered by sudden terrible rage or fear. Afterward, this man is as much astonished by what he did as are his comrades. Now ... when his rage or fear subsides, he feels nauseated. He may have to vomit the food he had no chance to digest ... and he may discover, to his disgust, that he has lost control of his bladder or bowels ... and shakes as if he had a chill! The cause? An overdose of adrenalin! (This same reaction can be reproduced in a calm man by injecting adrenalin under his skin.)

... Long-sustained, smothered stress can bring on a heart seizure. You have only to remember how your heart pounds when you get in an argument to sense why this is so. Studies show, in fact, that emotional stress is five times as prevalent in heart attack victims as in men with normal hearts. Yet not all stress is harmful ... far from it!

A man who is a man thrives on a reasonable amount of stress ... As that philosophic old character David Harum put it years ago: "A reasonable amount of fleas is good for a dog ... keeps him from brooding over being a dog!"

... Some men can relax within a few minutes after a situation is over; others cannot. Their over-mobilized bodies refuse to return to normal. As Dr. George B. Stevenson, internationally known psychiatrist, cautions: "The time to watch out is when tensions come frequently, shake us severely and persist...."

Transitory (and at first reversible) changes resulting from stress may lead to irreversible disorders.

Article #2: Application of Gymnastics to the Sick by Herbert M. Shelton

Exercise is often of more importance than changes in the food supply. This is essential not only as a condition prerequisite of assimilation, but as a means of directing with certainty and precision, just what parts and what functions shall receive the needed nutritive support. Pabulum has not the least intelligent and self-directive power, its flow is controlled by the demands of activity.

Food or nutritive support cannot in the least degree be forced upon inactive muscles and organs. These get their chief support by acting, for only in this way does the need of the support arise. To flood the system with an abundance of nutritive substances cannot increase its powers unless the necessary intra-cellular conditions for stimulation are present.

Such surpluses of nutrients accumulate as waste, due to crippled elimination, and become the source of greater weakness. Increase of strength is the complex effect of a number of essential antecedent factors, of which food is not always the most essential. We have seen numerous cases where there was an actual gain in strength while no food was being taken, though previous to beginning the fast these patients were losing strength on an abundance of "good nourishing food."

It frequently happens that the greatest need of an invalid is exercise, either local or general. In numerous cases this alone has resulted in complete restoration of health. Many invalids fail to recover health, because, although all the other factors are right, they cannot be induced to take sufficient or appropriate exercise.

Numerous methods are employed for the purpose of increasing the nutritive processes in local parts, as well as in the general system, but none of them are as efficient or as devoid of harmful consequences as muscular action. None of them are so prompt, none so localized, none so economical of vitality. Artificial agents and measures employed for this purpose occasion other actions and induce irrelevant changes and needless vital expenditure. These methods involve a harmful and uncompensated expenditure of the client's power.

Excerpted from Chapter 19—Exercise!

Lesson 96:

Corrective Exercises and Their Application

96.1. Introduction

96.2. What Is a Corrective Exercise?

96.3. Deformity Is Widespread

96.4. The Spine

96.5. Correct Postural Maintenance Vital to Wellness

96.6. Exercise—General

96.7. Questions & Answers

Article #1: Excerpt from Funk and Wagnalls New Encyclopedia

Article #2: Exercise

Article #3: Good Posture by Dr. Herbert M. Shelton

Article #4: Correcting Sensitivity to Light by Edwin Flatto, N.D., D.O.

Article #5: Words of Wisdom by Silvester Graham

96.1. Introduction

Humans were designed to live active out-of-doors lives, to forage for food, to seek shelter where it could be found and as need arose. They were structured to live among the trees and in the forest, to do physical labor for agricultural purposes, to tend to the harvest and to pick the fruit from tree and vine.

But humans were not designed to live in air-tight houses, to sit at a desk for hours on end, or to apply their minds constantly and continuously to solving multiple problems. Humans were not made to toil under electric lights or to sit passively for hours reclining in an overstuffed easy chair passively watching phantom figures flitting by on a television screen, all the while receiving multiple nerve impingements due to electrical and radiation impulses emanating from an electrical box and being transmitted through the ether.

Neither were humans designed to eat as the average person eats in today's world but, to the contrary, people were provided with certain digestive organs possessing well-defined physiological limitations and capabilities, organs made to process simple natural foods freshly gathered and served in the simplest of combinations, if combined at all.

Probably in no other country in the entire world has the available food been so altered and changed and in such a short time as in the U.S., although presently many countries of the world are fast imitating "The American Way," and reaping the same "benefits." Dr. Edmond Bordeaux Szekely in his The Book of Living Foods points out that, "From the starch-loaded, high-calorie fuel foods of our pioneer ancestors (who presumably needed strength to fight the Indians, who in turn won many battles eating only nuts and berries), to the "breatharians" of the 20s, ... our history has been studded with all kinds of nutritional facts and fancies."

As on many past occasions, the U.S. Government is again expressing dismay at the lack of physical fitness among children and young people in general. On all sides, even a casual observer of the current sad scene can see stuffed noses, curved spines, mouths dangling wide open, a lack of symmetry to childish bodies, sadly restricted by maligned organs and a veritable host of encumbrances of one kind or another. Hygienists have no lack of opportunity to do their best to correct that which obviously presents a major threat to the on-going vitality of our nation.

There can be no doubt that only a full application of all known Hygienic principles and total obedience to the biodynamics of our organic existence can save the human race from extinction and return it to its former pristine and perfect form. We have strayed mightily and willfully far from the physical beauty of face and form and lack the strength of the men, women, and children of ancient Greece. In no way do our children and young people bear any resemblance to the strong and straight offspring of the Mongols of northern China or even the young Romans who lived in earlier centuries;

and fewer yet adults who presently possess the strength and erectness of posture evidenced by the Greek dockworkers, for instance, of Sylvester Graham's time. Flat-footed, spines curved in and out and sideways, the men and women of today's world wend their weary way with stiffened muscles and osteoporotic bones.

It will probably take many generations of Hygienic living to return the human race to some semblance of what full health and perfect form can offer. We can only imagine such a time and place. However, the correct and consistent application of corrective exercises and a Hygienic lifestyle can at least improve the lot of some individuals who might otherwise suffer either now or at some time in the future from an ailment which, in the final analysis, might well be traced back to some deviation of the physical structure from the norm, such deviation being of either major or minor importance.

In this discussion, therefore, we will simply describe certain structural malformations giving, in some instances but not in all, the possible future negative consequences vis a vis the overall health of an individual who remains thus encumbered, and then present certain corrective measures which have been found to produce salubrious results in the past and which may prove of benefit in working with a particular client.

Obviously, there can be no guarantee that existing structural defects can be altered to such an extent and in such a manner as to return the body to a perfectly-normal state. There are always many determining factors that influence the direction, extensiveness, and effectiveness of physical therapy, just as there are in all remedial effort.

We refer to such factors as the overall health and vitality of a person, how fully s/ he understands exactly what s/he must do and why, how well s/he applies him or herself in the doing, mental attitude and natural intelligence, concentration on the task at hand, how well s/he lives his/her life in accordance with the universal laws of nature, the encouragement and familial support s/he receives, etc. Only in rare instances perhaps will total performance and total benefit be achieved, but even minor positive changes can add up, in the final analysis, to improved appearance and many years of more enjoyable and healthful living.

Because of the nature of this discussion, there seems to be no valid point in quizzing students on the lesson content. This lesson should therefore be used as a point of reference, among others which may be available, in planning corrective exercises for specific individuals having a well-defined structural defect which, in our best judgment, seems to limit their potential wellness.

96.2. What Is a Corrective Exercise?

96.2.1. How Do Corrective Exercises Differ from Other Kinds of Exercises?

96.2.2. The Physics of Corrective Exercises

Shelton defines corrective exercise as meaning the use of exercise to correct an anatomical defect or deformity, such as the size, shape, position, and so forth of some part or group of parts of the body that do not conform to the norm.

Among the types of defects or deformities which are subject to correction through exercise in varying degrees are the following: club foot, spinal curvature, bowlegs, misshapen fingers, poor posture, uneven shoulders, deformities of the toe, etc.; all, of course, to a greater or lesser degree depending on individual factors.

96.2.1. How Do Corrective Exercises Differ from Other Kinds of Exercises?

We can divide types of exercises into three main categories:

1. Hygienic exercises which include the more general exercise routines which are designed for Hygienic improvement of the health and vitality of an individual.

2. Remedial exercises are designed to affect certain desirable changes in persons afflicted with adverse physical results from poliomyelitis (less common now with improved sanitation than in former years), paralysis resulting from accidental or other injury, certain spastic conditions, respiratory ailments, and so on. Remedial exercises are usually done under the tutelage of a physical therapist and must be carefully monitored.

3. Corrective exercises are specific in kind, being designed and targeted for a particular area of the body and to accomplish a precise purpose. Corrective exercises can, Obviously be pushed more rapidly and more vigorously than possibly might be done with remedial exercises.

96.2.2. The Physics of Corrective Exercises

The proper use of exercises to correct a deformity or anatomical defect is based on certain well-known physiological facts and physical laws.

The physiological basis for the use of corrective exercises lies in the fact that while life exists there is change. The body is always in a state of organized flux. Every day cells die and every day new cells are born—all kinds of cells including bone cells but excluding brain and nerve cells.

Brain cells, once dead, do not replace themselves. We lose several millions of brain cells every day, never to be retrieved. Severed nerves cannot be restored but intact nerves, even though damaged, do tend to improve, albeit slowly, under careful Hygienic care.

In considering the physical basis for the effectiveness of corrective exercises we observe that the muscles of the human body have two main purposes:

1. To produce a desired movement as and when directed by the central nervous control mechanisms, and

2. To hold the bones in position both in rest and in movement.

Muscles are differentiated from the various and several ligaments which are simply sheets of fibrous tissue which connect two or more bones, cartilages, or other structures; or they serve to support the fasciae or muscles and retain organs in place.

Every muscle and each ligament has received a specific name and is registered in the complex volumes of medical nomenclature, but such precise terminology is not a necessary part of a Hygienist's training unless s/he so desires. There are many medical reference books to supply such information.

It should be remembered that it is the stronger muscles and their accompanying and therefore stronger tendons that become shortened, while the weaker muscles and their tendons become lengthened and weaker over the years.

Such changes are accompanied, in general, by a corresponding change in the length and strength of the ligaments and often, too, in the shape of the bone, and especially so in the ends of the bones where articulation occurs. Dr. Herbert M. Shelton provides an example of what may occur as when there exists a concave curvature of the spine, there simultaneously develops a shortening of the side muscles, tendons, and ligaments of the individual thus impaired.

In working with clients, it must be remembered that forcing is always contraindicated. Bones cannot be carried beyond their prescribed normal range of movement without causing injury to the ligaments attached to or near the joint being moved. It is these ligaments that bind the bones and permit their articulatory movement. Damaged and injured ligaments can prove extremely painful and difficult to heal.

It is the counterbalancing effect of muscles together with the constant turnover of cells that gives effectiveness to corrective exercises.

96.3. Deformity Is Widespread

96.3.1. What Causes Deformities?

96.3.2. The Most Common Deformities

There is widespread deformity among the populace today, some of it absolutely appalling. Just a few days ago we saw a striking example of inexcusable deformity in a fully-grown adult woman, in her middle years. She was exquisitely dressed, her coiffure had been arranged with great skill, cosmetics had been artistically applied, but the overall impression created by this woman was grotesque to an experienced eye. Her entire torso was out of alignment, a fact made very evident to us as she teetered by on her four-inch heels.

This woman's entire chest cavity represented no more than one fourth of her total body height, so small in size it was. She gave the appearance of two different women trying to exist in a single body! With such impaired respiratory capacity, her days of living will be severely curtailed. We doubt if very much could be done to correct this woman's structural defects at her stage in life. The older a person is, the more difficult it is to make changes and the longer it will take, all other things being precisely equal.

Another example cited by Dr. Shelton and one we can observe all too frequently in both children and adults is the size of the chest at full inspiration; that is, with deep breath. Only then is it extended somewhat close to the size it should be when fully empty! As many as 85 percent of the children sitting in the secondary school classrooms today have severely-limited chest capacity.

96.3.1. What Causes Deformities?

Deformity has its roots in many errors. Obviously, most of the damage is done by the mating of two physically-deficient parents who either cared not or had little or no knowledge of the possible consequences, long-term and/or short, of their sexual union; by the poor prenatal care and feeding of mothers; by the lack of exercises during pregnancy, during infancy and throughout childhood and by the physical restraints placed on children today who are foolishly kept indoors in classrooms for long hours sitting in unnatural positions at imperfectly-constructed desks and who receive limited and often inappropriate exercise.

Hygienists and physical therapists generally agree that most deformities are caused by one or more of the following:

1. Poor choice of ancestral heritage.

2. Poor health of parents.

3. Faulty nutrition before and after birth.

4. Continuing and long-lasting systemic fatigue due to many possible assaults, mental and physical.

5. General systemic weakness resulting from a plethora of physiological assaults of one kind or another, especially poor food choices.

6. Astigmatism that gives one an incorrect assessment of surroundings, both immediate and distant.

7. Impaired hearing, especially if in only one ear, a condition which may cause a person to turn his head to the source of sound in an effort to add visual response to the auricular.

8. Poor lighting that causes one to pull his torso away from a more normal stance and toward the source of light, often an occupational hazard.

Type of occupation as, for example, the hod-carrier whose one shoulder becomes wider and longer than the other and the bones which form it become thicker and more dense; or an interest or hobby as with the violinist who, after years of daily practice often extended for hours at a time, finds his left shoulder lower than the right shoulder and that the general alignment of the head, neck, shoulders, and arms is faulty.

Most deformities can and should be prevented through improved lifestyle. Where they exist, many, indeed most, can be corrected, especially when corrective measures are instigated at an early age, the earlier the better.

96.3.2. The Most Common Deformities

The most common deformities observed are:

1. Rounded shoulders.

2. Various forms of spinal curvatures including:

    a. Wry neck or torticollis in which the head is drawn to one side and usually rotated to some degree so that the chin points to the other side.

    b. Kyphosis, a term used to indicate an accentuation of the backward curve of the thoracic spine. Kyphosis is a condition which imparts a rounded or hunched appearance since the convexity of the curve is outwards. The degree of curvature, of course, will vary from individual to individual, with some being acute, others less so.

    c.   Lordosis, or the opposite thrust of the spine with an exaggeration of the forward curve of the spine causing the condition familiarly known as "sway back," or hollow back. Lordosis is usually accompanied by awkward movement of the buttocks in walking since the deformity often extends to the pelvic area.

    d.   Scoliosis, a term used to indicate the side-to-side curve of the spinal column with curvature either to the left or right to form either a C curve or to both the left and the right to form an S curve. The affected person tends to "list" to one side.

Any or all of the above deformities can be multiple in kind as, for example, a combination of both kyphosis and lordosis; or one or more can be combined with individual vertebral malformations and/or rotations of one or more of the vertebrae of the spine.

Spinal abnormalities sometimes appear at birth, perhaps during the growing years, but they usually just creep up on a person as he slowly deteriorates biologically over the years. Generally speaking, the above deformities will usually be the kind that will come to the attention of the Hygienists after they have been well developed.

Spinal abnormalities, which are far and away the most common, and regardless of how classified, generally develop silently and stealthily, without pain. It is interesting to note that perhaps as much as 30 percent of the bone structure can deteriorate before such deterioration can be detected by X rays.

According to the Scoliosis Research Society of the American Academy of Orthopaedic Surgeons, about 10 percent of the adolescent population have some degree of scoliosis. Parenthetically, scoliosis should not be confused with poor posture.

The Scoliosis Foundation states that "there are currently no medications to treat scoliosis, nor can its onset be prevented." Hygienists would agree that the condition cannot be "treated" with drugs but do not agree that such a deformity cannot be "prevented." The human body, like all living things, always tends to grow toward perfection when given the proper tools. We agree with the Foundation in saying that the treatment is mechanical, but we go further in that in any program designed to correct any deformity, it is necessary to employ all the known requisites of organic existence as and when required and as present capacity indicates, these used in conjunction with certain exercises specifically designed to correct the existing defect.

96.4. The Spine

96.4.1. Not Just a Cosmetic Problem

96.4.2. The Missing Ingredients

96.4.3. How to Detect Spinal Abnormalities

96.4.4. Typical Exercises Suitable for Mild Scoliotic Impairments

96.4.5. Exercises for More Severe Scoliotic Impairments

96.4.6. Exercises to Strengthen Abdominal Muscles

96.4.7. Exercises to Strengthen Side Muscles

The bony part of the spine is made up of a series of separate bones called vertebrae. In humans, the vertebrae are stacked "like a column of poker chips." They are held together by the ligaments.

The number of vertebrae vary, among different species of animals but, in man, the spinal column contains 33 vertebrae, as follows:

- 7 cervical vertebrae in the neck.

- 12 thoracic or dorsal vertebrae in the region of the chest or thorax. These provide the attachments for twelve pairs of ribs.

- 5 lumbar vertebrae in the small of the back.

- 5 fused sacral vertebrae forming a solid bone, the sacrum, which fits like a wedge between the hip bones.

Plus, a number of vertebrae which are fused together to form the bottom or base of the spine, known as the coccyx at the bottom of the sacrum.

During the fetal period, the spinal column forms a single curve with the convex surface toward the back. However, at birth, two main curvatures are present, both of which are concave forward. The upper curvature is located in the thoracic and the lower one in the sacral region. With normal development, two compensatory forward curvatures develop in the cervical and lumbar regions, just above the primary curvatures. These provide the resiliency which a stacked bone structure could not possibly provide. Unfortunately, as we have noted, a perfectly formed spine is a rarity, indeed, in today's world. As can be seen in the diagrams which follow, the vertebrae serve as protective housing for the spinal cord which functions in the transmission of ascending impulses from all parts of the total body up to the brain and of descending impulses and directives from the brain via the cord to all parts of the total body. This housing is known as the spinal canal. Peripheral nerves from many parts of the body enter into this housing and are affiliated with the main nerve cord. These transmit all manner of information from peripheral centers to the cord and thence to the brain and also appropriate responses from the cerebral centers back to the peripheral regions, and finally to individual cells. Every single muscular movement requires this transmission of information, the cerebral interpretation and the psychological and physical result(s) of the interpretation, the response.

96.4.1. Not Just a Cosmetic Problem

A spinal abnormality is not just a cosmetic problem, although that can be psychologically damaging in itself since it can lead possibly to rejection by one's peers particularly during the teen years and to depression and social isolation.

But, additionally, since all such irregularities tend to cramp all the abdominal and chest organs and can act. as an impediment to breathing, to digestion, and, in fact, to all bodily processes and will continue to do so throughout all of a shortened life, they should be corrected as early as possible and to the extent possible.

Unless mechanical corrective exercises and perhaps even braces are worn, the deformity can provide a seat for continued degenerative processes with later development of arthritis of the spine with increasingly severe back pain and disability.

The curvature tends to increase, and as it does it pushes down on the ribs attached to the spine. This in turn, narrows the chest cavity and restricts the ability of the lungs to expand. Thus, the lack of sufficient oxygen intake hampers full metabolic efficiency throughout the lifetime, which as we have noted, is usually shortened.

Dr. Hugo Keim of the Columbia University College of Physicians and Surgeons is reported to have said, "Telling a child with a scoliotic back to stand up straight is like telling a man with tuberculosis to stop coughing." Thus, most specialists insist on using the brace.

The most commonly-used brace, the Milwaukee, consists of "a leather or plastic pelvic girdle to which are attached three upright bars, one in front and two in the back. At the upper ends of the bars is a ring that circles the neck. A child wears the brace 23 hours a day, with an hour break for bathing, swimming or relaxing. Exercises are performed daily in and out of the brace. Total time in the brace averages 36 months, during which the child may take part in most of his usual activities." (Quoted from Parade, Oct. 28, 1979.)

If braces are used, they should be employed between the ages of 10 and 15, the period when growth tends to spurt, and scoliosis most commonly develops. Dr. Keim maintains that exercises are not sufficient to treat scoliosis, that using the brace is a "must."

Surgery is used in about one out of every 1,000 cases and is resorted to when bracing and exercises prove inadequate or when, in the beginning, it is obvious that other measures are required. Following surgery, the patient must wear a cast that may remain in place for as long as from eight to ten or more months.

At the Hospital for Sick Children in Toronto, a Dr. Walter P. Bobechko and his colleagues are said to be experimenting with the implanting of from three to six electrodes which are inserted into muscles of the back. During the night, while the patient sleeps, "mild electrical impulses are sent to the electrodes to activate the muscles, so they gradually straighten the curve." It is said that such treatment can only prove useful in young patients with at least two years' growth remaining and a curvature of less than 40 degrees.

96.4.2. The Missing Ingredients

All methods presently employed by the medical community depend solely on mechanical gadgets of one kind or another with the occasional administration of drugs to palliate symptoms of pain, to alter the mood when the patient becomes depressed, and/or to "biochemically balance" the mineral composition of the system. Little or no attention is given to the total spectrum of organic requisites or to the universality of the laws of life.

Even a beginning Hygienist knows that when any living creature fails to receive the tools of life, he will eventually, sooner or later, find that his health will decline, and his lifespan will be shortened in an amount determined by the extent of failure to meet the organic need. There can be no doubt that the body structure will be adversely affected.

Therefore, while the Hygienist would make full application of the laws of physics and his knowledge of the fact that all healing and repair must be self-instigated, self-regulated and self-powered, s/he would also employ all the known biodynamics of life, fresh air, pure water, sunshine, and warmth, all the psychological "pluses of life,"—in fact, all the many "tools" the body must have to straighten out and remodel young malformed spines.

Dr. Shelton in his book Exercise on page 262 says, "Lordosis is not difficult to correct, but the corrective work must be continued for a prolonged period." He goes on to state that this corrective work consists of training for proper posture, stretching the muscles and ligaments of the lumbar spine and strengthening the abdominal and psoasiliacus muscles (lower end of spine), all accomplished in due course, through the patient and persistent application of muscle stretching and working in specified patterns of movement, all of which, of course, must be pursued with full attention also being paid to all other biodynamics including revision of dietary practices when necessary, daily sunbathing in the nude whenever possible, extended periods of rest and sleep, and so on.

Yesterday, while at the printers, we began talking with a woman who had heard about our interests in matters of health. She told us that her fifteen-year-old daughter was afflicted with scoliosis but strangely, according to her, "No one seems to know much about it."

Upon inquiry, we learned that her daughter was receiving mineral medication in the form of multi-mineral capsules and a special pill "because she needs calcium." We asked her to what her doctor attributed her daughter's spinal abnormality and received the reply that "he said that no one knew what caused the condition and nobody knew how to treat it. She had come to the conclusion that her child would just have to live with it, meaning the scoliotic spine.

We suggested that possibly a Hygienist would be able to help her daughter and told her we'd be happy to recommend a good one to her and her daughter, one very knowledgeable about spines. We further encouraged her to study something about Natural Hygiene, that perhaps some dietary improvement might be in order. She laughed and said, "You know how these teenagers are today. I'll never get her off her hamburgers and coke!" And off she went, laughing.

Little did she realize that, in all likelihood, by such casual acceptance of the commonly-held belief that "nothing much can be done," she, in all likelihood, was condemning her child to a lifetime of low-back pain plus a multitude of allied disorders stemming from an impinged nervous system and an impaired digestive tract.

96.4.3. How to Detect Spinal Abnormalities

The following screening test has been devised by the Scoliosis Association. With the client standing straight, look at the back:

1. Is one shoulder higher than the other?

2. Is one shoulder blade more prominent than the other?

3. When the arms are hanging down loosely at the sides, is the distance between the arm and body on one side greater than on the other?

4. Does one hip seem higher or more prominent than the other?

5. Does the child seem to lean to one side?

Now, with the child bending forward, arms hanging down loosely and palms touching each other at about knee level, look carefully.

1. Do you see a lump in the back in the rib area?

2. Is there a hump near the waist?

If the answer is yes to any of these questions, professional examination and help is probably in order.

Other visual imperfections can also be noticed as, for example:

3. Does the client have a "swayback" (lordosis)?

96.4.4. Typical Exercises Suitable for Mild Scoliotic Impairments

1. Test your posture by standing with your back against a wall. Learn the mechanics of good posture by trying to straighten your back. Avoid a lazy slouched posture or a too rigid posture, either of which will tend to emphasize existing curves in the back.

2. Straighten the curve in your neck by standing tall with the chin slightly tucked in. Standing tall, consciously, is part of the Alexander Technique. Notice how it seems to re-align every part of the body, both internally and externally.

3. Tall girls and boys may try to look shorter by slumping. Most short people tend to have good posture with spines well positioned. Teenagers should be encouraged to straighten the curve in the lower back (swayback) by tucking in the stomach and tilting the pelvis forward (known as the pelvic tilt).

4. Tighten muscles in the buttocks, bending the knees slightly.

5. Stand behind a straight chair. Hold on to the back. Now assume a squatting position. Maintain this position as long as possible. Repeat for from two to five or more minutes several times a day.

6. At work or at home, sit on a straight-backed chair. Lean forward in the chair and lower the head to your knees. Maintain this position for at least one minute. Repeat, until you can hold the position for as long as five minutes. Notice how the back muscles are being pulled.

7. Use the slanting board several times a day. If a slanting board is inconvenient to use, as at work, simply lie on the floor and place both legs on a chair. Press shoulders back to floor. Maintain position for from five minutes (at first beginning) to as long as thirty minutes, after practice.

Many people think that just because the muscles on their arms and legs are strong and muscular, that the muscles on the back will be in a like condition. This is not necessarily so.

The muscles of the back should be thought of as being similar to the guide-wires that support a growing tree. If these wires are strong and kept taut, the tree will grow straight and be flexible but if, however, the wires are loose and mispositioned, the tree may not fare at all well, becoming crooked.

It is the same with the spine. If the tools for proper maintenance are lacking, the spine may become crooked with swayback or some other impairment developing. Therefore, it is important for both the back and the abdominal muscles to be strengthened in all persons, but especially when a scoliotic spine is evidenced. These back and abdominal muscles are the "guide-wires" to impart strength and flexibility to the spine.

96.4.5. Exercises for More Severe Scoliotic Impairments

These exercises may be performed in addition to those already suggested for milder impairments of the spine.

1. Partial bending forward while maintaining a straight back. Client may sit in a chair while performing this exercise. The number of repetitions (reps) will vary with the vigor of each client. Start with five.

2. Sit on the floor with legs extended out in front. Lean forward and touch toes with the fingers.

3. Lying on the back, elevate feet and legs to vertical position pointing the toes and trying to reach the ceiling.

4. Place client on a table with legs extended in front of him, the knees held straight. Stand in front of subject and grasp both wrists. Have client's feet push against your abdomen. Now pull the client forward and downward as far as possible. Repeat several times.

5. Lie on the floor with the hands behind the head, elbows on the floor. Keeping the knees straight, raise the legs and thighs to a 45° angle. Now, extend the legs outward in opposite directions. Bring back to position. Repeat several times. Relax. Elevate again, extend, etc. Repeat several times.

6. Lying on the back bring the knees up on the chest. Spread the legs apart as you straighten the knees, then draw the feet together. Repeat several times without resting the legs on the floor between movements.

7. Assume same posture as in Exercise 6, imagine a balloon tied on a string being suspended from the ceiling. Kick the balloon away from you, using both feet simultaneously.

8. Lie on the back on a table. Draw one knee up on the chest while the Hygienic therapist resists the movement. Repeat using other leg.

9. In same position as in Exercise No. 8, flex both thighs on the chest against the applied resistance of the Hygienic therapist.

10. Hang on bar. Raise the knees upward until they are at right angles to the abdomen. Hold for several seconds. Relax. Repeat.

11. Hang on bar. Extend legs outward and upward until they are at right angles. Hold for a few seconds. Relax. Repeat.

12. Hanging on a bar, flex knees as in Exercise Number 10 above. Now, straighten legs outwards. Hold. Relax. Repeat.

13. Simply hang from the bar in a relaxed position for a few seconds. Repeat several times.

96.4.6. Exercises to Strengthen Abdominal Muscles

As previously noted, it is just as important to strengthen the muscles of the abdomen as those 'supporting the spine in the back. However,/in this connection, it is important to choose exercises wisely.

Exercise, to be constructive, should not be easy but, on the other side of the coin, neither should they cause pain. If pain results from a particular exercise, that exercise should immediately be stopped. Pain is a body signal that injury has either occurred, or that one may be imminent. A wise precaution for therapists to follow is to do less than you should early on in working with a client. One can always add on, i.e., increase the intensiveness and/or the extensiveness of a particular muscle movement but, once an injury has resulted from the wrong kind of exercise or the manner in which a particular exercise was performed, then it is too late and further activity must be delayed until full healing has taken place, this sometimes requiring a prolonged rest—delaying progress. It is best always to keep in mind our "baby step" approach. Succeed with small successes.

The following exercises are suggested to strengthen abdominal muscles. They can be done in sequence or selections made to suit a special need.

1. Lying flat on the back on the floor, legs outstretched in front of you, point the toes and stretch to the extent possible. Relax. Notice the pull on the abdominal muscles. This exercise strengthens ligaments and muscles that lie vertically.

2. This next exercise may be done in three levels of achievement.

    Lie flat on your back with both legs and thighs straight. Point the toes of both feet and raise both legs. Lower and repeat.

The three stages of effort exerted in doing this exercise will depend, of course, upon the strength of individual muscles. It is not wise to attempt Stages 2 or 3 before gaining sufficient strength to perform Stage 1 with ease. After Stage 1 is accomplished, then the client may progress to Stage 2, and so on.

Stage 1. Have an assistant hold down the back while another assists the client in performing the upward movement of the legs. As strength increases, less assistance should be given.

Stage 2. The client places hands under the buttocks and lends support himself as legs are raised. An assistant may hold down the back in the early days of progression, but all assistance should eventually be abandoned as strength improves.

Stage 3. The client should perform this exercise unassisted.

3. Lying on the back, raise the right leg to a vertical position. Now carry the leg across the left leg as far as you can. The goal is to touch the floor on that side. Now return the leg to its former vertical position. Repeat. Do the same exercise with the opposite leg being raised and carried to the floor on the opposite side.

4. Lying on the floor with the feet hooked under the bed frame or with an assistant holding the feet firmly on the floor, with arms folded across the chest, raise body up to a sitting position.

This exercise may also be done in stages according to present capacity to perform, as follows:

Stage 1. Instead of placing arms in the folded chest position, place hands under the buttocks to add additional support to weakened abdominal muscles. Hygienic therapist lends assistance to the upward movement by giving back support.

Stage 2. Place hands under buttocks, feet firmly held by either an assistant or under bed frame or other restraint, raise body up to sitting position unassisted by therapist.

Stage 3. Hands folded across chest, feet firmly planted or held, with therapist assisting upward movement, raise to sitting position.

Stage 4. Perform exercise unassisted.

Stage 5. Lie flat on floor, arms extended fully behind head and on floor. Throw arms forward and at the same time, sit up. No assistance. In early days, it may be well to keep knees bent or even to elevate the legs vertically and use their pull to assist the body to attain the sitting position.

Stage 6. The difficulty of this exercise may be increased by clasping the hands behind the head and, without assistance, raising the body up to the sitting position. In performing this movement, the arms and shoulders should be held firmly back. Otherwise, this exercise has a tendency to encourage a rounding of the shoulders.

5. Twisting of the torso. Stand upright with feet slightly apart. Place hands on hips and focus eyes on a central spot on the floor. While performing this exercise, keep the eyes focused on this spot. Now, twist to the right as far as possible without straining, then to the right. Up to 20 reps. This is Stage 1.

    Stage 2. Focus eyes on a spot about halfway up the wall directly ahead of you; or, if out of doors, focus on some central object. Repeat physical movement, twisting to right and left, but keep the eyes on the one spot. Up to 20 reps.

    Stage 3. Focus eyes on a spot above in front of you on ceiling. Repeat exercise as above.

A dual benefit is received from this twisting exercise: stretching and firming of the horizontal abdominal and back muscles plus accomplishing the same for the eye muscles. Blinking the eyes after this exercise will help to relax the muscles.

96.4.7. Exercises to Strengthen Side Muscles

In correcting spinal imperfections, it is important to work also specifically on the side muscles. The following exercises are designed to stretch and strengthen these seldom-used muscles.

1. Stand erect, with the feet together and the arms extended over the head. Bend sideways at the waist, carrying the extended arms over slightly in advance of the head. Bend alternately from left to right but hold each bend for from 5 to 30 seconds. Keep the legs straight as you bend.

2. Rest weight of the body on the right bended knee. Extend left leg out to the side. Now bend the body to the right as far as possible without raising the left foot from the floor. Therapist should assist client in maintaining balance.

3. Repeat exercise no. 2 in the reverse position, resting weight on left knee and extending the right leg and bend to the left.

4. Lie on the right side on floor. Balance body with arms. Raise extended left leg until it is perpendicular with the body.

5. Repeat exercise no. 4 while lying on the left side. (Exercises numbers 4 and 5 may be increased in effectiveness by adding weights to ankles. These may be purchased at almost any sports store.)

6. Stand erect with a barbell of convenient weight suspended across shoulders and behind head. Bend alternately from one side to the other.

7. Rest the weight of the body on the extended right arm and on right foot. Place left hand behind head. Now lower the hips until they touch the floor. From this position, bring the body up and raise the hips until the body is arched. Lower and repeat. Therapist should support and assist on first doing this exercise and it should not be attempted until back, stomach and side muscles have shown progress.

8. Perform exercise no. 7 from the opposite side, resting the body weight on the feet, extending the left arm.

96.5. Correct Postural Maintenance Vital to Wellness

96.5.1. Pain

96.5.2. Sports Injuries

96.5.3. How to Keep a Straight Back and Improve Posture

96.5.4. If There Is a Back Injury, Certain Common Habits Should Be Overcome

The posture of the average American and also that of many others we have observed in our travels is in a sad state. Many deviations from the norm can be observed, especially in the natural curves of the spine. Postural defects are less serious than scoliotic ailments which represent degenerative changes brought about by incorrect habits of living. Postural defects can be more easily corrected than scoliotic abnormalities and in a shorter time.

It is important for the individual to maintain good posture for when the body parts are balanced and integrated, arranged naturally in a flexible manner, with energy and movement directed upward, the whole torso following—going with—the head, the entire body, its cells and organs and systems will be enabled to function more efficiently and in a more flexible manner.

When the body is balanced, correct nerve messages are relayed from one part to another, from one system to another system. There is better coordination and synchronization of part to part. When parts are correctly aligned, one to another, only those muscles which are essential to a particular action will be used to perform that action, thus saving precious vital energy. One can accomplish more and perform better and feel less tired than where the parts remain uncoordinated, poorly synchronized due to misalignment through carelessness or habitual slouching. In other words, when the posture is poor, we work against ourselves, we use energy that we need not expend to perform functional duties and movements just because everything in the body is not in its more proper position of balance. The systemic equilibrium is destroyed, tension pervades the body, even though we may not be consciously aware of such tension. This is exactly the same kind of tension (stress) that is radiated outwards in a leaning tower (as, for example, in the famous Leaning Tower of Pisa located in the Piazza del Duomo in the northeast part of the Italian city), or in a pile of bricks which have been incorrectly stacked.

Incorrect posture, in time, will lead to chronic low back pain, a condition which troubles many people today. There are many causes of poor posture: malnutrition, lack of exercise, occupational fatigue; emotional problems concerned with such things as family, financial security, sprains, disc damage, habits of daily living, etc.

When we consider that the average American spends countless hours every day staring at a television tube while sitting slouched down in an overstuffed chair, it is a wonder that we stand as straight and tall as we do and enjoy any degree of health!

96.5.1. Pain

Postural low back pain can be consistent and chronic and if we ignore the warning sign of early acute pain and do not begin a series of corrective measure, the aches and pains may become chronic, entering the vertical stage, until sooner or later, the back gives way.

Pain in the back develops when specific nerve endings are abnormally irritated and begin to send distress signals up the spinal cord to the brain's control center. Sometimes, the back muscles will receive instructions to go into spasm in an effort to hold the back immobile and quiet.

All of us are aware of the fact that there are innumerable nerve endings which intertwine and go in and out of the spinal cord. There are various conditions which can give rise to back pain such as were detailed above, these being both physical and/or emotional in kind. The worst enemies of the back are poor posture, a lack of exercise and overnutrition.

An increased lumbar curve as in sway back is indicative of a weak bony structure. Weak and flabby abdominal muscles (the familiar pot belly) deprives the back of its main support. Any overweight can add to back strain.

The average person when he feels pain simply takes a pill to get immediate relief. As Hygienists well know, such a practice is totally anti-health since chemical painkillers act to narcotize the nerves, to prevent the cerebral recognition of the systemic danger that is presently threatening the life process. The cause or causes of the pain remain undetected and, therefore, still working.

But there may be another and less apparent hazard in such a practice. Dr. Steven F. Brena, director of the Pain Control Center at Emory University in Atlanta believes that drugs become "associated with the pain itself, so the very act of popping a pill stimulates the feeling of pain."

It seems that, like Pavlov's dogs which salivated at the ringing of the bell, chronic pain sufferers may unwittingly learn to feel pain from the very drugs they take for relief!

In the Medical News Section of American Health for June 1984, Brena is reported to have said that "learning is important factor in any chronic illness." He believes that most people abuse pills. We should probably say that almost all people who use drugs, abuse them. Personally, we feel that painkillers should only be used in extreme cases, as in surgery or in certain advanced degenerative conditions when all other methods have failed.

Brena compares the central nervous system to a computer. It can be programmed to be pain sensitive, and the pain threshold lowered. (Emphasis by the authors.) He calls it "learned pain," a condition which creates further dependence on drugs. He cites the possibility that pain can become a physiological response elicited by the very drug taken to relieve the pain.

The possibility may exist that pain is not only a molecular cellular response, but also a psychological and perhaps even a social response, the "everybody-does-it" syndrome. At Emory's Pain Control Center, Dr. Brena attempts to retrain the central nervous system to raise the pain threshold, but he says it takes hard work. It also requires much systemic work to relieve pain.

Orthodoxy has not as yet learned the efficacy of fasting to relieve pain. If our students recall the case of Mike, our severely arthritic patient. After over fifteen years of high drug dosing to relieve his excruciating pain, he recently reported that he had just had two whole days during which he was totally without pain! Mike, our students will recall, has had two kneecaps removed as well as one elbow joint. Considerable fusing of his skeletal structure has made him almost, completely dependent upon others for his basic needs. What he has accomplished under great odds should inspire the most downhearted among us. A veteran, living alone except for the help of a university student, he has, with great determination over the past year fasted for short intervals and completely changed his dietary, has squeezed his rubber ball, has walked his corridor from bedroom to living room, faithfully and consistently, and is now beginning to reap his reward! Mike knows that the future is his to have, an unnarcotized future and one without pain.

Back in about the year 1945, Dr. Elizabeth injured her back badly. A heavy iron spring which helped to raise and lower a garage door gave way throwing her up in the air and then back on the concrete driveway. The pain was intense, but she refused all attempts to hospitalize her. She took as few aspirin as was possible. We were not Hygienists, yet!

Years later, when locking of muscles and the intense pain of arthritis descended upon her, the worst pain was felt at the site of this old injury. Of course, over the years, she had "favored" her back but in the late fifties, she began to notice that she couldn't walk either as long or as easily as she once had been able to do. Dr. Elizabeth, early in her career, had taught physical education as well as Swedish gymnastics. She had been a track star while in high school, took interpretive dancing while in college. The psychological effect of her disability obviously was intensely negative.

In the early sixties came the final episode which was to start us on our search for a "cure." By this time, Dr. Elizabeth had to hang on to another person to walk. If she got down on the floor, she had to have assistance to get up. She walked the floor night after night because of the pain.

It was then that we began a program of therapeutic exercise, learning about it and putting what we had learned into practice. Every night, Dr. Robert massaged her back, using open fingers along the spinal column, gently pressing along the lateral muscles outwardly.

As she lay on the floor, her legs were, at the beginning, lifted for her to a vertical position, and then lowered. Gradually she progressed through the exercises which are detailed in this lesson. She set herself goals to achieve and as she achieved one goal, she would move on to the next.

Let us see the sequence that took place with the bent-knee sit-ups. Her first goal was to perform a single sit-up without assistance. At first, her back had to be helped in raising to the sitting position. But the time came when she made it alone!

The next goal was to do 10 unassisted sit-ups with hands held under the thighs. When this was achieved, she placed her hands at her sides. The new goal was to do 10 sit-ups again. Then, to do 30! About two years ago, Dr. Elizabeth did 30 unassisted sit-ups holding her hands at her sides.

But she wasn't finished, yet! Her next goal was to accomplish 10 straight-leg sit-ups starting from a position where her arms were extended behind her on the floor. These were to be used as a leverage in achieving the sitting position. After about six months she was able to do 20 of these. She hadn't, as yet reached her final goal: to do 30 sit-ups with hands clasped behind her head, but she knew she'd get there one of these days.

Then, it happened! Another accident. Several months ago, she was out feeding her beloved birds. It was an unusually cold morning for Tucson. Having several appointments scheduled for that morning, she was in a hurry and caught her open-toed slipper in the curled hose which was rigid due to the overnight freeze. She went sailing through the air, landing on her right side, and skating along the gravel which tore at her muscles and ligaments.

For weeks, Dr. Elizabeth could hardly move. She took no pain killers in spite of the severe pain. Hot baths and occasional short fasts took away all the discomfort, but she was unable to do a single sit-up, to say nothing of most other exercises. But was she defeated? Not Dr. Elizabeth! Just the other day she did 26 bend-knee sit-ups, her toes tucked under the bed frame. She's off again with new goals beckoning down the road.

Incidentally, for females over the age of 60, those achieving bent-knee sit-ups in 90 seconds are awarded the Platinum Accolade. Dr. Elizabeth did hers in 60 seconds and she confesses to being over 70!

We have included this story in this lesson, not to brag, but to make a point. In working in the field of corrective exercises, patience and persistence will be rewarded.

In the legal world, there is an old saying, "Time is of the essence." This phrase is found in many contracts, especially those having to do with the sale or purchase of real estate. It means that within a certain time frame, the contract must be fulfilled and all legal obligations with respect to that particular contract must be fulfilled.

In correcting spinal or other physical imperfections, time is also of the essence but here the phrase must be interpreted differently. Corrective work cannot be hurried. The body will establish its own schedule and cells will be repaired according to a cerebrally devised master plan. The repairing and healing will take place methodically, generation by generation of cellular replication, as the body receives the proper tools—all of them. We refer, of course, to the biodynamics of organic existence.

It would be the height of folly, for example, too. expect recovery to occur with speed if proper-food be not eaten or should the impaired individual fail to obtain maximum rest, both physiological, mental, sensorial, and physical; or any other of life's basic needs.

It is this one element of time that is perhaps the most difficult of all principles for the novice Hygienist to grasp. Correcting defects in the physical structure requires the most time of all. It is slow work.

Generally, immediate results cannot be seen. They are not visible, they are often not even felt, but they are there! They take place internally, within and about the cell communities of muscles, ligaments, and bones. One generation of damaged cells is discarded, recycled, replaced by healthier cells, more efficient cells, cells that are less stressed. Time is of the essence! Patience and persistence in answering the body's basic needs will eventually occasion only salubrious results.

96.5.2. Sports Injuries

Failure to warm-up before exercising vigorously, failure to cool down following exercise, and not knowing how to perform correctly various stretching exercises are generally considered the most common causes of sports injury.

The most common sports injuries are soreness, side stitches, cramps, low-back pain, knee injuries, shin splints, tendinitis, bursitis, stress fractures, heel spurs, plantar fascitis, and common sprains.

Generally, incorrect stretching of muscles and failure to obtain sufficient flexibility and suppleness of muscles through sustained continuous and graduated exercise prove to be major factors in sports injuries; again, the failure to recognize that it takes time to develop physical wellness, including muscular wellness.

When muscles are stretched too fast, or in bouncy jerking motions, the body responds with the "stretch reflex," or the tendency of a muscle to contract instead of relaxing when stretched too quickly or forcibly. Therapists and sports experts suggest that all stretching, to be beneficial, should be done in slow, gentle movements not to the point where pain is felt. Stretches should be held at least fifteen seconds. Some recommend increasing the stretch time to as long as 30 seconds for maximum benefit.

Simple sprains are the most common back injury and often occur when muscles of the back or the ligaments are stretched or torn. Common activities that people generally don't even think about, when done improperly, can result in back sprains; simple everyday activities as bending, lifting, standing or sitting. This is why we emphasize in this lesson the need to proceed slowly when corrective exercises are introduced for any purpose.

Back sprains can also result from accidents as, for example, being wrenched when cars collide. Dr. Robert years ago suffered a severe back trauma when he swerved to avoid hitting a pick-up truck which carried two young children in its open back. He was grabbed by the passenger in his car at the same time. He suffered for several years before he eventually recovered.

Slipped or ruptured discs are uncommon but can cause severe pain and even complete disability.

Sometimes such slipped or injured discs can pinch the spinal nerves causing pain to radiate down the back of the thigh and leg—the "sciatica" pain. If the pinching continues, actual irremediable nerve damage can result. Osteoarthritis can be a major factor in back pain, especially in the late middle years. Spurs and sponging causes narrowing of discs with nerve impingements which cause the pain.

Male prostate problems and uterine problems in females, constipation, etc., are all probable factors which will influence the amount of pain felt.

Routine X rays of the back can only reveal bone changes and this only after there has been as much as 30% deterioration. They do not reveal sprains, slipped discs, etc. Other measures and tests may be required to identify a slipped disc.

96.5.3. How to Keep a Straight Back and Improve Posture

There are certain "Dos" and certain "Don'ts" that are applicable to sound body back mechanics. They apply when sleeping, sitting, driving, standing, walking and in lifting.

Sleeping Sleep on a mattress that you find comfortable. In general, most specialists in back problems agree that a firm mattress will supply the best support. Sleep on your side, in the fetal position, with the knees bent. Some persons find that sleeping on the back with a pillow placed under the knees provides the most comfort. Sleeping positions can often prove a moot issue since the average person changes his position many times during the hours of sleeping and does so without his conscious awareness of the fact. A good general rule of thumb, therefore, is to assume a comfortable position and just relax. Sitting Most chairs are an abomination. They are made to fit average people and actually there are few individuals who are "average." Therefore, most chairs are uncomfortable and stress the back.

Chairs should be low enough so that the sitting individual can place both feet on the floor with his knees somewhat higher than his hips. It is not wise to cross the legs at any time. If your sitting chair has legs that are slightly too long for you, you can elevate the legs by using a stool or have a carpenter or handyman make a correction in the height. Always sit firmly against the back of the chair. This will assist the spine to maintain a straight alignment.

Driving The car seat should be adjusted forward so that the knees remain bent. They should be maintained higher than the hips. The driver should sit straight and should drive well balanced keeping both hands on the steering-wheel. An elongated cushion placed against the back of the seat may assist posture since few car seat cushions are designed with correct posture maintenance in mind.

Standing If a person with back pain must stand at his work, he should stand with one foot up, changing positions often. If he is required to bend over, he should do so by bending with the knees while keeping the back as straight as possible.

We recall one housewife a number of years ago who had suffered much pain following a back injury.

While working in her kitchen and around the house, she made it a strict policy never to bend down to pick up an object or to obtain something kept in a lower cupboard. Instead, she would always do a deep knee bend while holding on to the sink or some other fixed object.

She told us that she had been amazed at first to find out just how many times she was required to do her "deep-knee act," as she called it, during the course of a single day.

However, she was well rewarded for this one simple discipline which she imposed upon herself. Her back gradually improved, and she found that the exercise helped her in other ways, too, since she began to enjoy greater vitality than she had known prior to the injury.

Walking When walking, one should maintain the "Tall, I AM Somebody Look." Let the head touch the sky and the entire body will have to follow. Tuck the chin in but keep the head slightly forward in an unstressed position. The pelvis should be slightly forward, and the toes should point the way—straight ahead!

Always wear comfortable walking shoes, preferably constructed of some sturdy, but porous material which will lend support but also permit gaseous toxins to escape. Walk at a fast pace, swinging the arms vigorously. This kind of walking, as opposed to leisurely strolling, will serve to strengthen back, side, and abdominal muscles as well as those of the extremities.

Lifting We have all heard the rules. I'm sure, about how to lift heavy objects, but how often we fail to abide by them. Therefore, perhaps it is in order for us to repeat them for the benefit of our students as they work to correct other people's errors. Perhaps the advice of our housewife will help us to remember them. Always bend with the knees, not with the back. Keep the back straight. Lift with your legs and hold the object close to the body. Lift only to the height of the chest. And always see to it that your feet are firmly planted on an even, non-skid surface.

If an object is heavy, get help. Don't try to prove anything by trying to lift or shove heavy loads and avoid shifting that can throw a person off balance and cause a sudden twisting of the body which can sprain or tear a ligament.

96.5.4. If There Is a Back Injury, Certain Common Habits Should Be Overcome

1. If you must lift a rather heavy object, make certain that the destination of the object, i.e., where you will place that object, is directly ahead of you. This will help you avoid twisting the body.

2. Don't try to lift anything above shoulder level.

3. Don't wear high-heeled or platform shoes. Any sudden throwing off balance might cause further injury. Additionally, when such shoes are worn, the center of gravity is thrown off the norm, thus rendering an individual more likely to lose balance. High heels also tend to cause organs to shift from their normal alignment, a state of affairs that sends silent stress signals tearing through the nerve pathways.

4. Don't forget to have the car seat adjust to YOU. Stretching for the pedals or for the steering wheel increases the curve of the lower back to cause strain.

5. When sitting in a chair, don't slump. Avoid leaning forward for any prolonged length of time. Arching the back in this manner is conducive to more pain.

6. If your mattress is uncomfortably soft, or it sags, or if the cushions in a favorite chair do not give full support to your injured back, make some changes. Without full support, an aching back will continue to trouble.

96.6. Exercise—General

96.6.1. Exercises Designed to Stimulate Circulation and to Stretch Tight Muscles

96.6.2. Exercises for Balance, Posture, Circulation, and Increasing Coordination

96.6.3. Exercise Planning

96.6.4. Teaching the Client How to Get the Most Out of Exercise

96.6.1. Exercises Designed to Stimulate Circulation and to Stretch Tight Muscles

Performed While sitting—

1. Sit well balanced on the floor with both legs stretched out in front of you. Pull knees up to chest. Relax. Touch head to the knees. Relax. Repeat. At first, you may not be able to bring knees all the way up or to touch them with the head. Persistence will soon pay off.

2. In same position, place the arms under bent knees. Now, straighten out right leg. Return to original position. Straighten out left leg. Return. Repeat, alternating legs.

3. In sitting position with legs stretched out on floor in front, bend forward from hips keeping the back straight with arms bent at elbows and held into side. Hold bent position, but do not bounce.

4. In same position as in no. 3 immediately above, spread legs apart and stretch down first to the right leg and then to the left, maintaining the straight back at all times. Hold the stretch position for the count of 5 each time before relaxing.

5. In the sitting position, place pillow under calf and rotate ankles of left leg, then the right leg.

Performed While Standing—

1. Clasp hands behind the back. Now straighten the arms, shoulders, and back. Breathe in quickly to the count of 4. Relax and breathe out to the count of 7. Repeat.

2. Raise arms to the front, breathing in as you raise the arms and exhaling as you lower them—as follows:

   a. Raise to shoulder height. Then lower to side.

   b. Raise above head, stretch to the ceiling. Let the eyes look at the ceiling. Lower to side.

   c. Raise above the head, turn the palms out. Lower to side.

   d. Start this exercise with 3 repeats and gradually add more as you feel comfortable.

   e. Place hands on sides directly in front of hip bones. Now bend forward to a horizontal position. Keep back straight. Feel the stretch in the back and legs. Bend knees slightly and then come up to straight position.

   f. With the feet slightly apart, elbows bent, rotate shoulders front to back several times. Reverse and rotate back to front.

   g. Deep knee bend. Just bend knees slightly. This will be sufficient to exercise many muscles without attempting the deep knee bend which may traumatize injured parts.

Performed While Lying on the Floor—

1. Lie on the back with legs straight on floor. Pull right knee up toward the chest. Hold in this position to count of 10. Be sure to tuck the chin in, do not let head fall backwards. Repeat with left knee.

2. Pull both legs up to chest and hold in this position with arms clasped around knees for a count of 10. Don't forget to breathe as you count.

3. In same position as in exercise two. 2, extend right leg up and forward into the air. Lower slowly. Repeat with right leg several times and then perform the same movement with the left leg.

4. Turn and lie on one side. Place hand under the head. Bend the bottom leg slightly. Now raise the top leg up and down, pointing the toes. Repeat several times.

5. Turn and lie on the other side and repeat the same exercise.

Performed on the Hands and Knees—

1. Get in position on hands and knees and relax. Now hump the back. Push it up as far as is comfortable. Relax. Repeat.

2. Same exercise as above, except as you arch the back, bring the head down. Now bring right knee in towards the head, then straighten leg out again behind you as you raise the head and straighten the back. Repeat several times with right leg, then repeat exercise using left leg.

3. Sit back on the heels. Now stretch out your arms and head on the floor in front. Hold for a few seconds, then return to original position. Repeat several times.

4. Lie on the stomach. Then place the elbows on the floor and clasp hands together in a fist. Place forehead on the clasped hands. Now straighten the right leg out behind and raise it upwards as high as you can. Lower. Repeat several times. Repeat with left leg.

96.6.2. Exercises for Balance, Posture, Circulation, and Increasing Coordination

Place feet together, arms hanging at the sides. Now, lift both arms over the head and, at the same time, bend the left knee up to the chest as high as possible. Hold a few seconds. Return to position. Repeat with right knee in the same manner. When comfortable doing this exercise, client should try to alternate, using first one leg and then the other while maintaining balance.

1. Stand with the feet together, one hand on the wall or a piece of furniture to lend support. In two even counts, swing the left leg forward and back. Keep the back straight, pull the abdomen up, and elevate the chest as the leg swings back. All the movement should be in the hip. Keep knee straight and the leg swinging like the pendulum in a clock. Repeat with other leg. Assistance in maintaining balance may be required by persons with severely weakened muscles.

96.6.3. Exercise Planning

In working with clients, it is always advisable to present the exercises in series; that is, this week do these, next week, another set, and so on. This will sustain interest by giving variety to the program. Clients should be advised to perform exercises, when possible, to music. The tempo of the music should be varied according to the age and condition of the participant(s). For example, for a class of older persons or when working with an older client who may not have exercised for many years, one might choose a melody like "Somewhere My Love" (Lara's Theme from "Doctor Zhivago"). As participants become more skilled, the tempo can be increased causing the exercises to be performed more quickly. However, remember that with corrective exercising, persistence is more important than the tempo. That is why we also recommend that the practicing Hygienist set up a schedule for his clients to follow.

A sample suggested schedule follows:

	Monday	Wednesday	Friday
First Week	Ex. A	Ex. B	Ex. C
Second Week	Ex. D	Ex. E	Ex. F
Third Week	Ex. A	Ex. E	Ex. C
fourth Week	Ex. B	Ex. D	Ex. F

The selected exercises should be typed out, xeroxed and Numbered A, B, C, etc.

On the fifth week, a new series may be given the client. Exercises should be selected keeping in mind the reason for a particular exercise. The exercises given in this lesson have been selected with certain definite problems in mind, such as posture, bent spine, weak back muscles, weak abdominal muscles, etc. There are many other possible defects that may present themselves to the Hygienic practitioner from time to time, and we have presented only the most common. The practitioner in working either with a group or with an individual must choose the particular exercises which, in his best judgment, will prove most conducive to good results.

96.6.4. Teaching the Client How to Get the Most Out of Exercise

There are several important rules to follow. When a precise schedule is formulated and presented to the client, s/he will be much more likely to do the exercises. S/he should be told to study your suggestions carefully and to follow them, if s/he wishes to secure the most good from the exercises. The following list contains suggestions only.

1. Make up an exercise chart and mark down the time spent doing the exercises and the precise number of repeats achieved.

2. Study the exercise routines, consult the recommended list given to the client by the practitioner. The practitioner should always demonstrate each exercise to the client and have the client do the exercise in his/her presence to be sure that full understanding of exactly what is involved in each exercise is achieved. If the client is unable at this time to do the selected exercisers) on his/her own,

some other person who may be called upon for assistance should also be present so that s/he may become familiar with each of the movements.

3. Set a regular time to exercise and follow a regular program each day.

4. Make, frequent check-ups on weight and improvements in sleeping, in eating, in ease of motion, etc. These may be recorded on the client's chart. All improvements should be brought to the attention of the client. These are the "successes" we have previously mentioned. They serve to encourage clients in their corrective work.

5. Exercise before meals, or wait at least one hour after eating, preferably two hours. Exercising before breakfast is a good practice.

6. Provide a suitable rug, floor mat or beach towel for the exercises performed while lying down on the floor.

7. Begin with a 5-minute exercise program and extend as endurance, vitality, etc., increases. Thirty minutes a day will prove sufficient for the average person. Even spending fifteen minutes every day with a half hour several times a week will be highly beneficial.

8. See that the ventilation is good. Keep the windows open while exercising or, better yet, exercise out of doors, except in very cold weather.

9. Wear loose garments made of open weave.

10. Exercise to music. Waltzes are excellent to start with, increase beat as strength and skill increase.

11. And, finally, exercise faithfully and follow instructions. Remember, that when a client first starts an exercise program, his/her muscles are usually weak and flabby. We recommend that everyone start out by exercising one day and then resting the next.

96.7. Questions & Answers

My daughter has been told that she has Scoliosis. Our doctor says that not much is known about this condition and that diet won't help, that the condition is inherited. The only thing he can do, he says, is to refer her to a bone specialist who will probably

put her into a brace, and she may have to wear this brace for a year or two. What do you think about all this?

How old is your daughter?

Fifteen on her next birthday, which will be in two more months.

Not having seen your daughter's condition, of course, I can make no specific recommendations nor offer any valid opinion as to what the full application of Natural Hygiene principles and practices might permit her body to accomplish, but I can say this: under full Hygienic care, her general condition would improve. It might well be that he would have to wear a brace for a time, but, with proper food, a lot of rest, and getting out in the sunshine and performing suitable exercises, her improvement would be much more rapid and, in all likelihood, she would not have to wear that brace for nearly as long a time as if she did not meet her systemic needs adequately as would be the case, no doubt, if she were placed under allopathic care, especially when the physician in charge fails to recognize the importance of a physiologically and biologically-correct diet. At age fifteen, she should not delay another moment to get started. Having a good posture at this important time of her life, may well determine the quality of the rest of her life.

My daughter has the same condition. Her spine is crooked forming an S curve. My husband and I are both Hygienists, but our daughter thinks we are way off the path. She won't eat anything but what the "crowd" eats and that's hamburgers, french fries, cokes and even beer when they party. What can we do?

There is little that you do except perhaps to lay it all out for your daughter. In this lesson, you have learned the importance of posture, how this crooked spine can influence adversely every single function within the body. Try to get your daughter to read this section and perhaps her future may become more real to her. In your own home, you can see to it that only good food is in the refrigerator. Learn how to prepare natural "delights" such as banana ice cream and you might hold a fruit party for your daughter's friends. Also, promise her a reward for good behavior after a certain short period as, for example, a theater party or a camping trip; whatever she would like to have or do most. Use this as an incentive. When you have done all this, you have done your best.

It seems to me that everybody has different ideas about how to tackle body defects; at least, physical, and structural imperfections. One chiropractor I know puts bottles of pills on

the chest of his patients and then recommends zinc or calcium or whatever to the client if there is some spinal malposition. Why are your methods any better than his?

I never knew health to jump out of a bottle of pills and magically into the body. Taking hundreds and thousands of pills can never straighten a crooked spine. The only possible means to correct a body defect which has been caused by a failure to meet systemic needs is to begin, and at once, to meet those needs and to move bones and muscles so as to balance the incorrect action of other bones and muscles. The correct diet and lifestyle will take care of the inside, the internal needs of the body, while the exercise and other Hygienic biodynamics will help the body to repair the defect to the extent possible, as determined by the age, present condition of the individual person and by how well he applies himself to his program.

Not everyone would be able to have the patience to correct structural defects since it seems to take so long.

We have a simple answer for this question. Without patience, knowledge, determination, and willpower, the unfortunate one must just learn to live with his defect! Furthermore, his/her life by the very nature of the life process, will be less enjoyable, less productive and curtailed in many ways—not a very enticing exchange!

Article #1: Excerpt from Funk and Wagnalls New Encyclopedia

The following excerpt from Funk and Wagnalls New Encyclopedia, Copyright 1979 is used to illustrate the complexity of structural movement so as to give us perhaps a better appreciation of the synergism that is involved even in simple structural manipulation. Excerpted from Volume 19, pages 118-119.

The human skeleton consists of more than 200 bones bound together by tough and relatively-inelastic connective tissues called ligaments. The different parts of the body vary greatly in their degree of movement. Thus, the arm at the shoulder is freely movable, whereas the knee joint is definitely limited to a hinge like action. The movements of individual vertebrae are extremely limited, the bones composing the skull are immovable. Movements of the bones of the skeleton are affected by contractions of the skeletal muscles to which the bones are attached by tendons. These muscular contractions are controlled by the nervous system.

The nervous system has two divisions, the somatic, which allows voluntary control over skeletal muscles, and the autonomic, which is involuntary and controls cardiac and smooth muscle and glands. The autonomic nervous system has two divisions, the sympathetic and the para sympathetic. Many, but not all, of the muscles and glands that distribute impulses to the larger interior organs possess a double nerve supply, in such cases the two divisions may exert opposing effects. Thus, the sympathetic and parasympathetic systems respectively increase and decrease heartbeat. The two nerve systems are not always antagonistic, however, for example, both nerve supplies to the salivary glands excite the cells of secretion. Furthermore, a single division of the autonomic nervous system may both excite and inhibit a single effector, as in the sympathetic supply to the blood vessels of skeletal muscle. Finally, the sweat glands, the muscles that cause involuntary erection or bristling of the hair, the smooth muscles of the spleen, and the blood vessels of the skin and skeletal muscles are actuated only by the sympathetic division.

Voluntary movement of head, limbs, and body is caused by nerve impulses arising in the motor area of the cortex of the brain and carried by cranial nerves or by those that emerge from the spinal cord to reach skeletal muscles. The reaction involves both excitation of nerve cells energizing the muscles involved and inhibition of the cells that excite opposing muscles. A nerve impulse is an electrical change within a nerve cell or fiber; it is measured in millivolts, lasts only a few milliseconds, and can be recorded.

Movement may occur also in response to an outside stimulus; thus, a tap on the knee causes a jerk, and shining a light into the eye makes the pupil contract. These involuntary responses are called reflexes. Various nerve terminals called receptors constantly send impulses into the central nervous system. These are of three classes: exteroceptors, those sensitive to pain, temperature, touch, and pressure; interceptors, which react to changes in the internal environment; and proprioceptors, which respond to variations in movement, position, and tension (especially important in doing corrective exercises. The Authors).

These impulses terminate in special areas of the brain, as do those of special receptors concerned with sight, hearing, smell, and taste.

Muscular contractions do not always cause actual movement. Ordinarily, a small "fraction of the total number of fibers in a muscle may be contracting. (One reason why it takes prolonged periods of time to accomplish desired results—The Authors.) This serves both to maintain the posture of a limb and cause the limb to resist passive elongation or stretch. This slight continuous contraction is called muscle tone.

Article #2: Exercise

An excerpt from The Genesis and Control of Disease by George E. Weger, M.D.

Those who exercise during the period of elimination (this refers to the Circadian Rhythm Cycles. The elimination cycle normally begins at about 4 a.m. and continues to, approximately, the noon hour—The Authors.) help to maintain muscular vigor, which appreciably curtails the period of recuperation. Exercises also stimulate the circulation and arouse lethargic cells so that these may more readily give up unusable waste.

An active, supple body can withstand shock, strain, and disease-building abuse to a degree that would wreck or kill the lazy, slow-moving individual. Exercise is just as essential as a rational diet. Dependable resistance cannot be attained without it. All people should exercise daily. The best way to cultivate the habit is to follow faithfully and methodically a regular, fixed program. This assists in the development of self-control and self-discipline, which are so necessary to those who wish to acquire poise and to become masters of self.

Only in the most profound states of enervation or in cases of inflammatory fever, or cardiac depression is positive exercise contraindicated. Moderate tensing of the arms, legs, abdomen, and neck can be done in bed in the prone position even during the fast. Patients are asked to do these tensing movements for periods of ten to thirty minutes depending upon the vitality and muscular vigor of the person. (See lesson on "Exercise in Sickness and Recuperation" for list of tensing exercises which can be used for corrective purposes while confined to the bed.) ... Willpower is necessary in order to make the start and go through with it.

... To obtain the maximum good, the muscular contraction should be positive, and the mind should be concentrated on every movement. Exercise done grudgingly is of little value. The benefit derived depends on the manner in which the movements are done rather than the time involved. Each movement should be emphasized and done with deliberation. To avoid holding the breath, patients are asked to count aloud, as follows: one, and two, and three, and four—and so on. All movements should be repeated to the point of reasonable fatigue as distinguished from overexertion.

It is suggested that patients try to awaken early enough in the morning to do this most necessary work before breakfast. If they do not, ready excuses are likely to come up that will cause it to be entirely neglected. The exercises should be repeated before retiring for the night. Some are advised also to do them in the middle of the afternoon.

... To each patient is given a chart explaining the movements that may be done in bed. These are very simple muscle-tensing and joint movements starting with the fingers and taking in the different joints of the upper extremities to the limit of their range of normal motion in flexion and extension in the following order: the fingers, hands, and wrists in flexion, extension, and rotation; elbows the same; shoulders, a sweeping motion in all directions with the arms fully extended throwing them outward from the body and then bringing the hands together on the return movement. Then the toes should be bent down and up, next the feet and ankles. A folded blanket should then be placed under the hips.

Knee and hip exercises are best obtained by the bicycle movement and also by crossing the extended legs past each other to and for. Next the blanket or pillow should be placed under the shoulders to allow the head to drop back: the head should be raised and lowered and swung and rotated in all directions. Next the muscles of the abdomen should be alternately tensed and relaxed and also kneaded with the fingers or knuckles. The position of the body should then be reversed with patient on hands or elbows and knees. The back should be alternately humped and swayed, and the entire body moved as far as possible forward and back. Swaying and twisting of the spine and torso may be done while sitting on the edge of the bed or on a chair or while standing. Many other movements may be suggested in cases where special advice is needed.

Article #3: Good Posture by Dr. Herbert M. Shelton

The upright position is man's natural one, but, due to many causes, the great majority of civilized men and women are stooped and round shouldered. "Old man's stoop" is the posture into which everyone is drifting unless his or her occupation or gymnastic activity is such as to counteract the tendency in this direction.

... Notice people as they walk, you will see that few walk well. Bad positions in sitting are so common we hardly notice them. Go into any school room and you will see boys and girls, go into any audience and you will see men and women, the majority of them, sitting in the most uncouth and unhealthy attitude. This is an indication of physical weakness, want of physical culture, and inharmonious development. The lungs are cramped and the stomach, liver and all of the abdominal organs crowded out of their positions.

Good posture is good form. Certainly, good posture is of as much importance as the correct pronunciation of words over which the schools spend so much time, while neglecting posture. Upon the upright attitude depends the usefulness of the senses, complete respiration, the ability to talk, speak or read with correct tone of voice, and the most efficient use of the body. Erect carriage is exceedingly important to health and vigor, as well as to best appearance:

Why are we so particular about the forms of our horses or dogs; why do we refuse to buy one with low head, limping gait, or half hipped appearance, with weak lungs and scraggy body, while we are willing to be and become all of these ourselves.

What is designated body mechanics has reference to the mechanical correlation of the various systems of the body, especially in reference to the skeletal, muscular, and visceral systems and their nerve supply. When the mechanical correlations of the body are most favorable to the function of its various parts, this is designated normal body mechanics. Any lack of correlation in any of its parts that hampers or impedes any of its functions represents a deviation from the norm or ideal.

Many deviations from normal mechanical correlation in the body result in visceral malposition's and in strain, thus resulting, not in disease, but in general impairment and enervation. To secure the best results in function in the body, all of its structures must be properly aligned and correlated. Those parts that are misaligned are under stress and strain at all times, hence wear down more rapidly than do properly aligned parts.

Dr. Skarstrom says, "Erect carriage, easy poise, and fine bearing, when habitual, signify perfect adjustment, weight distribution and balance of the different parts of the body. They represent economical distribution of muscular tension, a high degree and even balance of muscular tone, equalized pressure on the surfaces of joints and minimum tension on their fibrous structures. All this implies readiness for all kinds of action, elimination of unnecessary strain, conservation of energy.

Good posture also means the most favorable conditions for the internal organs as regards room, free circulation, relative position, and natural support. Thus, it makes for health and efficiency, as well as beauty and harmony.

... The precise degree to which faulty posture interferes with normal body function is not easily measured. There is, however, considerable evidence which shows that the stresses and strains produced by faulty posture, especially those assumed and sustained in work, are responsible for much pain, including "referred pains" and even functional visceral impairments. Ours is a day of stooped shoulders, relaxed abdominal walls and sagging viscera.

Lordosis of the lower spinal column is accompanied by kyphosis in the upper back and lordosis of the neck, the upper curves being compensatory. Changes in the curves of the spinal column result in changes in the attached structures thus throwing strain upon the supporting ligaments malposition's and sometimes crowding of the viscera, circulatory impediments, perhaps even nerve irritation from pressure.

Lordosis causes a forward tilting of the pelvis thus forcing the abdominal viscera against the front wall of the abdomen, the muscles of which become stretched and this under constant pressure. The attachments of the mesentery to the lumbar spine are also lowered by lordosis so that the intestines and other supported structures are permitted to sag and assume lower positions in the abdominal cavity. There is evidence that the liver may rotate forward and to the right thus stretching the common bile duct and perhaps, in some cases seriously interfering with bile flow. Ptosis of the kidneys, especially of the left kidney, results in traction on the renal veins. The pelvic organs are also involved in the general visceroptosis that results from faulty posture. The ovaries are ptosed, the uterus becomes malposed due to the weight of the sagging abdominal viscera resting upon it, varicose veins of the lower bowel and various impairments of the reproductive system are possible results of the impeded venous flow. The relaxation of the abdominal wall and the crowding of the abdominal organs in the lower abdomen and pelvis permits an increase of blood in the venous reservoirs of the abdomen, thus diminishing the blood volume. This pelvic and abdominal engorgement may also contribute to tumor formation.

Disturbed lateral (side) balance of the spinal column gives us unequal shoulders (one shoulder is lower than the other), a neck that angles in one direction or another above the shoulders or a head which is set crooked on the neck. Such defects of posture and evidences of poor body contour may result from a tilted pelvis, one leg being shorter than the other, or from habit.

... Proper posture is a normal by-product of healthful living and proper body activity. Nearly all of the activities of civilized life encourage the forward position of the head, arms and shoulders. There is a drooping or forward position of the head, a forward displacement of the shoulder girdle and more or less depression of the chest. This is not due to any inherent inability of the spine and associated structures to maintain the upright position. One writer says, "It is not correct to say that spines are not perfectly adapted to the upright posture; it would be more accurate to say that human spines were not evolved to withstand the monotonous and trying posture entailed by modern education and by many modern industries."

... The physical factors which determine posture are (1) the size and shape of the bones and their articular surfaces; (2) the relative length and tension of opposing muscles and fibrous structures; (3) the degree of localized muscular control.

The relative size or shape of ribs, clavicles, scapulae, and vertebrae, as indicated by the general configuration of the chest, shoulder and back, is largely a matter of nutrition and "heredity." However, their sizes are influenced to some degree by the use of these parts, especially during the growing period; for, use or exercise not only influences the size and form of the bones directly, through the demand made upon these by stress and pressure, but also, indirectly, through the constant tension on the bony segments from the resulting muscular tone. I have observed that well-nourished children are straight postured while malnourished children tend to let their shoulders and head droop and sag. I do not doubt that malnutrition is one of the chief causes of early faulty posture.

From Exercise! by Dr. Herbert M. Shelton

Article #4: Correcting Sensitivity to Light by Edwin Flatto, N.D., D.O.

Nature has designed our bodies so that muscles not in use will atrophy. Muscles that are constantly used will become stronger.

The mechanism of the eye which controls dilatation and contraction of the pupils is an automatic one. Those individuals who have developed a sensitivity to light should practice the following:

1. Forget to wear your sunglasses more often until you have found you don't need them.

2. Throw away the Venetian blinds, make dresses and tablecloths from your drapes, and take advantage of the natural sunlight in your home.

3. Try to do as much reading in natural light as possible. If the sun is too strong, cover the bottom half of the book with a black paper or cloth to avoid reflected glare from the printed page.

4. The following exercises are also recommended:

    a. Stand in a dark room and switch a 100-watt light bulb on and off at intervals of ten seconds.

    b. While standing in daylight (preferably before 10 a.m. or after 4 p.m. when the sun is at a slant) face direction of the sun and rotate the head from side to side, constantly blinking, and never looking directly at the sun. Try this exercise for no more than three minutes in the afternoon. As the eye muscles increase in strength, progressively increase the amount of time Until six minutes have been reached both morning and night. The exercise is not recommended for more than six minutes, twice a day. It is very important never to look directly at the sun, and should discomfort be experienced, the time period should be cut down. (Staring into the sun or staring at bright sources of light produces strain and should be avoided. In various eye diseases, such as glaucoma, detachment of the retina, iritis, it is advisable to abstain from sunning the eyes.) This exercise should be performed under the supervision of a qualified practitioner experienced in this type of therapy.

As another strengthening exercise for the eyes, face the sun with the eyes closed and slowly rotate the head from side to side. The warm, penetrating, and relaxing rays of the sun will strengthen and soothe the muscles of the eyes. This sunning of the eyes will also benefit upper and lower eyelids. It will also help overcome (in conjunction with dietary and systemic measures) sties, conjunctivitis, and blepharitis (inflammation of the eyelids—the authors).

From The Restoration of Health—Nature's Way by Edwin Flatto, N.D., D.O.

Article #5: Words of Wisdom by Silvester Graham

WORDS OF WISDOM from LECTURES on the Science of Human Life by Sylvester Graham

1. In a limb which is habitually and vigorously exercised, the arteries become much larger, and the muscle more fully developed, than in the corresponding limb which is little employed; and, on the other hand, if the same limb be suffered to remain inactive for a considerable time, the size of the arteries will be much diminished.

2. The habitual exercise of our body or limbs, therefore, in any particular kind of employment, enables us to put forth more muscular power in that employment, or one requiring the action of the same muscles, than in any other. Hence, one individual may excel in the muscular powers of his arms, another in that of the lower limbs, and another in that of some other part, according to the nature of the regular employment of each.

3. Exercise of the cerebral organs certainly does increase their activity and vigor, and unquestionably also it increases to a certain extent their size or volume.

4. To keep up this grand vital circulation, to give to all the vital functions, to give perfectness to all the vital changes, and to secure a proper supply of blood to every part and maintain the general health and energy of the system, EXERCISE, or voluntary action, is of the utmost importance. It greatly promotes circulation, and particularly in the capillary system, or the myriads of minute vessels which are so numerously distributed to every part of the body; it equally promotes respiration, causing full and deep inspirations of air, and a vigorous action of the lungs; and serves to impart vigor and activity to all the organs, and to secure the healthful integrity and energy of all the functions, and the symmetrical development and constitutional power of the whole system; and gives strength and agility and elasticity and grace to the body; and energy and activity to the intellectual and moral faculties. Indeed, exercise may truly be considered the most important natural tonic of the body. If it is wholly neglected, the body will become feeble, and all its physiological powers will be diminished; but if it is regularly and properly attended to, the whole system will be invigorated, and fitted for usefulness and enjoyment.

5. We have seen that every contraction of the muscles serves to exhaust their vital properties; and to replenish their exhaustion, a constant supply of fresh arterial blood is diffused throughout the muscular tissue in great abundance; and the more vigorously any part is exercised, the more rapidly and abundantly that part is supplied with arterial blood; and hence, the habitual, healthy, and vigorous exercise of any part, always serves to produce and maintain a full development of that part, and to give it greater power. Thus, if one arm is constantly and vigorously exercised, and the other remains wholly unemployed, the muscles of the former will soon be much more largely developed and far more powerful than those of the latter. Hence, the welfare of the whole system requires that each part should be duly exercised, and most especially in young and growing bodies, which are easily deformed and even dreadfully distorted by a neglect of voluntary action.

6. So far as voluntary exercise or labor is necessary to the most healthy condition and perfect functions of the human system, it is a blessing; and beyond that, it is in some measure an evil; for in proportion to the excess, life is always shortened, and the body predisposed to disease.

From constitutional necessity, therefore, if man takes too little voluntary exercise, he suffers; and if his voluntary exercise is excessive, he suffers. But happily, for the race, the sufferings from excessive labor bear no proportion to those which result from inactivity. A man may greatly abbreviate his life by overtoiling, and yet through the whole of his earthly existence enjoy1 comparatively good health, sweet sleep, and a cheerful mind; but he who suffers from want of exercise—and especially if with that is connected excessive alimentation and other dietetic errors—experience the bitterest and most intolerable of human misery.

The structure of society in civil life requires that many should be devoted to pursuits which are less favorable to health than the calling of the husbandman; and a large majority of these pursuits are of a nature which does not admit of sufficient active bodily exercise for health and comfort. To all such, therefore, exercise becomes a necessary part of regimen, and must be regularly attended to, or they must suffer. And yet, where it is mere matter of regimen, attended to because it cannot be neglected without suffering, it loses more than half its virtue. Exercise, in order to be most beneficial, must be enjoyed. The mind must enter into it with interest, and if possible with delight, losing the idea, of labor in that of pleasure.

Lesson 97:

Devising a Lifestyle That Includes Vigorous Activity

97.1. Introduction

97.2. Informal Exercise

97.3. Formal Exercise

97.4. Questions & Answers

Article #1: Exercise: A Hygienic Perspective by Ralph C. Cinque, D.C.

Article #2: Exercise: What Most of Us Forget

Article #3: Jogging and Other Vigorous Exercise

Article #4: Hiking Is More Than Just Exercise by Marti Wheeler

Article #5: Developing Your Arms

97.1. Introduction

97.1.1. What Is Vigorous Activity?

97.1.2. Is Exercise Unnatural?

"I'm too busy to eat."

"Sleep? Who has time for that?"

"I try to take a bath or shower on the weekends. I've got too much work to do during the rest of the week."

You won't hear people talk like this. Eating, sleeping, and bathing are all part of the normal person's daily lifestyle. Yet 63% of all Americans do not take part in another regular activity that's just as vital to our well-being and health—exercising!

Exercise is not a daily part of most people's lives. And that's very strange, especially when you consider that over 90% of all adults agree that proper diet and regular exercising would do more to improve health than anything that physicians or medicines could do for us (or to us).

Why isn't exercising more popular? Well, for one thing, exercise requires some hard work, a little time, and a good measure of self-discipline. You have to make room in your life for exercise and vigorous activity.

Once you put daily exercise into your life, the rest is easy. The difficult part is to first devise a lifestyle that includes vigorous activity. That is what this lesson is all about—how to develop a lifestyle for yourself or for your clients that includes regular exercise and daily vigorous activity.

97.1.1. What Is Vigorous Activity?

Almost everybody is active throughout the day. Performing our normal chores, doing our work, and running errands, even simply sitting, and reading requires a certain level of activity. Even in sleep, the body is still active, tossing and turning, using up to 60 calories per hour in this reduced metabolism.

Yet vigorous activity is needed by our lungs, our circulatory system, our muscles, and nerves for optimum health. Otherwise, we become sluggish. Bodily functions are impaired, the health of the organs deteriorates, and we suffer from poor sleep, digestive problems, constipation, and poor posture.

Vigorous activity is different from normal activity in that it makes our entire body work, strive, grow, and vibrate. It makes our breath quicken, our pulse race, and our heart pound. In short, it makes us feel alive.

97.1.2. Is Exercise Unnatural?

Thousands of years ago, there was no such thing as "exercise" or calisthenics or daily workouts. Life for primitive man was one of continual vigorous activity. He climbed trees for fruit, migrated 25 to 50 miles per day during the seasonal changes, and did a fair share of sprinting, running, and swimming just to avoid wild animals and his enemies.

Daily life was full of "exercising" for our ancestors, and their bodies remained supple, lean, and strong from just responding to the constant demands of survival and living out in the open twenty-four hours a day.

So, you see, exercise is unnatural. If man himself led a purely natural life, unfettered by the demands of civilization, he would receive a full range of vigorous activity that would keep the body in superior health. However, almost no one on this planet today has such a pristine existence. We sleep in buildings at night, "gather" our foods from supermarket bins, and ride in an automobile to a job that requires us to sit at a desk for most of our waking hours.

As Dr. Herbert M. Shelton has observed, "Some people often urge that the normal activities of life should supply all the exercise needed after maturity is reached. The reply is that the activities of civilized life are not normal."

Still, many people scoff at the idea that they might need daily periods of vigorous activity. They still see exercise or jogging or weightlifting as something artificial, unnatural, or abnormal. The real reason for their mistrust of exercise may be far simpler, however.

"It is often contended," writes Dr. Shelton, "that formal exercises are unnatural or abnormal, hence, of no benefit. But there is no difference between the contraction of a muscle in formal exercise and its contraction in what we may designate as primitive activities of life. There is no such thing as artificial contraction of a muscle. No exercise using spontaneous movements, whether in primitive activities or formal exercise, can be called artificial or unnatural. The objection to exercise seems to be the expression of that laziness that stems from a lack of vigor, the very vigor that exercise provides for."

Still, people resist the idea of devising a lifestyle that includes vigorous activity. As you deal with your clients and friends, you may hear an all-too common excuse: "I don't need to exercise because my job or my daily work provides me with all the activity I need."

97.2. Informal Exercise

97.2.1. Work Isn't Exercise!

97.2.2. But Don't Stop Working!

97.2.3. Rub-adub-tub: Exercise in the Bathroom

97.2.4. Office Calisthenics

97.2.5. Daily Life as Exercise

97.2.1. Work Isn't Exercise!

Exercising may be hard work, but hard work isn't exercise.

A common mistaken belief is that if you perform hard work or heavy labor at your job, then you don't really need to exercise during your nonworking hours. I remember talking to a city employee who repaired streets with a pneumatic drill or "jackhammer" all day long.

The man's forearms were immense knotted muscles that had been developed through years of holding a heavy jackhammer in place to rip up old asphalt pavement. His wrists were powerful, and he had a grip that made handshakes a must to avoid.

Yet when you looked past his arms, you saw a sagging potbelly, spindly legs, and stooped shoulders. His complexion was a dirty yellow, his eyes dulled, and his hearing almost gone from years of hammering at the pavement. Had his daily work kept him in good shape? Only the arms!

The sad fact is that most work performed today is not adequate, all-around exercise. "There are no less than 400 muscles in the body, each in need of regular exercise," writes Dr. Herbert M. Shelton. "The belief that the ordinary activities of life provide adequate exercise for the muscles of the body is a blind one. Anyone may readily see this for himself when he examines the limited extent to which his muscular system is used in his daily activities. Even in the man who performs manual labor, many muscles are neglected. Modern specialization, both in work and in play or athletics, neglects many muscles."

The busy mother and housewife who picks up dirty clothes and toys, straightens closets, and puts away dishes may be doing plenty of hard work, but very little significant exercise. Even a manual laborer such as a groundskeeper who mows, rakes, and trims yards for eight hours each day uses only a limited set of muscles.

Most work in the modern world, because of its highly repetitive, specialized, and limited nature, cannot supply the full range of muscular activity that is required for beneficial exercise. This is one reason why people find work and their jobs so tiring.

"Modern man," observes Dr. Shelton, "spends most of his working hours using but limited parts of his muscular system in specialized activities, and often using these only slightly, and so becomes but a caricature of a man. He is undeveloped, one-sidedly developed, and almost always lacking in vigor."

Exercise actually increases our vigor. Energy expended during proper exercise is quickly returned following rest and relaxation. Not only that, but a half-hour of intense and concentrated exercising can accomplish more conditioning than a full day of hard manual work.

In contrasting the benefits of selective exercising versus most daily labor, Dr. Shelton notes: "Greater strength and development and more symmetrical development may be obtained by appropriate exercise than by most forms of physical work. Actual tests have shown, for instance, that a few minutes of proper exercise daily will produce a greater increase in the size of the arms, legs, back or chest in a given time than work will do."

97.2.2. But Don't Stop Working!

Although more can be gained in an hour of structured and regular exercise than can usually be obtained from a day of regular work, we can still use our jobs as a form of beneficial exercise. After all, we spend the greater portions of our lives involved in some sort of productive labor. By using our imagination and becoming more creative, we can turn our regular daily jobs into mini-exercise periods all through the day.

Perhaps one of the most effective ways to devise a lifestyle that includes vigorous activity is to incorporate exercising into your daily job. This method is appealing because it doesn't take up much extra time. Since you're already working, you might as well be getting some form of vigorous activity. Let's look at a few case histories of people who have put the "exercise" back into their "work".

97.2.3. Rub-adub-tub: Exercise in the Bathroom

One group of people who need to exercise the most are those that seem to have the least time: young mothers and busy housewives. "Exercise?! After changing diapers, scrubbing floors, and cleaning out the garage. Just give me rest, thank you," said a young woman of three pre-school children.

Ann Dugan, a 55-year-old grandmother, however, disagrees. "You have to clean up the bathroom every day, and if you have to do it, you might as well make it productive," said Dugan, author of 12 books on exercise and weight training. She developed a series of "at-home" exercise that housewives can do while getting the necessary housework out of the way.

"You might as well toughen up your body while you're toughening up the bathroom," said Dugan, who also emphasized that her exercises can be done in homes, offices, cars, and airplanes. "With all the bending and stretching needed to get to high shelves, inside cabinets, and under furniture, it's easy to turn those movements into a tough workout."

For example, Dugan suggests that when you clean your bathtub, instead of getting down on both hands and knees, you can kneel on the right knee only and clean the tub with the right hand. This position causes the pectoral muscles to be used and the hamstrings to be stretched. By reversing the knees, you can achieve an equalizing stretch while giving the shoulder and chest muscles a workout.

Even cleaning a toilet bowl can turn into a beneficial exercise by using Dugan's "dip and-disinfect" method. The cleaner stands, facing the toilet bowl, with legs bent so that the hips are low. The thighs should be parallel to the floor, with the left hand braced on the water tank as you scrub with the right hand. During this scrubbing process, you should raise and lower the heels at least ten times. This modified form of the "squat" exercise is the same one that is used by weightlifters to develop their lower bodies and reduce fat around the thighs.

Of course, such intermittent exercising while doing housework cannot take the place of sustained and vigorous activity. Yet the extra bending, stretching, and flexing that may be done while at a regular job can help keep the body supple and ready for more intense physical activity later in the day or during the weekend leisure time.

97.2.4. Office Calisthenics

Some jobs, such as yard work, carpentry, construction, and farming, provide many opportunities for incorporating vigorous activity programs throughout the day. The construction worker may simply carry heavier and heavier loads while on the job to develop his musculature, while the farmer or gardener can take a shovel and hoe for an added hour of a combined exercise and work "workout."

Even the deskbound office worker can add activities to his daily job routine that will sneak in valuable minutes of vigorous activity. Here's how one Life Scientist got an hour's worth of jogging in without ever leaving his office building!

"I worked on the sixth floor in a large office complex and was behind a desk all day. My thinking became dulled and fuzzy from just all the inactivity. By the end of the day, I was so fatigued from the unnatural environment that I just couldn't drag myself out to a track where I could run in the evenings. Then one day I read that climbing stairs actually gave more of a cardiovascular workout than jogging for the same amount of time.

"I rarely ate lunch while at work, since I was sitting most of the day, so I decided to get some on-site exercising done. Like other large buildings, my office had hidden flights of stairs for a fire escape.

Almost everybody rode the elevators, leaving the stairways unused. That day I walked down to the bottom of six flights of stairs, and then ran to the top. Walked down, and then ran to the top again. After twenty minutes of this running upstairs, I was breathing very heavily, and my heart was pounding in my ears. I knew I was on to something good.

"Now everyday I'm out running up and down the stairs, sometimes three times a day in order to break up all the inactivity at my desk. I feel that I think much better after a period of stair-running. My only fear is that someday my co-workers will see me and think I'm running down the stairs because the building is on fire!"

Almost any job can be arranged so that small periods of vigorous activity can be performed. This is the easiest way and the first way that some people work exercise back into their daily routines.

So, remember, while work may not be exercise, you can put the vigor back into work by slipping in some exercise periods of your own.

97.2.5. Daily Life as Exercise

Besides the working hours, our lives provide us with many other opportunities for including vigorous activity periods.

Gardening, lawn work, planting and harvesting your own food, improving, and beautifying your natural surroundings—all of these outdoor activities increase our natural vigor and provide effective exercise.

Walking to our jobs or to the marketplace instead of driving provides valuable exercise while at the same time saving us money and conserving energy.

Performing our daily chores such as cleaning or sweeping at a fast rate of speed can turn a moderate work pace into a workout.

How can you determine how vigorous and effective your normal daily activities are? One way to determine the vigor required for an activity is to measure how many calories of energy are expended if that activity were done for an hour. For example, a moderate walk burns around 200 calories per hour, while a steady jogging run can use up to 500 calories or more in the same time. The following chart will give you an idea of how strenuous some of our daily activities, athletics, and exercises can be:

Activity	Calories Expended Per Hour

Sleeping	60
Sitting and reading	72
Sitting and eating	84
Sitting and knitting	90
Sweeping	102
Desk work	132
Playing the piano	150
Scrubbing floors	216
Walking (moderate)	216
Bricklaying	240
Ironing	252
Bowling	264
Swimming (leisurely)	300
Walking downstairs	312
Carpentry	408
Farmwork in a field	438
Mowing the lawn	462
Skiing	594

Handball	612
Running	630

Of course, merely burning up calories is not the point of exercising, and this chart should not be used to equate various activities. (For example, ten hours of sleeping at 60 calories per hour is not equal to one hour of jogging at 600 calories!)

What you can learn from the above chart is that normal daily activities can vary a lot in the amount of vigor that they require to complete. By selecting more and more of the more strenuous activities as part of your normal daily routine, you're getting more exercise into your life.

As you look for ways to turn your normal daily activities into mini-exercise periods, you'll discover more and more chores that can be done vigorously and with beneficial results.

As Dr. Shelton reminds us, "The total activities of the day, and not merely the short time spent in formal exercise, are involved in the development of the body; hence it is important that all activity be performed correctly and with a view toward improving the total organism."

97.3. Formal Exercise

97.3.1. Walking: The All-Around Exercise

97.3.2. The Three Rules of Exercise

97.3.3. Progressive Exercise: Setting Your Goals

97.3.4. Systematic Exercise: The Body as a Whole

97.3.5. Sample Exercise Regimens

97.3.6. Get the Habit!

No matter how good we become at including vigorous activities into our normal job and other daily routines, a formal exercise program is still an absolute necessity for radiant health.

This is where the difficulties begin. People resist making changes in their lifestyle, especially changes that may take up more time and require concentrated and dedicated physical effort. Mention to an overweight and sedentary adult that he or she will have to start running and lifting weights for an hour-and-a-half starting tomorrow and you'll probably lose a client.

Sudden changes in a lifestyle can be difficult, and even more so when formal exercise is viewed as hard work or distasteful. The first step is always the hardest, so it may be wise to adapt a sensible approach when either you or one of your clients begins making regular and formalized exercise a part of the daily routine.

Fortunately, there is an easy way of introducing exercise and vigorous activity into everyone's normal lifestyle. It's something that most people start doing after the first few months of life: walking.

97.3.1. Walking: The All-Around Exercise

Perhaps no form of exercise can be so universally recommended as a good brisk walk. Walking may be done safely by people of all ages and in all states of health. It requires no special equipment or location and is completely benign in its effects.

More importantly, walking is an exercise that can be worked into everyone's lifestyle, no matter how busy the schedule. Walk to work, walk to the store, walk to a friend's home, walk around the block, through the neighborhood, and across town. There is no other form of exercise that can be so safely and easily integrated into one's daily activities as the occasional walk.

For walking to be an effective form of exercise, generally an hour or more each day is required. This hour may be worked up to by splitting the time into two thirty-minute periods, three twenty-minute sessions, or even four fifteen-minute outings if the person is old or out of shape.

Unlike other forms of exercise, walking may even be engaged in right before or after a meal. Indeed, studies have shown that a walk after a meal aid in controlling the weight.

Although even slow and leisurely walking will have some beneficial effects, a brisk walk done at a fast clip will provide more benefits in a shorter time. "Speed walking" or race-walking (which is actually an Olympic event) can yield the same results as jogging for the same length of time and at a considerably less chance of foot or knee injury.

Walking not only benefits the legs and lower body, but it actually strengthens and firms the body, expands the chest and lung capacity, and corrects the posture from top to bottom. Chronic neck problems, including whiplash, have been gently corrected simply by regular and lengthy walking.

Yet for all the benefits of walking, few people make it part of their regular lifestyle. The automobile saves us time, but at a cost to our well-being. Any daily trip which is less than one mile should certainly be walked instead of driven. If you live within five miles of your job, then you may profitably walk to work by simply leaving your home 45 minutes to an hour earlier.

In Europe, walking vacations are quite popular. Each day you walk fifteen to twenty-five miles, seeing the sights as only you can on foot, and then resting in the evening at a hotel.

Primitive man was basically a walking, food-gathering creature. He migrated north to south, south to north, during the fruit-growing seasons, walking from berry bush to fruit tree, eating, moving, and receiving nourishment and exercise from his natural surroundings.

Not only may walking be used in a regular exercise program, it can also be part of an overall, health-restoring lifestyle. Consider the story of Milton Feher of New York City: "I was a dancer whose career was smashed by arthritis in the knees. An eminent orthopedist explained that I would never be able to dance again because cartilage in my knee had been destroyed through excessive ballet jumping. More than 20 chiropractic treatments made no difference. Nineteen injections failed to relieve me of my constant pain.

"I was a sorrowful ex-dancer as I hobbled miserably in Times Square one day, thinking of my dancing career that had been stolen from me. As I shuffled about, each step drawing pain, I started to pull my body up into a straight posture. I consciously aligned my body from neck to foot, relaxed, and then walked very purposefully in an erect manner, without tipping my head or trunk side to side.

"I felt no pain in my knees! As soon as I slumped or let my posture go, the pain returned with each step. For the next three years, I walked, walked, walked, all the time maintaining the best erect posture possible, yet without tension or strain.

"Now 15 years later, I can run 9 miles in the morning and lead vigorous dancing classes in the evening. The main source of my constantly increasing strength is a continuous improvement in the effortless straightening of my posture by devoted, regular walking for hours at a stretch."

There is no doubt that walking is an excellent corrective, as well as preventive, exercise. "I'd be out of business within a week," a chiropractor once told me, "If everybody would throw away their car keys and just walk. Almost all the complaints I see are from people who are too sedentary. Walking is the most natural way I know of adjusting and realigning the spine which obviates the need for manipulation."

Let's look a little closer at how daily walking as part of your lifestyle can not only strengthen you, but also improve the posture and tighten the abdomen.

Modern man developed his erect posture because he is a walker. Primitive man was round-shouldered, short-necked, and his head jutted forward, ahead of his feet. Through thousands of years of walking, man's spine and posture was gradually straightened.

When walking is neglected and is no longer part of your daily lifestyle, the posture is the first to go. As a person sits more and walks less, the head droops forward and pulls the spine with it. This slumping is then accelerated by gravity, and you become round shouldered, hunched over—much like the primitive caveman who once scampered on all fours.

Another side effect of neglecting walking and hence developing poor posture is that the abdominal muscles become weakened. Walking is an excellent "tummy tightener." The abdominal muscles are attached to the entire lower border of the front of the chest. They cover the entire abdomen and are attached to the upper border of the front of the pelvis. When they are strengthened and in good position by years of proper posture and regular walking, they prevent the organs in the abdominal cavity from slipping and sliding forward. The more they protrude, the weaker they grow as the muscles become stretched permanently. Strong abdominal muscles, insured by regular walking, hold you together to be more graceful, skillful, and stronger in all activities.

Regardless of the exercise program you now follow, walking should be a part of it. And if you have yet to develop a regular program of daily exercise, walking is the easiest and most effective way to begin.

The road to health is a simple one to follow—it's only two feet in front of you.

97.3.2. The Three Rules of Exercise

So far, you've learned how vigorous activity may be incorporated into your life through your job, your normal daily activities, and by simply making walking an important part of your daily routine. We've really said very little about a formalized exercise program, however.

To make sure that you get the type of intense activity that your body requires, it will be necessary to develop a daily exercise program. This program should become part of your daily lifestyle—something that you do without fail, just as you eat, sleep, and relax every day.

As you develop your regular exercise regimen, keep these three rules of exercise in mind:

To insure health and well-being, exercise must be

1. Progressive
2. Systematic
3. Habitual

97.3.3. Progressive Exercise: Setting Your Goals

Progressive exercise means that you progress from easy to more vigorous activity as your strength and capabilities increase. For example, if you start by lifting twenty-pound weights for exercise, then you should gradually increase the amount of weight lifted so that you might be using thirty or forty-pound weights as your strength increases. If you walk a half-mile each day, then perhaps increase the distance to a mile or two miles as your stamina develops.

For exercise to be effective, moderate demands must be made on the body. Since a healthy body responds so well to exercise, you must gradually increase the time and effort spent for each activity. On the other hand, do not make the mistake of thinking "a little is good, so a lot is better."

Dr. Herbert M. Shelton has observed that: "Progression in exertion should keep pace with the increasing strength and vigor of the body; it should be made step by step and not by leaps and bounds. Excessively prolonged exercise can be almost as injurious as violent exertion."

When we develop our lifelong exercise program, we must allow for progression. We must set and reach new goals. We must make sure that our daily exercise program allows for change and progress and that we do not become locked into the same routine series of activities that present no new challenges. At the same time, we must make sure that our beginning exercise program is not, overly ambitious, otherwise we may become discouraged or extend ourselves past the current limits of our capabilities.

To help you begin and plan a vigorous activity program, you should first determine your own maximum heart rate. You don't want to push yourself past this maximum rate; at the same time, you want to make sure that you are exercising intensely enough to raise your heartbeat rate to within a high, safe range of that upper limit.

The accepted formula for figuring out your own maximum heart rate is to subtract your age from 220. If you are 60 years old, then your maximum heart rate would be 160 (220 minus 60). If you're eighteen years old, then your maximum rate would be as high as 202. You can measure your elevated heart rate by first performing a few minutes of vigorous activity and then counting your pulse rate at the wrist or simply feel your heartbeat and count the beats for one minute (or more simply, count the number of beats for fifteen seconds and then multiply by four).

For safety's sake, some physicians recommend that you stay within 60 to 65 percent of your maximum heart rate when doing vigorous exercise. For a sixty-year-old, this would mean a pulse rate of about 96 beats per minute. On the other hand, Dr. James

A. Blumenthal of the Duke University Preventive Approach to Cardiology says that his older heart patients often safely reach 70 to 85 percent of their maximum rate.

Regardless of the upper limit you choose (60 to 85% of your maximum heart rate), you should work up to it gradually in a series of progressive exercises. Each week, extend the program either in time or intensity so that a slightly higher pulse rate is reached at the end of a vigorous exercise set. Remember that we are not in a race to health, but we should always feel that we are making a steady, strong progress in our daily exercise. With the rule of progression in mind, we should devise a daily exercise program that will allow for either increasing periods of time or intensity of effort while at the same time taking care not to be overly ambitious or unrealistic in establishing our goals.

97.3.4. Systematic Exercise: The Body as a Whole

The second consideration in planning a lifestyle that includes vigorous activity is that the exercise chosen must be systematic. Systematic exercise is simply an activity that conditions all areas of the body. For example, a combined program of running or walking along with weightlifting and bending and flexing exercises is a collection of systematic activities that call upon every muscle in the body.

Too often people choose only a single favorite form of exercise or sports, such as swimming or tennis, and use it to the exclusion of all other exercise activities. There is a danger in this because it is rare that any single form of exercise activity will provide the full range of movements that is needed to condition the entire body.

"But I like bowling! It's good exercise because I can do it in the winter as well as the summer and lifting that heavy bowling ball and tossing it down the alley sixty or seventy times a day gives me a good workout." The elderly woman was defending her favorite form of recreational activity—bowling—as sufficient exercise.

"But look at the muscles you use in your game," I responded. "You use only your right hand and arm to wing and release the ball, you go through the exact same range of limited motion, and the only parts of your body that get a workout are a few muscles in one arm and on one side of your body. Bowling is fine for recreation and relaxation, but it cannot qualify as an all-around life-long exercise activity. Now if you jogged down to the bowling alley each day with your bowling ball..." I began to joke.

She got my point. We must carefully select the exercise program to complement our other daily activities and work. As Dr. Shelton urges: "The exercise program should include movements that counteract the deforming tendencies of our daily work activities while at the same time exercising the unused portions of the body. Most of our sports, our different forms of work, and almost all of our daily activities are so one-sided and specialized that we become misshapen and underdeveloped."

To make sure that our daily exercise program is systematic, a few rules should be observed. First, there must always be at least a fifteen to thirty-minute period of vigorous conditioning, aerobic activity. This would include such exercises as jogging, brisk walking, intense swimming, fast bicycling, even repeated stair climbing or hill hiking. Whatever the exercise may be, it must make the heartbeat faster, the pulse increase, the breathing deepen, and the entire metabolism quicken. This pace should be maintained as long as comfortable, with an eventual goal of twenty to thirty minutes or longer. In the beginning, work up to such intense activity gradually. Increase your speed and time as your body responds favorably.

Second, there should be a period of exercise that stretches the many unused muscles of the body. Back bends, leg stretches, pull-ups, sit-ups, neck rolls, and twisting are essential for a well-rounded exercise program. An excellent series of such all-around exercises may be found in Dr. Herbert Shelton's book Exercise! Such exercises should be selected to balance out other daily activities and other exercise programs. For example, students and writers who bend over a desk all day should make sure that back bending exercises are used to compensate for the forward, stooped-over position assumed while reading or writing.

People who choose to run or walk as their primary exercise should also include a sequence of exercises to work the upper portion of the body, such as weightlifting or a racquet sport.

Third, there should be a final sequence of exercises or daily activity that requires coordination and balance. Many sports and recreational activities require hand-to-eye coordination, such as hitting a baseball, tossing a horseshoe, or even bowling a strike. While this type of activity does not provide the conditioning that vigorous exercising such as jogging delivers, it does help to relax and balance the mind. This group of exercises include most sports and athletics which, while fine ways to relax and play, should always be used in tandem with concentrated vigorous activities. Gardening, too, like sports and athletics, may also be classified as a relaxing and balancing form of exercise and activity that may be used to complement an intensive daily workout.

Using these three criteria, what might a daily program of exercise look like? Here are two Life Scientist's approach, one is a young man of twenty-four; the other is a sixty-seven-year-old woman:

97.3.5. Sample Exercise Regimens

Male, 24 years

Monday - Wednesday - Friday
Jogging/Sprinting (mornings) 45 minutes
Weightlifting, upper body 30 minutes

Tuesday - Thursday - Saturday
Swimming (summer)/Bicycling (winter) 30 minutes
Weightlifting, lower body (Thursday/Saturday) 30 minutes
Racquetball (Tuesday & Saturday) 30 minutes

Sunday
Soccer League Game 90 minutes

Every Day
Warm-up and Morning Flex-stretching 15 minutes

The above exercise program yields approximately one-hour-and-fifteen minutes to one-hour-and-a-half of activity per day. Notice that each day Usually contains activities that build both strength and endurance. In addition, he follows a daily stretching routine in the morning which incorporates selected exercises from Dr. Shelton's series of recommended exercises from the book Exercise! The racquetball games build upper body strength and coordination, while the weekly soccer game provides lower body conditioning. He usually breaks his exercises up into a morning and evening set of activities, about thirty minutes or so in length.

Female, 67 years

Monday - Wednesday – Friday
Brisk walking (mornings) 30 minutes
Walking/Hiking, slowly (evenings) 45 minutes

Tuesday - Thursday – Saturday
Gardening; digging, hoeing, weed pulling 2 hours
Swimming (summer) 30 minutes
Moderate walking (winter) 30 minutes

Sunday
Bowling 90 minutes

Every day
Stretching, yoga, sit-ups 20 minutes

An exercise program for an older person must be somewhat different than for a young person. Walking is used more as a form of exercise, athletics are not emphasized, and such recreational/outdoor activities as gardening are highlighted. Notice, however, that a full hour to hour-and-a-half of time is still allotted for moderately-vigorous activity that will use all the muscles in the body.

Whatever exercises you choose for yourself, always keep in mind that for a program to be truly effective, it must include vigorous activity that calls all of our muscles into play. It must affect the body as a whole; it must be systematic, thorough, and responsive to all the needs of the body, neither over nor under developing any part of the body to the detriment of the entire organism.

97.3.6. Get the Habit!

Remember that an exercise program should be progressive, systematic, and habitual. Perhaps that most important of these three for an insured successful exercise regimen is that it be habitual. If you make vigorous activity a daily habit, then you're sure to make progress and eventually exercise the entire body. On the other hand, if you don't perform your exercise set on a day-to-day basis, then it doesn't matter how difficult or thorough it may be.

The only way to devise a lifestyle that includes vigorous activity is to exercise at a fixed time each day. It may be in the morning before breakfast or at night before bed or even during your lunch hour. The important thing is that you schedule your vigorous activity at a standard, regular time and then do not deviate or make excuses.

Most people find the early morning hours to be the best time for regular exercise. By doing your exercises the first thing in the day, you can't ignore or postpone it, or conveniently "run out of time" later in the day. The most common reason an exercise program fails is that a person will skip it "for just one day" and then for two days, and three days, and finally he's no longer exercising but simply making up excuses.

If you make a firm promise to do some sort of exercise every day and at a regular time, then it will be more difficult to put off. "Lack of time," writes Dr. Shelton, "is perhaps the most frequently used explanation for avoiding exercise. Yet women may spend more time each day applying makeup than it would take to get some significant exercise, while men feel that it's more important to read the sports section of the newspaper than it is to actually be active and vigorous."

Lack of time is always cited as the excuse for not making exercise a regularly-scheduled part of the day's activities. No one, no matter how "busy" or important, cannot afford to make a small amount of time for so vitally an important an activity. Even the presidents of the United States, who certainly must be counted as among the "busiest" people in the world, find time in their packed schedules for regular exercise.

If you truly feel that your day is already so filled that you can't exercise on a regular basis, then try these tricks to get more quality time into your life:

1. Get up thirty minutes earlier or go to bed thirty minutes later. Use that extra half hour or hour at the beginning and end of the day for your own exercise period. The vigor and energy that such exercising provides will more than adequately compensate for that lost thirty minutes of sleep.

2. Skip breakfast or lunch and eat a piece of fruit later in the day in place of one of these meals. Use this mealtime period as an exercise period instead. (Isn't it funny that the same people who say they have no time for exercise always manage to make time for a full three meals a day?) Vigorous activity actually delays hunger since it brings fuel from the liver into the bloodstream, and you'll soon discover that a lunch hour spent exercising leaves you more invigorated than if you ate a heavy meal.

3. Keep an hourly schedule of what you do each day. Write down everything. Do you spend an hour watching news on television? Thirty minutes shopping? Ten minutes driving to the store? Write it all down. Now look and see how much

time/you're actually "wasting." You will have no difficulty finding an extra thirty minutes to an hour each day that could better be used by exercising.

People who say that they have no time for exercise are not thinking logically. If you exercise regularly, you'll live much longer and have years of added time to your life.

Exercising doesn't take time away; it gives you more time, better health, and a higher quality of life.

Besides lack of time, another obstacle to overcome in making exercising a daily habit is inertia, or just getting started. Kelly Kessing, a fitness and nutrition specialist in Philadelphia, has her own strategy for overcoming inertia.

"You've got to seduce yourself into going out there," she says. "For instance, if the idea of walking or running intimidates you, just don't tell yourself that you're going for a walk or jog. Don't pressure yourself. Put on your sweatsuit or walking shorts and a pair of comfortable shoes. Just say, 'Maybe I'll go for a walk or take a short jog, or maybe I won't.' Then just go outside to a park and start to saunter about. Maybe pick up the pace, and before you know it, you'll have slipped all the way into full-fledged exercise without feeling that you had to force yourself."

Another approach is to make a firm commitment to yourself. Write a note on your calendar or write on a piece of paper that "I will start my exercise program on Monday at 8 a.m." Then keep that promise as if it were the most important appointment in your life, because it is.

Another trick that some people use to make exercising a regular daily habit is to penalize themselves if they miss a day on purpose. For example, one Life Scientist has this unusual method to make sure he keeps his exercising promise:

"I have a jar at home that I stuff a $5 bill into for every day that I skip exercising. At the end of that month, I take whatever money is in the jar and send it to the American Cattlemen's Association. As a vegetarian, this is the one group that I would hate most to support. So, you see, I'm blackmailing myself. If I don't exercise, the only people who profit are the meat-producers. They've only gotten $10 from me this year. Any day that I think about blowing off my exercise, I think about giving my hard-earned cash to those days, and it always gets me out of bed."

So, whatever it takes—promises, schedules, or blackmail—make sure that your lifestyle includes the regular vigorous activity that you need for superior health and wellbeing.

97.4. Questions & Answers

How do I know if I'm getting enough vigorous activity in my life?

You should perform some activity that requires a concentrated effort of both mind and muscles. You should be breathing deeply, your heartbeat should be accelerated, and you should probably have a light film of perspiration, even in cool weather. You should experience this "conditioning" effect for at least ten to fifteen minutes, and preferably twenty to thirty minutes. After a vigorous activity is completed, you should still be in a state of accelerated metabolism (moderate heart and pulse beat, slightly deepened breathing) for another five to ten minutes.

As a practical rule, if you have difficulty sleeping at night, experience constipation, or feel continually fatigued and lacking in vigor, then you may also be sure that you probably are not receiving enough vigorous activity.

I'm fine on any exercise program—for the first two weeks. Then I find myself making excuses and finally I'm back to where I started, a weekend athlete. Any suggestions?

This is why it is so vital to make exercise and a vigorous activity period a normal part of your life—not simply something that you add to your day or do when you have "extra" time.

The most effective way to get exercise into your life—and make it stay there—is to do it as soon as you get out of bed. Before you eat breakfast, before you go to work, before you wake up the kids or read the paper, go, and exercise.

If you make exercise an essential part of your daily activities, at the beginning of the day, then you won't start to skip it. Most exercise programs fail because people try to work it into their schedules. Instead, revise and start a brand-new schedule. Treat that morning (or evening) exercise period as something you have to do; it's not an option, but a necessity.

You may have to be a little compulsive at first, and really (exercise your willpower and self-discipline. Reward yourself, punish yourself, but promise yourself that the time you have decided as your exercise period is sacred and will not be sacrificed according to whim or any other superseding responsibility.

Article #1: Exercise: A Hygienic Perspective by Ralph C. Cinque, D.C.

That daily exercise is essential to develop and maintain good health is one Hygienic principle upon which there seems to be universal agreement. Even the medical profession encourages regular exercise as a means of prolonging youthfulness and promoting cardiovascular well-being. The overall merits of regular exercise are fully recognized, and we have no need here to further expound upon them.

However, there exists a great deal of confusion regarding the relationship between exercise and health. Many people equate health with physical conditioning. The classical American model of male health is represented by a robust well-muscled physique, with erect posture, great strength, and power. Without necessarily deriding this ideal, I must insist that it is not synonymous with health. There is not always a direct proportion between the level of physical conditioning and the level of overall health. Physical conditioning is only one aspect of health. The best athlete is not necessarily the most healthy. The one who runs ten miles is not necessarily in better health than the one who runs only five, or one, or for that matter, none at all.

I once overheard a well-developed body builder relate to his companion that he was subject to occasional episodes of gout. Every few weeks one or the other leg and foot would swell up and produce agonizing pain. He would be crippled for days at a time and would have to resort to large doses of aspirin and other pain killers in order to obtain relief. This incident made a tremendous impact on me because this particular body builder had an absolutely splendid physique. His muscular development, his posture, his body weight, his carriage, his symmetry, and his proportions were virtually ideal. He had the physique of a Greek god. By all popular notions, he was a picture of health. Yet, it should be obvious to the readers of this article that his health was far from perfect. Gout does not develop without causes, and being well-muscled does not lessen its implications or severity. How ironic that in the process of building an admirable outward condition, he built a morbid internal condition. It is likely that his interest in body-building prompted him to follow a high-protein diet and to use protein supplements, liver extracts, etc., and that these practices were mostly responsible for the development of gout.

Although it is true that those who engage in regular physical activity achieve greater longevity than those who are largely sedentary, it has not been shown that superb athletes achieve greater longevity than those of moderate ability. With the exception of cardiovascular diseases, the incidence of degenerative diseases among athletes (such as cancer and arthritis) is approximately the same as for nonathletes. Lou Gehrig died of amyotrophic latoral sclerosis. Babe Ruth died of cancer. There have been many outstanding athletes who have died tragically of crippling diseases.

Acute diseases are equally as common among athletes. Many an athletic contest has been postponed due to colds and flus. Tennis star Jimmy Connors was recuperating from a month-long bout of mononucleosis right before the last Wimbledon tournament, and some have suggested that this was a factor in his loss to Borg.

Despite strong evidence to the contrary, the popular notion, today, is that exercise will insure us against disease. We are told that as long as you run every day, you can eat all the fatty meats you want and not develop atherosclerosis, for the running will keep down blood cholesterol and prevent arterial plaquing. We are told that playing tennis regularly will enable the body to "burn up" the caffeine and other toxic alkaloids of coffee and cola drinks, so drink all you want. Regular exercise will keep down blood pressure, so why cut out salt? Exercise diligently, perhaps excessively, and ignore every other aspect of Hygiene. That is the advice we receive from many of the "experts."

As Hygienists, we must stress the fact that exercise does not insure against disease, and it does not remedy disease. All it can possibly do is supply the body's need for activity. If the individual who exercises but ignores proper diet, fares better than the one who neither exercises or eats correctly, we can account for this by recognizing that the latter ignored two life essentials while the former ignored only one. Exercise does not undo the effects of dietary abuses, but a lack of exercise may compound the effects of dietary abuses.

The body has physiological needs that can only be met through vigorous physical activity. The development of muscular strength and endurance, a powerful heart, great respiratory capacity, vibrant circulation, thorough lymphatic drainage, and superb neuromuscular coordination all require the influence of regular exercise. However, from the standpoint of overall health, there is a limit to the amount of good that the body can derive from regular exercise. The body's actual physiological needs for exercise are not as great as some people believe. We do not have to become marathon runners in order to avoid cardiovascular disease. One can achieve high-level health without ever developing outstanding athletic capabilities. Of course, we have no objection to vigorous physical training, and we recognize that it is the only way to enhance performance. Possessing great strength, speed and endurance is practical and desirable even if it doesn't guarantee great health or longevity.

Vigorous exercise entails a tremendous energy expenditure. This expenditure is compensated for in the physiological benefits that we derive from exercise. The amount of energy that we can safely expend in physical activity depends upon the level of our overall health and vitality. The invalid, who is in great need of rest, can only engage in brief and mild periods of exercise without enervation. The seasoned athlete, on the other hand, may be able to perform amazing feats of strength and endurance without dissipation. It is difficult to designate arbitrarily what constitutes excess in the realm of physical activity because individual factors are the most important considerations. What is excessive for one person may be unproductive for someone else.

The initial effect of exercise is to deplete the body. The secondary and lasting effect, however, is to strengthen and build the body. This occurs while resting as the body prepares for future episodes of activity. Exercise must be vigorous in order to be effective. Slow walking, sauntering along on a bicycle, casually twirling the extremities—these activities are of little value. Subjecting the body to stress (within reasonable limits) is what exercise is all about. Exercise must be invigorating, strenuous, challenging and taxing in order to occasion dynamic physiological changes, only by placing great demands upon our bodies can we acquire great strength and stamina.

A short period of vigorous activity is more beneficial than a long period of mild activity. A short, but hard run will build greater power than a long, slow jog. It is also less depleting. Lifting a heavy weight a few times will build greater strength than lifting a light weight many times. A good exercise regime will provide for both endurance (the ability to sustain an activity over a long period) and strength (the ability to overcome resistance in a single instance), as well as speed and agility. A well-known jogging expert advised a woman recently to run slower in order to increase her jogging distance to ten miles. My advice would have been just the opposite, that is, to run a shorter distance harder, thereby deriving greater physiological benefits and less profound exhaustion.

Determining the best manner in which to train depends upon what one's objectives are. The person who is exercising for general health and fitness will have different goals than the one who is trying to achieve excellence in some particular sport. Obviously, one can only become a great long-distance runner if one habitually runs long distances. One can only become a great cyclist if one cycles regularly. Great swimmers become so only by putting in many hours in the pool. Developing outstanding capability requires participation far in excess of the body's physiological needs for activity. However, expenditures of this kind can be made without depleting the body as long as the individual gradually subjects his or her body to greater stress and makes a point to secure enough rest and sleep to fully compensate for the added exertion. For example, one could not attempt to run long distances (30 to 40 miles per week) while going to school full-time and working (as I once tried to do). It is possible to become progressively more enervated even as one's level of conditioning improves. However, for the individual with a less-hectic schedule, who is able to rest 9 to 10 hours every day, such a running program may be entirely constructive.

Unfortunately, many runners do overexert themselves of effects of excess vary from mild to severe strains and sprains. Pronounced physiological depression marked by weight loss, loss of libido, insomnia, amenorrhea in the female, and digestive disturbances have resulted from an overly-strenuous training schedule. These problems are usually resolved easily by securing more rest and curtailing one's activity. In some instances, too rapid progression is found to be the crux of the problem.

Which activities are best from a Hygienic standpoint? As always, we refer the argument back to Nature. Those activities that conform with physiological principles relating to joint motion and body mechanics are most desirable. Formal exercise is really just a substitute for natural activities that we would perform in a state of Nature. All natural activities require total body participation. When we run, jump, climb, swim, etc., our bodies are acting as a unit, even though certain muscle groups may be playing a predominant role. Such activities not only strengthen and condition us, they enhance body energy, coordination, balance, and freedom. By entailing a fluidity of motion, these activities enable us to avoid excessive strain and tension. In contrast, activities that entail rigid postures, isolated muscular efforts, and limited ranges of motion, may have the opposite effect, that is, to increase tension and to stress the joints and muscles.

Perhaps running is the most natural human activity, like deer, human beings are running animals. We are capable of running great distances smoothly, effortlessly and efficiently. Certainly, we are not aquatic animals and bicycles never grew on trees. Team sports are popular because of cultural influences, not biological inclinations. Running is considered to be the most superb exercise for strengthening the heart, lungs and circulation. It is not necessary to run great distances in order to derive these physiological benefits. Running 2 to 3 miles every other day is fully adequate to achieve optimal cardiovascular conditioning. Those who wish to run greater distances can do so, but no one should feel compelled to run longer than this for health reasons. Running sprints, running up hills, running upstairs and other variations are likely to be of greater value than just jogging. Running alone is not adequate for good conditioning. Such activities as vigorous calisthenics, weight training and gymnastics round out an exercise program that includes running. This is particularly important in regard to developing the upper torso and extremities, which are largely undeveloped by running.

When is the best time to exercise? Again, we must apply Hygienic reasoning. Eat when you are hungry. Drink when you are thirsty. Rest when you are tired. So, it would follow that you should exercise when you feel vigorous. It is a mistake to use exercise as a stimulant, to perk ourselves up through exercise when our bodies are actually calling for rest and sleep. A feeling of relative vibrancy should precede and occasion our workouts and not vice versa. If we feel languid, we should rest until our energies have been recuperated to the point that we feel like becoming active. If you happen to feel all washed out on any given day, it would be unHygienic to force yourself to exercise in spite of it. Just as we can rouse up an appetite by eating, even in the absence of hunger, so too can we rouse up a feeling of invigoration by exercise, but the latter is just as artificial as the former. Get in tune with your body and seek always to supply your body's needs as they fluctuate in the course of daily life. There is really no best time to exercise, just as there is no best time to eat. Some mornings I feel inclined to start running right out of bed, and I do so. Other mornings I feel no such inclination, so I postpone or cancel my usual run. Learn to live with a flexible schedule in regard to exercise, and for that matter, all aspects of Hygiene.

Can a person attain great athletic ability eating fruits, nuts, and vegetables? The answer is a qualified yes. I was introduced to Hygiene by two brothers, both in their 30s, who had been Hygienists for many years and who were excellent runners of marathon caliber. Eating Hygienically lends itself to greater athletic achievement, particularly in endurance activities. A high-alkalinizing diet, composed largely of fresh fruits and vegetables, enhances one's oxidative powers and one's ability to sustain muscular effort. On the other hand, such a diet promotes rather slender body build. I have never met a raw fooder with a "Charles Atlas" physique and doubt that I ever will. For one thing, the diet is too low in protein. Secondly, raw vegetable foods do not stimulate anabolism the way cooked foods do. Yet, lean muscularity may be closer to the biological norm for physical development than the immense size that we generally associate with classical body-building. It is unlikely that human beings in a state of Nature, living on the spontaneous products of the trees in a gentle climate, would tend to massive physiques. Peoples throughout the world who are known for achieving great longevity tend, as a rule, to be rather slender. Keep in mind that I do not object to weight training or body building, but only to the excessive bulkiness that many weightlifters develop.

Many Hygienists are too thin and underdeveloped. In most cases, barring pathological causes, this is the result of an overly-restrictive diet, both in regard to quantity and variety of food and to inadequate physical training. In all fairness, however, we must recognize that the paucity of outstanding athletes among Hygienists is due mostly to the paucity of Hygienists. Yet, Hygiene has not been without its talents. Among our practitioners, for example, Dr. Sidhwa is a first-rate long-distance runner. Dr. Burton is a prominent cyclist in Australia who competes regularly in grueling races. Dr. Benesh is a veteran physical culturist, who, at the age of 67, engages in weight training, running and vigorous calisthenics. The last time I visited him he said apologetically that he was running only six miles a day, but added quite candidly, "I try to take it at a fast clip." Dr. Shelton, himself was an outstanding weightlifter and had a rugged build that matched his personality.

What role does exercise play in the recovery of health? I believe that it plays a greater role than some Hygienists think. Unfortunately, many Hygienists are preoccupied with food and fasting. To them, life is one great cleansing. They live from one fast to the next one. Or they consume themselves in concerns over food in between. Purification becomes their greatest goal in life, elimination the ultimate purpose in living. They fail to see fasting for what is is—a temporary expedient that enables us to secure a foundation from which to build ourselves. The only contests they wish to enter are fasting marathons.

They never give their bodies a chance to enter a building phase. They deny themselves, by their imbalance, the opportunity to grow, to develop a physique, to acquire great strength, speed, and endurance. Instead of practicing Hygiene so as to live, they live so as to practice Hygiene—a most unHygienic endeavor. It is no wonder that such individuals remain weak, puny, and pedestrian in their lives.

Among feeble children, particularly, I have found exercise to be of greatest importance in building vigor and promoting growth and development. Those with weak digestion can derive much benefit from engaging in vigorous physical workouts. The role of exercise as promoting recovery in tuberculosis, and other respiratory problems, is well known. Exercise strengthens not only our muscles, but our entire organism, including our minds. It is possible that exercise has a more profound effect upon the organism than any other single Hygienic factor.

Article #2: Exercise: What Most of Us Forget

Exercise is defined by Webster's New World Dictionary as "activity for developing the body or mind." The average American has little difficulty meeting the latter but finds less and less time for the former—developing the body.

Day-to-day living develops the mind. Academician or laborer, wide-eyed child or wise old man, housewife or career woman, all of us are tested day in, day out with exercises for the mind. All the yesterdays of mental exercise, coupled with today's, strengthen, and develop the muscle between our ears.

Whether subtle—reading periodicals, listening, and watching the news, solving routine problems at work and at play—or applied, such as the efforts to become a better chess player by studying the masters of the game, our mind gets more than enough exercise daily. It is a natural activity for all of us.

Activity to develop our bodies, on the other hand, is not wholly natural. Although the body is in natural, constant activity throughout the day—even in sleep—vigorous activity needed by the body's circulatory system, its lungs and its muscles requires our willing commitment. No matter how old or in what state of health, there's a healthy form of exercise for nearly everyone. And an effort should be made by everyone to find that right exercise to develop the body.

If you, the Natural Hygienist and Life Scientist, are following the rules for natural health—a Hygienic diet, sufficient rest, and sleep, occasional supervised fasting and the proper amounts of sunshine and pure air and water—then a regular exercise program is a must.

Why is regular exercise so important? A long-standing, inactive body becomes sluggish. Bodily functions are greatly impaired and reduced. If you suffer from chronic fatigue, poor sleep, digestive disorders, shortness of breath after little exertion or poor posture (just to name a few symptoms) you are not exercising your body. You are depriving your body of the energy that it needs to properly maintain its natural, healthful functions. Reasonably vigorous exercise builds up the energy reserve our bodies need now more than ever in today's fast paced living. Taking appropriate and sufficient exercise daily keeps that energy reserve at its peak. The key to maintaining energy and maximum health is your blood circulation, both arterial and capillary. Without exercise, circulatory fitness is not possible.

Studies show that at age 25 blood flow has decreased 40% and decreases 60% by age 35. From an energy-level standpoint, then, the average American is middle aged at age 26 and all because we are sitters, we Americans. We sit on our way to work, at work and spend a major part of our free hours sitting, engaging only in a minimum of activity. Our endurance and stamina is stagnant as compared to primitive peoples who, all day long, lift and push and climb and more importantly, walk and run.

Regular exercise, then, provides us with a stronger heart and lungs, increased metabolism, better digestion, good sound sleep, the elimination of a multitude of physical ailments and especially with the energy to overcome stress. The question now is, what exercise is best for you.

First, find out how much exercise you can engage in by getting a proper physical. In some cases, it may not be possible for you to exercise at all. But that is a rare occurrence. Once you have determined how much you can exert yourself, your choices are many.

Walking, certainly, is the easiest and the least thought of form of exercise we can all do easily. A short series of calisthenics, cycling, jogging, dance exercises, isometrics and progressive resistance programs at health clubs are other choices. Swimming, tennis, volleyball, and golf are others. Yoga and martial arts disciplines from the Far East have a growing following in the United States, too. Whatever you choose as your form of exercising, there are some basic principles that you'll need to follow.

To be of any real value, your exercise should be a daily ritual, systematically performed. Mornings are the best times to engage in your physical activity and when your body needs it the most. A safe beginning is two to three sessions per week the first month and three to four the second month. Thereafter, as your strength increases, you can exercise more frequently.

Set aside at least 45 minutes each day for your exercise, allowing for a warm-up each time and a slowdown toward the end of your period. Take short rests during your sessions. Most of all, discover what works best for you. Exercise on an empty stomach is ideal. After meals, you should wait at least two hours.

For a well-rounded program, learn to do several types of exercise. This leads to a sustained interest in what you are doing as well as contributing to the developing strength, balance, flexibility, coordination, speed, and endurance.

Remember, there is no rule that says exercise has to be hard work. Look at all of the alternatives and what they can do for you. There's a healthy form of exercise for everyone. Many of you will be content with less vigorous exercise than others, which is fine so long as you are exercising regularly in order to build endurance, burn excess calories and strengthen your cardiovascular system.

Article #3: Jogging and Other Vigorous Exercise

Warm Up and Warm Down

Warm Up and Warm Down

Enlivening outdoor air, trees and other natural scenery, the exhilarating feeling of aliveness: These are some of the reasons why so many folks jog as part of their exercise program. Many people like to run in the morning when they arise; others prefer the afternoon after work before their evening meal. Dedicated joggers run morning and evening. Whenever you run, it is probably after a period of relative inactivity. So, unless you have been physically active before you jog, it is an excellent idea to warm up before jogging. It takes only a few minutes, and the results are well worth the time.

We run because we enjoy it, and we know it's good for our health. Let's enjoy ourselves now while we learn why it's important to warm up before jogging: Our circulatory system has to adjust to increased physical activity. Too sudden demands on the heart and the arteries are a strain on them. When we're relatively inactive, our heart beats slowly and arterial tension is low. Sudden violent exercise can easily cause unpleasant symptoms such as a painful throbbing in the side and front of the neck.

To do their work well the muscles must contain blood commensurate with the work they must do. The more work they do, the more oxygen they need and, as you now, the (red) hemoglobin in the blood supplies oxygen o all the body cells. When at rest, most of our blood is in our body cavities (head, chest, stomach, pelvis). Our venous and lymphatic circulations are relaxed.

When we exercise vigorously, as when we jog, most of our blood will flow through the muscles at a rapid rate and at high pressure. This increase in pressure and rate of flow begins at the start of vigorous exercise. The arteries of the body cavities, especially in the stomach, constrict, while the arterioles in the muscles and the vascular area of the skin dilate. Dr. Shelton says, "Such a vast circulatory adjustment cannot be made in a satisfactory way or sufficient to correspond to the amount of work demanded from the muscles if rapid or vigorous work is thrown upon the muscles suddenly." He also says that respiratory and eliminatory adjustments are best made by increasing the intensity and quantity of muscular exertion gradually.

Shelton says, "Nor is it desirable or even always safe to suddenly cease vigorous activity while in a state of high organic activity—the heart and lungs working hard, the glands working at high speed, the skin flushed and perspiring. The racehorse trainer acts wisely when he takes his horse, after the race, and walks him around a while, thus giving him exercise of progressively diminishing intensity until circulation and respiration have returned to nearly normal. Sudden cessation of vigorous activity throws as much strain upon circulatory adjustment as a sudden beginning of heavy work. It is best to decrease the quantity and intensity of muscular work gradually. Passive deep breathing may also be used to reduce organic activity."

To help you get warmed up or warmed down for exercise, here are a few exercises I saw in our local newspaper. Try them!

1. With, your feet a few inches apart, bend down and touch (or reach for) your toes. Then stand up straight, raising your hands high above your head ... then repeat this about a half dozen times.

2. Stand with your hands on your hips and your feet planted firmly. Twist the top half of your body until one shoulder points all the way forward ... then back to where it belongs

... then the other shoulder ... then back. Stop after about 10 swings.

3. Lie on the floor and stretch your arms and legs out until you look like and "X". Raise your legs, still spread out, all the way up and back until your toes touch your fingers. Do this about four times.

Happy jogging!

Article #4: Hiking Is More Than Just Exercise by Marti Wheeler

Hiking could become your favorite form of exercise. One reason why is because walking is easy. In case you're wondering what the difference is between hiking and walking, there's really very little difference. According to the dictionary, a hike is a long walk, especially for pleasure or exercise. (Of course, long is a relative term and so has little meaning unless we know long compared to what.)

At any rate, you can hike for both pleasure and exercise, among other things. Actually, do not hike "at any rate". Hike at a very fast pace. Walking cannot be very effective as a form of exercise if you don't walk fast. (Fast is a relative term, too, but here we mean relative to a person's ability. For example, a person just off a long fast might consider a moderate pace to be fast.) All the muscles of the body are used in walking, though the legs obviously benefit the most. Fast-paced uphill hiking provides as much exercise as jogging on level ground.

Hiking is healthful from standpoints other than that of exercise, however. It is an excellent way to obtain lots of fresh air, as well as a nice dose of sunshine. The mental wellbeing that results from a brisk walk cannot be underestimated, either. Enjoyment and appreciation of your surroundings can lift your spirits and make you glad to be alive—and healthy. There is something very uplifting about the feel of a breeze or wind on the face or body.

Such wholesome recreation is just plain good for us; Hiking is recreation on many counts. The scenery can vary from houses on neighborhood streets to woodsy settings, perhaps along a creek or river, to open fields or meadows. If you are curious or adventuresome, you may want to go exploring. If you are romantic, you may want to hike with a husband, wife, or lover. You may enjoy hiking with a companion, someone with whom you enjoy conversation.

If you are like many people and have less time in your life than activities you want to pursue, why not combine your exercise with your social life to make the most of your time? If you use your imagination, you will come up with many more ways to combine hiking with other pleasurable activities. Though it is preferable to walk free-handed, you can occasionally bring your camera and take photographs. You can sometimes bring a small backpack with some fruit and combine a hike with a picnic—a good combination! One last note on hiking: It requires very little equipment and no training or special skills. A comfortable pair of hiking shoes are an asset, though running shoes will also suffice in many places. If your inner ears are very sensitive, you may find it helpful to wear earmuffs or a hat or scarf that covers your ears if the temperature is below 65 degrees. Also, slacks, shorts or skirts with pockets are good to have. But all in all, you will need very little equipment for hiking. You don't even need as much energy and motivation as runners must have. Yet you can sure reap many benefits.

Article #5: Developing Your Arms

Are you a weakling? Can you do more than four or five pushups, even women's (modified) pushups? For some people, doing five pushups is pushing it. They are ready to stop at four if not before. (For those of you who are unfamiliar with modified pushups, they are done from the knees instead of from the toes. Otherwise, they are the same as regular pushups.)

The worst problem some people have when it comes to pushups is that they dislike or even despise doing them. But then it's not unusual for a person to dislike what they're not good at. You may want to develop your arms and upper torso without suffering, even if you're not a swimmer and dislike doing pushups. Here is a solution to this problem for weaklings who don't want to remain weaklings. Purchase a set of dumbbells, "a short bar with two identical spheres or with adjustable weighted disks attached to each end and used usually in pairs for calisthenic exercise"—Webster's New Collegiate Dictionary.

Start off with the lightest weights and do about five repetitions to start with. Then increase the number of repetitions in increments of five as you gain strength. You can do your weightlifting at the same time as other calisthenics, alternating between exercises for your legs, for your arms, and for your abdomen and sides so that the muscles in the various parts can rest somewhat between exercises. For example, you can lift both dumbbells from your sides, outward and meeting above your head, starting off with five repetitions and, in time, increasing to 10, then to 15 and to 20, etc. Then do 10 or 20 sit-ups, preferably on a slant board. So far you have exercised primarily your arms, then your abdomen.

Next lie down on your side and, with or without ankle weights strapped around your ankles, lift one leg 20 times (like scissors). Then stay in that position and lift it from your side up into the air and over your head several times. Do this same scissors exercise and dumbbell lift on your other side.

Continue exercising in this manner and lift the dumbbells in various ways. While lying flat on your back, lift from your sides with your arms as far away from your body as possible to a meeting point over your chest. Also, while lying on your back, lift from your sides with your arms beside your legs and then above your head.

These exercises are very effective, and your upper torso will develop as desired. You won't be a weakling anymore, even though your pushup ability may not improve. It will become much easier to open heavy doors, and turning the steering wheel on a car without power steering will be noticeably easier, too.

If you wonder why, you still can't do pushups after using dumbbells awhile, ask yourself if you can lift 50-90 pounds of dumbbells. When you can do that, perhaps you can lift about half of your body weight with your arms more than half a dozen times—and enjoy it.

Lesson 98:

Exercise Programs for the Healthy

98.1. Why We Should Be Vigorously Active

98.1.1. Life Is Activity

98.1.2. Quality of Life Is Determined by Vigorousness, Intensity, and Extent of Activities Cultivated

98.1.3. Fitness Essential to High-Level Health and Well-Being

98.1.1. Life Is Activity

Life is characterized by activity. Death is exemplified when all activity ceases.

Hence the quality of life is determined by the activity level of the organism.

98.1.2. Quality of Life Is Determined by Vigorousness, Intensity, and Extent of Activities Cultivated

If life is worth living, it's worth a lot more if lived at its highest possible level. For comparison, picture a sloven hillbilly who lives a life of indolence with a bottle of whiskey as his foremost companion. On the other side of the coin, consider an engineer who has a home, a wife, and children, who plays tennis and other active games, who has cultivated many arts, appreciates great music, and is involved in guiding his children to useful and active lives. Those who care about themselves, those around them, and about the kind of world they live in are obviously the kind we admire whereas those who are making no contribution to the world are despised.

Thus, you should undertake to encourage those whom you counsel to get involved in vigorous activities, especially constructive hobbies such as gardening, orcharding, flower-growing, etc., that absorb and develop a person culturally while at the same time eliciting a lot of vigorous physical activity. Physical activity is, in itself, constructive for it adds zest and quality to life as little else can. The enormous benefits outlined in this lesson will make that readily evident to you.

98.1.3. Fitness Essential to High-Level Health and Well-Being

While we can be fit without being healthy, we cannot be healthy without being fit. Anyone who tells you they're healthy very likely means they're not suffering from any prominent pathology. But, if they're not fit, it is obvious they're not healthy. And, as a rule, anyone who fancies him/herself as being healthy really is not. Hence it is incumbent upon you to determine the fitness and activity levels of your clients. And, likewise, to inspire your clients to undertake the activity levels necessary to achieve high-level fitness. This, in conjunction with other practices you'll move them to undertake, will build high-level health.

98.2. The Enormous Benefits of Exercise and Vigorous Activity

98.2.1. General and Specific Fitness Equip Us for Life

98.2.2. Increasing Capillary and Lymph Circulation

98.2.3. Maintenance of Life's Faculties at High-Functioning Levels!

98.2.4. by Developing and Using Energy, We Always Have an Abundance of Energy

98.2.5. Through Vigorous Activity We Develop Strength and Stamina!

98.2.6. Vigorous Exercise Develops Ability and Agility, Vigor and Vitality

98.2.7. Exercise Results in Better Posture and Profile

98.2.8. When You're Fit, You Devote More Time to Those Around You

98.2.9. Detoxification and Body Purity Are Achieved Through Vigorous Exercise

98.2.10. Bouncy Buoyant Feelings Result from Vigorous Activity

98.2.11. Vigorous Activity Eliminates Internal Conditions that Give Rise to Qualms, Worries, and Stress

98.2.12. Because Exercise Occasions Extraordinary Body Cleansing, Less Sleeping Time is Required for Regeneration of Nerve Energy

98.2.13. Vigorous Activity and a Cleaner Internal Environment Reduce Libido (sex drive) But Increase Sexual Capability and Intensity with Enhanced Enjoyment

98.2.14. Those Who Render Themselves Healthy and Fit Have a Better Self-image and More Pride But Tend to Less Ego Exhibition

98.2.15. Vigorous Activity Results in Better Functioning of All Faculties Including, Most Importantly, Mental Faculties and Emotional Well-Being

98.2.16. Regular Exercise Begets Perpetual Feelings of Exhilaration and Well-Being

98.2.17. A Vigorous Exercise Program Builds Greater Mental Powers and Alertness

98.2.18. Exercise Quells Food Addictions

98.2.19. Vigorous Activity Increases Capacity for Vigorous Activity

98.2.20. A Vigorous Activity Program Enables Us to Have Better Personal Control

98.2.21. While Involved in an Intensely Vigorous Exercise or Activity Regime, You Will Be Better Able to Face and Cope with Stressful Situations and Individuals

98.2.22. as an Active Person You'll Have More Poise and Stable Emotions

98.2.23. Regular Exercise Overcomes Constipation and Establishes Regularity

98.2.24. Your Nerves Will Be Steadier, Hence You Will Rarely if Ever Experience Edginess or Nervousness

98.2.25. Your Senses Will Be More Acute and Accurate

98.2.26. Exercise Enables the Body to More Quickly Heal Itself in Many Conditions

98.2.27. An Exercise Program Helps Overcome and Reverse Degenerative Conditions

98.2.28. Regular Exercisers Have Better Digestion

98.2.29. Exercise Will Eliminate a Headache

98.2.1. General and Specific Fitness Equip Us for Life

Becoming fit means developing the ability to do things. When you train yourself for a few tasks, your ability to master other tasks becomes much easier. When you become physically fit, it becomes easier for you to become skilled in areas other than those of your specific training.

As the joys of life derive from our abilities to perform easily and efficiently, it behooves us to undertake those steps to become fit generally as well as particularly. When we become generally fit, everything becomes better. It has been pointed out, as an example, that an unfit person is a much poorer sexual partner than a fit person with high energy and endurance. A highly-capable person makes him/herself happier by making his/her partner happier.

Just as learning to play one musical instrument makes it all the easier to learn to play yet another, so, too, becoming fit equips you to master other areas of living with commensurately less effort.

Truly, the broader our areas of mental and physical fitness, the more life becomes a joy to live.

98.2.2. Increasing Capillary and Lymph Circulation

Good capillary and lymph circulation is essential to complete nourishment, muscular development, high energy, thoroughgoing detoxification, rejuvenation, and greater mental powers.

Vigorous exercise is capable of conferring a plethora of benefits. This is accomplished in many ways. But the machinery that contributes to enhancement of body faculties is rehabilitation of the body's circulatory system.

It is said that the average person of 35 has already lost about 60% of his/her circulatory ability; at age 60, about 80%! This is bad news, of course. But there is a bright side: Most of us can regain most, if not all, of our circulatory potential!

We have within each of us about 60,000 miles of tubing that circulates about six quarts of blood. Most of this is in the form of capillaries, some so small that red blood cells must pass through in single file. Inactivity causes non circulation of blood through these tubes.

All cells are bathed in lymph fluid. The circulation of the lymph depends upon blood circulation and body activity. The poorer the blood circulation, the poorer the lymph circulation. Likewise, the more pronounced and forceful is blood circulation and the more vigorous the body movements, the greater the lymph circulation. Lymph circulation is necessary to bring nutrients from the bloodstream to the cells and, likewise, to take away cellular wastes from the cells to the veins.

You would do well to study the circulatory system so that you can better understand the enormous benefits of sustained, vigorous activity at least once daily to thoroughly ventilate the system with oxygen, to re-establish full circulation and maintain it for some six to ten minutes. It usually takes about six to eight minutes of continuous, vigorous activity such as jogging, swimming, biking, hard walking to achieve full circulation. And, of course, if the powers of life have declined, as it has in most of us, especially those whom you'll serve, it will be necessary to guide clients upon a gradually-accelerating course of vigorous exercise that will again rejuvenate the circulatory systems, both blood and lymph. Both are simultaneously benefitted upon exercising. And, as you'll discover, the reinvigoration of the circulatory system is the key to a flood of other benefits.

When you exercise vigorously, you place a demand upon your body for coping. More energy must be created, and more wastes must be removed, for increased metabolism calls for more nutrients, especially glucose and oxygen, and faster removal of waste products, especially lactic acid, and carbon dioxide. The brain causes the heart to pump faster to cope. More oxygen is processed from air by the lungs, passed to the arteries and circulated to the capillaries along with other nutrients. These are, in turn, passed through the capillary walls to the lymph and thence to the cells. The cells, in turn, pass their increased load of wastes back to the lymph which is passed on to the venous system which carries them to the lungs for removal (in the case of gases such as carbon dioxide) and thence to the liver and kidneys where more wastes are removed. Finally, the blood is pumped back through the lungs for new supplies of oxygen. And, of course, liver, and other organs have recharged the blood with more needed nutrients.

I hope this impresses upon you the absolute desirability of intense, sustained, vigorous activity for a period of from 20 to 30 minutes at least once a day and, preferably, two or three times daily. Not only can this take the form of jogging, swimming, or biking, but vigorous play as in tennis, badminton, basketball, etc. Heavier resistance exercises, of course, develop strong musculature as an additional benefit.

Not only should you indulge body rejuvenating exercise on a daily or twice-daily basis to make yourself exemplary, you should also profoundly inspire and motivate your clients to undertake an exercise or vigorous activity program. Only fasting and a change to a raw diet of mostly fruits can have a more dramatic impact on your clients' lives than the "magic" of a strenuous activity program.

98.2.3. Maintenance of Life's Faculties at High-Functioning Levels!

Exercise enhances your thinking power, revitalizes your body, and helps you to appear perpetually youthful! Exercise enables the body to revitalize itself and perpetuate a youthful condition into advanced years. An observer who went to Hunza stated that the women there appeared to be no more than 40 even though 90 years of age. And men of ninety were as active as 25-year-olds. What he was really saying is that Americans of

25 to 40 are in the conditions of ninety-year-olds! The Hunzas are very active and hardworking people.

To be sure, the best exercise program can be sabotaged by unhealthful practices. Thus fasting, a raw food diet consisting mostly of fruits, and ample sleep are crucial essentials in creating and perpetuating a youthful agility, ability, and appearance well into later years. Even conventional-living people who regularly exercise maintain youthful qualities as well as fitness into their 50s and 60s. Especially do we note this in tennis players, dancers, and other athletes who keep up their athletic activities. The virtues of exercise seem to prevail even over other practices that undermine well-being and health. Vigorous exercise creates the physiological capacities necessary to the successful conduct of all physiological processes. When operating optimally, there is almost no atrophy or loss of faculties or functions over the years until a natural death ensues. After all, the deer dying naturally was jumping and running like a youngster right up to the end.

98.2.4. by Developing and Using Energy, We Always Have an Abundance of Energy

More energy means more charm, better relationships, and altruism. Energy is the coin of life. As you've learned from the series of lessons entitled HIGH-ENERGY METHODS, you can order your life and program the regimen of your clients to be gradually more active until potential is realized.

The body tends to overcompensate or overdevelop to insure ability to cope with the demands made upon it. How many women, and men can start weight-lifting after seventy and win prizes? How many men and women can start running at eighty and win marathons? The truth is that most can achieve high performances if they set themselves to the task no matter what the age. As long as there's the spark of life, there's much unrealized potential. It merely has to be trained or developed.

Once the body has met the demands made upon it—as long as the correct regime of life is followed—we'll always have energy to spare. We'll have the energy to do the things that indolence and atrophy unfit us for. Once you have energy to spare, you'll find yourself going out of the way to help others.

You'll have the energy and disposition to spruce up, to be more voluble and expressive, to be better reasoned, in short, to be more attractive and charming. Exercise and other essentials of life properly observed can create the energies necessary to transform a grouch and a slouch into a live wire and lovable person. People who have lots of energy do favors for others, whereas those who have little of it must conserve it by resisting the demands of the world upon them.

When you boast a smile instead of a growl, you'll be appreciated and loved, esteemed, and looked up to. This immense benefit will stand you and your clients well if a vigorous exercise program and its life concomitants are appropriately implemented.

98.2.5. Through Vigorous Activity We Develop Strength and Stamina!

Just as the body becomes an organism generating more energy when the demand is made for more, we can also immensely enhance our strength and stamina. We can endure much longer without tiring or fatigue. We can face trying circumstances and cope with them easily and more facilely.

The principle of overcompensation or overdevelopment again comes to the rescue of those who adopt exercise as a way of life. You've witnessed or read of others who started lifting weights, even at advanced ages, and increased their ability to lift progressively heavier weights. You've read of, or witnessed, those who started running and progressively lengthened their time and distance until they attained marathon status.

You can do this too! And so can your clients! I count among our students some who were hopeless cripples by all standards, yet who started doing the exercises they could do and progressed until they ran, and speed walked even though they still limp or exhibit the vestiges of their disastrous accidents.

Staying power arises because we are not burdened by a toxic system and because we develop greater energy-creating capacities. A clean and efficiently operating organism has great endurance capabilities. Likewise, strength develops when a demand to cope with strenuous tasks is made upon the body.

98.2.6. Vigorous Exercise Develops Ability and Agility, Vigor and Vitality

Once you've started performing varied activities, your ability to perform yet other activities becomes all the easier. For instance, training to play certain instruments develops nimbleness of the fingers. Should such a musician then decide to learn typing, it is much easier than for a nonmusician. Moreover, speed and accuracy are also more easily realized.

Once you've developed fitness, your exuberant energy and ease of doing things translates into an agility that will surprise you. Perhaps you've felt lethargy and a disinclination to do things with flair and vigor. But, when you have energy to spare and increased abilities, you tend to do things with emphasis and embellishment—you do things with a flair that wins admiration, if not envy, from others.

The more vigorous your activities, the more vigor you'll have, for, in a word, vigor is a combination of energy, vitality and stamina. The same principle of overcompensation works to advantage in every area of your life.

Vigorous activity also enables your body lo rejuvenate or revitalize itself. Vitality may be characterized as roughly equivalent to nerve energy—the amount of nerve energy you have available to drive your engines with!

98.2.7. Exercise Results in Better Posture and Profile

People with lots of energy tend to walk with their heads high and their bodies erect. Those who have little energy tend to slump so as to expend as little energy as possible in activities. As you already know, debility breeds debility, whereas goodness tends to beget more goodness. Thus, the constructive role of exercise or vigorous activity becomes obvious.

When you have the energy to expend, you use it for ends that serve you better. And, in using energy, you maintain the basis for its enhanced creation, thus insuring the better usage you have made of it.

With more energy and an improved personal disposition, you will walk prouder, present an erect and confident profile to others and, as a result, be better respected and admired.

98.2.8. When You're Fit, You Devote More Time to Those Around You

By devoting time to others, you'll be appreciated more. Under the heading of altruism and better relationships we treated this aspect of an exercise benefit. However, this redundancy should be reinforcing.

With increased energy we are not reluctant to spend it in behalf of those with whom we're involved in life. We're more willing to do those little favors that take our energies, but, in reality, become investments in others. Inasmuch as humans are naturally altruistic being gregarious and cooperative in nature, your investment of time and energy helping others is usually well rewarded. Even if not, you've still the satisfaction of doing good deeds. Good deeds are performed for the pleasure of doing them, not necessarily with a view to future reward. In this world and time, however, most are imbued with little energy and an invidious attitude that disposes them to rip off those around them rather than contribute to their better well-being.

You'll be kind and considerate when you can afford to be! When being good to others involves an expenditure of energies you don't have, you'll tend to conserve them through defensive devices, some of them being withdrawn-ness, grouchiness to those who penetrate your wall with disagreeableness to all that threaten to make an inroad upon your energies or resources.

Having an amiable disposition is a virtue born of health and all that it encompasses. Even if it rewards you not, it is wise to be as human as you can and forebear the eccentricities of others with a philosophical understanding of where they're coming from.

98.2.9. Detoxification and Body Purity Are Achieved Through Vigorous Exercise

As you know, accelerated activity calls for increased blood and lymph circulation. The role of these two liquid transport systems is to insure delivery of nutrients (supplies) where and when needed and, as well, to take wastes away to the organs of elimination.

When circulation increases to meet an increased need for nutrient distribution to cells and the removal of their wastes, there are corollary benefits that are noteworthy. In a person with morbid materials in the system extraordinary to those generated by the activity itself, the increased circulation carries these out also. The body's tendency to do more than it has to in order to satisfy a need (the principle of overcompensation) works to our benefit.

Thus, sustained vigorous and strenuous activity of a few minutes or more accomplishes extraordinary body cleansing, thus unburdening us of previously uneliminated wastes and toxic substances. As poisons in the system are almost exclusively the responsible factors for debility, low energy, disease, and suffering, exercise thus bears benefits far beyond making us fit. Exercise or vigorous exertion keeps the system vital by keeping it unimpaired by the ordinary and extraordinary morbid materials that accrue from normal wastes and our predilection for ingesting unwholesome food and drink.

I like to think that daily vigorous exercise of a few minutes is the equivalent to a day of fasting though, to be sure, an occasional day of fasting plus exercise delivers inconceivably enormous benefits.

98.2.10. Bouncy Buoyant Feelings Result from Vigorous Activity

Performance is effortless and easy without noticeable flagging or fatigue. With supple musculature and ample energies, you'll find it a snap to breeze through your days. Quite literally, you'll float! There'll be a grace and springiness to your step that, perhaps, you've witnessed in athletes.

Without burdensome and impairing toxins within, activities will be untiring—without fatigue. Though other life essentials properly met are essential to this state, exercise or vigorous activity is the biggest key.

98.2.11. Vigorous Activity Eliminates Internal Conditions that Give Rise to Qualms, Worries, and Stress

Studies and researches have amply demonstrated that a regular activity program disposes us to less worry and fears. We become better able to cope with stressful situations. Stressful situations do not drain us nearly as much when we're healthy and fit as when we're already in a drained condition. The person who can cope does not wither on the firing line as much as the person who is not equipped to handle highly-demanding situations. What little nerve energy an unfit person has is quickly exhausted in emotionally upsetting situations, whereas individuals who have made themselves fit through exercise and healthful practices are ready for anything.

Most stress and worries arise from unstable and uncomfortable internal conditions that drain the body extraordinarily of nerve energy. These drains exhibit as fears and worries—fears that the demands of work and society cannot be successfully met.

Exercise, by keeping us fit and cleansed, does not dispose us to worries and qualms.

It enables us to handle most stresses "in stride".

98.2.12. Because Exercise Occasions Extraordinary Body Cleansing, Less Sleeping Time is Required for Regeneration of Nerve Energy

Yes, exercise helps our bodies to detoxify and thus it takes less sleep to regenerate nerve energy. Moreover, sleep is more efficient, that is, it is deeper and accomplishes its purposes more surely and more quickly.

In lesson 15 we learned about the role sleep plays. We learned that a morbid body is a disturbed body that squanders its nerve energies needlessly trying to cope with the disturbances to well-being occasioned by poisons within. The body thus struggles to eject them. But, with a constant stream of them being introduced into the body and, being unable to cope with the needs of ordinary waste elimination, the body becomes progressively more toxic until it initiates a "crisis of elimination" which we call a cold, flu, herpes, or other affection.

Exercise is salutary in keeping the body cleansed. When the body is pure—when it is freed of enervating factors, it does not squander as much nerve energy. Nerve energy not wasted does not have to be regenerated. Thus, less sleep is required.

Further, an undisturbed body can achieve deeper sleep levels for longer periods. The deeper the sleep, the more nerve energy the brain can generate within a given time.

You can reduce the time you need for sleep by a vigorous exercise program. As a result, you'll have more time for self-improvement, vocations, and avocations.

98.2.13. Vigorous Activity and a Cleaner Internal Environment Reduce Libido (sex drive), But Increase Sexual Capability and Intensity with Enhanced Enjoyment

Better sexual performance makes the sexual partner happier which, in turn, makes you happier. The more fit you are, the greater your capability of having a more exhilarating and satisfying sexual relationship. The sex act makes a heavy physical demand upon the body and its faculties. Fitness of a high order enables us to discharge the act with vigor and sensitivity. On the other hand, the demands are so great on the unfit that they frequently expend so much energy as to lose the blood supply to maintain an erection or become so exhausted as not to be able to continue. One of the foremost complaints of men I meet in the older brackets, even some relatively young (40s), is impotency. While impotency is primarily due to nerve impairment from toxicosis, it also stems from inability to execute due to insufficient oxygenation, insufficient blood supply, or other factors which a fitness program will remedy.

For those who complain of sexual inadequacy, both female and male, a Hygienic regime involving heavy exercise usually proves a boon.

A toxic body usually has its sex drive immensely heightened. This drive becomes psychologically imbued, especially in this day and age of sexual acculturization when one's sexual ability is a measure of one's stance in the world. When the body is toxic, there is an exaggerated "urge to merge" because the survival mechanisms of threatened organisms are intensified, including the reproductive faculties. Once this toxicity is decreased or removed, the organism normalizes, and the sex drive is consequently lowered. In the pasture a bull can be with 25 cows and pay them no mind. However, if one cow comes into estrus (heat), there's hardly a fence that will restrain the bull. In humans living naturally rather than under the condition of sexual acculturization where sex is recreation rather than procreation, libido in the male becomes attuned to female receptivity which, as a rule, is accentuated only by the ovulatory period.

In your practice, you'll come across many who are impotent, and even young men who are sterile. While I do not advise that you try to "deculturize" their intellectual disposition toward sex, I do suggest that you guide them to wellness and fitness in which case sexual faculties are usually rejuvenated—often with a vengeance! But, as their conditions improve and their ability to perform improves, there is a lessening of sex drive for the abnormal conditions that gave rise to a gnawing "urge to merge" no longer exist. There is frequently renewed bliss in marriages where one or both partners have previously become incapable and/or indifferent to sexual interaction. Just as a low-energy individual tends to defensive mechanisms that make him a slouch, a grouch, and unaltruistic—energy-conserving measures—so, too, does a sexually-crazed (acculturized) individual tend to refrain from acts he desires, but fears he cannot execute successfully.

You do not have to bow to the abnormal sexual compulsions that inhere in our commercial world and in a toxic populace. I suggest that you guide everyone to the highest level of health and fitness possible and let nature take its course. It's the rare person who is fit and healthy that will exhaust himself in pursuit of the pleasures of sex.

98.2.14. Those Who Render Themselves Healthy and Fit Have a Better Self-image and More Pride, But Tend to Less Ego Exhibition

As a chess player I've met many self-styled chess experts who "talk a great" game. When I attended my first chess tournament, I was intimidated by one who talked such a fine game that I was sure he'd take the tournament.

Imagine my surprise that, in the fourth round we were paired as undefeated players. I felt beaten in advance to have drawn this player. However, when we sat down to play, I found that we were playing in the open with visible pieces and equal opportunities. We played along standard book lines for perhaps fifteen moves when he made a move I deemed extraordinarily weak. However, not being sure, I pondered my next move for nearly ten minutes under such side (and snide) remarks by my opponent to observers and passersby that "that move has him floored". I could find no merit in the move despite my extensive considerations. So, I made the move that occurred to me almost immediately when he made it, having explored all the lines he could muster in response. As a result, his game collapsed, and he resigned within ten moves. This game proved to be an illuminating lesson to me:

People who talk a good game are bragging. If they can play a good game, they let performance speak for them rather than words.

In my fourteen years in the health field, I find that braggarts and boasters frequently fall flat on their faces under firing line conditions. I have employed hundreds of people and those who do a snow job on telling you how great they are usually do not begin to live up to their self-billing.

The point is again, that performers let their works speak for them, whereas jawboners substitute words and snow jobs for performance which is often mediocre.

Once you've achieved a high level of capability, that will become well-known. You don't have to "blow your horn" about it. With greater capability you develop more self-reliance. With self-reliance you have a better self-image, and this "pride of self" radiates to others as dignity and self-respect. You don't have to "put on a front" for self-aggrandizement. You can enhance your situation in all aspects by honest effort.

Exercise in conjunction with a healthful regime will strikingly upgrade your performance levels. Once you have the confidence that you can more than hold your own with others, you'll let your deeds speak for you rather than vain braggadocio. Your image of yourself will be so good that you'll be content to impress others with the results you get through performance rather than with words.

Improve your image through vigorous activity. Implore your charges to do likewise for the benefits of physical activity are innumerable and, as yet, still uncharted.

98.2.15. Vigorous Activity Results in Better Functioning of All Faculties Including, Most Importantly, Mental Faculties and Emotional Well-Being

A self-assured person is calmer, more self-disciplined and has great emotional poise. That well-being and sharper thinking comes from an exercise program is not new— research has shown that executives who regularly exercise vigorously, are more decisive and effective in directing others. Mental sharpness underlies the ability to think things through logically and formulate better courses of action.

It has been said that a sick body has a sick mind. Likewise, an improved body improves its mind also!

Your great thrust is to arouse in your patrons a desire for exceptional betterment. Inspire in them an envisagement of an ideal condition for themselves. Build in them a belief that they can realize the ambition thus engendered.

Then goad them into action to undertake the course necessary to realize their wishes.

You'd be surprised how effective you can be with others.

The key to achievement is the ability to perform the acts requisite to the result envisioned. Exercise (and the Life Science mode of life) will excellently equip your clients emotionally and mentally to realize the high goals you've inspired in them.

98.2.16. Regular Exercise Begets Perpetual Feelings of Exhilaration and Well- Being

Without inferring that, exercisers or the vigorously active are tranquilized zombies, I assure you that the regularly active do live in perpetual highs!

It has been well established that, after a period of running or vigorous and continuous activity, the body secretes noradrenalin or norepinephrine. This secretion occasions what is roughly the equivalent of what is popularly termed "second wind". In my own case I must run at least a mile or carry on steady work for at least ten to twelve minutes before I get "warmed up" and my work becomes effortless. I sort of float along at my work, being almost indefatiguable. Further, I am more sensitive to those around me and tend to be more cognizant of their needs. My thinking is sharper and more facile.

If I fail to exercise for a day, a relative dullness sets in though I'm still energetic. The second day without exercise does not cause untoward circumstances, but the inspired high is gone. Still energetic as usual, I no longer have the floating sensation. After two days of lapse without exercise, it is a chore to do my chin-ups, weightlifting, pushups, and other routines until I've "warmed up" again.

Recently an article appeared in most newspapers nationwide as follows: PUMPING IRON CAN HELP SHED THOSE BLUES! "Nonaerobic exercise, such as weight training, is just as effective as aerobic exercise in lifting the blues away, according to a new University of Rochester study. Forty-one moderately depressed women were randomly assigned to three treatment groups. In the first, participants ran on an indoor track four times a week for 30 minutes. In the second, they worked out with weights on a Universal gym for the same amount of time. In the third, they didn't exercise. At the end of the eight-week program, running and weight training were significantly more effective than no exercise in relieving depression, says assistant psychiatry professor Elizabeth Doyne."

Exercise, as you can see, causes the body to "drug" itself harmlessly, but helpfully, to better enable it to perform. The benefit of daily exercise for 20 to 30 minutes is thus established.

98.2.17. A Vigorous Exercise Program Builds Greater Mental Powers and Alertness

Increased problem-solving ability results from exercise. More oxygen to the brain helps it function better. Less toxins in the brain enable it to function at a higher level.

While I have stated that all faculties improve when an exercise program is observed, I still feel it wise to enumerate as many of those improvements as possible.

Experiments conducted by fasting students in a class resulted in sharply improved mentation, class participation and higher grades. Likewise, experiments with students who were given an exercise program slowly improved their grades over control students who did not participate. Both experiments were conducted in Chicago, one by Dr. Anton Carlson and the other by Thomas J. Cureton.

One of the most notable mental improvements in those students who got into an exercise program was alertness and greater ability to solve problems. Likewise, executives attest that they can solve business problems easier because of their exercise programs.

98.2.18. Exercise Quells Food Addictions

Of especial interest to those who are overweight is the fact that the urge to eat can be smothered by a short run, jumping jacks, or other vigorous exercise for six to ten minutes. Even genuine hunger, which is rarely experienced by most Americans, is overcome, and deferred for a while because of exercise. However, when hunger then comes, it is more intense.

98.2.19. Vigorous Activity Increases Capacity for Vigorous Activity

The more you exercise, the more you're able to exercise up to a point. Because of the body's propensity of exceeding the "demands made upon it in developing abilities and capacities, we're usually able to go a bit longer and exert a little harder with each succeeding exercise session.

98.2.20. A Vigorous Activity Program Enables Us to Have Better Personal Control

Yes, we'll be more controlled of self and faculties. Precise and accurate performances increase productivity and quality of production. Precision performers are less likely to have accidents and miscues.

98.2.21. While Involved in an Intensely Vigorous Exercise or Activity Regime, You Will Be Better Able to Face and Cope with Stressful Situations and Individuals

Perhaps Dr. Hans Selye demonstrated more graphically than anyone the power of exercise even though he made his experiments with rats.

He took four groups of rats. The first group he called his "fat cat rats" because they were permitted to loll around and eat all the food they wanted. No problems were posed for them at all. The second group also had all the food they wanted, but they were put on a vigorous exercise program. The third group was fed only every other day but permitted indolence like the first group. The fourth group was fed only every other day, but was put through a rigorous exercise program like the second group.

Then he started putting these rats through the stresses faced by humans. They had horns blaring, machines clanking, mazes to run, and vigorous activity to undergo to avoid contrived or obvious threats of calamity.

The result: Within 30 days all the fat cat rats were dead! Rats from Groups 2 and 3 had started dying. But, after 60 days, all the rats in group 4 were still going strong!

This demonstrates most dramatically the benefits of abstemious eating and vigorous exercise, especially within the context of a helter-skelter hustler-bustler society.

98.2.22. as an Active Person You'll Have More Poise and Stable Emotions

Your face will exhibit a smile instead of a gloomy expression. Hostility and intolerance will disappear. The ability to cope breeds self-confidence and a happy disposition.

When you have ample energy, strength, and endurance to fulfill your basic needs and a surplus to spare, you will be self-reliant. The ability to cope is developed concomitant with increasing energy levels, stamina, and fortitude.

When you are master of yourself and are aware that you can further improve yourself or prepare yourself for anything, you'll be happy. And happiness generates an amiable, radiant disposition, overcoming a low-energy, energy-conserving attitude of parsimony, reluctance, and grumpiness in conducting your relations with others.

You become more outgoing, helpful, and socially aware rather than demanding. This makes the difference between being appreciated and unappreciated by those around you, the difference between being popular and in demand and being deprecated and avoided.

98.2.23. Regular Exercise Overcomes Constipation and Establishes Regularity

Constipation is a national disease with over 90% of our people suffering from it chronically or occasionally. Exercise is a great boon for these people. However, a raw food diet of mostly fruits with adequate sleep and a regime that touches base with other life essentials are also mandatory.

98.2.24. Your Nerves Will Be Steadier, Hence You Will Rarely if Ever Experience Edginess or Nervousness

Nerves are irritated by body toxins, giving rise to unsteadiness, tics, twitches, muscle spasms, muscular constrictions, etc. When your body is cleansed, that helps a lot. Muscular rejuvenation helps make muscles more responsive to the exact commands of the nerves. And, of course, when not irritated, the commands of the nerves are voluntary and correct as received from the brain instead of being defensive reactions to a toxic environment.

98.2.25. Your Senses Will Be More Acute and Accurate

Your thinking will be sharper, clearer, quicker, and more correct. Your decision-making ability will be greatly improved with decisions that are more appropriate and productive of intentions. Your judgments will not only be better ones but, in time, exalted, which will earn you admiration.

Yeah, yeah! Exercise, self-mastery, and a healthful disposition will produce these qualities in you.

98.2.26. Exercise Enables the Body to More Quickly Heal Itself in Many Conditions

Exercise helps overcome pain and physical problems. When the body is required to cope with new demands, it tends to correct those problems that impede the performance demanded. Try and try again! Keep on trying and you'll find yourself mastering movements and tasks that seem impossible at the beginning.

98.2.27. An Exercise Program Helps Overcome and Reverse Degenerative Conditions

Degenerative conditions are remedied by exercise even though it cannot resuscitate lost, deranged, or damaged organs. However, it will develop residual faculties in many cases to compensate for lost or impaired faculties.

98.2.28. Regular Exercisers Have Better Digestion

Digestive problems will be quickly overcome if dietary improvements are also made.

98.2.29. Exercise Will Eliminate a Headache

If a headache is being suffered, a brisk run of ten to twenty minutes will so detoxify the body and cause the secretion of so many pain-killing substances as to cause its disappearance.

98.3. The Elements of a Well-Rounded Activity Program

98.3.1. Stretching

98.3.2. Warming Up

98.3.3. Intensifying Activities

98.3.4. Jogging, Running, and Sprinting

98.3.5. Biking, Hiking, and Swimming

98.3.6. Weightlifting or Resistance Exercises for Strength and Weight Gain

98.3.7. Coordinative and Training Exercises

98.3.8. Accelerating Activities for More Benefit in Less Time

98.3.9. Gardening and Constructive Activity

98.3.10. Hobbies and Work that Keep Us Vigorously Active and Fit

98.3.11. Games to Play for Exercise of Self, Mate, and Friends

A well-rounded activity program brings into use the entire body musculature, some 700 in number, from head to foot.

98.3.1. Stretching

Our day should begin with stretching! After a night of rest and sleep, the musculature should be slowly brought back to active status. There are hundreds of little things to do that stretch various body muscle systems. Undertake to learn stretching exercises so that you can use them daily, especially upon awakening. A book on hatha yoga is useful for discovering stretching exercises.

98.3.2. Warming Up

Stretching is for awakening musculature and, indeed, the brain, bringing it to a high state. Warming up consists in doing very light exercises to get the body minimally oxygenized and operable.

98.3.3. Intensifying Activities

Warming-up exercises should be heightened to the level of vigorousness and strenuousness. For instance, if we jogged 100 yards or so, did some squats, sit-ups, etc., to warm up with, we might intensify activities by jumping jacks, a short sprint, pushups, chin-ups, or something that takes advantage of the warming and puts a heavier demand upon musculature.

98.3.4. Jogging, Running, and Sprinting

These are all constructive exercises. It has been said that two-hundred yards of sprinting is worth a mile of jogging. However, that might be, I feel that both are good. I end a two-mile jog with a sprint of perhaps a quarter mile for, after the first mile plus I can sprint with abandon, whereas I cannot go but a short distance at the beginning.

98.3.5. Biking, Hiking, and Swimming

These exercises are elective as are others. Exercises chosen should suit one's inclinations and abilities. Exercises will widen your activity horizons in any event.

98.3.6. Weightlifting or Resistance Exercises for Strength and Weight Gain

Everyone should be put on some resistance exercises to greater or lesser extent. Legs, arms, and body musculature generally develop rapidly under weight-lifting with arms, legs, and body through squats, etc. Pushups and chin-ups are especially good at developing the upper torso while weights on the shoulder while doing squats produce general body musculature otherwise.

98.3.7. Coordinative and Training Exercises

Not only should you have a varied regimen of exercises, but you should adopt exercises that coordinate the whole body. For instance, skipping rope is not only a good warmup exercise, but it does marvels for developing body coordination. There are many other coordinative activities which you should cultivate in yourself and clients.

98.3.8. Accelerating Activities for More Benefit in Less Time

As mentioned, intensified activities such as jumping jacks, sprinting and faster pacing or regular exercises place a greater demand upon the body that causes the same exercise benefits to accrue in a fraction of the time. It bears repeating that perhaps a few hundred yards of sprinting is worth a mile of jogging though, to be sure, a jog should be accelerated to running and huffing and puffing all-out sprinting at the end. An intense, continuous demand upon the body for six minutes or more generates the many benefits heretofore cited. Of course, it is advisable to precede intense sustained activities with 15 to 20 minutes of stretching, warmup calisthenics, and moderate exercises such as swimming, jogging, and biking.

98.3.9. Gardening and Constructive Activity

While all vigorous activity is constructive if it does not injure, there are some that are very beneficial. Gardening, which creates a food supply, is soul-satisfying as well as physically/mentally constructive. I suggest that you and your clients start gardening, orcharding, and beautifying your grounds as much as possible. Remember, even indoor gardening is constructive, for plants remove some aerial poisons while reoxygenating the air.

98.3.10. Hobbies and Work that Keep Us Vigorously Active and Fit

There are many hobbies that require much and varied physical exertion, especially shop work involved in making things. Your and your clients' inclinations will dispose you to a hobby. Keep in mind that a hobby should never be permitted to substitute for exercise. It should be in addition! Both the hobby and the exercise go better with each other.

98.3.11. Games to Play for Exercise of Self, Mate, and Friends

Few exercises are as beneficial as social exercises. As gregarious beings, humans thrive best while interacting with each other. Thus games like tennis, badminton, volleyball, baseball, and other vigorous noncontact sports are ideal forms of recreation. Play that meets both physical and social needs has a certain advantage over solo efforts though, to be sure, solo efforts permit of cogitation and reflection that build character and strength of purpose.

98.4. Questions & Answers

Will exercise correct hiatal hernia?

A hiatal hernia is an opening in the diaphragm that permits organs on either side to protrude through. In Dr. Shelton's book, Exercise, we learn how to cope with abdominal hernia very slowly through graduated exercises. I don't see any reasons why relaxed musculature of the diaphragm should be any less responsive to an exercise program.

Over the years I've received letters from individuals who were once overweight and said that the drastic weight reduction experienced in undertaking a Hygienic regime of raw diet and exercise also overcame their diaphragm problems. How long have you had this problem?

Nearly three years.

How much do you weigh now?

242.

Are you willing to undertake a raw food dietary and exercise program kicked off with a fast to help restore normalcy?

If that's what it takes.

How do I get my four-year-old son to be active? He's way overweight, being nearly 70 pounds. We have no neighboring children. He just sits and watches TV all day long, eating freely of his father's snacks. What should I do?

I suggest that you unplug the TV and remove father's snacks. I suggest that you and/or your husband take the youngster for walks, play ball with him, and otherwise get him involved. It might even pay for you to transport him to the nearest children's playground where he can participate actively with other active children, though, to be sure, at that weight he's in no condition to do more than walk. I suggest that you put him on an all-raw diet of mostly fruits as well as take him for walks. That, more than anything, will help him lose weight to the point he can be more active. What he needs more than anything is parental participation as well as identification with peers. Praise for activity accomplishments will encourage him to win more praise. There's much you can do. Explore your circumstances. A ruined child bespeaks parent failure. I'm happy you want to remedy this situation, and I'm sure the desire will give rise to a solution.

You sound like exercise will create Utopia for us. I'm about sixty pounds overweight. I've read lots that says exercise would help me get down to a normal weight and that would be heaven for me, but I've heard very little about all the other good things you say. Aren't you putting us on just to get us to do this thing?

All the benefits I've spoken of have been gleaned from researches and published literature during my past 14 years as a student of the health scene. And I've experienced many of the benefits cited for myself. Why should I lead you on? Why not try a vigorous, regular exercise regime and find out for yourself." Open up your ears and eyes to those who do. You'll be surprised that, indeed, exercise is one of the primary keys to a personal Utopia.

Can I lose weight by exercise alone? How soon can I expect to go from 227 to 125?

Yes, you can lose weight by exercise alone, but there are many considerations. First, if you exercise extensively even without a change of diet, your hunger will be considerably lessened as a result; you'll lose weight not only because you eat less, but because you'll burn up more calories. However, I doubt that you'll ever lose 102 pounds unless you get to the point where you're exercising at least two hours per day, something you can do. And then it takes more than a year. I've read of a case where a meat-and-potato-diet gal lost over 125 pounds within a year-and-a half and became a marathon runner as a result. But it's better to edge your diet over to more and more raw foods in conjunction with your exercise program. All raw will occasion drastic weight loss without much regard to your exercise program and food intake, though an exercise program and lowered food intake are always constructive.

How do you expect me to exercise if I never feel like it? You've said that you really shouldn't exercise if you feel against it. I never feel like it.

I've said that exercise makes you feel good. I've said that old practices make you feel progressively worse. How do you expect to feel like exercising unless you start exercising? Just start exercising regardless of how you feel. Do it because you know you must. Start off by fasting for a week or two. Go on an all-raw diet. Start walking vigorously and work that up to a jog, and then punctuate it with running and sprinting. The first thing you know, you'll be looking forward to those daily stints. You'll find your exercising period to be moments that give you some time to cogitate, and you'll discover you're cogitating more intense and productive while out jogging and running, even just walking. That which activates your body tends also to activate your mind. Do it and you'll be rewarded. Don't get roped in on a "which comes first, chicken or the egg" deal. Just do it because you know you have to force yourself to.

What you've said means everyone could become a real super person. If that's true, why isn't exercise pushed by the powers that be in this country?

If you've read the media, you find that the powers that be advise you to see a physician before undertaking any exercise program. And a physician is as likely as not to advise against it. Further, there's lots of adverse publicity about exercise and lots of pooh poohing of it. But, also, there's much publicity and much urging to exercise. Exercise is getting a better and better press. But there are many factors that militate against exercise, notably the sick diathesis that derives from your debilitating and slavish addiction to energy-draining foods. Pushing junk foods is far more profitable for industry (the powers that be) as a whole than pushing fitness. After all, the junk food

623

industry; the medical trades; the drug industry; the liquor, beer, wine, soft drink, cigarette, and other industries constitute a powerful quorum that despoils us. Enlightened consumers don't patronize them, and an exercise program scuttles them. Perhaps that's the reason only about a third of the country is active.

Lesson 99:

Restructuring the Way We Produce our Foods Part I

99.1. Having Enough Food for Our World

99.2. The Quality of Our Food Is Determined by the Quality of Our Soil

99.3. Questions & Answers

Article #1: How Vitamin and Mineral Content in Food Decreases Step-by-Step

Article #2: Saving Open-Pollinated Seeds by Margaret Flynn

Article #3: Hand Pollination of Squash by Richard Grazzini

Article #4: The Spirit Speaks

Article #5: Origin of the World's Basic Food Plants

Article #6: You've Just Been Poisoned by Mike Benton

99.1. Having Enough Food for Our World

99.1.1. Sharing the Harvest—Starvation and Malnutrition in the World

The old man stopped for a moment to rest as the sun began to sink on the horizon. He shared a laugh with old Rob, the mule, as he wiped the sweat from his brow. Another day of plowing done, and maybe it will rain.

We're a long way from this quiet twilight hour on a small farm when we stare down the long brightly-lit aisles of a "modern" supermarket, and we're also a long way from our own roots. We now live in a society where we can actually pass through life without growing a single carrot or piece of fruit. All Life Scientists should become as involved with life in all its aspects as they possibly can. Hopefully all of us have experienced the joy and wonder of planting a seed and watching it bloom and bring forth its gift to us: life. It is truly miraculous to behold the transformation of life that occurs when food is ingested and it becomes a part of our very being.

Like air, food is a miracle; it is also a union of nature's creation and human effort. When food is available in sufficient quantities, we tend to take it for granted, like the air we breathe. World leaders come and go, astronauts circle the earth in the space shuttle, but without the farmers and harvests, all else would be meaningless.

In the twentieth century, only one out of two people works in agriculture (the majority are women). In the past, the vast majority of people who ever lived were farmers. More than 20 centuries ago, a Chinese poet wrote:

"When the sun rises, I go to work, When the sun goes down, I take my rest, I dig the well from which I drink,

I farm the soil that yields my food,

I share creation, kings can do no more." And so, it is.

In the midst of an era of persistent hunger and poverty, this fertile earth could produce more than enough food to meet our needs today and for the foreseeable future. Yet many people cannot afford to buy food; others are denied their ability to produce it because they have no access to land, seeds and tools. Others face erratic weather conditions, poor soil, and a scarcity of water.

Two-thirds of our exported grain goes not to feed starving children, but to feed hungry animals raised for meat that is too expensive for hungry people to buy. Many areas of the world have the capacity to feed themselves but their cropland is being used to grow cash crops for export to the developed world.

99.1.1. Sharing the Harvest—Starvation and Malnutrition in the World

Population increases by exponential growth or multiplication; a system variable can continue through many doubling intervals without seeming to reach significant size. But in one or two more doubling periods, this size can be considerable. After 4,000 recorded years of human history (in the Bible), world population grew to an estimated 300 million people by 1 A.D. and reached a billion in the early 1800s. By 1930 (about 100 years later), the population had already doubled to 2 billion. Within another 30 years, another billion was added, reaching about 3 billion in 1960. Fifteen years later (1975), it was about 4 billion. From mid-1982 to mid-1983, world population rose by 82 million. In 1983 the estimated world population was between 4.6-4.7. billion (twice the global population of 20 years ago) and will probably reach 5 billion by 1986.

Today about 75% of the world's population live in the "underdeveloped" nations, 40% of these in extreme poverty. Political and economic pressures are rising in many nations. Countless refugees migrate, hoping to find salvation in a new country, just as our ancestors did when they came to this new world. Often those who themselves have next to nothing reach out to these refugees and offer shelter; others are not so pure in spirit and greet refugees with hostility, or even drive them away. Most Americans have, for the most part, been fortunate and have not really ever suffered from starvation, but as human beings we must ask ourselves how we would feel if the hand reaching out for help and a morsel of food were our own, and we were turned away.

Statistics indicate that a person born in the richer, industrialized countries will consume during a lifetime 20 to 40 times as much as a person born in Africa, Asia, or Latin America. Another statistic says that the average American consumes 2 1/2 times as many pounds of food over a lifetime as the average Asian, eating about 30 tons in a lifetime compared to an Asian's lifetime total of about 12 tons, which is mostly in rice. Westerners average almost 5 tons of meat, 1 1/2 tons of sugar (not including cakes, pastries, and ice cream) and 12,000 eggs. Asians consume about 1/4 the sugar and "only" about 500 pounds of meat, fish and eggs combined. (East/West Journal, November 1982.)

A study on meat consumption gave the following figures: New Zealanders consumed the most meat worldwide—about 229.1. pounds of meat per person in 1982. The United States was second with about 222.2. pounds per person. We have already discussed how vegetarianism can help in alleviating world hunger—again, cropland would be used directly to feed the people, not indirectly to feed animals to feed people. We have seen that people are frugivorous by nature, and so land used for animals as food is both wasteful and contrary to our biological heritage (to say nothing of cruel, as far as the use of animals for food is concerned).

In the middle of the earth's bounty, over a billion of us—that is 1 out of 4 members of the human family—go hungry. Fifteen to twenty millions of us die from hunger every year. That is 41,000 of us each day, 28 of us every minute, 21 of us children. In Africa alone, 4 million children may die this year and next from starvation and malnutrition. Humanity has never lived without hunger, its oldest and most lethal enemy. Ours is the first generation that has ever had the possibility of calling forth a world in which hunger may be ended. What is lacking is not technology, but the individual and global will to take necessary actions to preserve human lives and our precious environment. Meanwhile, while 1 of 4 of us go hungry, and 41,000 of us die daily from hunger, at least dogs with wealthy owners on the Cote d'Azur in France are getting by. A news item (May 14, 1984) reports that a gourmet restaurant for dogs featuring 3-course meals costing up to $15 and "served on real china" just opened recently. (I read of a similar restaurant in New York a few years back.) The restaurant offers a selection of cheeses from Holland and France, elaborate main courses, and a pastry cart. Some examples of the plat du jour are "a selection of beef filet with artichoke," or "fish mousse with skimmed milk and fresh green beans." The dogs are served by white-coated waiters "under the supervision of a veterinarian, a profession dog handler, and a dietitian." It used to be that dogs were thrown table scraps, but perhaps now a few starving people could apply for jobs as waiters there and hope for a few table scraps themselves! Fifteen dollars would buy dinner groceries for a whole family, if this family were "worthy" enough to receive the same generosity bestowed upon these dogs.

The World Conservation Strategy was published by the International Union for the Conservation of Nature and was the result of three years of research and discussion involving more than 450 government agencies and over 100 countries. It was "launched" on March 1980, in London and 32 other capital cities across the world. A summary of the strategy appears in the April 1980, Not Man Apart. However, it fails to recognize the naturally retrogressed and humanly overexploited state of the biosphere and of the present 8late-interglacial soil, and does not emphasize remineralizing soils, reforesting large areas or establishing biomass energy plantations, or restoring the earth's poverty-stricken ecosystems. It is more concerned with "conserving" than rebuilding but does say that most countries are too poorly organized even to conserve, that severe soil degradation is already a critical problem, that deserts could soon adversely affect 630 million people, that tropical forests were quickly becoming extinct—and that time was "running out." Because there is less and less to conserve in the first place, nowadays, it is now imperative that we rebuild our environment, while there is still some time left to do so. Conservation alone is not enough.

These times are characterized by a great awakening of the human force all over the planet, as more and more people become more and more conscious of the human potential for higher evolution. This is seen in the many popular movements, grassroots communities and local organizations that are flourishing everywhere. This world force is a new kind of leadership that can unify the expressions of groups and organize for action. Leadership from, and of, the group—and from the "least" among us—is the hope for change in our time!

The elimination of poverty is the ethical issue of our time, said John Sewell, President of the Overseas Development Council (Washington, D.C.), who says, "some 100 or more years ago, the idea that trade in human beings should be abolished was one that struck reasonable and rational observers as a political impossibility, yet that issue became the moral problem of that time, and eventually trade in humans was stopped. And I would guess that my children will wonder why we are not about our task faster in the last part of the twentieth century, when we have both the knowledge and the wherewithal to deal with global poverty."

R. Buckminster Fuller devoted his attention to the need for integrity in the world in the last months of his life before he died at 87. "Human integrity," he said, "is the uncompromising courage of self-determining whether or not to take initiative, support, or cooperate with others in accord with all the truth and nothing but the truth as it is conceived of by the divine mind always present in the individual."

As of 1983, 73 countries have "ended" hunger, at least as a basic, society-wide condition. This was true of no country on the planet in the year 1900. By 1940, it was true of only nine. It is clear that the individual—each one of us—is the key to realizing these, and future, achievements. When famine struck Biafra in the late 1960s, $6 million was raised in the U.S. for relief. It took more than a year. But in March 1980, $42 million was raised in only five months to aid Cambodia. On a global level, the growth in responsiveness to emergencies has been equally dramatic, and today, world response to emergencies is faster, more generous—and more effective, when it begins with the assumption that the purpose of aid does not end with temporary relief, but that its purpose is to find the resources for food-sufficiency within the situation. Recently, a Canadian nongovernmental organization called Inter Pares ("among equals") invited Third World farm leaders to live with their Canadian hosts; they had joint meetings and worked out solutions to mutual production problems. Successful education projects in every industrialized country show the same truth: We share one planet, and our opportunity is to succeed together or not at all.

Crop yields are usually assumed to be continually increasing, but former USDA researcher Lester Brown documented that chemically-induced yields were falling or leveling off in the U.S., China, France, and elsewhere (The Worldwide Loss of Cropland, 1978, Worldwatch Paper No. 24). Pollution by pesticides and fertilizers, and potential deterioration in climate or weather, are not taken into account when predicting higher crop yields. Brown says that major improvement in the food supply for the world's poorest populations isn't likely if things continue as they are, and what improvements do occur "will require an increase of 95% in the real price of food." (p. 415). Those who think that today's agricultural methods will increase crop yields in the future also think that food production will only increase fast enough to meet rising demands if world agriculture becomes "significantly more dependent on petroleum and petroleum-related inputs" (again, this would increase the real price of food over the 1970-2000 time period), but it is obvious for ecological reasons that it is now time for a world transition away from petroleum dependence, though it is uncertain how this will occur.

Meanwhile, farmer's costs of raising and maintaining yields have increased rapidly; yields will increase more slowly than projected. These yields also assume a (roughly) 180% increase in fertilizer use. These fertilizer projections are intended to apply to a full package of "yield-enhancing inputs," including pesticides, herbicides, irrigation, etc. Not enough emphasis is being placed on the fact that there are only 2 1/2 inches of the original glacial deposit left in the topsoil, and there is no more on the way up. (We'll talk more about this later.)

Because we have not fully recognized the natural operational principles of the earth's ecology and applied these principles in the key areas of our lives, we have brought ourselves to the point where we must now courageously face the totality of our problems.

99.2. The Quality of Our Food Is Determined by the Quality of Our Soil

99.2.1. Mother Earth: Our Soil and Giver of Life

99.2.2. Erosion

99.2.3. Farming in the United States Today

99.2.4. Poverty and Hunger at Home

99.2.5. Is Big Really Better?

99.2.6. The Fox is Guarding the Chicken Coop

99.2.7. Demineralization of Soils Worldwide Variations in Mineral Content in Vegetables

99.2.8. Chemical Fertilizers and Pesticides

99.2.1. Mother Earth: Our Soil and Giver of Life

99.2.1.1. Soil Structure

Good granulation or crumb structure of the heavier soils is essential for good results. Sandy soils show little if any granulation because their particles are coarse. With soils containing a substantial percentage of clay, working them when wet results in destruction of the granular structure. Tillage also tends to break down the structure of many soils. Alternate freezing and thawing, or wetting and drying, and penetration of the soil mass by plant roots are natural forces that favor the formation of soil granules, or aggregates. Such aggregation is developed most highly in soils near neutrality in their reaction; both strongly acid and strongly alkaline soils tend to run together and lose their structural character. (Organic Gardening, Rodale.)

99.2.1.2. Porosity

Pore spaces may be large, as with coarse, sandy soils or those with well-developed granulation. In heavy soils, with mostly finer clay particles, the pore spaces may be too small for plant roots or soil water to penetrate readily. Good soil has 40-60% of its bulk occupied with pore space that is filled with either water or air. Too much water slows the release of soil nitrogen, depletes mineral nutrients, and hinders proper plant growth. Top much air speeds nitrogen release beyond the capacity of plants to utilize it, and much is lost. (Organic Gardening, Rodale.)

99.2.1.3. Soil Groups

Sandy soils: Gravelly sands, coarse sands, medium sands, fine sands, loamy sands

Loamy soils: Coarse sandy loams, medium sandy loams, fine sandy loams, silty loams, stony silt loams, clay loams

Clayey soils: Stony clays, gravelly clays, sandy clays, silty clays, clays

Sand particles are gritty; silt has a floury or talcum-powder feel when dry and is only moderately "plastic" when moist, while the clayey material is harsh when dry and very plastic and sticky when wet.

As we said, the ideal structure is granular, where the rounded clusters of soil lie loosely and shake apart readily. (Organic Gardening, Rodale.)

99.2.2. Erosion

Soil erosion rivals oil dependency as a threat to the economic progress of the world, according to a report issued in February 1984, by the Worldwatch Institute. "Under pressure of ever-mounting demand for food, more and more of the world's farmers are mining their topsoil, d soil erosion has now reached epidemic proportions; its feet on food prices could ultimately be more destabilizing than rising oil prices." Half of the world's cropland is losing topsoil faster than nature can replenish it. In the Soviet Union, an estimated half-million hectares of cropland are abandoned yearly because they are so severely eroded by wind that they are no longer worth farming. (State of the World—1984, Worldwatch Institute's analysis of global trends.) The report paints a grim picture for other resources, including forests and water supplies.

The main loss of soil occurs by sheet erosion, that is, each time it rains, the runoff water removes a thin layer of surface soil. As the topsoil becomes thinner, miniature gullies appear. After most of the surface soil is gone, gullies become the main problems.

There is usually a clear difference between topsoil and subsoil. Subsoil is finer textured, more plastic, and lighter in color than topsoil. Erosion is classified as follows:

No apparent erosion. All or nearly all surface soil is present. Depth to subsoil is 14 inches or more. The surface may have received some recent deposits as the result of erosion from higher ground.

Slight. Depth to subsoil varies from 7 to 14 inches. Plowing at usual depths will not expose the subsoil.

Moderate. Depth to subsoil varies from 3 to 7 inches. Some subsoil is mixed with the surface soil in plowing. Severe. Depth to subsoil is less than 3 inches. Surface soil is mixed with subsoil when the land is plowed. Gullies are beginning to be a problem.

Very Severe. Subsoil is exposed. Gullies are frequent.

Very severe gullies. Deep gullies or blowouts have ruined the soil for agricultural purposes. (Rodale Press.)

There is a direct relationship between erosion and a soil's ability for intake of air and water. When the soil surface becomes compacted, the danger of erosion increases, while the intake of water and air decreases.

Agriculture Department programs have been under heavy criticism because of severe erosion problems nationwide. One recent federal report said erosion was increased by the payment-in-kind program (which paid farmers who had surplus grain for not growing more) because many participants who were required to plow up fields to qualify for the program did little to protect the soil. In addition, congressional critics have charged that farmers were putting more of their fragile farmland into production to boost their acreage in government programs.

Overoxidation of humus by tillage exposure also increases CO_2 in our atmosphere. Tillage exposure permits the oxidation that releases carbon to the air and, simultaneously, decreases the carbon storage the humus provides in the soil mantle. Forests conduct more photosynthesis worldwide than any other form of vegetation. Photo-synthesizing plants are our source of oxygen. When we harvest forests, extend agriculture onto soils high in organic matter, and destroy wetlands, we speed the decay of our precious humus heritage (Lesson 50).

Some soil scientists say that under the best conditions nature can build topsoil at a rate not faster than 1.5. tons per acre each year, and under some conditions, the rate is only .5. tons per acre per year. About 2/3 of U.S. cropland is experiencing a net loss of topsoil. From water-caused erosion (and wind erosion, such as on the Great Plains) we are losing topsoil, on the average, five times faster than nature can build it, even under the best conditions.

Soil conservationist Neil Samson explains the problem in his 1981 book Farmland or Wasteland. He says to think in terms of the acre-equivalents of farmland productivity we lose each year through erosion. Losing a thousand tons of topsoil on one acre— equivalent to six inches of soil— would destroy the productivity of most cropland. He says that well over one million acre-equivalents of farmland productivity are lost yearly. Over 50 years, this could amount to 62,000,000 acre-equivalents.

The government estimates that 43% of land planted in row crops in the Corn Belt is highly susceptible to erosion; plowing up fragile soils that should have remained pasture and will only produce a few harvests is like the "slash-and-burn" technique of jungle agriculture.

Most conventional farms in the Corn Belt grow corn and soybeans year after year, without the rotation with small grains and legume hay so important to the organic farmer. In addition to nutrient building, these crops help to reduce erosion by covering the ground with a living mulch and binding the soil with their roots, thus protecting the fields from the destructive forces of rain and wind that are destroying American cropland faster than at any time during our history.

Corn and soybeans have brought the best price in the export markets, but these two crops are linked to the highest rates of soil erosion. Planted in rows, they leave part of the soil exposed, unlike grasses or clover which cover the ground entirely. Soybeans have shallow roots that also leave soil more susceptible to erosion. Crops of small grains (oats, barley) and hay (alfalfa) have less cash value, but these crops are grown close together—this reduces surface water runoff and erosion. Because many farmers plant the same crops each year instead of rotating them or letting the earth lie fallow, the soil further loses its ability to rebuild itself. Chinese farmers have tilled the same land for at least 40 centuries. In America, farmers may wish to conserve the land they farm, but the economic forces at work do not "reward" soil conservation in the short term, so many farmers do not invest in soil conservation.

99.2.3. Farming in the United States Today

The United States currently exports one-third of its annual agricultural harvest, growing enough to feed about 240 million Americans, plus 120 million people abroad.

In 1980, the Rodale Press initiated the Cornucopia Project to document where the

U.S. food system is vulnerable and to suggest how it could be transformed into one that maintains high productivity and also conserves its resources. The book Empty Breadbasket? is a report on the results of that study. Here are some of its findings:

- The size of the average U.S. farm has tripled since 1920.

- In 1978, 1% of farm owners controlled 30% of the land.

- The average molecule of processed food travels 1,300 miles before being eaten. (One of the first things I remember hearing in my transition to natural foods was that it is considered better to eat foods that are grown within several hundred miles of where one lives, the logic being that foods native to the area, those surviving in the climate where one lives, contain the nutrients best suited to maintain health in the climate of the particular area. Of course any food that is fresh is certainly always superior to any processed—or sprayed, or otherwise altered—food, and contains more vitamins and nutrients, but all other factors being equal, you might want the bulk of your diet to consist of fresh foods local to your area, if you are able to obtain fresh, organic produce that is grown close to home, with nonnative foods used to supplement your diet.)

- Every year, enough topsoil is eroded to cover to a depth of one foot Maine, New Hampshire, Vermont, Connecticut and Massachusetts.

- About 15% of American cropland is irrigated—and on that land is raised 25% of the total value of U.S. crops. An estimated 25% of the groundwater used is being removed faster than it is replaced.

- America's farmers use an average of two pounds of pesticide and 120 pounds of synthetic fertilizer per acre of cropland per year. These chemicals lead to contamination of soil and water, destruction of wildlife populations and health problems for soil workers.

- It takes 10 times more energy to produce a calorie of food today than it did in 1910.

- In short, the study concludes that the U.S. agricultural system is productive but not sustainable, either economically or ecologically.

Much farmland is lost to urban growth, as cities spread; as the cash value of their land increases, some farmers sell to developers.

When the prairie grasslands were turned and plowed, a long line of ecosystems (that stretched back 30 million years) was broken. It had been a wilderness that supported migrating water birds, animals, and the native Americans. In the short run, the European crops grown by the "new" Americans would out-yield the old prairie, but they were not looking ahead. We have discussed over and over the intricate workings of the body, and how interference with nature's ways eventually distorts these workings. Imposing manmade chemicals on our systems, and altering our natural bodily rhythms by improper lifestyles, disturbs our balance. The new farmers forgot one important fact: the prairie is a polyculture. Crops are usually grown in monocultures. Whereas the prairie has many perennial plants, agriculture relies heavily on annuals, but species diversity is the key. There are millions of microscopic life forms, and nature prefers polyculture, not annual monoculture. We are also gambling foolishly with our chemical fertilizers, for if we could see on a microscopic level, we would see that life is much more intricate than a few calculations and "fertilizer" additions. Mechanical disturbances of the prairies, and chemicals, may make "weed control" effective, but the farm will be weakened in the long run as, soil compacts (increasing erosion), crumb structure declines, soil porosity decreases, and the loss of a "wick effect" (of pulling moisture down) lessens. Monoculture decreases the range of invertebrate and microbial forms. Even crop rotation doesn't give enough diversity when compared to the greater diversity that was in the prairies originally, and monoculture results in the loss of botanical (and thus chemical) diversity above ground. Plants are weaker and invite insect pests or disease. (Insects are also better controlled if they have to spend some energy looking for the plants they evolved to eat among many species of polyculture.)

Organic farming methods attempt to take more of nature's plans into consideration, and work with nature, not against it. There are an estimated 30 to 50 thousand organic farms in the U.S. When Chinese farmers were forced to move south and east because of deforestation and destructive agricultural practices, they had to relearn how to farm. For

40 centuries Chinese peasants have been developing a culture that survives because it return everything to the land.

99.2.4. Poverty and Hunger at Home

A report in January 1984, showed that demand for emergency food or shelter increased in the United States last year in 95% of the cities surveyed, despite an improving employment picture in 70% of the cities. Even in America, there are thousands of homeless people who sleep in streets, alleys and abandoned cars. Chicago estimates that there are 25,000 people in their city alone who "don't even have a ragged hut or camping tent to call their home—an indictment of us as a people," says the mayor.

President Reagan's task force on food assistance announced in January that it could find no evidence of "rampant hunger" and saw no need for new assistance programs. But the Citizens Commission on Hunger in New England said its Harvard-based members and staff conducted five months of field investigation and reviewed every public and private study of hunger in the United States done since 1980 to support their statements about the national dimensions of the problem. Their report calls on Congress to increase funding for federal programs that affect hunger, saying that all the evidence gathered showed an increase in poverty and hunger over the past five years, and that hunger in America is no longer confined to the traditional poor or to ethnic minorities—they have been joined by other Americans who were not poor and not hungry several years ago. The hardest hit are poor infants and young children, the elderly, (especially those on fixed incomes) and families with an unemployed breadwinner.

99.2.5. Is Big Really Better?

Now that so much of our nation's farming is done on a larger scale than ever, with more complex machinery, can we expect a better food product at the end of the line? Sad to say, we pay in more ways than one for "progress," and we pay the most dearly when the end result of food processing is a drastic decline in nutritional quality. Even the best our supermarkets have to offer—fresh produce—is less tasty and healthful than organically-grown, sun-ripened produce. Anyone who has ever eaten both a commercially-grown strawberry and a sweet, juicy homegrown one, sun-ripe, can tell you about the difference in taste. Anyone who has eaten a vine-ripened tomato will cringe at the watery tastelessness of green-pulled tomatoes so common in supermarkets—there is simply no comparison. This is aside from the obvious advantage that organic produce is free from pesticide residues.

As to processed foods, we've discussed all their negative aspects in detail in earlier lessons and are by now quite familiar with them.

A 1983 newspaper article on food additives reads like this:

"Let's say that you ate bacon and eggs for breakfast, with a muffin and jam on the side." (Let's hope you didn't, but to continue ...)

"For lunch, you downed a hamburger with ketchup, some pork and beans and a cola. And for dinner you munched on tossed salad with Caesar dressing, gnawed on barbecued ribs and french fries and slurped ice cream with butterscotch syrup for dessert."

"That feast would have filled your belly with about 150 food additives, many with frighteningly unpronounceable names—jawbreakers unknown before scientists started fiddling with food in the post-World War II era."

Still, the chemical companies try to save face by constant efforts to convince the public that only "safe" additives are used in food. Recently I saw a pamphlet put out by Safeway Food stores entitled "Additives: Why Are They In My Food?" and I couldn't resist the temptation to hear what sales-pitch they'd come up with! Let's take a look:

- First of all, "additives make it possible for the shopper in the family to do the shopping only once or twice a week." (I manage to do this while just eating fresh foods, but we'll go on ...)

- "Additives keep our food, supply fresh and consistent." (Unspoiled, perhaps, but fresh?)

- "No longer is it necessary to slave over a hot stove, all day, every day." (No problem there for us raw fooders.)

- However, the statement that really caught my attention, lightly stated, and casually tossed in there with all the others, leaving me with a somewhat eerie feeling, was: "And, if we all wanted fresh, there just wouldn't be enough to go around."

Is that the good news or the bad news?

99.2.6. The Fox is Guarding the Chicken Coop

The pamphlet goes on to tell us, among other things, that "in 1971 the Food and Drug Administration (FDA) began to review all 'Generally Recognized as Safe' (GRAS) additives. Most of the substances which have passed through this screening process have been reaffirmed as safe and remain on the list." (Those that aren't were undoubtedly consumed by countless unfortunate individuals until this point.) "Substances not listed as GRAS and substances new since the 1958 Food Additives Amendment must be safety tested under the manufacturer's auspices and approved by the FDA. Manufacturers submit the results of all of their tests to the FDA. If they indicate the additive is safe, the FDA establishes regulations for its use in food." Are we really to believe that the manufacturers of these chemicals can be trusted to keep our best interests in mind if they are "safety-testing" their own additives? We can be sure that the safest foods are foods with no additives at all: fresh, raw foods, as nature delivers them to us.

A final note on ethics, or lack of ethics, as the case may be (excerpted from Acres U.S.A., May 1984):

It was discovered that "the International Biotest Laboratories in the United States had falsified results of some long-term pesticide tests so that some pesticides may have appeared to be less hazardous than they really are (though the company shredded records after the scandal broke). The scale was large: in about 10 years IBT did more than 20,000 tests for some 200 companies and was responsible for about 1/3 of all pesticide toxicity and cancer testing done by government and industry."

Please review "The Case Against Commercially-Grown Foods," of Lesson 49.

99.2.7. Demineralization of Soils Worldwide

In Lesson 49, nutrient contents of organically-grown foods are compared with those of chemically-grown foods, and it was found that the foods grown by organic methods had higher contents of nutrients, as well as better flavor.

In the summer of 1977, a corn crop was grown on soil that was mineralized with glacial gravel crusher screenings and tested with corn from the same seed grown with chemical fertilizers. The gravel-mineralized corn had 57% more phosphorus, 90% more potassium, 47% more calcium, and 60% more magnesium than the chemical-grown corn. The mineral-grown corn had close to 9% protein, which is good for a hybrid corn, and all the nitrogen in the mineral-grown corn (whose content in the food is the indicator for protein) came from the atmosphere by biological processes and was in the amino acids of the corn protoplasm. None of it was raw chemical nitrate, the precursor of the carcinogenic nitrosamines. No pesticides were used and there was no insect damage.

Microorganisms can reproduce abundantly only when all minerals are present, along with plant residue to supply carbon needs for energy and protoplasm compound building, plus nitrogen, oxygen and sea solids from the air, and (of course) water.

The chemical-grown corn of 1977 had substantially less mineral content than corn listed in the 1963 USD A Composition of Foods Handbook of nutritional contents of foods, but the mineral-grown corn of 1977 was substantially higher in mineral content than the 1963 Handbook's corn. Most people are now consuming food with less mineral content, and then further destroying what nutrients are left by processing, cooking and otherwise altering food. Then, with improper eating habits, overeating, bad food combinations, and so on, they reduce the value of their food even further.

Firman Bear of Rutgers University did a study on trace element contents of vegetables, published in the 1948 Soil Science Society of America Proceedings. His study shows the significant fact that foods that may look the same actually have huge variations in mineral content, and thus their health-promoting value. A chart summarizing his findings was reproduced in Acres U.S.A. (1977), as follows:

In a 1977 paper, John Hamaker compared Bear's data with the USDA's 1975 reprint of the 1963 Composition of Foods Handbook. He says that the Handbook only gives data for a single trace element (iron) and says: "but it is a very significant element. A comparison on a part-per-million basis with Bear's highest and lowest, followed by the Handbook average, is as follows: snap beans 227, 10 and 8; cabbage 94, 20 and 4; lettuce 516, 9 and 14; tomatoes 1938, 1 and 5. In the Bear study, if one trace element is low in all vegetables, then all the other trace minerals are low. Therefore, the average of these vegetables in 1963 were no better supplied with trace minerals than the lowest in 1948. It has been 14 years (now, in 1984, 21 years) since the 1963 studies. The USDA ought to have upgraded its information and included much more trace element information. Instead, they copied the old 1963 Handbook tables and put them out in a fancy new cover in 1975. An honest set of figures on trace elements would show a lot of zeroes on a part-per-million basis and would damn chemical agriculture for the monstrous fraud it is. All of our food should be as good or better than the best found by Firman Bear. Such standards can be and must be obtained very quickly if we are to survive."

A September, 1980 letter from the USDA said, in part, "Revised sections of Agriculture Handbook No. 8 covering cereal grains and grain products, fruits, vegetables, legumes, nuts and seeds are all underway, with publication dates scheduled for 1981-1982." It would be interesting to see what these revisions reveal, and if they are, indeed, honest.

The United Nations Food and Agriculture Organization (FAO) Soils Bulletin No. 17 is entitled Trace Elements in Soils and Agriculture, dated 1979. It gives data similar to Bear's in showing the wide variations in extent of soil mineral depletion. It notes the biologically essential nature vitamin "therapies." We have discussed the futility of using "supplements" in earlier lessons.

Variations in Mineral Content in Vegetables

	Percentage of dry weight	Milliequivalents per 100 grams dry weight					Trace Elements	
	Total Ash or Mineral Matter	Phosphorus	Calcium	Magnesium	Potassium	Sodium	Boron	Manganese
	SNAP BEANS							
Highest	10.45	0.36	40.5	60.0	99.7	29.1	73	60
Lowest	4.04	0.22	15.5	14.8	8.6	0.0	10	2
	CABBAGE							
Highest	10.38	0.38	60.0	43.6	148.3	53.7	42	13
Lowest	6.12	0.18	17.5	15.6	20.4	0.8	7	2
	LETTUCE							
Highest	24.48	0.43	71.0	49.3	176.5	53.7	37	169
Lowest	7.01	0.22	6.0	13.1	12.2	0.0	6	1

	TOMATOES							
Highest	14.20	0.35	23.0	59.2	148.3	58.8	36	68
Lowest	6.07	0.16	4.5	4.5	6.5	0.0	5	1

Voison looks at the relation of cancer to soil depletion and imbalance in Soil, Grass, and Cancer: Health of Animals and Man Is Linked to the Mineral Balance of the soil (1959). According to Voison, "the dust of our cells is the dust of the soil," and "animals and men are the biochemical photograph of the soil."

1. Trace Elements in Plant Physiology (Wallace, 1950) says that the relation between cancer and the soil may be readily understood by a look at the four types of cell processes known to be subject to the balance of trace elements: synthesis and breakdown of tissue structures. energetic processes ("oxido-reductions"). regulation of nervous stimuli. detoxification of cellular poisons.

These processes refer to the actions of about 5,000 soil-dependent enzyme systems, all of which can be disrupted or prevented by element deficiency, imbalance, or drugs, pesticides, radiation, etc. (Knight, 1975.)

Billions of dollars a year are spent on efforts to "find 'cures' for cancer," but very little, if anything, is spent on efforts to remineralize the soil and save it from chemical abuse! With the same money used yearly for cancer "research" about 15 million doctors could obtain a round-trip ticket to the Hunza region, to observe the peoples' good naturedness and superior health. How many doctors really want to learn why the ten-bed hospital for about 40,000 Hunzacuts is practically empty all the time? How many "researchers" would be out of a job if people learned how to prevent sickness and had no for "cures"?

Schauss, an experienced criminologist, counselor, and director of the Institute for Biosocial Research says:

"Eskimos and Native Americans living in very remote territories on indigenous food supplies in the Stewart Islands of Alaska, who had been physically and psychologically healthy for centuries, experience the degenerative diseases and moral decay so prevalent in western culture when the foods (not specified) from that culture are allowed in. Crimes are subsequently committed for which these 'primitive' cultures didn't even have words in their language to describe; the words had to be invented."

As we said, virtually all of the subsoil and most of the topsoil of the world have been stripped of all but a small quantity of elements. In the Hunza region of the Himalayas many people live to a fine old age and stay healthy and vigorous. The valley's soils are

641

irrigated with a milky-colored stream from the meltwater of the Ultar glacier. The color comes from the mixed rock ground beneath the glacier. Ten thousand years ago the

Mississippi Valley was fed and built up by runoff from the glaciers. Illinois had a deep deposit of organically-enriched alluvial soil that resulted in a long period of luxuriant plant growth, but when the settlers plowed the valley, they didn't find topsoil that would give the health record of the hunzakuts. Ten thousand years of leaching by a 30-inch mal rainfall is the difference. There are several other places in the world similar to Hunza, such as the Caucasus Mountains in Russia, where 10% of the people are centenarians. There are glaciers in the mountains. Wherever people attain excellent health and maximum life, there is a continual supply of fresh-ground mixed rocks flowing to the soil where their crops are grown.

Robert McCarrison (Director of Nutrition Research in India years ago) did extensive studies on nutrition, health, and deficiency-diseases. After observing the magnificent bodies of the people of the Hunza Valley, their sound teeth, strength, longevity, intelligence and happy dispositions—human health almost to perfection—he gave Albino rats the diet of the Hunzas. Then he gave other colonies of rats the diets of disease-ridden cultures on the Indian Sub-Continent. He found that the rats would duplicate the health of the people eating the diets: perfect health and contentment on the Hunzas' food, and the disease of the Madrasi on the Madrasi food.

Working seven years among the Hunzas and Sikhs, both good gardeners and farmers, he never found a case of stomach ulcer, appendicitis or cancer. It was his finding (already in 1936) that: "it seems clear that the habitual use of a diet made up of natural foodstuffs, in proper proportion one to another, and produced on soils that are not impoverished, is an essential condition for the efficient exercise of function of nutrition on which the maintenance of health depends," and combined with healthy bodily activity, "is mankind's main defense against degenerative diseases; a bulwark, too, against those of 'infectious' origin."

In 1948, J. I. Rodale, the well-known organic agriculturist, published The Healthy Hunzas, which revealed how the world's healthiest people annually add to their soils the mixture of stones finely ground by the local Ultar glacier, together with the abundant organic matter produced by these highly-mineralized soils. (Little animal manure is added as the Hunzas keep few animals.) Rodale stressed the great value of adding the wide variety of rock to soils in a "ground-up, flour-like form" by using the most efficient modern machinery (p. 100). He also pointed out the danger of adding imbalancing single rock types, and concluded his chapter, "Rock Powders," by giving major credit for the Hunzas' outstanding health, longevity, and intelligence to the glacial rock powder, their provision for perpetual soil fertility, and high-quality foods. Rodale was emphatic that we in the United States begin to utilize the billions of tons of rocks of all kinds, and apply them—equivalent of the Hunza sediments—to our lands, in a powdered form.

Sir Albert Howard, (often called "the father of organic agriculture") also described the Hunzas in his 1947 book The Soil and Health, and he too observed the Hunza Valley's glacial silt fertilizer, and the powerful evidence suggesting that "to obtain the very best results we must replace simultaneously the organic and mineral portions of the soil."(p. 177)

In the next lesson when we continue to tie in the links between soil demineralization and climate changes, we'll be talking about the Ice Age. Scientists have offered various theories on what causes the ice ages to recur every 100,000 years, and many of them used to think that they were caused by changes in the earth's orbit around the sun (Milankovich's theory). Recent computer modeling (by a man who has been the foremost modern exponent of this theory, John Imbrie at Brown University) has finally cast serious doubt on the validity of Milankovich's hypothesis, because Imbrie says that the most sophisticated recent of the minerals for health of soil-building microorganisms, plants, and humans, and says that widespread deficiencies now exist. Soil zinc deficiency is documented for 12 European countries, as is boron for nearly every European country. It also makes note of the danger of trying to correct soil deficiencies by adding purified single elements, due to their toxicity (for example, boron has been used as a weedkiller).

Nowhere is soil remineralization considered in the bulletin, but it does say that generally from two to six times more of the main nutrients are taken annually from the soil than are added by mineral fertilizers. Crop and manure residues return some of them, but a negative balance of these nutrients likely remains.

As for trace elements, on page 1, the FAO soils bulletin says that deficiencies in these elements were first reported in the late 1800s, and that extensive areas of the earth's soils are no longer able to supply adequate amounts to plant life.

• Furthermore, several factors are causing an accelerating exhaustion of the available soil supply: weathering and leaching stimulation of increased yields by one-sided NPK fertilizing decreasing use of natural fertilizer materials compared with chemicals increasing purity of these chemicals used to stimulate growth

The bulletin doesn't provide any solutions, but it does state the problems that need solutions, saying "trace elements are not regularly applied to the soil by the use of the common fertilizers. Their removal from the soil has been going on for centuries without any systematic replacement." (p. 1).

In Mount's The Food and Health of Western Man (1975) he said that 66% of American college women had low-to-absent iron stores. The 2nd World Symposium on Magnesium held in Montreal in 1976 said there was "a grave danger of magnesium deficiency in foods consumed in the developed countries." The Ecologist (12/79, p. 317) said that "cancer, arteriosclerosis, and heart and bone diseases are implicated as resulting from such deficiencies." A 1979 South African study showed 89% of the cancerous regions had poor soils, whereas 66% of cancer-free regions were on comparatively rich soils. (Life Scientists know that there are other factors involved as well, such as improper lifestyle and eating habits, exposure to environmental toxins, and so on, but these studies also point to factors as basic as the soil itself as contributing to dwindling health.) Trace Elements in Soil-Plant-Animal Systems (Nicholas, 1975), shows continuing findings by researchers of "new" essential elements for human health, and shows that deficiencies can be expected to result in breakdown of the physiological functions where the element is involved. They say that there are now 14 known trace elements essential for animal life, and most or all of them are essential for soil microorganisms as well. In order of their discovery as essential, they are: iron, iodine, copper, manganese, zinc, cobalt, molybdenum, selenium, chromium, tin, fluorine, silicon, nickel and vanadium; also boron for "higher plants."

Weston Price wrote a book entitled Nutrition and Physical Degeneration (1945, 1975) that gave his findings from many years of studying people of cultures and lands worldwide. He proved how rapidly individuals and entire peoples degenerate physically, mentally and morally when their diet changes from natural whole foods from fertile soils to the refined and nutrient-poor foods of modern societies. Price was a dentist by training, and found, among other things, that people suffering from tooth decay were ingesting deficient amounts of vitamins and less than half the minimum requirements' of calcium, phosphorus, magnesium, iron and other elements. He also said severe malnutrition was a primary cause of juvenile delinquency and violent criminal tendencies.

In his chapter "Soil Depletion and Animal Deterioration," he says:

"In my studies on the relation of the physiognomy of the people of various districts to the soil, I have found a difference in the facial type of the last generation of young adults when compared with that of their parents. The new generation has inherited depleted soil ... The most serious problem confronting the coming generations is this nearly insurmountable handicap of depletion of the quality of the foods because of the depletion of the minerals of the soil." (p. 392)

We might note that this serious problem was being talked about almost 40 years ago. Metabolic Aspects of Health: Nutritional Elements in Health and Disease by John Myers, M.D. and Karl Schutte, Ph.D. (1979) also stressed the widespread incidence of soil mineral deficiency; the innumerable forms of diseases brought on by these deficiencies, including psychobiological imbalances; that dozens of known human enzyme systems are absolutely proven to be keyed to soil elements, including zinc, boron, cobalt, manganese, barium, nickel, copper, magnesium and more; and the great need for the natural balance of these elements via the food supply. Schutte, the botanist, shows that the same principles apply for health disease/insect-resistant plant growth.

The exact relations between the many soil elements and cancer, atherosclerosis and hypertension haven't been defined, but Myers and Schutte say that it is now clear that they can also be associated with imbalances in the trace elements supply, which keys the normal enzymatic activity of the cell. (p. 193)

The Hunzakuts are virtually free of cancer, but in the U.S., one out of every four people will develop cancer in their lifetimes (Eckholm and Record, 1976). Gus Speth, Chairman of the Council on Environmental Quality, announced in 1980 that the incidence of cancer rate jumped by 10% from 1970 to 1976, whereas from 1960 to 1970 it "only" increased 3%. Science News (vol. 110, p. 310) says: "Diet can have a dramatic influence on the prevention and treatment of cancer." (How long have you and I been saying this?) He goes on to say that "spontaneous regression of cancer, for instance, appears to have resulted from a change in the balance of trace elements."

Remember, there is a difference between getting these trace elements naturally in foods and trying to manipulate the body through all manner of haphazard, random version of the Milankovich theory (Imbrie's) is capable of explaining only the smaller, climatic changes associated with minor fluctuations in glaciation, and these, only for the past 150,000 years or so—beyond about 350,000 years it seems to have little value in predicting any of the climatic changes we now know about. So with astronomical causes more or less ruled out, the great ice age cycle must be caused by something here on earth. This is where John Hamaker comes in.

John Hamaker was trained in mechanical engineering at Purdue. He became interested in climatology only after thinking about the environment for many years, watching it deteriorate from neglect and abuse. He got first-hand information on the danger of toxic chemicals while working as an engineer for Monsanto in 1940 (we'll mention Monsanto again later, so we can make a mental note of the name), long before the rest of us got the bad news from Silent Spring. After serving in the army for five years during WWII and coming out a captain in the reserve, he went to work designing oil refinery machinery in Texas. But he began to feel sicker and sicker, and realized that he had to get out of that toxic environment.

He bought a farm in east Texas, and "learned about really worn-out soil—and the mess that chemicals make on farmland." He noted that his cows kept as far away from agricultural chemicals as they could, and wondered if they were smarter than people. Later he moved to Michigan, where he is now retired. For many years he has been doing experimental work on a ten-acre farm outside of Lansing.

During the late 1960s, while thinking about big questions like the health of the soil and man's relationship the earth, he began to read every book and scientific tide he could get his hands on about climate and soil and the health of plant life, and he believed he then understood what causes the ice ages to come and go with such predictability.

Why, he had wondered, are the winters getting colder, the summers hotter and drier, the storms and tornados increasingly frequent with every decade? What forces on earth are large enough to cause such global changes?

When he looked at these steeply rising curves, another curve came to mind: the exponentially rising curve of carbon dioxide (CO_2) in the earth's atmosphere. This CO_2 is well-known (we'll talk more about this too in the next lesson), and many scientists link it to the greenhouse effect that traps warmth radiated off the earth from the sun and increases the temperature all over the globe, but there is no consensus as to when this global greenhouse effect could be large enough to cause such changes. In spite of the very large increase of CO2 that has already occurred, the earth seems to be in a cooling phase in recent decades (more details next lesson).

Apparently Hamaker saw what no one else did: that the greenhouse effect is occurring differentially—primarily in the warmer latitudes, which get the most sunlight (the poles don't get any sunlight for six months out of the year, and very oblique rays the rest of the time), and that the pics have already been heating and drying up for the last few decades, that consequently the northern latitudes have been getting colder and wetter, and that the increasing temperature differential between the two has taken on a life of its own and is accelerating the whole process.

John Hamaker tells us:

"I have observed the things of the world for almost 66 years. The luck of the genes equipped me to observe and learn. I had the highest mechanical aptitude test score in a class of 110 students majoring in Industrial Engineering at Purdue University (class of 1939). In a Motor Maintenance Battalion of 650 men and officers in WWII, I had the highest army test score. So, I became a "90-day wonder" and was discharged with a superior officer rating. In every engineering office where I have worked, the jobs requiring the most synthesis generally wound up on my drawing table. On the four occasions when I could not work because of chemical contamination, I have either worked on the problems that affect humanity or I have spent time on inventions. I have found that the solutions to the problems of the economy and the environment can be found by the same rigid attention to facts and established principles which yield solutions to problems of machine design.

In my 66 years I have seen more history made than any generation has seen before. Now it appears that I will see one more thing—the end of civilization as we know it during this interglacial period. For 10 years I have known that the soils of the world were running out of minerals and that glaciation was inevitable. For 10 years warnings and the solution have been ignored by people in government.

I don't think I care to see the tragedy which is scheduled to unfold in this decade."

In The Survival of Civilization, John Hamaker tells us that "failure to remineralize the soil will not just cause a continued mental and physical degeneration of humanity but will quickly bring famine, death and glaciation in that order."

Glaciation is one way of remineralizing the soil. Large amounts of plant life's carbon moves (as carbon dioxide) into the atmosphere, as the plant life dies out. We then see what is now happening: the carbon dioxide's greenhouse heating effect is causing large amounts of evaporation from the tropical oceans. Hamaker describes the resulting process as follows: Cold polar air moving over the cold land areas displaces this lighter, warm, wet air from the tropics, forcing the warm air to flow over the warm oceans toward the northern latitudes to replace the cold air, be cooled, lose its moisture to snow and descend over the land mass. The massive cloud cover will result in "huge amounts of cold air being generated, from which ever-increasing amounts of precipitation occur. Every winter must be worse than the last. At some point winters may carry over into summers and destroy crops with frosts and freezes. Numerous temperatures from 32 to 40°F were recorded in the summer of 1978 from Michigan to the Rockies. Cold waves can cause major crop losses in Canadian or Eurasian grain crops, which are mostly at the latitude of Michigan or farther north."

Chemical agriculture uses soluble chemicals that are either acidic or basic, but which have the final effect of acidifying the soil, destroying the soil life, using up the organic matter and, in the end, leaving the soil useless. Because choice soils have been almost fully demineralized in the 10,000-11,000 years since the last glaciation, the popularity of chemical agriculture has grown. However, chemicals, unlike microorganisms, will dissolve the carbonates and a few other rocks completely, liberating some of the remaining useful elements, so that enough microorganisms grow to support a crop growth, but the crop gets a short supply of an unbalanced protoplasm. The crop is then more prone to disease. Bits of useless demineralized skin (cell membrane) weathered from the stone are ignored by the microorganisms as they build the granular, capillary soil system that provides aeration and water retention to the soil. Percolating water carries the bits of subsoil down into cracks under large particles of unused stone. The cracks are caused by drying of the soil. The percolating water washes used material off the top of the unused stone, leaving a space into which the stone can rise when wetting of the soil forces the unused stone upward by the amount of material sifted under it. So, in 10,000 years, 8-10 feet of glacial deposit has been cycled to the topsoil, demineralized by the soil life, and has descended back into the subsoil to form a dense clay. As we said before, there are only 2 1/2 inches of the original deposit left in the topsoil, and there is no more on the way up.

We must provide minerals to the soil or glaciation will happen again!

99.2.8. Chemical Fertilizers and Pesticides

In The Survival of Civilization, John Hamaker has the following things to say about chemical fertilizers:

Plant and animal digestive systems will readily pass water into the plant or animal. If toxic compounds are in solution in the water, they too pass readily into the plant or animal. Water-soluble chemicals used in the soil (and in foods and beverages) are dangerous. Any toxic substance can enter a plant or animal with the protoplasm if it has been taken in by the microorganisms. So, anything other than the natural balance of elements and the natural organic compounds produced from them by the microorganisms is damaging to the entire chain of life. The continued buildup in the biosphere of nonbiodegradable synthetic organic compounds is destroying humanity by alteration of the genetic compounds.

As we said before, chemical farming depletes the organic matter in soil. Chemical fertilizer may release enough elements to grow sufficient microorganisms to feed a weak crop, but when the chemicals are used up (on weak soil this often happens before the crop matures if chemicals are inadequate or too fast in dissolving), the production of microorganisms virtually stops. Then too, the stalk is often taken with the grain (or vegetable, etc.), limiting the utilization of the few available minerals in the decreasing supply of passivated stone particles still in the soil. A look at mineralized organic gardens shows that organic farming methods are, by far, more beneficial.

"Farmers who returned corn crop stalks to the soil have the highest yields, maintaining a better reservoir of carbon and nitrogen in the soil to supply the crop. Unfortunately, the acid in NPK is constantly dissolving organic matter and inorganic material from the soil. With an estimated 30 to 50 percent of the acidic component of NPK winding up in the rivers, it is obvious that a lot of the fertility elements are going the same way."

"In the 50s and 60s, the agricultural 'experts' were helping the fertilizer industry by recommending to the farmer that dumping the barnyard waste into a pond was more 'economical' than spreading it back on the land, because the same amount of fertility elements could be 'obtained more economically from NPK fertilizer.' They learned the hard way that crops won't grow without organic matter, so now they say the organic matter is required to 'buffer' the soil. Technically, a buffering agent is one that tends to neutralize an acid or a base. Crop residue won't do that, but if it is put into the soil and there are any minerals at all present, microorganisms will multiply. Obviously, the basic elements in the protoplasm are the most available elements in the soil for buffering the acidity in NPK. If the rains are gentle, the dissolved protoplasm may be reconstituted into new organisms before it is leached or eroded into the river. And that can take place only if there are enough basic elements in the soil so the microorganisms can find what it takes to bring order out of chaos. The natural mixture of elements is geared to natural conditions—not to the absurd practice of deliberately acidifying the soil. Basic elements would have to be added to the natural mix to compensate for the manmade acid."

"Nitrogen is the most acidic component. If I can get 60 bushels per acre of wheat without nitrogen fertilizer, why should farmers buy it from the chemical companies?

"Phosphorus should be left where found because those deposits contain large amounts of fluorides. The agricultural soils are now badly contaminated with fluorides. Fluoride levels in food are increasing. Cattle concentrate the fluorine in their bones. When the bone meal is used in pet foods, fluorosis results. Do we wait until the overt symptoms of fluorosis show up in half the population before we stop this nonsense?"

"There is plenty of phosphorus and potassium in the natural rock mixture* and at a much lower price. If a farmer uses 200 pounds of a 15-15-15 NPK fertilizer, he gets about 100 pounds of gravel dust* per acre. (*Rock mixture and gravel dust will be discussed again in the next lesson. River gravel screenings—to add to the soil to remineralize it—can be purchased for under $6 a ton!) The gravel dust in the NPK fertilizer costs about 75 cents, but the fertilizer is priced at $25 to $30. (Editor's note: these were prices at the time the book was written, several years ago). What the farmer pays for is five paper sacks and me chemicals, neither of which he needs, and sooner or later the chemicals will destroy the land—some 'bargain'!"

"The USDA's Conservation Service has finally come to the conclusion that we are not going to continue the habit of eating much longer. They base their conclusion on the following: we had 18 inches of topsoil a couple hundred years ago; now we have only several inches of topsoil. The U.S. is losing 6.4. billion tons to erosion every year. All of the soils are eroding, and 1/4 of them are eroding at a destructive rate."

"How widespread is the practice of using gravel dust as the filler in a sack of NPK, I do not know. In those areas where gravel screenings or sand has been the most economical filler available, the dust has probably been used for years. I suspect that it is now a general practice because all soils have been largely stripped of some elements, and there is no cheaper way to add them."

"Generally speaking, the fertilizers, as exemplified by 'Eco-Agriculture,' use a mixture of minerals in combination with a compost or compost-like material which is high in nitrogen and carbon."

"Organic farming, as advocated by the Rodale organization, concentrates on organic matter plus specific fertilizers such as greensand and granite dust."

The chemical NPK will accelerate erosion. Eco-Ag and organic methods will slow the rate of erosion and maintain better balance of elements in the soil. None of them are supplied in amounts sufficient to build-up the mineral supply in the soil. All of them are partially dependent on the dwindling availability of the small amount of gravel and sand remaining in the soils. They work best on the strongest soils."

"All three fertilizing methods are dependent on annual applications. If anything were to interrupt the production and distribution for one crop year, we would starve to death in large numbers."

"None of these will sustain our food supply indefinitely. They will also not do the all-important job of removing excess CO_2 from the atmosphere. They are all too expensive. We must have a bulk production and distribution of gravel dust, or its equivalent. Without it there is no future for civilization."

" 'Hazardous Substances and Sterile Men' is the title of a powerful condemnation of the chemicals industry in the September 1981 Acres U.S.A. Ida Honorof has summarized research on this subject. In 1981, 10-23% of American males were sterile (very unlikely to father a child). In 1938 only 1/2 of 1% of males were sterile. According to this research, in 30 years, half of the males will be sterile, and 67-83% of all birth defects are caused by men—the chances of causing a deformed child to be born increase with the quantity of chemicals in the sperm. Ten chlorinated chemicals alone have been found in the sperm. Birth defect rates in the United States are believed to be about 6%—

it seems only a few years since that estimate was 3%. Many of the chemicals contaminate our food supply. One statistic says that 94% of food has pesticides in it.

"If people keep eating the poisoned foods of chemical agriculture, there will be more cancers, deformities, stillbirths, and as many different ailments as there are parts in the body. Either we stop the manufacture of organic chemicals which are not readily biodegradable, or we destroy ourselves."

"The balance of nature, in part, means that for every living organism there is a predator, so that no organism can populate the earth to the exclusion of all others. Our asinine, conceited view of ourselves as 'masters' of nature has led us to make a wreck of the balance of nature. We are paying a high price and we will continue to pay for a long time, even if we turn quickly to a rational concept of our role in the natural order. I have seen radical improvements in the ecology on two small plots of land when the poisoning was stopped, and minerals applied to the land. Perhaps nature can rather quickly reestablish the animated part of the balance of nature."

John Hamaker

99.3. Questions & Answers

What can we do to lessen starvation and hunger in the world?

If you want to lessen hunger in the world, look around you. Many cities have some types of food distribution programs and/or "soup kitchens" (places where people can go for a meal). You can support these programs, or if your area does not have them, perhaps you can become involved in getting them started. If you prefer even more direct action, you can "adopt" (figuratively speaking) an elderly person or persons, and/or a family. In every community there are people who need help—just look or ask around, and you will find them.

If you go on vacation in another country, you may want to meet some of the residents of its small villages and spend some of your money into their local economies instead of just spending it all at a modern hotel in a big city. Your life will be enriched by the experience, to say nothing of learning a whole lot more about life and other cultures than you would back at the hotel! When you return home to the U.S., you will know someone real that you can send a "care package" to now and then (clothes or household items, etc.). This is easy to do, and a needy family in an impoverished area will really appreciate your thoughtfulness. When you send a package directly to someone you know abroad, you'll know exactly what they need and "who is getting what"—when funds are sent to "traditional" charitable organizations, they keep something for their operating expenses, and you may not be as sure about how much finally reaches anyone, or how the money is actually being used. (I once saw a group asking for more money "to provide medicine for children." They'd be better off with fruit or other fresh food, and clothing!) I went with friends to a tiny village on the Mexican seacoast once, and every few days we brought boxes of fruit and vegetables for the family we stayed with; each time, the next day there'd scarcely be a banana left over—the children loved fruit. Unfortunately, if we'd just handed money to their father, he'd have probably gotten a few bottles of liquor since he liked to drink—we just brought food and other things like laundry soap, batteries, candles—things the family used daily. (We did give Mom some money now and then; she used it for the family.) The day we left; we tucked a 1,000-peso bill into her hand. At the exchange rate then, this only amounted to about 10 dollars for us (an easy gesture), but for a woman who didn't work outside the home (there were no paying jobs for women in their village), this was like a windfall (it would also go further there than its equivalent $10 would go here in the United States).

Along with many beautiful memories, this was the gift these people gave to me: the chance to be on the giving end for a change, to feel as if I could actually make some difference in someone else's life—as much a gift to me as anything I could have ever given them. For we are truly fortunate when we are able to give, and this also means giving of ourselves as well as of our possessions. When we reach out to other members of our human family abroad, we draw our world family closer, we strengthen the bonds. We exchange a mutual gift, that of increased understanding, and of a vision of a world in greater harmony. We are indeed brothers and sisters—our mirrored smiles tell us this, even when we "don't speak the same language", At last we become real to each other.

Another note on the joy of being able to give to people wherever we may be someone once told me that members of the so-called "beggar caste" of India also had their "special life purpose", their purpose being to allow others to be givers (the givers thus being given a chance to enhance their own spirituality by an act of giving). This concept returns the dignity owed these "beggars" as human beings; it sees beauty in every person.

Come to think of it, I remember the strategy used by some elderly women in the marketplace of Casablanca, Morocco, one that was quite ingenious. When the vendor gave you your change and you reached out for it, you'd suddenly be aware of another hand stretched out alongside your own, making it a bit awkward to "pretend you didn't have any money" (to say the least), but at least you were guaranteed an immediate increase in your level of spirituality!

When you are at home, remember too, as we said, that hunger may be as close as a mile from your house.

Pressure your local leaders to take real action against hunger. Sometimes "surplus" food is just held in storage, or even dumped—I once saw a news item on TV showing perfectly good oranges being dumped to "keep prices normal" (they didn't want too many oranges to "flood" the market!). It is immoral to keep this food from hungry people.

Another way to alleviate hunger around you may be as close as a few friends who live on a tight budget—invite them over more often for meals. Share the harvest.

If you can't find someone who is hungry, you aren't really looking. Remember, most people are much too proud to ask or tell you, so you need to be aware and sensitive to others' needs.

Years ago, I was staying in the Canary Islands off the coast of Africa, in a small boarding house, and a young woman lived in the room next door with her three children. Every day she went to work and, although the landlady (who lived downstairs) looked in on them now and then, the little four-year-old girl was really in charge of her younger brother and sister. Once I saw her peel potatoes, light the gas burner on the stove, and fry them, and I must admit, it was the first time I'd ever seen a four-year-old cooking completely on her own. One day I went in to offer her an apple and she said no. Three times I offered it, to no avail. When I went back to my room and mentioned this to my roommate, she said, "just go in there and set it on her table". I was skeptical, having assumed the child just didn't want the apple, but I did so anyway. A minute later she'd finished eating it.

The "moral" of this story is, not only will some people not ask for anything, but they may even refuse something you offer, because they "don't want to be a burden to you." When you ask, "do you want this?" or "do you need this?", they're very likely just to say no, out of pride, whether they do or not. So, keep your eyes open and assess the situation. The idea is not to make someone feel like they are accepting "charity"—no one really wants to be in this position. There's always a way around these delicate situations. Let the person know that you "have extra and can't possibly eat it all yourself," i.e., they're doing you a favor by taking it off your hands. There's a subtle difference.

The following was excerpted from Mother Jones magazine (September/October 1981), by Loretta Schwartz-Nobel:

"I found her by accident, trying to crawl out of her doorway and down the broken concrete steps in an effort to get food. She was 84 and living alone in an abandoned house in Philadelphia. That afternoon in 1974 I went with my seven-year-old daughter Rebekah to our local supermarket and bought food for Mrs. Roca. In the months that followed it became a habit to take several bags of groceries to her each Saturday afternoon. Rebekah thought of it as the best part of our week. Another woman, Julia, also in her 80s, lived nearby. Once she had tried to go to a local supermarket, but tripped and fell in the gutter, and lay there until a little boy stopped and helped her. The next time she tried, someone grabbed the bag of groceries on her way home and ran off."

I saw a TV documentary one night on the elderly in Chicago—some of them were being shuttled to and from the store in a bus because they were such easy targets for muggers. These people helped to build our country, and this is their "retirement dream"—these are their "golden years"—having to go to the store in a group because it is dangerous to attempt it alone.

A young boy interviewed on TV discussed his way of helping others—one night he saw a documentary on "street people" of his city and asked his parents to take him to see them. They were a bit hesitant but did so. Now he checks on the street people daily, bringing food, clothes, and so on. (In fact, other people began leaving boxes of things at his house, too, for distribution.) This boy sees these people as people, not "street people," and his father said that, while an adult keeps a distance, his son would touch these people or hug them—he now knows all the "regulars" there by name. A man on the street wrote a letter that was read on the show, and he sums it all up better than I ever could:

"One day I was so tired of living that I decided to end it all. Then something happened— that day I looked up into the eyes of a young boy, who smiled at me and handed me a blanket. That day, not only did I fall in love with this child, but I fell in love with life again, because my faith in humanity was restored."

Unless we've known true hunger and need, it's difficult to understand what it's really like to "live on the edge," but we can be sure of one thing: every morsel of food we give to anyone, in nourishing a fellow being, adds to life, and what can we do on this earth that is of greater purpose and joy, than to add to life? Let's recall, in our humility, that each morsel of food given to us by life and the powers that be is a miracle—we are all receivers as well as givers—we should never take this miracle for granted.

Article #1: How Vitamin and Mineral Content in Food Decreases Step-by-Step

In this lesson we have seen that there is more than one way in which food loses vitamins and minerals, but that most of our food is subjected not only to one but to a combination of assaults on its nutritional value, as indicated below:

• Food is grown on minerally-depleted soils in the first place.

• Plant breeding of hybrid seeds, and crop management, result in another measurable decline in protein and vitamin/mineral content.

• Pesticide spraying leaves poison residues in our food.

• Food processed by any of the techniques mentioned in the lesson (irradiation included) further decreases its value. (Note: It wasn't specified whether fresh food could also be irradiated before being shipped to food processors; only irradiation of food destined for the produce stand in our stores was discussed. However, it is conceivable that some food could be irradiated to keep it "fresh" longer for the food processors as well, in which case it would undergo two assaults in this step alone.)

• As if all the above steps do not reduce the life in our foods enough, much of our food is then cooked, spiced with condiments, salt, etc., smothered in sauces, and, to top it off, eaten in excess and/or in improper combinations, washed down with beverages that dilute our stomach's digestive enzymes, and often eaten in a hurry, and/or according to "the time of the day" instead of true hunger, and sometimes in a state of mind that is not conducive to good digestion.

We are paying dearly for our ignorance, indifference, and lack of good conscience, because we are destroying more and more of the life factor within our foods each time, we alter them further from their natural, fresh state.

How can we expect food that is virtually dead to sustain life? It has been said, with reference to vegetarianism vs. meat eating, but this also applies in the case of lifeless, foodless foods, that: "from life comes life, and from death comes death."

The choice is ours.

Article #2: Saving Open-Pollinated Seeds by Margaret Flynn

Drying Seeds

Beans

Broccoli

Chinese Cabbage

Corn

Cucumbers and Cantaloupes (Muskmelons) and Watermelons

Eggplant

Gourds

Lettuce

Okra

Peas

Peppers

Potato

Pumpkins and Squash

Radishes

Spinach

Sunflowers

Tomatoes

Hot Water Treatment of Seeds

Germination Testing

Cleaning Seed

Isolation and Purity

One of the first things to remember when saving seeds is never plant all your seed from one stock. Always save some in case anything should happen to your crop.

You need to be aware that cross-pollination of seeds can occur from other vegetables in the same family, or from other gardens within about 1/4 mile.

It's best not to save seed from just our largest tomato, for example, but to save seed from the smallest, largest, earliest, and latest fruits. Equal amounts of these four types of seeds should be mixed. In this way we will have a much greater genetic diversity in our seed samples. We should look at the whole plant too, not just the fruit. Select several plants to save seed from, those with characteristics you want for your next year's plants: size, flavor, earliness, ability to survive a short season (where applicable), disease-resistance, drought-resistance, insect-resistance, lateness to bolt, trueness to type, color, shape, thickness of flesh, hardiness and storability. All these factors can and should be selected for.

Temperature and moisture extremes, especially in combination, can cause damage to seed before harvest. For example: an early sustained freeze while the seeds still have a high moisture content. It is best to have dry weather before and during harvest, so that the seeds can dry on the plant and remain dry.

Drying Seeds

When drying and storing your seed, you want its vigor to stay as high as possible so that seeds will germinate rapidly with good disease-resistance. Vigor is destroyed by high temperature and high moisture during storage. Seeds can be dried on a screen or on wax paper in the sun, by sealing them in an airtight container with silica gel (until they reach the proper moisture levels for entry into storage), or by putting them in your oven with the pilot light on and the door cracked.

(WARNING: Damage to seeds will begin at temperatures of 96° F or more. Even at the very lowest setting, an oven temperature can vary enough to damage your seeds.)

Seeds must be completely dry before you store them, and they should break instead of bending (less than 8% moisture). Store seeds in a completely airtight container at as low and constant a temperature as possible. Put each variety of seed in an envelope and write the name and year on each one. Put these envelopes into any glass jar that has a rubber gasket lid that can be screwed down tight enough to make the container airtight and moisture-proof. Homemade gaskets can be cut from old inner tubes.

Adjustable channel-lock pliers can be used to screw the lids on as tight as possible.

Black electrical tape can be used to seal questionable lids.

Another possible container is a flat bag that has laminated walls of paper/foil/plastic. It can be sealed with a Seal-A-Meal or sealed with an iron set on "wool" applied to the open end of the bag for three seconds. (The sealed edge can later be cut off and the bags reused.) They can be put directly into the freezer and take up less space than jars; they are also inexpensive.

Your containers can be kept in a freezer with no damage to the dry seeds. The next best place is a refrigerator, and the next is any cool area where the temperature will remain as constant as possible. When you take the container out of the freezer, you must let it sit out overnight to come to room temperature before you open it. If you don't, moisture will condense on the cold seeds and your effort to dry them will have been wasted. Do not leave the container open for any length of time, and don't go into it too often because temperature fluctuation is not good for the seeds. If you store your seeds by this method, they will hold their vigor for up to five times the period shown on viability charts.

We discussed reasons for saving nonhybrid, open-pollinated seeds, what to consider when choosing plants for saving seeds, and how to dry them. Let's look at some more detailed information on specific vegetables.

Beans

Phaseolus vulgaris contains common bush or pole beans, whether used for green snaps, green shell or dry. They are self-pollinating before the flower opens, so there is very seldom crossing. Sometimes you'll notice variation or oddities in the seed that may be due to a genetically unstable variety or a difference in conditions such as a change of soil pH or wetness at harvest rather than to any true crosses. You can plant varieties of Phaseolus vulgaris side by side.

Phaseolus coccineus are "runner beans." You can tell these when they come up because they develop with their two seed halves under the ground. Their flowers are self-pollinating, but bees or bumble bees and hummingbirds work them heavily and thus cross them. You should either grow only one variety of runner beans or separate two of them by at least the length of your garden.

Mark a few of your best plants, and let the pods dry out completely on the plant, weather permitting. When most of the leaves have fallen off, pull the plants and hang them under cover to finish drying. Small amounts of seed can be shelled by hand; for large quantities, make sure beans are thoroughly dry, crush or thresh pods, separate the beans from the chaff by winnowing in the wind; label, and store.

Weevil eggs are almost always present under the bean's seedcoat and can ruin your seed in a few months. They can be killed by placing the thoroughly dry beans in a tightly sealed jar and freezing them for at least a day.

Broccoli

Broccoli produces seed its first season (unlike the other biennial members of the cabbage family) if you sow it early enough that plants are quite large by the long days of summer. However, it crosses readily with cabbage, kale, brussels sprouts, cauliflower, or kohlrabi, if any of these are flowering within 1/4 mile. Don't cut flower heads for food that you are saving seed from.

Chinese Cabbage

Brassica pekinensis is a cross-pollinating annual. It will not cross with any of the cabbage family but will cross easily with other varieties of Chinese cabbage. It sends up a seed stalk which forms a pod that will turn brown when mature. If you plant more than one variety of Chinese cabbage, the isolation distance is 1/4 mile. The rest of the method is the same as with lettuce.

Corn

Corn is wind-pollinated, so any corn (sweet, popcorn, ornamental, dent, flint, etc.) will cross very easily with other corn. To keep corn "pure," you must grow it 1/4 mile from any other corn, or hand-pollinate it. Corn is very "plastic," so by observing and selecting carefully you can gradually determine characteristics your future crops will have. Let ears you are saving seed from ripen on the stalk until husks are dry, pick them, pull husks back, tie several husks together by the husks, hang in a dry, well-ventilated place until completely dry, shell, save only completely formed kernels, and store. (An early and late variety can be planted side by side if the early one stops pollinating before the silks of the late one begin to emerge.)

Cucumbers And Cantaloupes (Muskmelons) And Watermelons

These all belong to different species and will not cross with each other (bug gherkins cross with cukes, muskmelon with casaba, and watermelon with citron). They are all insect-pollinated, so different varieties of each of the three will cross easily among themselves. If you are going to save seed, grow one variety of each. (Remember that with vine crops and any other vegetable that crosses very easily, that if you have any neighbors within 1/4 mile who are also growing that vegetable, you would be wise to try to supply them with your seed.)

Let a few of the earliest maturing well-formed fruit become completely ripe (cukes turn golden yellow, muskmelons crack at the stem, watermelons have a deep hollow sound when thumped). This ruins cukes for eating, but with watermelon and cantaloupe, the seeds are mature when they are ready to eat. Scoop out the seeds, wash them gently to remove pulp (a sieve may be used), and let them dry. totally on a piece of foil. Keep them separated and stir them occasionally so they don't stick together. When completely dry, label and store. (Remember, seeds are dry when they break instead of bending.)

Eggplant

Pollination is like peppers, so separate varieties by the length of your garden or with a tall crop. Leave the best fruits on several of your plants for as long as possible, and when fully mature, scrape out seeds, separate from the pulp, dry and store.

Gourds

Legenaria siceraria are hard-shelled bottle gourds with evening-blooming white flowers. They don't cross with vegetables in the squash section, edible varieties include: Cucuzzi (also called Italian Edible Gourd and Italian Climbing Gourd) and Guinea Bean Gourd (also called New Guinea Bean and New Guinea Buttervine). Saving seeds of squash, pumpkins and gourds is the same as with cucumbers (except that summer squash varieties must be left on the vine much later than the eating stage, until the shell is quite hard).

Lettuce

Lettuce is self-pollinating with little chance of crossing. Select several of the firmest heads or best leafy plants which are slowest to bolt (send up their seed stalks). When seed is fully developed, pull plants, and hang them under cover to finish drying. Crush pods, separate seeds, label, and store.

Okra

Okra is self-pollinating, so you can grow more than one variety with little separation. Leave at least two of your best plants completely alone. When pods are dry, but before they open enough to drop seeds on the ground, shell them and save.

Peas

Peas are self-pollinating, but cross slightly more easily than beans. So, if you grow two varieties, separate them by the length of your garden or with a tall crop. Everything else is the same as with beans.

Peppers

Peppers are mainly self-pollinating, but insects may cause some crossing in varieties planted closer than 1/8 mile. When growing more than one variety of peppers (or if sweet and hot), separate them by the length of your garden or with a tall crop to keep them from crossing (and sweet peppers from becoming hot). Select several of your largest and best peppers from your best plants. Let them ripen on the plant until red and starting to soften, scrape out seeds, dry and save.

Potato

Potato varieties don't cross since tuber divisions are really just clones. Crossing between potato flowers affects seed balls, not the roots. Select a few of your best-looking plants that are surrounded by healthy plants to save for seed. Never keep potatoes for seed that show any sign of scab. You might be able to increase your production by planting small (egg-sized) whole potatoes, since they are less apt to be badly sprouted and often produce a vigorous plant more quickly than cut potatoes. If planting small whole sprouted potatoes in spring, don't damage the big sprout on the eye end of the potato since this will produce the most vigorous plant. You can just break most of the other sprouts off. Some people think that yields are improved by planting sprouted potatoes. Plants sometimes emerge in just a few days (sometimes two weeks) ahead of non-sprouted potatoes. Dig potatoes when the vines begin to dry up— when the soil loses its shade, it gets hot, and your crop may be damaged. Washing/not washing doesn't seem to affect how well your potatoes keep. After drying in the shade for only a few hours to toughen their skins, they are ready to store, the colder the storage temperature the better (34°-40°F). It's been said that burying them in dry sand is the perfect way to store them.

Pumpkins And Squash

These are insect-pollinated and cross very easily. All pumpkins and squash belong to one of four species of the genus Cucurbita, so when saving seeds, plant only one variety of each of the following species:

Curcubita Pepo includes summer squash, all true pumpkins, varieties that are both bush and long vined; stem and branches both have five sides and spines. Includes all acorn squash (Des Moines, Ebony, Ebony Bush, Jersey Golden, Royal, Table King, Table King Bush, Table Queen, Table Queen Bush, Table Queen Ebony, Table Queen Mammoth), Black Beauty, Casserta, Cheyenne, Chiefinei, Cinderella. Includes all of the cocozelles (Green, Vining), Connecticut Field, Cozini. Includes all of the crooknecks (Dwarf Summer, Early Summer Golden, Early Summer Yellow, Golden, White Summer), Crystal Bell, Delicata. Early Cheyenne Pie, Fordhook, Fordhook Bush, Fort Berthold, Golden Centenial, Golden Custard, Golden Oblong, Hyuga Black, Jack O'Lantern, Kikuza White, Lady Godiva, Little Boo, Lunghissimo Bianco Di Palermo, Mammoth Gold. Includes all the marrows (Boston, English Vegetable, Green Bush Improved, Long White, Vegetable, White Bush, White Vining Vegetable), Naked Seeded, New England Pie Pumpkin, Omaha, Panama, Perfect Gem, Pie Pumpkin, Royal Bush. Includes all the scallops (Benning's Green Tint, Early White Bush, Early Yellow Bush, Long Is. White Bush, Mammoth White Bush, Patty Pan, St. Pat, Summer Bush, Yellow Golden), Small Sugar Pumpkin, Spaghetti Squash, Spookie, Stickler, Straightneck, Early Prolific, Streaker, Sugar Pie, Sweet Dumpling (Vegetable Gourd), Table Gold, Thomas Halloween, Tricky Jack, Triple Treat, Uconn, Winter Luxury, Winter Nut, Youngs Beauty, Vegetable Spaghetti. Includes all zucchinis (Black, Burpee's Fordhook, Burpee's Golden, Dark Green, Gold Rush, Gray), and any of the small Hard-shelled, Striped and Warted Gourds.

Cucurbita maxima have very long vines and huge leaves, stem is soft, round, and hairy. Alligator, Arikara, Atlas, All banana squash (Blue, Giant, Orange, Pink, Pink Jumbo), Bay State, Big Max, Big Moon. All buttercups: Blue, Bush. All delicious: (Golden,

Green), Emerald, Essex, Estampes, Gilmore, Gold Nugget, Greengold, Guatemala Blue, Hokkaido Green, Hokkaido Orange. All hubbards (Baby, Baby Blue, Chicago,

Chicago Warted, Warted Green, Warted Improved), Hungarian Mammoth, Hungarian Mammoth (Cornell Strain), Ironclad, Kindred, King of Giants, King of Mammoths, Kuri Blue, Kuri Red, Mammoth Chili, Mammoth King, Mammoth Whale, Mammoth (Genuine), Marblehead. All marrows: (Autumnal, Boston, Orange, Prolific), Plymouth Rock, Rainbow, Red Estampes, Show King, Sibley, Silver Bell, Sweetmeat, Tuckernuck. All turbans (American, Golden, Turks), Victor Watten, Winnebago, Yakima Marblehead.

Cucurbita Moschata has large leaves and spreading vines, and a smooth five-sided stem which flares out as it joins the fruit. African Bell, Zizu Gokwuase, Alagold, Butterbush. All butternuts (Baby, Early, Eastern, Hercules, Ponca, Puritan, Waltham, Western), Calabaza (Cuban Squash), Calhoun, Cangold. All cheese (Large, Long Island), Fortuna, Futtsu Kurokawa, Golden Cushaw, Hercules, Kentucky Field, Melon Squash (Tahitian), Patriot, Peraora, Ponca, Tahitian (Melon Squash), Virginia Mammoth, Wisconsin Canner.

Cucurbita mixta was formerly included with C. moschata and has similar characteristics. Chirimen, the Cushaws (except Golden Cushaw which is C. moschata), (Green Striped, Solid Green and White), Japanese Pie, Mixta Gold, Tennessee Sweet Potato.

Varieties within a species (one of the four groups) cross very easily, but don't worry about crossing between species. Crosses between different species are hard to make and their progeny are so highly sterile, that crosses by natural means are unlikely to cause concern. You do need to consider pollen from neighbors' gardens contaminating your efforts at keeping pure seed strains if they are within 1/4 mile. Otherwise, you can use these lists to keep four varieties of, pumpkins/squashes pure (one from each species). If your aim is purity (and/or if you are sending seeds to the Seed Savers Exchange) and you do have close neighbors, you need to hand-pollinate. Otherwise, you could lose in one season what someone else has spent a lifetime of gardening to develop or preserve. (If you are afraid that a squash you are growing might have crossed, remember you won't see the variation in that summer's fruit. Grow it again to check it. If it has crossed, you'll see the variation when you grow the seed from the fruit that crossed.)

In an experiment to determine at what point there was the greatest number of fertile squash seeds, they found it to be 20 days after the fruit is fully mature—a 20-day after-ripening period when the seed actually improves in the fruit after you pick it.

Radishes

Radishes are insect-pollinated, so grow only one variety. Choose several of the largest, earliest roots to save seed from. The seed pod on the seed stalk will turn brown at maturity. At that point, pull the plants and finish drying under cover.

Spinach

Spinach cross-pollinates and has very fine pollen that is carried long distances by the wind. It only crosses with other varieties of spinach, very easily. Plant one variety only for purity in seed strains. Save seed as with lettuce.

Sunflowers

Sunflowers cross easily with wild sunflowers, making them unsuitable to save for seed. Some people call this home-saved seed that is "running out"—seed doesn't really run out, but if you don't take the right precautions, a gradual process of undesirable crossing over several generations can make the seed of some vegetable varieties practically worthless.

Tomatoes

Tomatoes are over 98% self-pollinating, but even such a slight amount of insect pollination over a number of seasons may be enough to destroy the characteristics that made the variety unique. Don't grow tomato varieties side by side if you want to save seed from them. Remember, don't just save seed from your largest tomato. For better genetic diversity, save seed from the smallest, largest, earliest, and latest fruits. (This would only be twice the work if you saved seed from the earliest and also a large fruit at the beginning of the season, and the latest and also a small fruit near the end of the season). Mix equal amounts of these four seeds.

Select well-formed fruits from a few of your best plants and let them ripen on the plant beyond the edible stage until they are getting soft, but not to the point where they are going bad. Squeeze seed from several fruits into a glass, add some water, let the mixture ferment at room temperature for several days, stirring vigorously several times daily. After a couple of days, the good seed will be on the bottom and bad seed and pulp will float on the top and can be washed away. This fermentation is said to kill several seed-borne diseases (many people use this method to separate seeds from pulp whenever seeds are embedded in soft fruit). If you don't want to use this process, squirt the seeds into a sieve and rub them with your fingers against the sieve under running water. Pick out or work all the pulp through the sieve and keep working seeds until the whole batch is really clean. Then spread them thinly and separately on wax paper. When they are completely dry, label and store.

All of the above vegetables are annuals, which grow and develop seed in one season. Biennials don't produce seed until the end of their second growing season. Biennials are the root vegetables (carrots, onions, leeks, parsnips, rutabagas, salsify, beets, turnips, celeriac and winter storage-type radishes), the cabbage family (cabbage, broccoli, brussels sprouts, cauliflower, and kohlrabi), parsley, celery, kale (or borecole), collards, endive and Swiss chard. All these vegetables (except salsify and endive) are cross-pollinated, so to save seed and keep it pure, grow only one variety of each and only one member of the cabbage family, since they all cross. Select good-sized roots or firm heads to save seed from, dig them before frost, keep them in cool storage over the winter, replant them the following spring and they will bear seed that summer. If your climate isn't really severe (or with hardy roots like turnips and rutabagas) you may be able to just mulch them heavily over the winter, take the mulch off early in the spring and let them go to seed. Carrots will cross with wild carrots (Queen Ann's lace) if your garden is surrounded by meadow. Swiss chard, beets, mangles, and sugar beets all cross. Celery and celeriac cross. Turnips and beets and broccoli will behave as either an annual or biennial depending on the climate, they are grown in.

Hot Water Treatment of Seeds

This is a method for controlling the seed-born phase of diseases such as black rot and black leg in the cabbage family, bacterial canker, and target spot in tomatoes, and Septoria spot in celery. You'll need an accurate thermometer, electric fry pan, large saucepan, kitchen sieve and paper towels. Try a practice run without the seeds. Heat some water to 50°C. Pour a little into the warm electric fry pan, fill the saucepan 2/3 full and set it in the fry pan. Regulate the temperature either by late the temperature either by turning up the fry pan or taking the sauce pan out of the fry pan. When you can maintain 50°C, pour in the seeds, stir until they are all wetted and not floating, then stir gently throughout the whole process. Treat broccoli and Brussel sprout seed for 20 minutes at 50°C, cabbage for 30 minutes at 52°C, cauliflower for 25 minutes at 52°C, celery, and pepper seeds for 30 minutes at 50° C, and tomato for 25 minutes at 55°C. Then sieve the seed and spread it on paper towels away from direct sunlight, dry and store them.

Germination Testing

If you want to test the viability of your seeds, especially if you intend to exchange them with the Seed Savers Exchange (in fairness to fellow members), you can take 10, 25, 50 or 100 seeds for each variety, roll in a damp paper towel, put in a plastic bag, and put it in a warm spot. Count the sprouts after 7-10 days. Seven sprouts per 10 seeds is 70% germination, etc. The idea is to be sure that at least some of your seed will sprout; it's better to find out you have more to learn about saving seed than to have you or an exchange member waiting next spring for your seed to come up.

Cleaning Seed

Seeds that are harvested wet can be cleaned by floating off the light (and weak) seeds, hollow hulls, and other debris. This works well for tomatoes (after fermentation), peppers, eggplant, melons, and squash. Remove seeds from fruit, ferment if required, add water, and stir vigorously. Good seeds are heaviest and sink; the rest of the debris floats and can be poured off. Repeat this four or five times or until the water poured off is free of debris. Rub wet seed over a sieve to remove attached pulp, rinse again, and dry.

Seeds that are harvested dry should be rubbed and winnowed to remove chaff.

Isolation and Purity

We have used isolation and planting only one variety of cross-pollinating crops to maintain pure strains, but it should be noted that even self-pollinated plants may cross if conditions are just right. If your aim is absolute purity and you are saving seed from more than one variety of a self-pollinating crop, separate varieties by at least a row or two of another crops.

Thanks for saving seeds!

Article #3: Hand Pollination of Squash by Richard Grazzini

Excerpted from one of the Seed Savers Exchange catalogs.

This year I looked at about 150 different varieties of squash. A few were commercial hybrids or commercially available standards, but most were heirlooms. On the other hand, some of the heirlooms were obviously crosses of two (or more) winter squashes, or winter squashes and summer squashes. If you grow squash for seed, PLEASE hand pollinate or grow only one variety of each species. You could wreck in one season what someone else has spent a lifetime of gardening to develop or preserve.

To keep varieties of squash from crossing and to make them come "true", you must self-pollinate them by hand. First, in the late afternoon or evening, find both male and female flowers that are unopened, but firm and yellow (the female flower has a small "baby" squash below it). These will open overnight unless they are sealed. Wilted yellow flowers have already opened—don't use them. The flowers you will be using the next morning must be sealed so that bees don't do your pollinating for you and bees are early risers! I usually seal with 1" or 2" masking tape placed around the top third of the flower. The next morning, wait until the dew dries and then pick the male flower. Remove the petals from both male and female flowers. Swab the pollen-covered part of the male flower on the stigma of the female flower. A glassine envelope should be ready to use (so the open flower is not exposed for too long). Cover the female flower after pollination with the glassine envelope and hold it in place with a wired label which closes the glassine envelope and labels the pollination all in one step. This will let you keep track of your hand-pollinated fruit all during the summer until harvest.

That's it, except for removing the glassine envelope after three to five days. If the envelope is not removed, more often than not the fruit will rot. Always make as many hand pollinations as possible. Some fruit may rot at any time, and you can lose a variety because you quit one flower too soon. Self-pollinating a naturally-crossed crop can lead to what's called "inbreeding depression" or a loss in plant vigor. Luckily for those of us who like to work with squash, squash don't seem to show any inbreeding depression. Watermelon and cantaloupe can be hand pollinated just like squash. The flowers are smaller and not as easy to manipulate. You may have to use tweezers, but it works.

Article #4: The Spirit Speaks

I have never once deviated

In my love for you.

From the moment you were conceived

I have loved you with a love

Changeless

Endless Irrevocable.

There has never been a day, an hour, an instant

When I was not with you

Loving you.

I nurtured you as a seed

Enfolded you as a child

Strengthened you as man.

I was an invisible shield over your head

Though you knew it not.

I am still that invisible shield!

With infinite care I attend your wounds,

Govern your heartbeat

Remove the wastes that do not belong.

I sleep not at night.

When you close your eyes

Yielding at last more fully to my care I go to work

And heal, as far as I can

The ravages of your insane, inexplicable self-activity.

You imagine in your blindness

That you can love or not as you choose,

Condemn, criticize, hate As you choose.

Fortunately for you I have no such choice.

I am true always to the solemn dictate of love.

I respect to the last the covenant I made

When I came into the world.

Yet I know too that you cannot survive

If you continue to fight against me,

Ignoring my government

Preferring strange impulses of your own choosing.

Rejecting me you reject love.

This is why you are always looking for love

But never find it.

Just when you think you have it Love

Like a bird Flies away.

Your songs, art, literature, all sing

This vain and fruitless quest

For a love that will never change

A love that will never die

A love that is ever new.

Turn to me Acknowledge me

Accept me

Love me

And you will know such love

Here and now.

Together we will restore the world

To order and to beauty.

—Origin unknown

Article #5: Origin of the World's Basic Food Plants

Old World Centers

New World Centers

Almost all of the world's basic food plants originated in a few relatively confined areas of the planet, close to the equator, named Vavilov Centers after the renowned Russian plant breeder and geneticist N. I. Vavilov. Although these areas remain the sole source of all natural food plant varieties, they are rapidly being urbanized, and much of the agricultural land is being planted with patented hybrid seeds developed in Europe and the U.S.

Old World Centers

1 ETHIOPIA

Banana (endemic) Barley

Castor bean Coffee

Flax Khat Okra Onion Sesame Sorghum Wheat

2 MEDITERRANEAN

Asparagus Beet Cabbage Carob Chicory Hops Lettuce Oat

Olive Parsnip Rhubarb Wheat

3 ASIA MINOR

Alfalfa Almond (wild)

Apricot (secondary) Barley

Beet (secondary) Cabbage

Cherry Date palm Carrot

Fig Flax Grape Lentil Oat

Onion (secondary) Pea

Pear Pistachio Pomegranate Rye

Wheat

4 CENTRAL ASIATIC

Almond Apple (wild) Apricot Broad bean Cantaloupe Carrot Chickpea

Cotton (G. herbaceum) Flax

Grape (V. vinifera) Hemp

Lentil Mustard Onion Pea

Pear (wild) Sesame Spinach Turnip Wheat

5 INDO-BURMA

Amaranth Betel nut Betel pepper Chickpea

Cotton (G. arboreum) Cowpea

Cucumber Eggplant Hemp Jute Lemon

Mango Millet Orange

Pepper (black) Rice

Sugar cane (wild) Taro

Yam

6 SIAM, MALAYA, JAVA

Banana Betel palm Breadfruit Coconut Ginger Grapefruit

Sugar cane (wild) Tung

Yam

7 CHINA

Adzuki bean Apricot Buckwheat Chinese cabbage

Cowpea (secondary) Kaoliang (sorghum) Millet

Oat (secondary) Orange (secondary) Paper mulberry Peach

Radish Rhubarb Soybean

Sugar cane (endemic) Tea

New World Centers

8 MEXICO-GUATEMALA

Amaranth

Bean (P. vulgaris) Bean (P. multiflorus) Bean (P. lunatus) Bean (P. acutifolius) Corn

Cacao Cashew

Cotton (G. hirsutum) Guava

Papaya Pepper (red) Sapodilla Sisal Squash

Sweet potato Tomato

9 PERU-ECUADOR-BOLIVIA

Bean (P. vulgaris) Bean (P. lunatus) Cacao

Corn (secondary) Cotton

Edible roots (oca, ullucu, arracacha, añu) Guava

Papaya Pepper (red)

Potato (many species) Quinine

Quinoa

Squash (C. maxima) Tomato

10 SOUTHERN CHILE

Potato

Strawberry (Chilean)

11 BRAZIL-PARAGUAY

Brazil nut

Cacao (secondary) Cashew

Cassava Mate

Para rubber Peanut Pineapple

12 UNITED STATES

Sunflower Blueberry Cranberry Jerusalem Artichoke

Article #6: You've Just Been Poisoned by Mike Benton

Pesticides and Your Health

Why Is This Happening?

Poisons for Profits

Deadly Bananas

Foreign Killers

What Can You Do?

Economic Action

Political action

Consumer Action

A Good Diet Can Help!

Fight Back!

Have you had a headache recently? Maybe you've felt tired or nervous or irritable for no particular reason. Or has there been some pain somewhere in your body, but you didn't know just where?

Well, consider yourself poisoned pesticide poisoned, that is.

You may be a victim of pesticide poisoning if you've experienced any of these symptoms lately: fatigue, aching bones, headache, indeterminate body pains, chronic tiredness, mental confusion, fever or other "cold-like" and "flu-like" symptoms.

Many times, you may be poisoned by pesticide residues in your food and just not realize it. Pesticide poisoning goes virtually undetected by doctors because they rarely recognize the symptoms for what they are. Since you may not have become immediately sick after eating pesticide-contaminated food, you may not connect your negative feelings with the poisons you just ate.

While few people do know that many aches, upsets, and illnesses are pesticide-related, over 500,000 people each year are seriously poisoned by pesticides each year—over one every minute.

Another 5,000 people die each year as a direct result of pesticides. Up to 5 million or more cases of pesticide poisonings go unreported or undiagnosed each year.

Everybody in the world—no matter where they live or what they eat—have pesticide residues throughout their body. That's right—you've been poisoned!

Pesticides and Your Health

Pesticides seem especially damaging to the liver and spleen. Blood disorders such as leukemia, anemia and "tired blood" have increased with their use of pesticides. More leukemia cases are reported in the farm states that have had the highest amount of pesticide spraying.

Liver disorders such as hepatitis, jaundice and other ailments have skyrocketed with pesticide use. "It is now believed," says Dr. W. Coda Martin, "that the greater number of hepatitis cases may be caused by DDT on the leaves of green vegetables."

In 1969, Miami University did a study on cancer patients. A random selection of terminal cancer patients revealed that they had exceptionally high pesticide residues in their liver, brains, and fatty tissues.

Although we can't blame all our nation's ills on pesticide use, pesticide poisoning is real. Stillbirths, miscarriages, and deformed babies occur most where pesticide use has increased the most rapidly.

Why Is This Happening?

The government is doing a miserable job of keeping pesticides out of our environment. Agribusiness aggressively promotes the use of these poisons for profit—even when they know they are killing people! Does this sound incredible, do you still believe that people are crying "wolf"? Well, read on.

Poisons for Profits

In 1977, workers at a pesticide plant in California discovered that they had been made sterile due to exposure to DBCP (a pesticide). Some of the companies making this poison suspended production while the government investigated. One company, called Amvac, did not.

Amvac told its stockholders that although DBCP had suspected "carcinogenic and mutagenic" properties, they would continue to sell it. They explained: "It was our opinion that a vacuum existed in the marketplace that (we) could temporarily occupy...(and) with the addition of DBCP, sales might be sufficient to reach a profitable level."

Finally, after two years that it was determined DBCP did indeed cause sterility, the Environmental Protection Agency banned its use in this country. So, do you think you're safe? Nope. Read on.

Deadly Bananas

Although DBCP is now banned in this country because it is believed to cause cancer and sterility, there are no restrictions on selling this pesticide to foreign countries.

Banana plantations in Costa Rica, Honduras and Ecuador buy DBCP from us. They use it to kill soil-dwelling worms that attack the bananas. Then they ship the sprayed bananas back to the United States where you eat them.

Foreign Killers

Imported produce is more likely to be highly poisoned than food grown in our country. The reason? "Americans eat with their eyes," a Mexican agribusinessman said. "They won't buy a fruit or vegetable with any insect marks or blemishes, so we spray them heavily. About four times as much spray as we use on our domestic crops. No insects ever touch that food."

And probably neither should you.

Strawberries from Mexico often have residues of 60 or more pesticides. A single head of imported lettuce had 11 different poisons used on it.

Bananas from Central and South America had 45 "allowable" (by FDA standards) pesticides plus 25 prohibited pesticides and 37 additional poisons that are not normally detected by FDA tests. Mexican tomatoes had 53 "allowable" pesticides, another 21 banned pesticides, and an additional 28 unidentifiable sprays and poisons. The FDA frequently finds mysterious, unknown poisons in imported foods no doubt illegal pesticides that were manufactured and sold by the United States.

The FDA rarely seizes these poisoned food shipments or refuses them entry. Instead, they remove a small sample of the food for testing and send the rest to the marketplace. By the time they run the test and discover the deadly pesticides, the food is already in your stomach.

During one recent 15-month period, half of the imported food identified as heavily pesticide-contaminated was sold without penalty or warning to the American public.

The government is not protecting you. The pesticide manufacturers certainly won't protect you. It's up to you.

What Can You Do?

You cannot avoid pesticide poisoning. By now, the waterways, the soil and the rain are so polluted by them that it will take at least 20 to 40 years to eliminate them from the environment even if we start today.

Is it hopeless? Do we have to sit back and allow ourselves to be poisoned for someone else's pocketbook? No. You can take actions today that may save the lives and health of all the people and wildlife on this planet. Here's how:

Economic Action

As much as possible, boycott the giants of agribusiness who are chiefly responsible for pesticide production and use. Buy local and organic produce as much as possible. Support the small, independent grower.

Tell your local grocery store that you want more homegrown and unsprayed produce. Spend your dollars wisely so as to give little support to the food industries that use poison for profits.

Political action

Let your congressmen at the state and federal levels know about your deep concern for the pesticide problem. Write letters, emphasizing that their actions in this one area will greatly determine how you will vote.

Protest the exportation of pesticides to other countries. These poisons find their way back to your dinner table. Insist that federal agencies be more responsive and stringent in monitoring pesticide levels. Tell your representatives that you want more funding for environmental protection agencies.

A list of consumer action groups that are lobbying for stricter pesticide control is included with this article. Contact them for additional information about how you can help.

Consumer Action

You can consume less pesticides by growing your own food. If you have extra room, grow additional poison-free food for friends and relatives. However, realize that pesticides are now throughout the environment. Rains carry deadly poisons from around the world and deposit them in your garden. Even homegrown and organically grown food is now being pesticide contaminated due to our polluted waterways. You can't run away anymore from the problem—it's being brought home to you, like it or not.

If you can't garden or raise your own food, grow sprouts. These are virtually poison tree food and may be had fresh all year round. Sprouting dried seeds and grains can help you consume less supermarket poisoned foods.

A Good Diet Can Help!

Yes, you can eat certain foods and avoid others to reduce your pesticide poisoning. By wisely choosing your foods, you can consume up to 100 times less poisons than the average person. Here's how:

1. Avoid meat and dairy products. Pesticide residues are 16 times to several hundred times higher in meat and milk products than in fresh fruits and vegetables.

Animals must eat 16 pounds of plant material to produce one pound of flesh. The poisons in the feeds and plants are concentrated in the fat and vital organs of the animal. When you eat the meat, it's like getting a super-concentrated dose of pesticides. The pesticides that are bonded in the animal fat is even more difficult for the body to handle than the pesticides found in the fruits and vegetables. When pesticides are subject to heating as well (as in the cooking of the meat), additional dangerous chemical changes occur.

The former secretary of Health, Education and Welfare, Robert Finch, said: "If strict enforcement of pesticide residues in meat, dairy products and eggs existed, I fear we would have to become a nation of vegetarians." Actually, the fear should be that we won't become a nation of non-meat eaters.

Although DDT contamination of fruits and vegetables has now slightly decreased since the limited 1973 ban, pesticide poisons in livestock, poultry and fish have steadily increased. Animal fat is a storehouse of poisons. The more fat in your diet, the more poisons. It's that simple.

Remember too that it is now impossible to consume any dairy food in any form and not receive dangerous levels of DDT. High-fat dairy products are, of course, the worst.

2. Limit or reduce grain products. Grain farming is most conducive to heavy spraying and mono-crop farming. After a few years of continual spraying, the grain fields become saturated with high doses of pesticides. The safest grain to eat is wild rice. Corn and wheat are among the heaviest sprayed.

Buy organic food or grow your own. Obviously if you grow or buy unsprayed food, you'll get less pesticides. Remember, however, that as long as there are pesticides used anywhere in the world, your food will still be contaminated. The only sure way to prevent pesticide poisoning is to make certain that these chemicals are not released into the environment in the first place.

3. Use careful food preparation. You can remove some surface pesticides by washing them with a harmless soap to remove oil-based poisons, vinegar or lemon juice to remove alkali-based sprays, and soda for acid-based sprays. Make sure all such washed produce is then cleansed with water (preferably distilled to avoid other contaminants).

You can peel some fruits and vegetables (especially waxed produce). You should remove outer leaves of green vegetables.

Once again, however, these are not sure protection measures. Most pesticides are not on the surface of the food but are throughout the entire system of the plant. The poisons may be entirely intercellular, and none may be on the surface at all.

4. Avoid most imported produce. Food that is imported has often been more heavily sprayed and with poisons banned in this country. This is not always true, however. For instance, many foreign countries will not let U.S. produce come into their country because of the poisons we use. Oftentimes, the food you get inside these countries is safer than what is grown inside the U.S. It's just that to produce high-cosmetic produce for Americans, the foreign countries heavily spray their export crops.

5. Avoid produce that receive the highest amount of spraying. This is often difficult to determine, as pesticide use is not consistent for any crop across the country. In general, "soft" fruits which are more prone to insect attack will usually be more heavily sprayed than those foods with a naturally protective layer or skin.

6. Don't worry. Strange advice after all these warnings, but you should realize that at this time, it is impossible to avoid all pesticides. Worrying does no good anyway; action is what is needed.

If you follow a good diet, you can be protected from most of the harmful effects of pesticides. For instance, uncooked foods present less of a problem to the body as it tries to separate the poisons from the food. If you cook your food, you're creating chemical bonds with the poisons that may present difficulty. A little poison on your fresh fruits and vegetables won't hurt you as much as the high amount of poisons most people get in the typical high-fat, high-meat American diet.

Fasting can help your body eliminate the pesticide poisons by burning up those fat deposits where the residues are stored. As these poisons are released during the fast, you may experience the usual symptoms of pesticide poisoning—nausea, headaches, irritability, etc. It's uncomfortable but fasting and/or the eliminating of this body fat may be the only way of ridding yourself of the pesticide load.

Fight Back!

Remember, you don't have to sit back and be continually poisoned. You're not helpless. You have to take action. You're fighting for your life.

No one is immune from pesticide poisoning. We are killing the birds, the animals, the children, and all life on our planet by the crazy, unjustifiable use of deadly pesticide poisons.

We have a chance. There are still people—people like you—who believe health, life and well-being are more important than a few extra dollars for a poison manufacturer or for the chance to eat an "unblemished" apple.

But you can't wait any longer. You've got to fight back—now —because with the next bite you eat, you've just been poisoned.

Lesson 100:

Restructuring the Way We Produce Our Foods Part II

Article #1: Tropical Rain Forests: Earth's Green Belt

100.1. Introduction

"The Sky is Falling!" ... or is it?

"The Sky is Falling!" ... or is it?

Once upon a time there lived a storybook character named Chicken Little, who said the sky was falling—this is about as cheerful as most of the news we're subjected to nowadays, and if it appeared as tomorrow's newspaper headlines, it probably wouldn't even raise many eyebrows in comparison. (It'd make a nice National Enquirer headline!) In gathering material for this lesson, I was soon saturated with one piece of "bad news" after another—certainly no shortage of negative environmental factors to be found, and I began to wonder how I could ever present both the good and the bad sides of the story without sounding like a "doomsday prophet"! Yet, reality is made up of both sides. So, before going any further with our discussion on ecology, let me clarify what my intentions are in opening our Pandora's box of world problems. I'd much rather be the bearer of good news, so my purpose in this lesson is a dual one: to admit our mistakes honestly and still count our blessings, the good news being that we're finally discovering the limited scope and potential of self-consciousness, and evolving to an awareness of the broader scope and potential of our collective (or universal) consciousness, i.e., what we do to others, we do to ourselves. We are creating our mutual destiny daily, and what we create also depends upon the strength of our will to live. Since negative attitudes are self-fulfilling and self-defeating, please keep your chin up when reading this lesson. Its purpose is also not to attempt to predict future events, climates, or cataclysms, but to evaluate our world as it is and could be. The question is not so much whether the sky is falling, it is whether we will let ourselves fall. If we give up hope, and throw in our cards early in the game, we give up our destiny as well. My purpose in writing this lesson is to present the rose in all its beauty and to smell its sweet fragrance, but to watch out for the thorns. I hope the lesson will inspire you and challenge you to discover and create a beautiful future for all of us.

When we see the reality of what is happening to all of us, the total picture can't help but stir up many mixed emotions. Few of us enjoy speculating on potential destruction/ devastation of our planet. We want to be positive and cheerful and would almost rather not hear the bad news at all, but there's also a difference between the bad news given by the broadcaster with little emotion and the bad news that comes with suggestions as to how changes can be made and how we can help ourselves—the latter news is motivated by a desire to help humanity. We can listen and learn from Hamaker, for example, and should get over our resistance to confronting reality. Not only does it keep us ignorant, but avoidance of the truth does nothing to change the situation. When we have a flat tire, we know that we'll have to fix it—a temper tantrum or flood of tears might fit the mood of the occasion, but they won't fix the tire. It's the same with world problems. When we're faced with the complexity and seriousness of our total world reality, the tendency is to become overwhelmed at first. This is only natural. After grudgingly adding up all the environmental factors involved, in our minds, we can't see our earth's state of health without an overwhelming sense of urgency that so much needs to be done—like looking at stacks of dirty dishes the morning after a party, only we have a lot more to clean up on earth. Where to begin? What can "just one" person do? Well, it becomes apparent what "just one" person can do if we look at the world around us—we're already doing it now, every day, all together at every moment, and the continual combined impact of all human action/interaction at once on the globe is no small matter. What "just one" person can do (and does) amounts to a lot since we're all doing it at the same time, and it adds up even more quickly when everyone is doing it constantly.

Our collective energy is just as capable of healing as it is of destroying. Once we imagine what we can do with this incredible healing power if our collective energy is used in a positive way, we have but to realize our fullest potential by living it. Unity and harmony will bring a new dimension of growth to our collective human energy. If we could but see the heights our spirits will reach when we build together, we would shun the depths our spirits sank to with pettiness, violence, and destruction. We would outgrow these primitive rituals—we have no use for them in our quest for a better world.

We must pass through the "crisis point" and bypass the emotional traps that keep us from changing what we dislike, by misdirecting and draining our energy: anger, blame (of self and others), revenge, guilt, self-pity, fear, confusion, delusion, anxiety, wishful thinking, depression, apathy, and inertia. All of these traps can become obsessive; they immobilize us; and, in fact, we often confuse the emotions themselves with actual action. Strong emotions drain us physically as well as mentally, giving the impression that we've expended a lot of energy (we have, but it was misguided and wasted). Emotions do not act—we act—our feelings are incapable of acting on their own (aside from their mental effects). We often resort to them because they offer immediate "satisfaction", an outlet or channel for our feelings—they become harmful when used in excess or to harm others. What is needed is action, after the reaction, not more expenditure of energy in the reaction itself. All time spent wondering "what if?" and "why?" is better used doing something or changing something, or even watching your garden grow or simply smiling at someone.

If we try to submerge negative images into our subconscious minds, we'll never be able to bury them deep enough as long as they exist. Just as with the Pandora's box, as long as the problems remain unsolved, keeping the lid shut won't make them go away. Ostriches have devised an ingenious way of dealing with "scary things they'd rather not see"—if the enemy approaches, they merely bury their heads in the ground—unfortunately, what we don't see or don't know can also hurt us. If we avoid looking at our problems, because we don't want to see the "enemy", how will we know our enemy? We need to know the enemy in order to keep one step ahead of its grasp. Refusing to look at the world as it really is, is like our avoiding mirrors when we have a pimple—we'd rather wait until it goes away. Is that what we're planning on doing with our world problems?

Once upon a time there was a happy ending for every story, and like breathless children listening to a fairy tale, we anticipate the book's final moment of magic and salvation in just the nick of time. Are we lured by the thrill of danger that comes with our defiance of Nature, and thereby daring our life source to react to our defiance? We'll be sadly disappointed when we discover that the knight isn't coming on his horse to carry us off to safety at the last minute, and it's time we realized that the horse has been waiting for us all along in an empty pasture, for it is we ourselves that are meant to be the heroes in this story. We've been writing this one altogether, all our lives, and it's about time we paused for a moment to read the chapter on psychic numbing. We get "tired" of bad news, try to harden ourselves, desensitize ourselves so as to feel less pain, to feel less vulnerable. This is understandable considering the harsh realities we face at times, but it is also a type of psychic defense mechanism we've adopted to deal with our environment—we try to "adjust" our reality to our own particular tolerance level. Whereas we find the ostrich's defense mechanism ludicrous, our amusement should fade when we realize we're doing exactly the same thing with our numbing mechanisms.

Sensitivity is our best defense against numbing apathy— the less we close our eyes to truth, the more we see. Sensitivity can also help us deal with insensitivity around us— we can imagine how little an insensitive person feels because we know how much we feel, as sensitive persons. People of the strongest character, courage, honor, clarity of perception, vision, and greatest physical strength, are often the most sensitive persons around. The more sensitive you are, the more you experience in life.

A bird can't fly until it jumps out of the nest. As we busy ourselves in our nests, rearranging furniture and curling up in front of the fire for a cozy nap, we sometimes hear the distant rumblings of change on the horizon. The thought of jumping from our nest disturbs us, but if we want to feel the freedom of spirit possible in our lives, we'll have to take a chance someday. The light of a new dawn is breaking on the horizon. It's a good day for learning to fly.

100.2. Water, Water Everywhere?

100.2.1. We Don't Miss the Water till the Well Runs Dry. . .

100.2.2. The Lawn

100.2.3. Landscaping

100.2.4. Other watering

100.2.5. Showers

100.2.6. Sinks

100.2.7. Toilets

100.2.8. in the kitchen

100.2.9. Laundry

100.2.10. Around the house

100.2.11. Odds and ends

100.2.12. Soil Drainage

100.2.13. Drought

It can easily cost 500 to 2,000 gallons of water to produce a typical American meal. According to Rep. Tony Coelho (D., Calif.), agriculture accounts for 80% of all water consumption in America. It takes the use of 408 gallons of water to get one serving of chicken to a dinner able, 12 gallons for one 8-ounce baked potato, 18 gallons for one serving of green beans and 6 gallons for a salad. A dinner roll takes 26 gallons of water, plus 100 gallons for the pat of butter on it. That adds up to 570 gallons for one "conventional" meal. A steak alone costs 2,607 gallons of water. On the average, it takes about 1,630,000 gallons of water to feed one American for a year. (Parade Magazine, Sunday newspaper supplement, 3/25/84.)

It must be obvious that water is, indeed, a very precious resource and one that is all too often taken for granted.

Soil water has three forms: hydroscopic, gravitational, and capillary. Hydroscopic water is chemically-bound in the soil constituents and unavailable to plants. Gravitational water is water that normally drains out of the pore spaces of the soil after a rain, and if drainage is poor, it is this water that causes the soil to be soggy and unproductive. Excessive drainage, on the other hand, makes capillary water run short sooner, and plants suffer from drought. Plants depend on capillary water for their supply of moisture, so the ability of soil to hold water against the pull of gravity is important. Organic matter and good soil structure add to this supply of water in soils. Plants can't extract the last drop of capillary water from soil since the attraction of soil materials for it is greater than the pull exerted by the plant roots. The point at which these two forces are equal is called the willing coefficient of a soil, that is, the percentage of water in a soil when water loss from transpiration exceeds renewal of the water by capillary means. Medium-textured loams and silt loams (because of their faster rate of movement of moisture from lower depths of the root zone, and the fact that they can bring up moisture from greater depths than either sands or clays) provide the best conditions of available (but not excessive) soil moisture for best plant growth. (Rodale Press)

The following excerpts on water come from The Survival of Civilization, page 22:

"The microorganisms in a rich soil build the soil to take in rainwater and hold it in storage. The proper proportion of water in protoplasm is 90%. It is important that protoplasm be maintained as a dilute solution. Water evaporates from the leaves of the plant, concentrating the protoplasm solution. It is characteristic of water solutions that the water of the more dilute solution will pass through a membrane into a more concentrated solution. This force of osmosis is very powerful. It is the force that moves the water to the top of a sequoia. Water is, of course, necessary to all cells in order for them to function. Cells have a way of opening up and engulfing the very large molecules of protoplasm. Since the cells are alive and expend energy, they probably pass the I molecules or its components from one cell to another until it reaches the part of the plant where it is needed. If dry weather depletes the water held by the soil and the microorganisms to the concentration of the water in the leaf cells, all protoplasm feeding stops and growth is arrested.

"Irrigation is not the answer to water shortage problems. If all farmers irrigated, the underground water supplies would soon be depleted (as they are in the process of becoming now). The answer is to keep feeding microorganisms until the aerated zone is 18 to 24 inches deep and capable of holding all the rain that falls until the excess can seep into the subsoil and reach the underground aquifer, instead of running off the surface and taking the soil with it. It will take a decade or two for roots and earthworms to deepen the topsoil significantly below plow depth.

"Nitrogen from the air is the ultimate source of most of the nitrogen in the protein compounds of the microorganism protoplasm, the solid matter of which is about 2/3 protein. It is not, however, the principal source of crop-growth nitrogen. The same is true of carbon, which is the dominant element in all organic matter. The leaves take in CO_2 and give off oxygen, retaining the carbon for the necessary carbohydrate construction and for energy requirements. When the plant dies, it goes into the soil or on the soil where it is used as a part of the food supply of various soil organisms. Eventually it is all carried into the soil, principally by earthworms as they combine leaf mold with minerals ground in their gizzards to produce microorganisms. Their castings are almost all microorganisms, and a source of protoplasm not overlooked by the hair roots of plants. Since the rye plant has been estimated to have a root system seven miles long, it is apparent that plants can do a lot of searching for protoplasm. The root tips grow a lot faster than microorganisms can move, so the microorganisms are easy prey to roots. When in intimate proximity to the cell, the flow of protoplasm begins.

"The root cannot take in the cell membrane of the organism. The membranes are held against the root by the pressure of other cells forced against the root by the diffusion pressure between the microorganism cells and the root cells. Soon the older root cells are all plugged with microorganism cell membranes, which subsequently turn the brown color of all mature roots. The root functions simply as a pipe, while the rapidly growing white root tips continue to devour cell protoplasm. "If the protoplasm of the root cells gets too dry, then the protoplasm intake must stop because osmosis requires that the more concentrated solution in the microorganisms must flow toward a more dilute solution in the plant cells. For this reason the root tips (which can take in soil water) constantly remove water from the zone where they are feeding, and the water is moved upward toward the leaves, keeping the cells saturated and evaporating the excess.

"The intestinal tract of all animals works essentially the same way, except that the microorganisms and their food supply are inside Intestines and the protoplasm compounds feed into the intestinal wall where they are picked up by a blood vessel system for sorting out in the liver. Excess water passes readily through the system and is ultimately evaporated from the sweat glands or extracted by the kidneys and excreted in the urine.

"Nature has used just one basic design for all the living organisms with variations as required by each type of organism."

As we said in our section on chemical fertilizers and pesticides, plant and animal digestive systems will readily pass water into the plant or animal, so if toxic compounds are in solution in the water, they too will pass readily into the plant/animal.

"We see, then, that the rate of production of microorganisms will be high if: the soil contains a large surface area of available elements; a large supply of plant residue for carbon and a little nitrogen; plus, the nitrogen that many organisms can take from the air as the air breathes in and out of the soil with temperature changes; water and the other necessary factors from the air."

We have seen that the key to achieving crop growth depends on a delicate balance between minerals available/absorbed, water, climate, and so on. It must be obvious by now that we cannot just "dump chemical fertilizers onto the soil at random and pour lots of water onto it," and expect to match nature's achievements! Irrigation is not the same as natural rainfall (i.e., rain as it should be, not acid rain) in the first place; in the second place, most water is full of chemicals by the time it flows through our taps.

100.2.1. We Don't Miss the Water Till the Well Runs Dry. . .

We will also talk about drought later in this section and again in our section on climate later on in this lesson. Barry Slogrove (ecologist) says the Southern hemisphere is suffering droughts like never before because of the transfer of cloud cover across the equator to the north—this is visible on satellite photographs. The results are felt in Australia, which has the worst drought in human history, and also in Africa, which has also suffered severe drought. The rain volume may be the same, but the precipitation patterns are different, which means that less moisture actually gets into the soil. (Slogrove also maintains the view that an Ice Age is on the way.)

In 1984, much of Texas suffered under heavy drought and in the Austin area, water use during the spring of 1984 far exceeded previous spring consumption (and exceeded peak use in the summer of 1983). To encourage public awareness of water use, the newspaper published water consumption figures daily. Voluntary water conservation was at first in effect (each day, households whose last number of their street address is the daily given number may water their lawns on that day—this amounts to watering every fifth day only). Mandatory water conservation began after three consecutive days at 150 million gallons usage. In Corpus Christi, Texas, mandatory water rationing to limit lawn watering and car washing began July 1 in this drought-plagued city. The new ordinance, carrying a fine of up to $200 for violators, was to continue indefinitely until the Nueces River watershed was replenished. (Alice, Texas, also instituted mandatory rationing in May.) Corpus Christi had called for voluntary water conservation in May, but officials said that residents didn't heed the request.

The following tips on conserving our precious water supplies were offered by the Austin newspaper, suggestions which can be put into practice by all Americans to save water and to increase consciousness so that water won't be taken for granted and wasted so often.

100.2.2. The Lawn

Water deeply and infrequently to get a good root structure, which can't be achieved by frequent shallow waterings. Water long enough for water to seep down to the roots. Check soil before watering; if it springs back when you step on the grass, it doesn't need water yet. Water during cool parts of the day, and don't water while the wind blows, because wind increases evaporation. Oscillating sprinklers are among the least efficient because they spray many thin streams of water high in the air. Use sprinklers that make big drops and keep the water close to the ground. Among the better sprinklers are the smaller versions of sprinklers used by golf courses or park operators, which rotate, sending pulses of water in a circular pattern (Rainbird makes these). Try a drip hose in odd-shaped areas. The least evaporation occurs when water is applied directly to the ground with a perforated hose or other drip irrigation method. Don't water the gutter—arrange hoses and sprinklers so the water doesn't run onto concrete. Even in instances where it appears the water is running off a sidewalk onto a lawn, a large part of the water evaporates. If you have an automatic sprinkler system, set the timer to operate between 4 and 6 a.m., when demand on city systems is at its lowest. Don't scalp your lawn. Set your mower to cut no lower than 1 1/2 inches; better still, 2 inches. Taller grass holds moisture better. A rule of thumb is not to cut more than 1/3 of the height of the grass. If planting new sod or grass, prepare the soil with compost so water won't run off (the same idea works in gardens).

100.2.3. Landscaping

Use native trees and shrubs that are hardiest in your area. Put a layer of mulch around trees and plants. Not only does this conserve moisture and keep the soil around plants cooler, but it also adds nutrients if leaves are used, have some weeds for insects and balance (polyculture), but not so many that they are taking too much water away from vegetables.

100.2.4. Other watering

Don't use a hose as a broom, to "sweep" sidewalks and driveways, etc. Use a rake or broom. Use a bucket or a water can to water hanging plants—using a hose to go from basket to basket wastes more water than makes it to the plants. Cut down on car washing (if nothing else, for the sake of your paint job), and wash with a bucket of soapy water, using the hose only for rinsing. Put a nozzle on your hose.

For almost every outdoor job, you'll save water by using an attachment that lets you turn the water on and off at the end of the hose rather than at the faucet. (Don't forget to turn the faucet off when done.) Wash your car at a commercial car wash, since the high-pressure equipment used by most will wash your car in less time and with less water than most people use at home.

100.2.5. Showers

Showers usually take no more than 1/2 as much water—sometimes less—than bathtubs. If you don't have a shower, you can still save several gallons of water simply by reducing the water in your tub baths by a few inches.

You can check your use by plugging the drain during a shower and comparing the water level with your normal bath. Also, bathing and shampooing at the same time cuts water use. Take a shorter shower. Most showers use 6 to 10 gallons of water per minute. If you install a low-flow shower head, that can be cut to 2 1/2 to 4 gallons per minute, and the new shower head will pay for itself within a few months.

100.2.6. Sinks

Use aerators in sinks. Aerators which are made to screw into most standard faucets will cut your water flow. Check faucets for leaks. Even a small drip from a worn washer can waste more than 50 gallons of water a day—steady drips can waste hundreds. When brushing your teeth, turn off the water until you rinse your mouth. (Children can be helped to develop this habit while still young.) When shaving, partially fill the sink to rinse your razor rather than rinsing with running water.

100.2.7. Toilets

Cut down on the number of flushes. An old-style toilet can use five or more gallons per flush! Frankly, that's a lot of water for a cupful of urine. Newer models use 3 1/ 2 gallons per flush or less. Cut the water level in the toilet. Fill two one-quart bottles with water and replace the caps. Put them in the tank, to reduce the water used per flush. Don't use bricks for this because they will crumble and possibly damage the toilet. You can also reduce the level of water with the toilet's own equipment. Many have adjusting screws. In older toilets gently bend the float rod downward to reduce water level. Check for leaks. Add a few drops of food coloring to the tank. If the color appears in the bowl in a few minutes (without flushing), you have a leak. Common sources of leaks are that the water level in the tank is too high or that the flapper ball and other parts are worn. Some plumbing supply stores and many stores that specialize in energy conservation sell inexpensive devices such as plastic water dams which will help reduce the amount of water used in each flush.

100.2.8. in the kitchen

Don't rinse the dishes with running water. If you have two sinks, fill one with hot rinse water. If you have only one sink, buy a small plastic tub for rinsing or gather washed dishes in a rack and rinse them when done with a spray device or by pouring water over them. Don't rinse vegetables with running water. Rinse them in a partially filled sink or pan. Cooking with less water, such as by steaming, saves water and retains more vitamins in the food. (Of course, we might note here that not cooking retains even more vitamins!) Those who use garbage disposals are encouraged not to cut the disposal on (with water running all the while) for every little scrap, but to let them accumulate a bit—better still is to compost your scraps, of course. Dishwashers use about 25 gallons of water per load. Not only is this wasteful, but some people don't even fill the dishwasher with dishes each time. Any housewife who had to walk several miles for water and haul it back to the house would definitely think twice about using 25 gallons to wash dishes, that's for sure. Some new dishwashers have cycles that use as little as four gallons of water, but I still wouldn't promote the use of dishwashers. (Again, think of all the dishes and pots and pans you'll save washing on a raw food diet ...)

100.2.9. Laundry

Use the washing machine for full loads only. Each load requires as much as 35 gallons of water — (some older machines actually use as much as 59 gallons). Try hauling that from a well. If you must wash only a few pieces, do it by hand. If you replace your machine, be sure to buy one with adjustable water levels. If you have a small family, consider a European-style, front-loading machine, which uses far less water than top loaders. If you live in a city, washing clothes, cars, etc., can be done on week-days since the heaviest demand on the water system tends to be on weekends. Check for leaks. In many older homes, the washer isn't located in the most convenient spot, which means that leaks can go undetected for weeks. Use cold water when possible.

100.2.10. Around the house

Turn down the hot water thermostat. High settings can waste water because you turn on more cold water at the faucet to mix with the hot. Check your buyer's guide or ask the store where you bought the appliance if you don't understand the range of settings on the dial. (If you don't know where the thermostat is, find out before an emergency.)

Evaluate your inside plant-watering schedule—check before watering—many plants die from overwatering as well as underwatering.

Insulate hot water pipes. The less time it takes for hot water to reach the tap, the more water you save. Check for system leaks. Turn off all faucets, then check your water meter. If it continues to run, you've got a leak.

Even if you don't live in an area that is prone to drought, it would be well to adopt as many water-saving habits as possible, because water is wasted needlessly, and is being used faster than nature can replace it in many places. As we said, children can be encouraged to develop a conscious attitude toward natural resources from the very beginning so that their conscientious habits become second nature to them—this is always easier than making the change later on in life. The next time you and your children brush your teeth, imagine that you live in a country where you must go to a distant well and carry your water home. How much water would you use in a day for all your needs? Could you imagine carrying that extra gallon or two that each of your family members lets run down the sink while brushing their teeth? It would then become apparent how wasteful this really is. Nor could you afford to carry the extra few gallons that run down the drain each time you rinse your hands, a glass, or something to eat. These all add up—if you're fond of mental exercise, you may want to calculate your average daily household water use in gallons and multiply by 365 for a year's use. You'll be amazed.

100.2.11. Odds and Ends

Use dishwashing detergent sparingly. I've lived for months in areas where our dishwashing consisted of rinsing dishes in streams without even using soap at all, and the only available water was, of course, cold water. Since dishes were rinsed right after eating, there was certainly no real food decomposition yet, and we all remained as healthy as ever. Most people seem to think they need "lots of suds", but soap residue is unhealthy—and more suds also mean more water for rinsing. If dishes have been sitting a few days, soaking them first will help, and a pad that is "scratchy" but made not to harm dishes (such as those sold for Teflon surfaces) can be used to get them clean with very little soap.

If children want to play in the sprinkler in the hot summer, put it somewhere where the water can serve a triple purpose: water the grass, entertain the kids, and serve as their shower/bath that day. Many of us in today's society have become so "clean" conscious that we actually shower and bathe too often for our real needs, especially if we "scrub daily with soap". This destroys the skin's natural oils and protective bacteria—while many people believe that their "cleanliness will protect them from germs/illness", it is more the opposite that is true: they'll be hardier if they don't attempt to "sterilize" their bodies. For freshness sake, we may take a quick shower/rinse with a loofa sponge or washcloth. As children, my 2 sisters and I often took our baths all three at the same time—another way to save water.

If everyone were to develop even the minimal suggestions given above for conserving water, billions of gallons of water would be saved constantly with very little effort, i.e., just by cutting wasted water use alone. Imagine the following savings:

Gallons of Water Used	Households that change	Gallons of water saved
59-gal. washing machine to 35-gal. one	1,000	24,000 gal. each time
	1,000,000	24,000,000 gal. each time
Not running a gal. of water down the drain while brushing teeth	50,000,000 people	50.000.000 gal. daily
Fixing a drip that wastes 100 gal. daily	1.000,000 people	100,000,000 gal. daily

Miscellaneous: 5 gal. of water saved daily by any change made	10,000,000 people	50,000,000 gal. daily

We can see how quickly this all adds up!

100.2.12. Soil Drainage

Many soils in the world have only enough water reaching the drainage layer to keep small streams flowing at intervals of 6 or 8 feet; the rest of the gravel layer has become infiltrated by clay, and the gravel has begun to rise toward the surface. We are in the process of losing the drainage layer on a worldwide scale. The destruction of the drainage layer has been further intensified because some farmers have installed toxic plastic drain pipes a few feet below the surface in order to short-cut the percolating water and thereby further dry up the drainage layer.

Over 25 years ago, John Hamaker dug a pond in East Texas, and along 250 cut into the base of the hillside, there were only 2 or 3 sand channels where the water was still coming down the hill—all the rest had been sealed up by clay long ago. The water simply penetrated the 8" of sandy loam, to the dense clay beneath it and drifted downhill—an ideal set-up for sheet erosion if anyone tried to plow the land. Topsoil there eroded in heavy rains. There is a penalty for failure to maintain the drainage layer.

When lands begin to fall off in yield, they usually cease to have useful productivity in a few decades, and no amount of agricultural chemicals can bring that production back or keep it from dropping to a lower yield—at this point, the unused, fine rock material has stopped coming up from the subsoil because there isn't anymore. During the few decades when the soil collapses in yield, the fine material is used up and the major part of the surface area of rock is gone, i.e., the availability of elements has all but ended. This is why remineralization, as discussed later in this lesson, is needed—not random chemical "fertilizer" application, which is either unbalanced and/or lacks elements needed for proper growth of microorganisms, and thus, plant life itself.

All underground water eventually drains into a stream bed, or lake; it then comes up in springs at a lower elevation or runs directly into the ocean. The point is that the capacity of the subsoil drainage layer in any area has been geared to the annual rainfall and water penetration under natural conditions. When we alter the amount of water reaching and being maintained in the drainage layer, we are in trouble. If we decrease the amount of water by losing it to surface run-off, we will lose water and therefore sand and gravel from the drainage layer. This sand and gravel cannot be replaced. Arid soils have very little drainage layer left, simply because a drainage layer which isn't kept full of slowly flowing water will clog up with fine, worn-out particles which will eventually displace the drainage sands and gravels and lift them to the topsoil. The sea salts carried in by infrequent rains accumulate in the soils for lack of sufficient water to establish drainage systems and thereby flush the salts back to the ocean. When dry lands are irrigated, they tend to become water-logged for lack of drainage. The salts dissolve and are left on the surface when surface moisture evaporates. The best use of arid soils is to put them back into grass, the way most of them were when the land was settled. With remineralization, more and better grass can be grown for animals. Many remineralized arid and semi-arid lands could also be afforested with valuable drought-resistant trees and shrubs (e.g., pistachio, jojoba). The water left in the underground reservoirs should be reserved for people and livestock. The refill rate of the reservoirs is much too slow to support irrigation, as shown by steadily-falling water tables in most exploited areas.

The mineral requirements to support the growth of soil organisms (hence plants) are a natural balance of the available (to the microorganisms) elements in the total mixture of the rocks on the top layers of the earth's crust, and the natural balance of the elements dissolved and suspended in sea water brought with the clouds. The mineral balance of salted soils must be restored by remineralization and by allowing large quantities of plant refuse to go back into the topsoil. The plant refuse would provide the carbon requirements of the microorganisms; the gases in the air and water complete their food requirements.

100.2.13. Drought

The Ethiopian drought is a forewarning of widespread regional water crises in the 1990s that could rival the energy crisis of the last decade, according to a study by the Worldwatch Institute. Falling water tables and dry riverbeds indicate a widespread overuse of water resources, and if current trends continue, fresh water in many areas may become a constraint on economic activity and food production over the coming decades. In the United States, areas where excessive withdrawal of underground water supplies threatens its future availability include the High Plains from Nebraska to Texas; the Colorado River basin, particularly the areas around Phoenix and Tucson; the Florida and Pacific coasts; and much of California. The report cites statistics from the U.S. Geological Survey estimating that the Ogallala Aquifer, used for irrigating one-fifth of

U.S. cropland is now half-depleted under 2,200,000 acres of Texas, New Mexico, and Kansas. Rising pumping costs and falling well yields associated with the depletion of the Ogallala are causing farmers to take land out of irrigation. Still, most officials continue to take a "frontier approach" that looks to dams and other multibillion-dollar diversion projects as a solution, failing to see the unfortunate irony in the situation. While the government pays farmers to idle rain-fed cropland in an effort to avoid price-depressing surpluses, farmers are exhausting a unique, underground water reserve to grow these same crops. The government is encouraging waste of water from the Ogallala by giving farmers a depletion tax break based on the drop in the water level under their land. Instead, says World watch, the government should be taxing that water use.

If we continue to ignore warning signs of future water shortages and close our eyes to the waste and overuse of decreasing water supplies, we will pay dearly for our indifference. We need not imagine what our lives would be like without water—we need only look at the suffering people in Africa to see the stark reality of what extensive drought can do. Television brought the starving, emaciated bodies of drought victims into our living rooms in 1984, and it is a painful sight, but one that we must face up to. Thousands of people have been reduced to skeletons as the drought takes its toll.

In the African country of Mauritania, not only must they cope with the severe drought plaguing 6ther African countries as well, but they must also cope with the spreading Sahara desert—one government official says the parched and rainless country "could disappear from the map in 10 years and become only sand." The Sahara is literally pushing southward; crews along a key highway passing through 690 miles of Mauritania wage a daily battle with the desert, trying to keep the road clear of wind-blown sands. Crops are gone after being withered by a drought that has affected some areas since 1969 and covered by the shifting dunes of the Sahara. With two-thirds of its land already swallowed up by the desert, Mauritania now produces only about 5% of the food it needs. Cereal production used to average 100,000 tons annually but was estimated at 15,000 tons in 1984. The government is trying to, drill holes for water in the countryside to slow the rush to the towns. Vast herds of cattle (about 80%) have died or have been driven into neighboring Senegal for grazing (Senegal agreed to allow up to 300,000 animals to graze there), but now Senegal is also suffering from a drought. Although it defies all laws of common sense to keep cattle in areas so dry that even human beings can scarcely find enough to eat (and many don't), these people are raising animals because they've done so as long as they can remember; they don't know any other lifestyle. (If we are tempted to pass judgment, let's look at our own Society— we've certainly made enough environmental errors ourselves, wasting resources for rapid gains that result in long-term losses. Being more educated, what excuse would justify our own lack of foresight?) Some Mauritanians have goats, and donkeys are, of course, a necessity for those who depend on them for work. The nomadic way of life has been a tradition for many people here. In the past, during the worst times of drought, nomads moved to farming areas, then returned to their old way of life when pasture became available. International aid agencies now argue that there is no longer sufficient grazing land or water to sustain a nomadic life, and the U.S. embassy's 1984 economic report said there was no question that Mauritania's centuries-old nomadic way of life has been irreparably damaged. Nevertheless, those who can survive as nomads still cling to life and try to continue on as best, they can. In all these countries affected by the drought, Africans struggle to survive with a severe shortage of water, limited resources, and less opportunities for education than we have here. Their courage should be a lesson to all of us who have been blessed with advantages that we far too often take completely for granted. Some of us panic at the mere thought of missing a single meal or consider ourselves unfortunate if we can't afford a new outfit of clothes. Some of us would even feel underprivileged if we couldn't own a yacht. As a nation of consumers, we pride ourselves on our "high standard of living" and are dazzled by a vision of "progress" that has led many of us to become obsessed with "success", this

694

success being measured in terms of our wealth and possessions. Swept along in the tide, inundated by commercials in the media urging us to "buy more", we tend to forget that what we perceive as a normal way of life here in this country is very rare in most of the world. In Lesson 53 we mentioned that our country uses more of the world's natural resources than any other country; our "high" standard of living is more expensive than we may care to admit.

Objectively speaking, we may be accused of being selfish. How do we justify this use of natural resources? Are we using them to better the lives of all our brothers and sisters around the world, to make the world a better place for all human beings to live in? Or are we using them to add to our own comfort, and patting ourselves on the back for our technological marvels, choosing to forget that millions of people in the world are still hungry? We have a right to survive, to secure the things that we need for our survival in this world—this is true. But if we already have 6 pairs of shoes and find ourselves gazing longingly into a store window at "just one more pair" we might stop and ask ourselves why we want to have more than we need. What is it within us that keeps us unsatisfied? Why do we never seem to have enough?

We've trailed a bit off the subject of water here, but it is time to see ourselves honestly in the mirror. It is time to appreciate the things that we have, because it is too easy to forget where all these things come from if we don't stop for a moment to realize how precious water and all our natural resources are, and to do everything in our power to appreciate them and conserve them all, before "the well" runs dry.

100.3. Ecology and Climate

100.3.1. Deforestation

100.3.2. Carbon Dioxide—Global Climate Changes—Weather Patterns

100.3.3. Warmer or Colder?

100.3.4. The Glacial-Interglacial Cycle

100.3.5. "Hope Springs Eternal"

100.3.1. Deforestation

The earth's remaining forest cover is being destroyed by human exploitation at an almost unbelievable rate: about 50 million acres a year, or 50 acres per minute. Trees are cut down by hungry people to get fuel or a few more crops off demineralized jungle soils, and the lumber business takes its own heavy toil. Our forests and jungles must be saved. Our rain forests have been called "the lungs of the earth", because so much of the earth's life-giving vegetation is contained in them. The present level of carbon dioxide over "normal" levels will increase 50% in the next decade. Many jungles are now living off the minerals in the decaying wood of dead trees, but they are usually in areas of high rainfall, and if minerals are added to the decaying organic matter, the trees will increase their growth rate and be immensely valuable in taking up and storing carbon from the atmosphere.

When water evaporates, oxygen is released into the air. Photosynthesizing plants are also a source of oxygen; leaves of the trees absorb carbon from the air and produce oxygen, releasing it into the air. We are disturbing the whole oxygen-carbon dioxide balance of our biosphere with our unwise activity.

Volkswagen Foundation has about 300,000 acres of former virgin forest land in Brazil, that is now used for an expanding cattle export operation involving deforestation at an average 13,000 acres per year (Grainger, 1980). Weyerhauser Corporation has 6,000 square kilometers of timber concession in the fragile rain forests of Indonesia (Myers, 1979).

• If the jungles are not saved, John Hamaker says we have no chance at survival, and that they cannot be saved unless croplands of starving people are remineralized. Rain forests have been virtually eliminated from most parts of West Africa, Southern Asia, and the Caribbean. The world's forests are also affected by climatic extremes, soil degeneration, insects, diseases, worsening climate, air pollution and acid rains—fires also ravage our forests, especially in dry seasons and times of drought. As more forests burn, a cycle of destruction actually takes place, because forest fires contribute to adverse conditions that, in turn, accelerate the destruction of more forests. In forest fires, not only are more precious trees lost, but destruction occurs on all these levels: climatic stress (including record heat and drought) when trees burn, carbon dioxide increases in the atmosphere, so pollution—and acid rain—are increased (they're already caused by burning fossil fuels and by auto/vehicle and industrial exhausts/emissions) deforestation and spreading deserts chronic insect and/or disease epidemics

Data on tropical forest fires is scarce, but it is reported that the nutrient-poor soils and highly carbonaceous (mineral-poor) vegetation there burns quickly when moisture is withheld for a time. Wide-scale drought and acid rains not only lead to destruction of forests; they can also lead to more tropical forest fires. At present rates of human deforestation and desertification, most researchers say these forests are scheduled for virtual extinction in 15-30 years.

The April 1961, American Forests magazine warned of the explosive fire situation building up in U.S. Forest lands—this was already 23 years ago.

	1964-1975	1976-1978	% Increase

Average # of fires per year	119.000	207,000	74%
Average total acreage burned per year	2,720,000	3,612,000	33%

"War Technology Comes to the Forests", by J. A. Savage, was printed in Friends of the Earth's Not Man Apart (December 1980) and described how the U.S. Forest Service is adapting technologies used in Vietnam to "modern" silviculture. In addition to the arborcide Agent Orange, flame-throwers and bombs of napalm-like jelly are used to achieve a "clean burn" of all the "debris" left after clearcutting. With these methods, no "slash" (from the slash-and-burn technique) is left, only "charred dirt". I assume their "clean" overlooks the damage to the environment and toxicity of the chemicals involved. In 1984, nationwide publicity of Vietnam veterans who had been exposed to Agent Orange revealed its effects in victims and their children; I hope the U.S. Forest Service isn't making more victims.

American Forests (March 1969) said that in a few years all varieties of trees were dying in a tract of forest in the Adirondack Mountains, except for hemlock and tamarack. Insects that attacked the trees multiplied greatly in the same span of time. The same thing that happened to this forest land is happening in all of the forests and jungles. The last of the minerals have come up in the forest lands, as in the croplands. Over the last 30 to 60 years, the finer fraction of used rock has been turned into subsoil, greatly reducing the surface area, and therefore, protoplasm production. Because these compounds build health, and resistance to disease and insects, the trees become easy prey to parasites. Acid rain (heavy in the northeastern states) has wiped out the last of the carbonates, resulting in excessive acidification of the soil. The lakes of that region have also been acidified. When acidity of water and soil drops below about pH 5.5, it begins to kill off various kinds of microorganisms. Only a few acid-tolerant organisms can survive, and only a few acid-tolerant trees and plants can survive on the poor quality and quantity of protoplasm which the soil provides. No amount of pesticides can stop this dying in a forest—only immediate aerial remineralization can save what's left of it.

In September 1961, W. Schwenke presented a paper on "Forest Fertilization and Insect Buildup". The paper described work done in the previous nine years at the Institute of Applied Zoology at the Forest Research Center, Munich, Germany. The work was based on the observation that forest parasites had greater population density on poor forest soil than on more fertile forest soil, and on the observation that forest soils can be improved by fertilization. They used 1/2 to 1 1/2 tons per acre of limestone plus a light application of NPK. This minimal soil remineralization cut parasite population from 30 to 50%. On some of the oils the effect was still observable nine years after the application. The increase in growth rate produced a value hat far exceeded the cost of fertilizing the soil. Limestone probably has a broader range of elements to support living organisms. This was shown by the observed fact that the lasting effect of the fertilization depended on the minerals that were in the soil before fertilization.

Severe deterioration of tree foliage and declining tree growth are also being observed throughout the Ohio Valley (AP news, April 16, 1984). The damage is a result of air pollution more acidic than the acid rain believed to be destroying freshwater life in the Northeast, according to a scientist who studies the valley trees. Dr. Orie Loucks said the decline can best be explained by the cumulative impact of over 20 years of stress from a combination of air pollutants. One important pollutant was the sulfate emitted from power plant and factory smokestacks. The acidity of the sulfate particles exceeds that of battery acid, he said. The major difference between the air quality of the Ohio Valley and that in the Northeast, he said, is that the sulfate content of the air is significantly higher in the Ohio Valley region (which includes Ohio, Indiana, Pennsylvania, West Virginia, and Kentucky). For some years forest deterioration has been reported in parts of the Northeast and other areas of the world—now Loucks has found that tree damage may be even more severe in the Ohio Valley, where there is a heavy concentration of coal-burning power plants that lack devices to clean emissions. The region is also believed to be the source of much of the acid rain now falling over the Northeast and Canada.

States in the Ohio Valley have been resisting legislation aimed at curbing acid rain through programs requiring modifications of power plant smokestacks, because such measures would mean higher costs for public utilities—but it's now obvious that the cost to life is far greater in the long run. In August 1984, New York became the first state to pass a law to curb acid rain, with legislation designed to reduce smokestack emissions 30% in the next decade. State environmental officials said the cost of the program, including pollution control devices, would add from $2.40 to $4.80 to the monthly utility bill for the consumer by 1991. Which of us would not gladly forfeit the price of a movie or a few magazines, if it would mean better air quality for everyone?

As we said, acid rain also comes from sulfur dioxide from lignite and coal-burning power plants and nitrogen oxides from auto exhausts and factories. It changes chemically in the atmosphere before falling to earth, killing freshwater life, and damaging crops and forests. Acid rain has destroyed fish populations in 200 lakes in the upstate Adirondacks (many lakes have become so acidic that no life can exist in them) and, as we said, has damaged millions of acres. Congress must adopt legislation to require a nationwide reduction of 10,000,000 tons of emissions.

Lewis and Grant (Science, 1/11/80) also present some frightening statistics. On the Colorado section of the Colorado Divide where there is very little industrial pollution in the direction of the prevailing wind, the pH of all precipitation still dropped from 5.43 to 4.63 in just three years. Neutral pH is 7.0. Hamaker says that since the CO_2 curve is almost vertical at the year 1995, we can go back 20 years to 1975 for the start of the 20-year critical period (to be mentioned in a moment) and not be off by more than a couple of years. The pH then must have been about 6.

Acid rain occurs "naturally" in some places—in the Canadian arctic, natural fires in exposed lignite coal beds produce tremendous amounts of sulfur oxides. These chemicals fall to earth, rendering nearby lakes as acidic as lemon juice. Studies of the Greenland ice cap show that acidic depositions on the earth's surface have been rising since the beginning of the industrial age, with the greatest increase occurring since the 1940s. Central Europe seems hardest hit. Forests are dying throughout Czechoslovakia, Poland, and East Germany. In West Germany, 3,700 acres of woodland died from 1978-1983, and 200,000 acres were seriously damaged, the most vulnerable being dense, pure stands of conifers between 20 and 40 years old that will probably not survive another 10 years (Bernhard Ulrich, German biochemist, 1983). Mr. Ulrich estimates that almost 5,000,000 acres of German forest soils are at the threshold where toxic aluminum will begin its lethal work. Industrial emissions drift from England to Scandinavia. The industrial Ruhr and Rhine area in Germany affect most of central Europe, and Russia (the largest burner of sulfur-bearing fuels) is also polluting Finland. America's industrial Midwest helps render the rain acidic in virtually every state east of the Mississippi; much of the Midwest's emissions join those from Canada, acidifying eastern Canada and threatening its fish and forests—two of its chief resources. In the U.S., only some of the Rocky Mountain states and parts of the Southwest enjoy healthy rains of pH 5.5. or more. Crops and temperate zone vegetation cannot grow on acidic soils, so the large number of dead and dying trees in our forests is attributable both to increasing soil acidity and decreasing quantities of available elements. Dead forests burn easily with a hot fire which oxidizes large quantities of atmospheric nitrogen. Lewis and Grant found that the oxides of nitrogen were dominant in the acidic precipitation. The more trees die and burn, the more the soils become acidified, and the more trees must die. There are also a number of mildly acidic gases released from burning wood. These, plus the acidic gases from volcanism (volcanic power or action), are nature's way of bringing on glaciation.

Man's fossil fuel fires are also a big factor in the destruction.

Belgian scientist Genevieve Woillard showed that the final changeover to sub-arctic climate and vegetation (to be discussed later) took only 20 years at previous interglacial to-glacial transitions, as recorded in the undisturbed pollen deposits of Grand Pile, France. In Woillard's study, the change in vegetation was from hazel, oak, and alder to pine, birch, and spruce—that is, a change from warm-weather to cold-tolerant trees. But even more significant: this change is from nut-bearing trees to trees that can't yield a proteinaceous crop. That translates to mean a decline in soil minerals to the point where there are insufficient microorganisms in the soil to grow proteinaceous trees.

It now appears that the 20 years for the change in vegetation can be shortened because of industrial pollution; we are actually speeding up the deterioration process on all fronts, by the sum total of all our environmental errors. Hamaker said: "Judging from the CO_2 curve, we are actually 5 years into such a period." (This was at the time his book was written.)

The Amazon Forest is the largest tropical rain forest left in the world, but it is paying a heavy price for "progress". Deforestation of large tracts (such as Volkswagen's aforementioned tract) is causing a change in the region's climate, something climatologists have warned of for some time. A change in the region's water balance seems to be the result of increased runoff due to deforestation. If so, the long-predicted regional climatic and hydrological changes expected as a result of Amazon deforestation may already be beginning. Increased flooding is the first sign of damage to the Amazonian ecosystem. A heavily deforested area has developed along the edge of the mountains in upper Amazonian Ecuador and Peru during the past 10-plus years, the result of large slices of forests being cleared for roads, housing, and other development, all of which are exposing the land to increased runoff and erosion. Scientists have found that runoff is increasing in the area while rainfall patterns remain the same; this is caused by interference in the process of transpiration—trees take up moisture that falls and send it back into the air. Now that the trees have been eliminated, the recycling process has been curtailed to an extent that the report warns "might eventually convert much of now-forested Amazonia to near desert." Note: While in most areas (such as the North American Great Plains or Western Europe) most of the rainfall represents moisture blown in from the sea, about half of the Amazonian rainfall is water that is recycled within the basin. Thus, in tampering with the balance of ecology in the Amazon rain forest, one tampers with its rainfall cycle as well.

Since population and farming are concentrated along the Amazon's seasonally flooded river margins, scientists warn that the magnitude of damage is potentially great and say that the "rapidity with which relatively-limited forest destruction (which has since increased) appears to have altered the Amazonian water balance, suggests the need for planned development." This is obviously an understatement—planned reforestation and remineralization are also needed to save the Amazon area, before going about any so-called "planned development". When viewing the earth via satellite, you can literally see the moisture that swirls and sweeps outward from the Amazon area—it covers such a large area that it is seen as a giant moving form that takes on a life of its own—rapid development in the Amazon not only tampers with local ecology, it also affects areas farther away that would normally be affected by these huge, moving atmospheric systems of the Amazon.

Throughout the Third World, unchecked erosion is washing away valuable topsoil. Reforestation could stop the process, aid in CO_2 removal, and aid rainfall cycles—it must be a top survival priority. Because it can take years for reforestation's results to be felt, local governments and villagers have been reluctant to take on what appear to be long-term, labor-intensive projects, but they are failing to realize what failure to do so will mean to their ecosystems.

Researchers are working on what they call a "miracle tree", the Leucanna leucocephela, which is an extraordinarily fast-growing, all-purpose, self-fertilizing tree, used for both fodder and timber. Under ideal conditions it reaches a 10-inch circumference in one year.

Arbor Day began in Nebraska in 1872, when more than one million trees were planted to help prevent erosion and moisture loss in a state with few trees. Within two decades, 100,000 acres had been turned into forested preserves. Arbor Day is now a legal holiday in four states and is celebrated in all the states, but please don't wait for Arbor Day to plant trees—do so whenever you can. Fruit trees are especially needed everywhere.

Over 100 countries grow tobacco; flue-curing about 2,500,000 tons annually uses about one hectare of trees for every ton, amounting to about 12.5% of 18-20 million hectares of trees cut yearly, which means about 1 in 8 trees is axed just for drying tobacco! Cropland used for tobacco should be used for growing food instead.

100.3.2. Carbon Dioxide—Global Climate Changes—Weather Patterns

The increase of carbon dioxide in the atmosphere is our most urgent problem. John Hamaker drew a carbon dioxide curve projection in 1979 and said that unless we gained control of the curve shortly after 1985, by 1990 the rate of breakdown of the environment would be occurring much faster than we could repair the damage. However, in order to gain control by 1985, we would have had to start in 1980 to have a fully operating program of soil remineralization, pollution reduction, and so on. As of 1985, few people took seriously what the curve was saying—nevertheless, Hamaker hasn't given up hope for humanity's survival, even though he's also considered the possibility that "if we were to start to work in the next few months, we could have less than a 50% chance of success". He's written countless letters and says three world science organizations finally agreed to meet in 1985—he thinks action is long overdue, with "nature just beginning to show her teeth". While we wait around for statistics and more data, the power of centralized wealth is holding us to a system of soil destruction. World leaders, concerned with what they must do to get re-elected (if they are indeed elected), merely serve the interest of a wealthy minority that controls an economic system that is ruining our lands, keeping millions of people poor and/ or in debt, keeping our countries in debt, and threatening our very survival with destructive weapons, aggressive foreign policies, and decisions that continually compromise the quality of our environment.

The Global 2000 Report to the President was commissioned in 1977 by President Carter and finally released in July 1980, as a three-volume work of over 1,000 pages. The report's findings aren't represented as predictions, but as depictions of conditions likely to develop if there are no changes in public policies. Some of its findings on CO2 were:

- CO2 emissions will increase to 26 to 34,000,000,000 short tons per year, roughly double the CO2 emissions of the mid-70s.

- 446,000,000 hectares (each is 2.47 acres) of CO2-absorbing forests will be lost.

- Burning of much of the wood on 446 million hectares will produce more CO2.

- Decomposition of soil humus will release more CO2.

By June 1979, the percent of increase of CO2 over an assumed "normal" level of 290 ppm was about 15%. In 1985, it could be 18%. By 1990, it could be 22% (50% more than it is now). Yet we go on bringing carbon out of the ground and putting it into the atmosphere.

John Gribbin (New Scientist, 4/9/81), noting the intensification of worldwide forest destruction and fossil fuel combustion, reports that the present annual CO2 increase has jumped to 2 to 4 ppm, and "is increasing rapidly today, in 1981". (Hamaker's CO2 curve projection could even prove conservative.)

"The Role of CO2 in the Process of Glaciation", published in April 1980, was written as a concise explanation of the glacial process which could be understood by the

U.S. Congress, at a time when the CO2 problem was just being recognized by some of its members. It appears in Hamaker's book and refers to the relationship that has been virtually never considered by the hundreds of researchers of glaciation, starting with the first "Great Ice Age" theory of Louis Agassiz in 1837 (Imbrie and Imbrie, 1979).

This excess carbon dioxide is causing what is known as "the greenhouse effect "because carbon dioxide behaves like the glass in a greenhouse, permitting the sun's rays to reach the earth, but not allowing the heat to escape. The effect is like that of a "thermal blanket" around the globe. As a result, some scientists think that the earth will become warmer, but others, including John Hamaker, say that it is now getting colder. All scientists now agree that carbon dioxide levels are too high, and with acid rain, forest fires, deforestation, and trees dying from soil demineralization, CO2 levels continue to increase. Nature will complete her necessary cycles and go about her own self-healing processes, just as our bodies do. We'd do well to understand her cycles and healing crises better, and offer help instead of waiting for chronic illness to set in. We tend to forget that the earth is very much alive, and a living being/entity (albeit a large one!)— it regulates itself as surely as our bodies do. Because we need the earth to survive, its state of health is very fundamentally—and really—speaking, as important as our own.

I'll present both the warm and cold predictions to show how complex climate "analysis" becomes—all environmental factors interrelate to affect it. Having considered their total impact on our ecology and weather, heard both sides (warm/cold) of the story, and watched worldwide weather trends these past years, my intuition tends to believe scientists who say the world is cooling. In any case, we can't deny that our planet is being manipulated (and often assaulted) on all sides daily by millions of its inhabitants. Some of these assaults are very serious; we discussed long, periods of time that some radioactive waste materials remain dangerous in Lesson 53—this is only one example. Life Scientists know of chemical medicines adverse effects in the body. Can you imagine how our planet's health is affected and weakened by millions of daily assaults on its body?

The saying "do unto others as you would have them do unto you" is not just a suggestion on how to be "nice". It says, in essence, that what you do unto others you do unto yourself—more and more we see how true this is. Now we must also do unto our planet as we would have our planet do unto us, for what we do to our planet, we do to ourselves.

100.3.3. Warmer or Colder?

Before continuing, let's clarify the fact that scientists who see the world as cooling do not necessary dispute the greenhouse effect's warming potential in and of itself—some see a preliminary warming as part of an "energy booster" or catalyst in the Ice Age transition process: the tropics do become hotter/drier as precipitation increases farther north, but increased cloud cover and other factors, to be discussed later, lead to increased cooling conditions.

Let's take a look at the two opinions ... warmer or colder:

In the fall of 1983. the federal government, based on an Environmental Protection Agency report, said that a "dramatic warming of the earth's climate could begin in the 1990s because of the greenhouse effect, with potentially serious consequences for global food production, changes in rainfall and water availability, and a probable rise in coastal waters". The report said that "levels of $CO2$ in the air created by burning of fossil fuels could result in an increase of 3.6. degrees Fahrenheit by the middle of the next century and a 9-degree rise by 2100, representing an unprecedented rate of atmospheric warming".

"It's going to have a very profound impact on the way we live," said John Topping, staff director for the EPA's office of air, noise, and radiation. "Some of the effects will be beneficial; some will be detrimental. But our ability to accommodate them will depend much on our planning beforehand. Temperature rises are likely to be accompanied by dramatic changes in precipitation (more rainfall in some areas, more drought in others) and storm patterns and a rise in global average sea level," the study said. "As a result, agricultural conditions will be significantly altered, environmental and economic systems potentially disrupted, and political institutions stressed."

Stephen Seidel, one of the authors of the report, said that milder winters and much warmer summers by the 1990s may no longer be unusual. The report said the trend will occur regardless of what steps are taken to reduce the burning of fossil fuels.

The study said a warmer climate would raise the sea level by expanding the oceans and by melting ice and snow now on land. An increase of only two feet "could flood or cause storm damage to many of the major ports of the world, disrupt transportation networks, alter aquatic ecosystems and cause major shifts in land development patterns". The warming is expected to be greater at the North and South Poles and less at the equator, the EPA said. John Hoffman, head of strategic studies for the agency, said "New York City could have a climate like Daytona Beach (Florida) by 2100".

A major report issued in 1983 by the National Academy of Sciences said that the approaching warming of the earth "is reason for concern, not panic". The report warned, however, that a warming trend and decreased precipitation could "severely affect" the Texas gulf, Rio Grande, upper and lower Colorado River regions; California; and other Western regions. One projection in the report shows a possible reduction in water supply of nearly 50% when the full force of the warming phenomenon is felt after the year 2000. The tone of the academy warning was less urgent than the EPA's, stressing the need for "more intense research". However, the academy found that since (in their opinion) there is no politically or economically realistic way of heading off the greenhouse effect, strategies must be prepared to adapt to a "high temperature world." The EPA report said that even a total ban on coal would only delay the process for a few years, and said that, because the CO2 in the earth's atmosphere retains heat rather than permits it to escape into space, thus creating the greenhouse effect, the buildup of gas will be accompanied by a rise of global surface temperatures, most likely in the range of 2 to 8 degrees F. These projections are roughly similar to those in the EPA report; it is expected that this rise will be accompanied by "rapid climate change, including changes in rainfall patterns, as well as a rise in the sea level of over two feet".

Some additional notes on the greenhouse effect are of importance:

Recent investigations have established that other man-made pollutant trace gases may increase the greenhouse effect by another 50% (Flohn, 1979; Kellogg and Schware, 1981). These gases come primarily from burning vegetation, release of industrial halocarbons (freons), and the denitrification of nitrogen fertilizers in the soil. The Greenhouse Effect by meteorologist Harold Bernard, issues a strong warning that the heating effects alone will likely be devastating to humanity due to increasing climatic stress; agriculture in particular will suffer greatly. He cites increasing storminess with tornados, hurricanes, floods, searing "dust bowl"-type droughts, water depletion, and massive forest fires if we continue on the fossil fuel route, presenting a whole bank of reasons against doing so.

The last few years have seen dramatic changes in precipitation—more rainfall in some areas, more drought in others— but these are also part of the weather forecast given by scientists who say the world is cooling. Apparent warming trends could be superseded by cooling trends in the long run, if we are due for transition into a glacial period.

Systematic measurements of atmospheric CO2 began only as late as 1958 (Calder, 1975). Most climatologists seem fond of repeating the dangerous oversimplification of CO 2's greenhouse effect, that is, that the earth will warm up as a result.

In a 1977 paper, Hamaker asked, "How Rapidly is CO2 Increasing in our Atmosphere?" In 1977, a National Academy Sciences panel on energy and climate provided a frightening statistic (Charles Keeling, Science, 9/2/77). Keeling said there'd been a 13% rise since the Industrial Revolution began. Alarming is the fact that five of this 13% had occurred since 1962". That same Science article discussed the oversimplified computer models of CO2's "general warming" effect and stated that there are some scientists who "privately suggest" that because of "complex feedback phenomena ", global cooling could result.

Hamaker says that even if the average temperature of the atmosphere is getting warmer, it is false to assume polar ice will melt and temperate zones will move toward the poles. According to Hamaker, "the experts have given us a time scale for weather changes that is longer than we have. Many things are operating at once to affect climate. They all have long overlapping time lags so that we cannot say that this happens, then this, and then this. But the first stage of glaciation, which is initiated by a change from temperate zone to northern latitude types of trees, and by dying of tropical forests, is here now."

Hamaker says "the theory that the world will get warmer is based on the absurd idea that the earth's average temperature depends solely on the sun's energy and the heating effect of atmospheric CO2. On that basis these scientists have projected a rise in temperature in the next century when the CO2 has doubled, so they have drawn a line tangent to the recorded curve and ending up in the next century." He disagrees with the projection, saying that nature is clearly drawing a curve that is constantly increasing at an accelerating rate of increase, and the scientists have merely decided that nature must change her ways to suit their predictions.

The time to stop the onset of glaciation is before it starts, because it starts with the destruction of agriculture. Hamaker says that we must act now, before our technological capacity to remineralize the soil is lost in the chaos of a world of starving and dying nations. As we said, climatic cycles and factors may overlap, but we can identify a point in the whole climate cycle at which the temperate zone climate is destroyed, and we stop eating! We can chart the CO2 content of the atmosphere and know whether we have enough minerals in soil and water. The CO2 curve is showing us that the time of no temperate zone could be approaching. We must remineralize the world's soils and put carbon back into the earth as fast as we can to reverse the CO2 curve and bring it back to a safe level.

Hamaker says that scientists predicting a warming also aren't taking into consideration the role of life in and on the soil in demineralizing it in a period of 10,000 to 15,000 years, depending on the amount of ground rock supplied by the last glacial advance, nor do they all understand the earth's tectonic system and its role in determining the weather. The climate cycle is a by-product of the entire life system, all of which rests on the expenditure of atomic energy in the tectonic system. There are two energy systems which are powerful in comparison to other factors (such as sunspots, Milankovitch's theory, or the alignment of planets in space)—the effects of these other factors may be noted, but they don't substantially alter the glacial process—both of the primary energy systems use the energy in the atom. One is the sun and the other is the tectonic system.

The earth constantly intercepts the sun's energy. If the energy incident to the earth at the higher latitudes is deflected into space instead of being absorbed at ground level, the total amount of energy available to warm the earth is decreased by that amount. During a glacial period, the total amount of sun energy reaching the earth is decreased because the CO_2 (from the tectonic system) directs a heavy cloud cover to the polar latitudes. The clouds have a very high albedo, that is, ability to reflect the sun's rays back into pace.

The tectonic system constantly removes materials from the mantle of the earth, separates the compounds containing a balance of elements useful to living organisms, and moves them into the mountains or into the atmosphere. Compounds containing elements not required for life processes are consigned to the core or are recycled to build the basic ocean floor at the ridge.

Everything on earth is totally dependent on the tectonic system; if it were to run out of fuel, the earth would be cold and lifeless like Mars. Climate is directly controlled by the discharge of carbon and sulfur oxides by the tectonic system. Now that mankind has a hand in adding CO_2 to the air (and making other environmental errors), climate is also affected by the human factor. There is a scarcity of minerals on the land and in the sea, further contributing to the CO_2 buildup in the atmosphere as more and more CO_2 is supplied by the tectonic system and less and less is put back into the earth's crust by the living organisms. All these factors overlap and affect climate. We can say that the minerals (those available to microorganisms) and the carbon released by the tectonic system can be monitored—and thus, theoretically, can be controlled to some extent—we still have much to learn in this area, but we can and do have an effect on climate.

The burning of temperate zone vegetation will carry huge quantities of CO_2 into the atmosphere. In the zones of latitude where the sun's rays are most intense (the equatorial region), CO_2 holds the sun's heat at the surface of the earth, increasing surface temperature and providing the energy to increase the evaporation and to move the massive cloud cover to the polar regions; CO_2 has no heating effect at the poles in the winter when it's dark 24 hours a day. The warm, demineralized ocean can't take up the CO_2 as fast as it is being put into the air, and decreasing plant life and less trees also mean less CO_2 is being converted. We cannot allow the CO_2 increase to reach the point of no return—that is, the increase in CO_2 from the tectonic system and our own input must not be allowed to exceed the capacity of the remaining forests and sea life to remove the CO_2. When the minerals are too few to support enough life to hold down the CO_2 level, the level begins to rise and the death of the temperate and tropical zone forests swiftly initiates the air flow pattern which brings glaciation to polar latitudes and extreme, killing heat and drought in between.

When air gets hotter, its atmospheric pressure decreases. It's then easier for the cold air moving down over a cold land mass to displace the warm equatorial air and force it to move poleward over the warm ocean to replace the cold air moving toward the equator. This is the normal air circulation pattern impressed on the west winds. During glaciation, when there is an extensive ice field, there is no summer because the refrigerated air from the ice field maintains the temperature differential required to carry the clouds to the northern latitude. Thus, there can be unusually large masses of hot air in the equatorial latitudes and unusually large masses of cold air in the polar latitudes. Glaciation, or for that matter, anything else on earth, can't take place without an expenditure of energy. Without a buildup in CO_2 and hence temperature, glaciation cannot happen.

Hamaker says that the average temperature at the start of a glacial period must be higher than the interglacial temperature and must remain higher until the cooling effect of the ice sheets starts bringing it down, but says this won't help agriculture: the southern temperate zone will have excessive heat/drought; northern/temperate zone: summer freezes and frosts; cloud cover lowers the temperature and increases the quantity of cold air which flows south over the land masses. With early cold snaps and longer, colder winters, the temperate zone will become a part of the subarctic zone. The summer frosts/ freezes, short-growing seasons, drought and violent storms, rapidly diminishing soil minerals, and increasing rain acidity will destroy the world's grain crops; we can't grow grain in the subarctic. Growing seasons have already been shortened and interrupted by freeze damage. (The local areas to survive will be the few near the equator that are blessed with a constantly renewed supply of basic minerals sufficient to maintain a neutral soil in spite of the acidic rains, says Hamaker in Survival of Civilization.) We've already seen indications of these patterns. He says we can stand cold winters for some time, but not if they carry over into summers to destroy crops and trees. Cold waves, just a few degrees lower in temperature, can cause major crop losses in Canadian and Eurasian grain crops that are at the latitude of Michigan or farther north. Hamaker says food production in the northern hemisphere in 1980 had lost about 20% of potential because of adverse weather (drought/ heat in the U.S.; cold, wet weather on the Eurasian continent; and, in the southern hemisphere the growing season started with drought in Australia, Africa, and South America). He fears that famine could begin soon, that it could be a few years away; 1978 and 1979 fruit and vegetable losses in California, Texas, and Florida, as well as winter crop losses in 1983/84, show what could happen to crops in the years just ahead.

Anyone interested in studying the whole glacial process in more depth is urged to read Hamaker's book—there is an entire section on the tectonic system, plus more details on the role of CO_2 in glaciation and many other facts and figures on the glacial process, including the period of glaciation itself. Our space in this lesson requires us to focus more on the transition period from interglacial (warm) to glacial (cold) so that we may become more aware of signals observable during a change to glaciation.

Let's take a look at what some other scientists who foresee a cooling have to say about the energy expenditure required for glaciation; we've seen that scientists agree, in general, on some information about past glacial periods and our present interglacial, but they don't all agree on why glaciation happened. What force could bring such a change about? We've said that Hamaker saw the greenhouse effect as occurring differentially: the increasing temperature differential between warmer (hotter/drier) and colder (colder/ wetter) latitudes has taken on a life of its own and is accelerating the whole process. When the supply of minerals ground from rocks by the last glaciation is used up in the soil, this exhaustion of soil minerals by the life in and on the soil initiates a whole chain of events which results in restocking the soil with minerals and a new proliferation of life.

David P. Adam of the U.S. Geological Survey, a longtime student of glacial periods, has emphasized that to understand their causes, one must solve the "energy problem" they present. His Quaternary Research paper (1976, "Ice Ages and the Thermal Equilibrium of the Earth (II)") shows that an essential requirement to begin and sustain a glacial period is an increased transfer of (excess) energy towards the glaciated regions, and that energy is in the form of moisture. This is of course precipitated largely as snow, thus forming the initial perennial snowfields and subsequent ice sheets. He states that some increased energy source must therefore be invoked to sustain these vast energy transfers, yet he does not consider in his paper the fact of excessive CO_2's solar heat-trapping effect as the possible "booster" for providing this increase of effective energy, which, as Adam points out, is "required to fuel a continental glaciation".

In a personal communication to Hamaker, David Adam agreed that Hamaker's theory (CO_2) indeed fulfills the requirements of providing the glacial energy fuel. Yet, surprisingly, David knew of no one in the history of modern Quaternary research who had postulated a CO_2-glaciation relationship, perhaps due to the relative state of infancy of modern CO_2/climate studies, but he said there was one well-respected climatologist who had presented an explanation of the basic glacial process very similar to Hamaker's, Sir George Simpson of Britain. He was first to point out that the glaciation that characterizes an ice age can't come about by a general cooling of the earth's atmosphere—because some source of increased energy is required to transport poleward the huge amounts of moisture which make up the glaciers. Most climatologists now agree, because a decrease must lower the mean temperature of the earth's surface (especially in the tropics), decrease the equator-to-pole temperature gradient, and distinctly lower the moisture content of the atmosphere. He realized that it's obviously paradoxical to expect fulfillment of certain fundamental requirements for glaciation (intensified equator-to-pole temperature gradients, stepped-up atmospheric circulation, and increase of poleward heat and moisture transfer) with a declining surface temperature, especially in tropical regions.

John Hamaker, while unaware of Simpson's theory, was apparently the first to correlate the basic heating and circulation principles operating at glacial initiation with the soon-to-be-infamous" differential greenhouse effect. Other recent warnings on this differential heating effect have come from Lester Machta (head of National Oceanic and Atmospheric Administration (NOAA) Air Resources Labs), saying that CO_2 could indeed cause the massive cooling cloud coverage and cooling at the poles, and from Justus (1978) of the Congressional Research Service: "If the earth's temperature rises, the water vapor content of the atmosphere is likely to rise. A rise in water vapor would quite likely increase the fraction of the globe covered by clouds. Such an increase could cause the amount of primary solar radiation absorbed by earth to fall." In a document prepared for Congress (" Weather Modification: Programs, Problems, Policy, and Potential," Chapter 4), Justus says: "In geological perspective, the case for cooling is strong. If this interglacial age lasts no longer than a dozen earlier ones in the past million years, as recorded in deep-sea sediments, we may reasonably suppose that the world is about due to begin a slide into the next Ice Age." (p. 153.)

Hamaker says that failure to remineralize the soil will cause continued mental and physical degeneration of humanity and quickly bring famine, death, and glaciation, in that order.

The majority of the world's people fall into one of these categories: those who are aware of problems and take action; those that are angered by problems but talk or worry about them and don't take action; those who just give up hope; those who trust in the system, right or wrong, problems or no problems; those who are just plain indifferent to problems; and even those who are unaware that problems exist at all!

Most people probably think that the last ice age was "a million years ago", but the fact is, it ended only about 10,000 years ago—a few seconds in geological time. Everything that we know in terms of our "civilization" has taken place in that brief span of time since the earth last warmed up. The potential global climate changes that face all of humanity could re-arrange everything on the planet and affect every living creature on earth more than any other ecological issues in question—even beyond such crucial concerns as world peace—for the issue here is whether we want to have a world at all in which to live in peace. We must make the ecological changes necessary for survival. Because most of the subsoil and topsoil of the world have been stripped of all but a small quantity of elements (by time, water, erosion, chemical fertilizers, pesticides, and so on), Hamaker says man can stay on this earth only if the glacial periods come every 100,000 years to replenish the mineral supply—or if we get smart enough to grind the rock ourselves and apply it everywhere on soil that is depleted. Glaciation is an acceleration of the normal process of using evaporated water to carry excessive heat energy from warm zones to cold zones, and the greenhouse effect (of an increase in atmospheric CO_2) is to increase cloud cover over polar latitudes. The clouds have a cooling effect as well as providing the snow for glaciation. The energy is dissipated in arctic space. Glaciation occurs whenever the soil minerals left by the last glacial period are used up and the plant life (forests are the major factor in CO_2 control) can no longer regulate the carbon dioxide by growing faster in response to its increase in the air.

100.3.4. The Glacial-Interglacial Cycle

The glacial-interglacial cycle was revealed by numerous workers in many fields of Quaternary research as of the 1970s. (The Quaternary is the present geological period including the Pleistocene epoch and the Holocene—recent—epoch, the present interglacial in which we now live). A National Academy of Sciences (NAS) publication, Understanding Climate Change (1975) says: "The present. interglacial interval—which has now lasted about 10,000 years—represents a climatic regime that is relatively rare during the past million years, most of which have been occupied by colder, glacial regimes. Only during about 8% of the past 700,000 years has the earth experienced climates as warm or warmer than the present. The penultimate interglacial age began about 125,000 years ago and lasted for approximately 10,000 years. Similar interglacial (warm) ages—each lasting 10,000 (+2,000) years and each followed by a glacial (cold) maximum averaging 90,000 years—have occurred on the average every 100,000 years during at least the past half-million years. During this period, fluctuation of the northern hemisphere ice sheets caused sea-level variations of about 100 meters."

This NAS publication concludes that: "If the end of the interglacial is episodic in character, we are moving toward a rather sudden climatic change of unknown timing. ...

If, on the other hand, these changes are more sinusoidal in character, then the climate should decline gradually over a period of thousands of years." All factors considered, Hamaker doesn't think we have that long.

Paleoclimatologists agree that the major warm periods (interglacials) that followed each of the ends of the major glaciations (cold periods) have lasted from about 10,000 to 12,000 years, and that, in each case, a period of considerably colder climate has followed immediately after these intervals. About 10,000 to 10,800 years have now passed since the onset of our present period of warmth, so the question certainly arises as to whether we are really on the brink of a period of colder climate. The 100,000-year cycle of glaciation is now recognized as occurring with regularity, so, technically speaking, we could be due for another ice age "any time during the next 1,200 years". As we said, though, signs that signal the changeover or transition from temperate to colder climate are already in evidence and increasing due to our environmental errors.

Most scientists are noncommittal, but those who are beginning to express concern say that these signs mean that we may be much closer to the first stages of the next ice age than anybody would like to think. Let's review some of the signs we've already talked about:

We have already seen that the earth's total soil microorganism and earthworm populations have been dying back over the recent centuries and decades due to soil demineralization, and so the earth's plant and tree life has been forced to die back—known as "retrogressive vegetational succession" in the literature of ecology. Deserts (now growing at a rate of 15 million acres per year) are generally a final stage of this retrogression process. Our abuse and neglect have reinforced this desertification, as it has deforestation. Soil demineralization (with acid rains accelerating the devastation) is causing the increasingly rapid sickening and dying of whole forests. The massive death and burning of the forests is signaling the "teleocratic" or end phase of our present interglacial period. Svend Th. Andersen saw the broad picture of glacial/interglacial stages and said that the interglacials were stable intervals between the glacial stages of disturbance and chaos. The vegetation had a chance to develop until the new glacial released its destructive forces. He divided the interglacials (warm intervals) into four broad phases:

1. Protocratic phase. At the start of warm intervals, open forests of pioneer species entered—these were quickly-spreading trees and shrubs with unpretentious requirements to climate and soils. Birch, pine, poplar, juniper, and willow were most important in Denmark, Andersen's home.

Mesocratic phase. The soil had developed a high fertility, and plants of rich soils reached maximum frequencies. Immense forests covered great portions of the earth in the last mesocratic phase (from about 6,000 to 3,000 B.C.) Some of these trees, such as oaks, were reported to be often of remarkably large size; these are found preserved in now-degenerate treeless peat soils in England and elsewhere. The phase is dominated by trees such as elm, oak, lime, hazel, ash, hornbeam, and alder, growing on stable mull soils which Dr. Johannes Iversen (State Geologist, Geological Survey of Denmark), showed to eventually begin to retrogress. Iversen tried to find out at what point in the interglacial the retrogressive vegetational succession starts, and said it is "when the yearly disintegration of the plant debris no longer keeps pace with the fresh supply from the living plants, and consequently a layer of 'mor' (raw humus) is accumulated on top of the mineral soil". "Mull" humus has a richness of available minerals; "mor" is acidifying humus. He studied soil conditions and said that, from the point approximately 10,000 years ago commonly accepted as the beginning of our present (warm) interglacial, it took about 3,700 to 4,500 years for the first of the glacially deposited raw mineral soils of basic or alkaline pH to "mature" and then go into a gradual "irreversible" degradation/depletion. Iversen says this degradation process is characterized by reduced soil organisms, earthworms dying out, and by the vegetation regression that comes when soil is depleted and lacks minerals. Andersen and' Iversen have similar descriptions of this process. In these mull soils, of roughly 6000 to 3000 B.C., the leaching of the soil salts is to some extent counteracted by the mixing activity of the soil fauna and the ability of the prevailing trees and shrubs to extract bases from the deeper soil layers and contribute them to the upper layers during the decomposition of their litter. However, a slow removal of calcium carbonate will bring the soils into a less stable state, where the equilibrium may be more easily disturbed. This leaching of calcium carbonate (lime) is shown to be so significant to the topsoil ecology because, according to Andersen, "the leaching of soil minerals other than lime will be insignificant, until the calcium carbonate has been removed". With this gradual leaching, the mull forest could not maintain itself, and with the lapse of time, caused itself a depauperization and acidification of the upper soil layers, which extended so far that the dense forest receded, and more open vegetation types expanded. The changeover from mineral-rich mull soils to acidifying mor soil conditions begins in the mesocratic, and with the gradual demineralization of formerly calcareous soils, growth of impenetrable hardpans and soil life die-outs follow. This creates shallow topsoil's susceptible to drought or being easily swamped; and this infertile state leads to takeover by heathlands, peat bogs, and trees with ability to survive on acidic soils—spruce, pine, birch, poplar, etc.

2. Oligocratic phase. This condition becomes prevalent in this phase and is brought on as a result of degeneration of soils. The increasing podzolization, characterized by increased demineralization and acidity, continues up through the telocratic (end) phase. (Podzolization is a process of soil formation, especially in humid regions, involving principally leaching of the upper layers with accumulation of material in lower layers and development of characteristic horizons; specifically, the development of a podzol. Podzol: any of a group of zonal soils that develop in a moist climate especially under coniferous or mixed forests and have an organic mat and a thin organic-mineral layer above a gray leached layer resting on a dark alluvial horizon enriched with amorphous clay.)

3. Telocratic (end) phase. The final interglacial phase is the time when the demineralized soils begin to be removed. The rigorous conditions at the end of the interglacial are reflected by an increase in allochthonous mineral matter, no doubt due to increasing surficial erosion.

The information in virtually every textbook on soils, forestry, or ecology leaves no doubt that the present world civilization is at least deep into the oligocratic phase. Andersen's work also shows that the Scandinavian lakes and soils reflect a close parallel development from basic to acidic conditions—again, many thousands of lakes there, as well as in other parts of the world, are now already acidified into lifelessness from acid rain. Rapidly accelerating worldwide erosion rates are evident; the figure in 1981 was already 6,400,000,000 tons of topsoil lost per year to erosion.

These facts, along with increasingly rigorous conditions imposed by the weather since at least 1972, very strongly indicate that the telocratic end phase may indeed have begun. As we said, the final changeover to sub-arctic climate and vegetation has been seen to have been made in only 20 years in other interglacial to glacial transitions.

What other changes come with the end of a period of interglacial warmth? From studies of sediments and soils, George Kukla agreed that "major changes in vegetation occurred at the end of the previous warm period. Deciduous forests that covered areas during the major glaciations were replaced by sparse shrubs, and dust blew freely. The climate was considerably more 'continental' than it is now, and agricultural productivity would have been marginal at best." George Kukla and Julius Fink studied interlayered soils exposed in excavated brickyards of Czechoslovakia. Seventeen major cycles of glacial loess deposition (loess is mixed rock dust and silt ground by the glaciers and swept by the winds) and subsequent interglacial soil "decalcification" (and overall demineralization) over the last 1.7. million years were revealed. The interglacial soils are shown to have supported the deciduous forests native to northwest and central Europe until in some way they died off and gave way to the steppe vegetation of a chilled, wind torn glacial desert with blowing dust. Loess always returns to cover the demineralized soils. Then, again, over the centuries, the loess becomes mostly consumed by the soil formation and development process.

The cycle of glaciation is complete when the supply of minerals ground from rocks by the last glaciation is used up and glaciation occurs again. Whereas plant life normally removes all excess CO_2 from the atmosphere by growing faster as CO_2 increases, it can no longer do so, since it gets its cell protoplasm from the soil microorganisms and, as we know, the microorganisms start dying too when insufficient elements are available to them.

A conference was held at Brown University in 1972 with paleontologists, sedimentologists, stratigraphers, paleoclimatologists, and others, entitled The Present Interglacial, How and When Will It End? They strongly confirmed the 100,000-year average glacial-interglacial cycle, and many stressed the fact that we should be at or close to the end of the present interglacial.

The search for causes of the Ice Age began over a century ago, and Hamaker says the answer literally lies beneath our feet: progressive soil demineralization of the earth's soil mantle causes an eventual collapse of the global carbon cycle. The cycle is: soil remineralization -> interglacial soil demineralization -> vegetational succession and collapse -> the glacial process -> soil remineralization

Hamaker also believes the large increase in earthquakes can be attributed to the steadily increasing weight of snow and ice cover pressing on the molten layers just underneath the earth's crust, causing shifting and slippages. He notes that the sharp rise in major earthquakes began about 10 years after the climate began to get noticeably colder beginning in 1940. He also predicts a steadily-increasing incidence of volcanic eruptions, for the same reason, and suggests this has already begun in the last few years.

Glaciation usually comes at a time when the earth's tectonic system has fired up volcanic activity by feeding ocean floor into the continental heaters, mostly located in the Pacific "ring of fire". Volcanic action releases larger amounts of liquified gases trapped in the molten rock. Carbon dioxide and sulfur dioxide are the main gases released, and both cause the greenhouse effect, resulting in our present "100-year cold cycle". These cycles vary in their time interval, intervals being determined by the pressure in the tectonic system. Carbon dioxide from decaying and burning mineral-starved vegetation is then added to these volcanic gases—together, they initiate the change from interglacial to glacial climate. Acidic gases from volcanism and burning forests can then stifle life on earth by leaching the few remaining basic elements into the subsoil. In this way the change from interglacial to glacial conditions can be made in 20 years (Nature, G. Woillard, 1979). Hamaker says that man may have moved the present glacial process! forward in time by 500 years by the continued pouring of CO_2 into the air, by acidic gases and acid rain, and by forest; and jungle destruction by people seeking lumber and fuel or farmland ... the 20-year change period can also be shortened. Hamaker estimates that the beginning of a 20-year changeover period from interglacial to glacial conditions was about 1975. If this estimate is accurate, then tremendous weather changes should have begun by that time, signified by growing intensification of all storm effects, including unusually heavy rains and snows, record cold and heat, drought, hail, tornados, etc., all symptomatic of increasing temperature and pressure differentials, greater evaporation of moisture, and an overall speeding up of global atmospheric circulation.

Iversen warns us that in former interglacial epochs, the anthropogenic factor was negligible; i.e., man's impact on nature was less dramatic than it is today.

According to Hamaker, all the requirements for glaciation are now in place and accelerating in intensity at a very fast pace: CO_2 increases; precipitation pH moves toward intolerable acidity; earth's soils (demineralized) can't support a strong, healthy plant/ forest cover; the carbon of the soils and trees is being transferred back to the atmosphere in huge amounts as carbon dioxide gases. As the primary infrared heat-trapping "greenhouse effect" gas, CO_2 excess causes the sustained overheating of the vast oceans (especially tropical oceans), thus causing the sustained evaporation increase required to nourish the polar regions with the "food" of glaciers: water, snow—and keep them shaded from melting with clouds. This increase of glaciation is now occurring and has been since about 1950, so, although some scientists expect a warming from the greenhouse effect, the rise isn't being found over the last century—on the contrary, the earth seems to have been cooling in recent decades. The polar ice field is expanding and growing in northeast Canada (more on this in weather section), and pressure is rising in the tectonic system, indicated by the accumulation of lava flows along the ridges, and by increased volcanic activity. We're in the high-pressure part of the "ocean floor feeding cycle", which has occurred about every 100 years, at least for a few centuries.

It's certainly not a good time for CO_2 to rise!

100.3.5. "Hope Springs Eternal"

Scientists tell us of a glacial/interglacial cycle of 100,000 years, and say we are now about 10,000 to 10,800 years into a warm interval that can last from 10,000 to 12,000 years. Some scientists also say there is a "magnetic pole reversal cycle" of 200,000 to 1,000,000 years and that, since the last one took place about 710,000 years ago, we could be "due" for one "sometime in the future". As of 1984, there hasn't been much talk among the general public about Ice Ages or magnetic pole reversals; if either of these possibilities do exist, even remotely, as calculated by scientists, one would expect at least some debate on these issues to have hit the national/international media by now.

There are several explanations for the apparent lack of awareness. For one thing, countless brilliant minds go into fields totally unrelated to science, so Ice Ages and pole reversals aren't necessarily familiar to them. Then, within the field of science, scientists specialize, usually in one specific area of research, often depending on the project(s) they've received funds and grants for. They may be experts on one particular subject, but unfamiliar with either fields of science (even related fields) or even with other areas of study within their own fields. They may have spent years refining a certain body of knowledge and focusing on one aspect of one branch of science. This narrows down the number of experts available on any given subject, let alone that of glaciation or magnetic pole reversal. Most scientists accept as fact many things they don't have the time, knowledge, or money to prove for themselves, relying on research done by other scientists to fill in the gaps. This means the number of informed people who could "accurately" predict art onset of another Ice Age is quite limited anyway. Within this number of informed people there are: scientists too busy working on something else to become involved in speculation about an Ice Age; others uninterested one way or the other; some who have considered it, then given it no further thought; others who may have speculated on when it could come, but don't want to give their opinion because they don't want to make a mistake or prefer not to contradict scientists who think the world will warm up; others who don't want to alarm the general public (or perhaps fear causing "mass panic" or migration?); and finally, there might be a few who are willing to make a statement. As we said, this will be a rare person, one with courage of convictions, faith in his/her calculations, enough concern about humanity to bring something of such epic proportions out into the open, and nerve to contradict other scientists' theories, such as theories of scientists who initiated the Environmental Protection Agency report and the National Academy of Sciences report. Anyone who disagrees with them has to prove his own theory and discredit theirs—somewhat comparable to a single doctor challenging the entire American Medical Association— it happens, but this is probably considered an awesome task, one many professionals would undoubtedly prefer to avoid if at all possible, having their "careers" and reputations" to think about.

Scientists and experts need more than knowledge and facts—they also need intuition, the ability to synthesize what they know into an overall picture from all the little random bits and pieces of information. Beyond book learning, they need sensitivity and awareness, consciousness, and creativity. Educated experts often lack some of these qualities needed to make good judgment and a proper diagnosis. We can see, in light of the above "analysis", that it could indeed be possible for the general public to miss something of such magnitude, even if it were true.

John Hamaker puts it this way: "It may seem incredible that up to now this work could have escaped becoming common knowledge, at least to workers in agriculture, forestry, geology, climatology, and other such immediately-related fields. Apparently the many diverse pieces of the glacial/ interglacial climate cycle 'puzzle' had to be gradually discovered through various disciplines over decades, before at least enough pieces were evident to be joined in a coherent picture by a trained ecological thinker."(John Hamaker in this case.) Yet now everyone may see for themselves the truth in his synthesis.

He continues: "Congress has evaluated the CO2 problem on the basis of a consensus reached by 'specialists'. They freely admit that they do not know what causes glaciation yet say the average temperature must drop several degrees C before we can have glaciation simply because they have evidence that it does get much colder during glacial periods. They ignore the fact that, historically, glaciation has alternated with interglacial periods on a roughly 100,000-year cycle and the fact that glaciation is due. Do they think that crop soils turning to deserts (due to erosion and soil demineralization, etc.), and weather catastrophes we've observed, are all just coincidence? They haven't thought about soil and its relation to glaciation, nor the role of the tectonic system in the glacial process.

"The people charged with the responsibility for the CO2 problem are simply not trained to solve problems. They are trained to be observers and have done a creditable job of that. But the job of making a rational synthesis of the facts as a basis for Congressional action ought to have been assigned to engineers and physicists, both of whom have been trained to work with the facts and laws of Nature. The fault lies at the higher levels of education, which have neglected the necessity for interdisciplinary education and action in favor of specialization."

The meteorologist Harold Bernard, who also warned of CO2 increases and effects on climate, wrote a chapter "We Can't Put Weather in a Test Tube," which criticizes scientists' incorrect assumptions, inaccurate modeling techniques, and ignorance of important processes through lack of knowledge. It is clear that the interglacial soil demineralization is one such process they have ignored. The knowledge is. now freely available.

Let's consider a parallel that Life Scientists are very familiar with by now. The concept of the body as self-healing and the body of knowledge found in the Life Science philosophy both follow the laws of common sense, of Nature, and of logic. We need only try it for ourselves if we want "proof", since Truth is self-evident. We have come to accept as obvious the fact that live food (uncooked fruit, vegetables, nuts and seeds) imparts the most perfect state of health possible. We have experienced our bodies' self-healing powers and learned about fasting as a means of allowing our bodies the chance to rest and divert all their energy into healing. We have decided that medicine and herbs interfere with the body's self-directed healing actions, and that suppression of symptoms (which are manifestations of the healing process going on) likewise interferes with the body's innate wisdom. We have found that health is produced only by healthful living and that sickness will vanish only when cause is removed (not when symptoms are suppressed). That about sums it up in a nutshell.

What I'm getting at is this: if all the above is so obvious to us, why isn't it obvious to the countless doctors and "health" professionals all over the world? Why is it obvious only to a few people? How can something be true and not be recognized by more people? All we can say is, truth is still truth, in and of itself, even if not one single person sees it. Truth doesn't need believers in order to be true; it doesn't need followers or majority acceptance in order to be valid. Truth doesn't have to wait for everyone to catch up. The earth was still round when everyone believed it was flat, despite what "everyone" thought. Microscopic life existed long before we saw it in microscopes; it didn't have to wait for us to see it in order to exist. If we are sliding into another Ice Age, and the scientists who foresee its arrival are correct, an Ice Age won't need our approval or belief in order to be a reality, that much we can be sure of.

Of course it would be easier for our own "practical purposes if some of their calculations we are "off ." After all, many so-called scientific theories have fallen by the wayside throughout the years, as new knowledge superseded old knowledge. Even the "world is flat" theory fell prey to the test of time. Whereas truth is truth despite what people believe, knowledge may or may not be true despite what people believe. Even if it isn't true, it may be paraded around as fact for years, centuries, or even indefinitely.

In the meantime, many people continue to believe what they're told, looking to "experts" for answers and depending on them for knowledge; it's not a foolproof learning technique, but it's often the best they can do. So, when the experts themselves make mistakes, it doesn't matter how big their herd of followers is—but, of course, many people are influenced by the size of the herd when choosing their beliefs. They feel safety in numbers and prefer the comfort and "security" of a large herd. If "everyone else" believes something, it must be true, says their inner logic, or if nothing else, they'd still rather be with the majority. There is an alternative to joining herds and following experts: intuition. If you can trust your intuition, you are fortunate. As a free thinker, you can ask yourself what your intuition tells you about the world's current situation, the state of our environment, weather patterns, and Ice Ages. I've tried to present various opinions on these subjects, but I don't presume to have all the answers.

My intuition tells me to keep an open mind, and not to give up hope. If the observations and premonitions of the scientists who see the world as cooling are correct, I for one would rather have had a hint ahead of time than be surprised at the last minute! At least this leaves us with the option to take action, and to try to survive on this planet. It's been said that we don't fail until we give up trying. Hope is our strongest ally—it reinforces our will to live. Without it, we are lost, for without hope, nothing matters anymore.

So, even if an Ice Age were approaching during our lifetime, we would still have hope as our "open door". For one thing, we have the potential for change. Some people believe that there is a future that can be known in the present (often called destiny), but that, at the same time, there is still our free will—a powerful force that can change or alter "what is meant to be". This gives us control over our "destinies" and the ability to create the lives we choose. As we said in an earlier lesson, we ourselves are responsible for our states of being; we underestimate our power as individuals when we believe that random outside influences alone shape our lives. Ironically, though, there is also some element of "chance "in life that can weave its influence into what we are busily creating; while we often tend to define things in simple dualities of yes and no we actually have yes, maybe, maybe not, and no. We can predict that something will or will not happen, and we can be very sure that it will or will not happen if we are accurate. Even so, the fact still remains that, beyond our free will or any so-called destiny, there are also other powers and forces of life in the universe that can enter into every situation and coincide with any variables involved, and these sometimes alter the outcome or cause slight variations between what we expect and what actually happens. For this reason, when considering the return of an Ice Age, we can still allow for the possibility, however small, that something completely unpredictable at this present time—some unforeseeable factor—could still come to pass, something we cannot even conceive of or envision with our present knowledge or awareness. This is not to say that we should resort to an escapist mentality or rationalize our way out of solving our serious environmental problems by using the excuse that "a miracle could happen" as a justification for inertia—this would be wishful thinking and sheer delusion! We're merely trying to show that everything that happens in life is affected by the intricate interworking's of many multi-faceted forces, and that this includes our attempts to predict specific global climate changes. We've attempted to speculate on the past and present factors pertaining to Ice Ages, so now we're considering future factors, which, of course, also lead us to the unknown. Technology and scientific knowledge that we use daily and now take for granted were unimaginable to people a century ago, so it is conceivable that someone could still discover an energy force/source that is presently unknown to humanity or find a new technique for cleaning and restoring the environment or invent something that we can't even imagine that would change our world or its course of events. We can hope that our ingenuity will prove itself once more; we've gotten ourselves into our present world state—maybe we can get ourselves out of our problems, as well. There is a tremendous growth in spirit evident all over the planet—we ourselves can perform the miracle of increased awareness—with a quantum leap in consciousness, we could save ourselves by realizing what must be done before it is too late.

It has been said that our strongest instinct is to survive. When I finished reading Hamaker's book, I began to see our world ecology as a whole and realized the importance of seeing our environmental problems collectively, as they interrelate, rather than individually. There's an old expression that comes to mind: "Couldn't see the forest for the trees." We've been looking at the trees so long that we've forgotten what the whole forest looks like. Few things can make us appreciate life more than the realization that it can end. The suggestion that time could run out for our planet forces us to reassess our values as human beings. Where are we going? What are we doing to our environment, our source of life? What are our real priorities? Ask anyone who's ever been told s/ he would have "only 3 months to live". The first thing that happens is a total overhaul of priorities, a total rethinking of what the person can still do. Time becomes more precious than ever before. Energy becomes focused as never before. Life is no longer taken for granted. I guess we never wake up until after we've been asleep. Let's hope we wake up in time—it seems we've ignored the alarm clock already.

Even if we are "let off the hook" somehow and an Ice Age is averted or postponed, or its timing was miscalculated to some extent, we still have some very important moral decisions to make regarding our ability—and, moreover, our will—to revitalize the world for our continued survival on this planet, because we are still left with our CO_2, soil, water, and other pollution problems, and as long as we continue to put money and technological "advances" before the welfare of humanity and our ecosystem, we still have our greed to deal with. And we still have to figure out a way to keep from destroying ourselves in nuclear war.

718

One way or the other, we have to get together worldwide and face the problems that we ourselves have created. We call ourselves civilized, and we want to believe that we have advanced and evolved, but an honest appraisal of our collective self-portrait reveals that we are painting ourselves into a corner every time we compromise our ethics and assault Nature's principles. We cannot hope to survive if we destroy our planet, because it is our source of life, but we must also understand that our survival is just as surely threatened by the destruction of our basic human values— love for humanity—and that we now have a profound need to revive and restore these basic values. Only by realizing that we co-exist—what we do to others (both psychologically and environmentally) we do to ourselves—can we expect to rally on the large scale necessary at this point for our survival on this planet.

It's obvious that we've been born into a time of incredible challenge, so let's meet this challenge with all our strength—and with a smile—for as always, life continues amidst the chaos. We must see the world as we want to be, as it must be for our survival, and use this positive image to create this world. The key to our survival lies in visualizing and acting for our survival over and over again until it becomes a reality. Every time another individual loses hope and gives up, our survival as a group is also threatened, because the force of our collective will to live is diminished once again. Every time our basic values of faith, hope, and charity are abandoned, the quality of life on earth is tarnished for everyone, and if we continue on a collision course with Nature, life on earth will only become more miserable. Without love, food, natural resources, and an environment clean enough to support life, people everywhere would have little to live for or to look forward to. We create our reality, and if this is the reality we choose to create, humanity as a whole will despair, and it doesn't take a genius to imagine what will happen if no one cares. As surely as we need faith, love, and action, we need hope.

Fear is the lock and laughter the key to your heart.

—Stephen Stills

100.4. Politics of Food Production

100.4.1. The Land of the Free, and the Home of the Brave

Since countless members of our human family are already hungry or starving, it is imperative that we find solutions now. Anyone who has ever grown a garden knows the disappointment of losing some plants, whether to a hungry forest animal or to an early frost and seeing the work of months of tender care vanish before their eyes. A neighbor's cows got past a broken fence once and visited my garden; every corn plant was reduced to stubble and all my salad greens were lost to their hearty appetites overnight—months of growth were gone. Anyone who has ever planted a small fruit tree and watched its slow, steady progress, knows that it takes years before fruit will be harvested. It takes time to grow all food, and nothing can replace growing time when a crop is lost.

We may think we have enough food today, but we've long been pushing our luck, by pushing Nature time and time again and tampering with our environmental quality. We can no longer refuse to acknowledge and deal with our environmental and agricultural problems, and with the profound impact their combined effects have on our ecosystem and food supplies. We are dangerously out of touch with reality if we think we can defy the laws of Nature indefinitely with no consequences. We can't just "wait for the weather to improve", because the atmospheric carbon dioxide which is destroying temperate zone climate is increasing at an accelerating rate. Everyone who has ever studied the CO_2 problem has warned that the result of permitting the rise of CO_2 would be to alter the weather in ways which would be destructive to agriculture. Meanwhile, while our use of fossil fuels is increasing, our forests and jungles are fast disappearing. All this is a sure prescription for mass suicide.

What, if anything, are our world governments doing about all this? Our politicians should have begun programs for soil remineralization and biomass solar energy 15 years ago. We would now have major growing machinery and equipment industries related to food and fuel, and a better food supply with more mineral content. But what can we expect from an elective system that lets the Farm Bureau and the corporate structure buy candidates at election time? This makes the legislature and the executive branch putty in the hands of corporate interests. The situation is the same at the federal level. Congress dispenses (out of our pockets) palliatives by the hundreds, but if we suggest solutions to problems that conflict with corporate interests, they start squeaking like mice. Ralph Nader says that 80% of the time Congress comes down on the corporate side of an issue. It really takes massive public demand to make them listen if they listen at all.

Our ancestors came to this country to be free and independent—we are being manipulated by the power of centralized wealth, and our system of soil destruction threatens our agricultural and technical civilization. The devastation of the biosphere is seldom perceived as the ultimate threat to survival because, for many people and their governments, this issue is overshadowed by what they imagine to be more immediate concerns: war, poverty, sickness, the energy crisis, inflation, unemployment, drought, famine, and so on. What they don't realize is that the failure to conserve and rebuild living resources is closely linked to the worsening of these other problems.

Soil remineralization is a priority now. We were once blessed with an abundance of natural resources, but we have squandered them over the years; and we must now redirect our energy, money, and resources into positive, peaceful enterprises that will benefit all of humanity and life on this earth.

We can no longer wait for our governments to "take action"—nor can we depend blindly on systems, authority, scientists, experts, professionals,, specialists, doctors, or someone else in general, for our existence and survival. We cannot wait for someone else to care about our survival—it is we ourselves who have to survive. We are responsible for our own lives.

100.4.1. The Land of the Free, and the Home of the Brave

We, the people, are the government. Imagine you're a passenger in a car and the driver falls asleep just as the car is heading toward a cliff. Earlier in this lesson we mentioned some of the different types of people who make up our world. Let's listen to what they have to say, as the driver loses control of the car:

- Those who're unaware that problems exist: "What a fantastic view!"

- Those who remain indifferent to problems: "So what if we go over a cliff?"

- Those who trust in the system, right or wrong: "It's not the driver's fault that we're heading for a cliff—after all, his intentions were good."

- Those who give up hope: "Too late now—I'd better cover my eyes!"

- Those who recognize problems but are all talk and no action: "Maybe the driver will wake up in time! Whatever happens, it's the driver's fault—I'm not to blame!"

- Those who are aware and take action: "I'd better grab the wheel and steer for my life!"

What would you do?

If our leaders, "experts", or drivers of our vehicles are asleep at the wheel, and we see the cliff coming, we're not going to have time to "think things over", evaluate more scientific facts, wait for the driver to wake up, or wait for a new driver. We will have to act with all the survival instinct within us, on a moment's notice.

Are we ready?

Article #1: Tropical Rain Forests: Earth's Green Belt

South America Caribbean Central America South Asia Africa Southeast Asia Australia Pacific Islands

Left in peace, rain forests would ring the Equator with vegetation wherever days are hot, and precipitation is high. But farming, ranching, logging, mining, and roads have greatly reduced their actual range.

In central Africa and Amazonia huge tracts remain largely untouched, but rain forests have been virtually eliminated from most parts of West Africa, southern Asia, and the Caribbean.

In 1980 the U.S. National Academy of Sciences estimated annual loss at 20 million hectares (50 million acres). The World Wildlife Fund speaks of 25 to 50 acres a minute. A 1982 study by two United Nations agencies reported 7.5. million hectares lost each year.

Estimates vary so widely largely because of different criteria. To biologists, loss means either conversion of primary forest—say, to agriculture, pasture, or tree plantations—or modification, implying biological impoverishment through selective logging or shifting cultivation. To foresters, loss means deforestation—the removal of all tress.

A world survey of rain forest status appears below.

South America

BRAZIL

Earth's largest rain forest little disturbed except for fringes of southern Amazonia and areas in the east. Small chance of major losses in the west for the near future.

PERU

Vast area covered by undisturbed Amazon forest. Farm settlement expected to become more extensive in next decade or two.

COLOMBIA

About one-third forested, mostly in Amazon region, some along Pacific coast. Efforts to colonize have been slowed.

VENEZUELA

Large tract in south barely touched. Smaller areas in north heavily cut, converted to ranches and farms.

GUYANA

Most of population lives along coast. Little threat to forest. SURINAME

Virgin rain forest covers most of country, much protected by parks and reserves. ECUADOR

Large forests along Pacific already gone, oil exploration and agriculture encroach on Ecuadorian Amazonia.

FRENCH GUIANA

Population lives along coast. Little pressure on undisturbed forest of interior. BOLIVIA

Not much exploitation of forests yet. But government has begun roads, farming, and ranching.

Caribbean

Most island forests long ago reduced to remnants after heavy exploitation by dense populations. Small tracts survive, for example, in the

DOMINICAN REPUBLIC, TRINIDAD AND TOBAGO, and PUERTO RICO, where a U.S. national forest protects 104 square kilometers.

MEXICO

Shifting cultivators, timber harvesters, and cattle ranchers encroach on the country's last rain forest area on the southern border with Guatemala.

Central America

A strong trend toward cattle ranching on this highly populated isthmus has greatly reduced primary forests, now believed to be two-thirds removed. Small areas found in the Peten region of northeastern GUATEMALA, the Mosquitia Forest of eastern HONDURAS, parts of eastern NICARAGUA, southern BELIZE, the national parks of COSTA RICA. and much of PANAMA.

South Asia

INDIA

Patches of forest along the western Ghats and on Andaman Islands disrupted by landless poor, forest farmers, and logging.

BANGLADESH

Narrow belt of rain forest in Chittagong region heavily exploited by hill tribes. SRI LANKA

Small tract on southwestern and central parts, largely disrupted by logging and slashand-burn farmers.

Africa

ZAIRE

Holds Africa's largest rain forest (nearly one-tenth world total), parts of it now secondary growth. Some clearing by slash-and-burn farmers in south, but vast areas still undamaged by mainly rural population.

GABON

Almost entirely forested, with exploitation just beginning. CAMEROON

Extensive disruption of large forest areas—especially in the southwest—by timber companies and slash-and-burn farmers.

CONGO

Forests in remote northern and central regions still undisturbed. Some logging in south.

IVORY COAST

More than 70 percent of primary forest at turn of century now cleared. Rest may be gone within a decade. Timber harvesting intense. Forest farming increasing rapidly.

LIBERIA

Very little primary rain forest left due to shifting cultivation. CENTRAL AFRICAN REPUBLIC

Rainforests in south. Little pressure from small population. NIGERIA

Most forest disrupted by dense population and a century of logging. Small areas remaining in south expected to be exploited soon.

SIERRA LEONE

Very few forest areas undisturbed by cultivators. EQUATORIAL GUINEA

Almost totally forested. Little loss expected. GHANA

Little or no virgin forest remains. About half removed during last 25 years by forest farmers. Remnants found in the southwest.

GUINEA

Small area still covered with rain forest in the southwest. BENIN About three fourths of original forests left, but heavily disrupted due to strong pressure of growing population.

ANGOLA

Small rain forest concentrated in north. MADAGASCAR

Much slash-and-burn farming. Only fragment of eastern rain forest still survives.

Southeast Asia

CHINA

Rain forests along southern coast largely disturbed, though a few areas are protected.
INDONESIA

Contains largest rain forest in Asia (nearly one-tenth world total), but much harvested already. Log production multiplied sixfold during 1960s and 1970s. Farmers and transmigrant settlers also eliminating large forest areas.

MALAYSIA

About two-thirds of lowland forests on peninsula heavily logged, converted to oil palm, rubber plantations. Large forests on Borneo also being harvested.

PAPUA NEW GUINEA

Largely covered by undisturbed rain forest, much inaccessible to logging companies. Full forest harvesting under way in small areas on north coast. Half of population forest farmers.

PHILIPPINES

Large timber companies harvesting remaining rain forests, less than a third of what existed 30 years ago. Clearing by rural poor also severe.

BRUNEI

Mostly covered by rain forest, much undisturbed. Revenues from oil taxes take pressure off timber cutting as source of foreign exchange.

Only pockets of forest survive in Indochina, mainly in southernmost THAILAND, lower BURMA, southern KAMPUCHEA, and parts of the Mekong Plain in VIETNAM.

Australia

Fragments of primary forest remain along east coast of Queensland. Other lowland forests heavily cut for timber, sugar plantations, mining interests, and dairy farms.

Pacific Islands

Rain forests found on southeastern side of FIJI. Major areas allocated to timber companies. About three-fourths of SOLOMON ISLANDS also forested, most in terrain too steep to harvest.

Lesson 101:

Harmonizing Society, Culture, and Lifestyle to Save our planet

101.1. Introduction

101.2. Life

101.3. Liberty

101.4.................... And the Pursuit of Happiness

Article #1: "Who Is at Fault?"

Article #2: Radiation Hazards

101.1. Introduction

101.1.1. Age-Old Excuses for Inertia

Now that we've completed the mind-boggling task of trying to Condense earth's ecology and its millions of interrelated life processes into two lessons, we can breathe a sigh of relief. In these three "survival" lessons, I found myself in a predicament: I wanted to be comprehensive enough to cover a wide range of environmental (and other) issues related to survival, but because of the overwhelming abundance of related subject matter and limited space. I was forced to "dilute" a lot of material in order to keep things from getting out of hand! I also realized that many of us are already familiar with many of our earth's problems and didn't want to overburden everyone with a deluge of "the same old" negative facts—but by summarizing them and viewing them as a whole (the only real way to look at them) we see them in a new and different way.

The more we perceive the broad spectrum of reality, the more enlightened we become, and the more we can share knowledge with others. Heroes, like the person who happens along at just the right moment to pull a drowning child from water, are everywhere—just waiting to be asked to lend a hand. There are few human instincts more beautiful than true heroism—without compassion, this would be a cold, hard world indeed.

Because potential heroes are everywhere, just waiting to help, our task is to start asking and to know what to ask for, to spread the word among the people. We must be sensitive enough to paint the picture truthfully, and strong enough to do so without such fear and gloom that peoples' psychic numbing mechanisms pop up to block everything out. Despite our aversion to bad news, most of us would appreciate being told we were standing in the path of an oncoming bus, and once people know they 're needed and what they must do, heroes will come forth one-by-one.

As destructive effects of our industrial age become more apparent, and as we see our once-pristine environment deteriorate and more deadly weapons accumulate among our green hills and valleys, places we dreamed of calling home are threatened, damaged, or destroyed. We feel betrayed, and we're grouping together more and more to protect our lives and those of our children—our very survival now depends on this cooperative endeavor.

This lesson wraps up our discussion on survival and taking charge of our destiny, but of course by no means ends it—rather, it leaves us all with the ultimate challenge: the actual taking charge, the doing, the harmonizing of all our knowledge, faith, hope and love into a force strong enough to save our planet.

By survivalism, we mean the positive spirit of cooperation of all beings toward preservation of life. Let's make it clear from the start that our concept of survival in no way includes those of any so-called "survivalists" who advocate stocking up on guns and/or "survival" food. Nothing could be farther from our image of survival. A self-serving approach not only does nothing to help life on the planet or to clean up the environment so all life thrives; it is also based on the absurd delusion that one can "protect" oneself in the first place in a world where life itself cannot survive. We are the earth—it is our larger form, our larger body. If we are to survive, our earth must also survive. Our goal is total well-being, for only with total wellness can the parts themselves be well and flourish.

Those who plan on guns to "fight over what's left" would be sadly disappointed at the reality of such a world anyway and would be like rats fighting over the last morsel of food in a cage: trapped together. Their fear and terror in the world they would create would far exceed any fear of hunger, or even death, that we could ever know. Even death in our world of life would be preferable to so-called "life" in their world of death. But let's reserve such thoughts for last-minute realities and resorts, because we must concentrate on survival of life instead!

If we were in a darkened room and the door were opened just a crack, the light would stream in, and even if the door were closed again, we'd never forget that light. So, it is with truth. If we want to know what's on the other side of the mountain, we can wonder and speculate, or we can climb to the top and see for ourselves. It's more work, but well worth the effort. We don't even have to be "experts" to see truth for ourselves, nor to appreciate life and contemplate its wonder, even when our "knowledge" is limited. All of us have this special gift: wisdom, instinct and intuition don't depend on book learning!

It is not, therefore, "who" we are or how much we "know" that determine our ability to contribute—it's what we do with our thoughts, intuition and energy that matters as far as evolution and change are concerned. If you doubt this for a moment, take a look at what some so-called people of "wealth, influence, power or brains" do with their lives and for others—and at what they do not do. Some of them merely perpetuate the problems in our world.

Imagine being near a large fire and surrounded by people of knowledge, wealth, influence, and power. The fact remains that the only things you really need to put out the fire are water and action.

101.1.1. Age-Old Excuses for Inertia

We've heard them all by now. These are but a few of our favorites:

- I overslept.
- I'm too busy.
- It's too late.
- I don't have time.
- I'll do it later (tomorrow, and so on).
- Someone else will do it.
- It's Monday (Tuesday, etc.).

- It's not my fault.
- It's not my problem.
- Call me when it gets really urgent.
- Don't call me, I'll call you.
- I need time to think it over and ask the "experts" more questions.
- I don't care.
- I don't know how to help.
- I can't ...

101.2. Life

101.2.1. Human Nature: The Mind and Evolution of Consciousness

101.2.2. Dreams

101.2.3. "A Penny for Your Thoughts"

101.2.4. The Life Force

101.2.5. What Time Is It?

101.2.6. "Time Is of the Essence"

101.2.7. Vegetarian Thinkers

101.2.1. Human Nature: The Mind and Evolution of Consciousness

We may observe the brain in its physical form and learn about its function, yet much is still unknown about how our mental processes actually work, leaving many unanswered questions about our perception and states of consciousness, and how they evolve from the "convergence" and "merging" of our physical and nonphysical realities. Some of us are at least aware that a healthy body and mind go hand in hand, and that deviations from physical health promote deviations from mental health as well.

Some scientists say that the left side of the body controls the right side of the brain, and that this right hemisphere is closely linked to feelings; emotions; intuition; subconscious thought; instinct; innate artistic, musical, creative tendencies; and so on. The right side of the body controls the left side of the brain, which is linked with rational thought, analysis, conceptualization, logic, and cognitive (conscious) thought. The right relies on the left for speech; its messages are verbalized by the left. Studies of serious worriers show they have an overactive left side of the brain compared to nonworriers (worriers also exhibit a lower level of alpha-wave readings—a measure of how relaxed a person is). Scientists are still not completely certain about all the specific areas of the brain; for example, the frontal lobes are still considered by many to be the most mysterious part of the human brain. Mild electrical stimulation of other parts of the brain makes people move a finger or hand, turn their head, or see flashes of light, but it is harder for researchers to link this vast, "silent" area to particular movements or sensations. When lobotomies were performed—by the 60s they more or less went "out of style" (thank goodness)—changes later evident in their victims suggested that the frontal lobes control such important qualities as self-awareness, initiative and the ability to plan to synthesize. The left frontal lobe seems to process information about shapes.

Eugene d'Aquili, a psychiatrist interested in the link between philosophy and neurobiology, says that strong feelings activate a certain part of the right hemisphere of the brain ("which instantaneously comprehends wholeness"), thus boosting our minds into a "separate" reality. He says some individuals report the altered state he calls "Absolute Unitary Being" in which "time stands still," and they see only the totality of a given situation or psychological reality and have a sense of absolute and complete unity—of self, of cosmos—caused, he says, by the "occipital parietal region on the right practically obliterating the rest of the brain, perceptually." He says this experience can result in a religious or agnostic feeling (depending upon individual interpretation), but that everyone who goes through it is absolutely certain that the transcendent, absolute realm of things does exist. He says "since most psychiatrists and medical doctors really know very little about mystical states;" they often refer people to him. For example, he sees people who "don't seem to have actual thought disorders, but are unbalanced by a pervasive negative feeling, in which life and the universe are seen as purposeless; they aren't clinically depressed or 'disturbed,' but they want relief, relief from their belief that the state they're in is ultimate reality—their misery makes them wish to be taught to think it illusory so they can survive."

According to d'Aquili, for those who have experienced "both" realities—the reality of the daily world/objective science and the reality of transcendent unitary being—the problem is not reducing one to another, since these people say they "know" both are real, but rather to "reconcile what they perceive as two drastically different perceptions of reality."

We discussed states of consciousness somewhat in Lesson 90, and may want to review this section briefly before continuing here. It is precisely the wrongful perception of our physical, mental/psychological/spiritual/collective states of being as drastically "different" that has led to the intense confusion many people feel in today's times of introspection and transition into greater awareness. Upon closer scrutiny we see that together they make up our total being and are parts of a unified whole, just as night and day seem "drastically different" but are linked inseparably into one complete cycle. Until we understand and accept this concept of total unity, we'll remain confused at our scattered feelings and find it difficult to integrate all our thoughts, feelings and experiences into some semblance of order and understanding—a sense of wholeness. Remember, integrating our thoughts isn't necessarily defining or categorizing them; rather, it is allowing them to flow, synthesizing our impressions into an experience we can understand and view as a whole. It's best to allow our intuitive subconscious much more freedom and space in our minds because our conscious thoughts so often crowd them full. There is a subtle balance to be found, and the more complicated our minds become, the more we need to find this balance for ourselves, for our own peace of mind. It's ironic with today's constantly-increasing input of news, information, people, faces and other distractions, that the more dispersed we become, the more we also risk dissipating our precious life energy. Our "busy" nature can keep us out of focus if we don't learn to deal with our accelerated lifestyles. Each of us has a different solution to juggling input and output, but we can all benefit from an overall simplicity, by learning how to get to the point of clarity so that we see the whole picture through all the layers and layers of ideas.

As we said in Lesson 90, we must also avoid becoming so fascinated with "mental gymnastics" and so involved with analyzing our conscious, rational thoughts that our subconscious intuitive messages are unable to "penetrate" all the layers to reach us! We are sometimes so swept away by our passionate desire to "expand" our consciousness that we become wrapped up in the techniques themselves and can miss obvious truths amidst all the pomp and circumstance. It's as if we have a luscious ripe peach in front of us, and we spend hours looking for a plate to put it on so that we can eat it when all we really have to do is put it in our mouths, so simply.

We often overlook the simple things in life because we're dazzled by the so-called complex ones. Our world of gadgets and "scientific" facts and figures encourages us to expect complexity and to seek truth with fancy equations. We've come to expect much ado about nothing and everything, and it's human nature to be curious—we all learn that famous word at about age 2: why? It is probably one of the most frequently asked questions. We want to know.

Stanley Bass once said that early Life Scientists/Hygienists viewed life as encompassing the totality of a person's being, including the mind and the spirit, but that in the 1920s the writers began to leave out more of the inspirational, "spiritual" (meaning of the spirit) aspects of Natural Hygiene because we were entering the "scientific" age, and Hygienic doctors didn't want to be considered "quacks" or strange people. He felt that this was a shame because it is inspiration that makes people change, more, than facts in black and white.

Although I came across his above statements only recently, from the very beginning of my writings I've had an uncontrollable urge to include the nonphysical realm of our minds and spirits in our discussions, not only because they are such a strong part of everyone's being and reality, but also because once the dietary truths we've learned have become a habit, we still need somewhere new to go. As we've said, once we change to a pure diet/ lifestyle, a growth in consciousness is inevitable, so the more we understand our minds, the better off we'll be. There is a gap or void left when we try to attend "only" to our physical needs, and I'd be more than happy to try to fill it.

Curiously enough, most of us nowadays are up-to-date on political figures and movie stars, the newest car models, the latest in art or literature—whatever we happen to be interested in—but still relatively little is said (in comparison) about the psychic energy of our minds; and those of us interested in it often find a lack of information on this subject, in contrast with the wealth of facts available on television, airplane engines, or simple arithmetic, for example. People hint at this energy, but there doesn't seem to be much general consensus on "scientific" explanations of non-physical phenomena of the mind—psychic energy doesn't seem to be taken for granted yet, at least not in the sense that something like television is taken for granted (although television also involves waves invisible to the naked eye and concepts beyond the physical reality that most of us are familiar with). The reason we have television is that people shared their knowledge until scientific concepts and technological aspects were put together. Pieceby-piece, bits of information and parts were assembled until television became a reality. Until we share our knowledge about what goes on in our minds, our understanding will remain limited. It's only when we synthesize knowledge that patterns emerge.

Perhaps we have experienced unusual intuition, precognitive dreams, or other nonphysical phenomena, but don't know who to share them with. After all, not everyone is open-minded; we may hesitate to speak about such things to just anyone. Until more of us open up and become aware that these phenomena do exist, and talk about our experiences, these phenomena will remain unrecognized or largely misunderstood. I doubt that the "cavemen" were already talking about tax reform, molecular biology, or their blood pressure—most of the "reality" we take for granted in our lifetime has taken years to develop into its present "form." A car would be as unexpected and "miraculous" to a primitive person as extrasensory perception is to some of us today. As more individuals come forth with their stories, our understanding of nonphysical reality will be broadened and become "second nature" to us—we'll consider it as normal and as basic as part of our being as breathing, eating, sleeping, and so on. Over the years we've gained a general understanding of how our bodies work; although many people are still off-the-mark nutritionally, most of us know some basic facts about physiology—for example, if we scratch ourselves and something red appears, we know it is blood from our veins, and the thump, thump we feel on our chests is a heart beating within. We take these things for granted now, but we must admit that our bodies and their contents would be very mysterious to us if we didn't already have these years of knowledge behind us.

It's unfortunate that pioneers of the mind, consciousness and the nonphysical realm have been mislabeled and misjudged so often, and that they have at times even mislabeled themselves because they didn't understand their vision or unusual insight. Whenever a person has been different from the "majority," s/ he has often been called abnormal as well, if not crazy or any other number of descriptions considered "fitting" by peers. If we weren't so judgmental and concerned with comparing ourselves to others and others to ourselves, we could use the simple word "different" as a substitute for all these other words—it's certainly a nicer way to say "eccentric."

101.2.2. Dreams

"You may say that I'm a dreamer, but I'm not the only one."

—John Lennon

We spoke of unusual dream experiences in Lesson 90 but might add a few notes on this dimension of consciousness, since it accounts for approximately 1/3 of our lives and is obviously much more than a "sleeping fantasy." Just as people didn't begin to explore the ocean until they had boats, and that vast watery mass remained a mystery, so too have we been limited in our exploration of our minds and dreams, for want of a "vehicle" to take us there, or more appropriately, the understanding we need to operate a "nonphysical vehicle" in a nonphysical reality. Dreaming is but one such vehicle.

Some of us have begun to cross the boundaries already and are becoming more familiar with the mind's "dimensions." Others of us have arrived but aren't sure what "country" we're in; some of us are still looking for a parking place or haven't even left "home" (our physical body) yet. Just as gifted children are often assigned extra learning projects at school when their special intelligence is recognized and go on to advance more rapidly than their classmates, so too must those gifted with exceptional sensitivity go into the uncharted territory of the mind long before others. Just as any mathematical or scientific formula was first devised by one (or several) inventive mind(s), so too are we pioneers of the mind discovering new worlds beyond the physical, beyond the tangible things we can see, hear, smell, taste and touch. If such realities, waves and energy—all quite invisible to the naked eye—didn't exist, we wouldn't have satellites, radios, microwaves, and so on. Before these realities could be "harnessed" for our physical world, someone had to have intuition and believe in what they could not see. We must transcend our physical world and believe in things we do not see with our eyes before we can expect to understand the nonphysical realities in our world.

In a "lucid" dream, a dreamer is actually aware that s/he is dreaming, and can sometimes even control or influence the dream. Most people don't connect their waking and sleeping realities consciously, but lucid dreamers can do so. This has been verified in sleep labs by scientists studying dreaming and sleep.

Dr. Stephen LaBerge taught himself and others to wake within dreams and believes that lucid dreaming can change the quality of our lives. ("Think of the value of being able to imagine vividly anything you can conceive of, and then to experience it," he says. "That would free us from so many restrictions.") LaBerge, who began as a student of chemical physics, first found references to lucid dreaming in the literature of Tibetan Buddhism—then, spontaneously, he experienced a lucid dream. As he studied the limited scientific literature available on lucid dreaming, he realized he'd had such dreams as a six-year-old. After finding a "technique" that worked for him, he was able to recall about 21 lucid dreams a month. In order to prove that he was actually controlling his dreaming, he decided to send a signal with his eyes while dreaming. In the laboratory, he was wired to a complex research polygraph (a polysomnograph) and fell asleep prepared to send the prearranged Signal to the researcher monitoring the machine. The lucid dream came after seven hours, and he decided to give the signal. The researcher saw the recording pens move on the polygraph, and this experiment was repeated successfully many times. However, because LaBerge knew that even the paralyzed muscles of active sleep twitch occasionally, he set up the polygraph to record the electrical activity of the muscles of his wrists. Then, during a lucid dream, he clenched the left fist of his dream body four times, the right fist once, and the left twice more. The polygraph showed the pattern: he had spelled out his initials, S.L., in Morse code—lucid dreaming became a scientific fact. Recent studies show that about a third of the population probably experiences at least an occasional lucid dream.

La Berge says the first step is remembering your dreams. Then, when you can succeed in incorporating a pre-sleep suggestion into a dream (if, for example, you tell yourself you want to see your hand in your dream and manage to do so), you have crossed the "boundary" and are able to connect both your waking and sleeping realities and states of consciousness. Those of us who don't feel "disciplined" enough to use techniques to arrive at these experiences can be assured that if we are meant to experience them, we will—one way or the other! I've had lucid dreams and precognitive dreams on many occasions without "trying"—they just happened (probably long before I recognized them too!). Those who benefit from trying "techniques," however, should do so.

LaBerge says dreams can be a workshop of creativity and growth. While dreams are often what he calls "repetitious melodramas" where we "confine ourselves by habit to a prison of self-limitation" (I suppose if we do so in our waking lives, well do so in our sleeping lives), lucid dreaming, he says, "presents a way out of this sleep within sleep." For example, a lucid d reamer caught in a nightmare could choose either to escape it or to attempt to resolve the fears behind it. Neither choice is available in ordinary sleep. Many of us have experienced nightmares in which we wished so strongly to wake up that we did—these were lucid dream experiences too, because we were aware that we were dreaming at the time.

LaBerge says that lucid dreaming might also offer psychological support to the handicapped; while awake, the paralyzed can't walk, but in their dreams they can dance and fly, helping them go beyond their physical handicaps in their inner lives.

As Stephen LaBerge says: "Your waking life is brief enough as it is. If a third of it must be shortened by sleep, do you want to sleep through your dreaming too?"

If we can learn to "combine" or blend our waking and sleeping realities, we have a whole new dimension open to us, a new opportunity for increased understanding and awareness. We can then make the conscious decision to go beyond our physical reality and bodies into the nonphysical realm, and potentially, find information there (as discussed in Lesson 90) that we aren't finding in our normal physical ("awake/conscious") world. We should use every tool we can, whether it be physical or mental, to increase our awareness. Dreaming is overlooked by many of us as an option for enhancing our lives, and as the wonderful flight from our bodies' physical boundaries that it is: a chance to feel our (spirit's) existence beyond our physical body ...

101.2.3. "A Penny for Your Thoughts"

We also have a lot more options in our waking lives than many of us even realize. I'd like to share some excerpts with you from the May 1984, issue of Acres, U.S.A., from an interview with Dr. Phil Callahan (an internationally famous entomologist and ornithologist who was also a navigation and electronics specialist in the 1940s). Several topics were covered, one of which was a brief mention of the circuitry of the brain. When asked about thought transmission and how it might take place between husband and wife or close relatives, Callahan says:

"You have, say, a mother in the U.S. and a son, say, in Vietnam, and suddenly the son is hurt or wounded, and she knows it instantly. This has been verified in war after war after war. One of the best verifications of ESP (extrasensory perception), in my opinion, is case reports of things that take place during traumatic experiences in war. The son's electric circuit brain is very much like his mother's—he has 50% of her circuits. Therefore, his brain puts out a lot of energy. If you can scan the earth from a satellite with 10 to the -17 watts, there is no reason why your brain isn't putting out much more than that: In fact, your brain is probably putting out, I would guess, 10 to the -12 watts and 10 to the -17 watts is less. Yet you can take a TV picture and turn something from a satellite into a TV picture with 10 to the -17, and that is a trillion, trillion, trillionth of a watt. Your brain putting out 10 to the -9 or something like that is certainly a stronger signal and would go around the world 40 times. Of course, signals do go around the world in nature. You have what you call Schuman Resonance. Schuman Resonance is when you have harmonics from lightning bolts that go around the world at about 8 to 20 cycles, and who knows what they are controlling. You have thousands of lightning bolts all over the world, and the ionosphere above and the earth below act like a big hollow cavity. So, you get these frequencies trapped in this hollow cavity, and they go around and around. You can tune in to them. Nikola Tesla did this. He sent waves around the world. He was no doubt utilizing the Schuman Resonance to do it. He was ahead of his time. Schuman Resonance wasn't even discovered until about 15 years ago, but Tesla was doing this back in the 1890s."

Electroencephalograms measure the activity of brain waves; it is now obvious to scientists that these waves exist and show various levels of "energy." Many believers in thought transmission/reception probably think that it depends on the level of sensitivity, awareness and receptivity of the individuals involved, at this point— recognition of thought transmission/receptivity may now depend on these things, but the actual transmission/reception most likely occurs constantly, whether we are "aware" of it or not—just as our blood moves through our veins whether we are aware of it or not, our thought wavelengths can move out through space independent of our realization that anything is happening at all! Believers have been aware of this phenomenon for ages, but many people are still skeptical; perhaps they don't have firsthand experience with it or know someone who has—anyone who has experienced such things needs no convincing. I've recognized (and even experienced) verifiable thought transmission/ reception often enough to be a firm believer. Even when such an event happens once in a lifetime, it will alter one's outlook on life as few other experiences can. Truth is self-evident.

We already know we can "harness" waves that we can't even see to make a picture appear on a television screen, or to make songs come over the radio, but some of us still doubt that thoughts can be transmitted or received. Just because we can't "explain or understand all the physics" involved—or don't have enough awareness yet to control them ourselves to much extent—doesn't mean that thought transmission doesn't exist. We've already seen that many things exist outside our awareness of their existence. For example, microscopic life certainly existed before we saw it in microscopes!

Nowadays we readily accept the reality of TV waves, radio waves, telegraphic signals, microwaves, and so on, but a century ago people would have scoffed at such ideas (or perhaps labelled their proponents as "witches"); enlightened persons might have been open-minded enough to agree that these ideas were at least conceivable or perhaps possible "in the future," with more knowledge available. People today also readily acknowledge the following (and other) realities: that grooves on a record (or a thin, shiny tape in a cassette) will result in music; that X rays take pictures of things we can't see with our eyes; that radar sensors pick up objects; that cameras "make pictures"; that laser beams can, among other things, burn holes in objects; that computer chips we can barely see will hold thousands of bits of information; that we can talk to people thousands of miles away on the phone; and that the power of the atom (also "invisible" to us) in nuclear power has the ability to destroy our planet! How's that for an example of immense physical power in an element so small we can't even see it!

In our waking, conscious lives we learn what we want to learn, and advance (or degenerate) at our own individual rates; so, it is with mystical dimensions. Just as an infant sitting in a car (who may someday learn to drive) is content for the time being to fidget with all the knobs, buttons, and switches at random (sometimes to the chagrin of Mom and Dad), so are we when it comes to our level of understanding and awareness. We have a lot to learn, but the knowledge and insight we need to "grow up" are within us, as well as without. Remember too, that just as with any skill of any kind, abilities in interpreting "paranormal" reality definitely vary; some mistakes or errors in judgment are to be expected, even from gifted persons, and some charlatans can be expected as well, just as with any talent or creative ability. We're taking our baby steps into the world of the psyche, finding out that our spirits aren't limited to the physical realm, as our bodies are.

"Suspended in the physical, and yet, I am beyond this skin, these eyes, and cannot quite forget."

We have but to imagine how free we can be in our spirits—we've only just begun. Just as a baby looks around at everything with that "so-this-is-where-I-am" look, we too are now in awe of our newfound dimension of consciousness and reality and wonder how far we can go here. That we can contemplate life in all its marvel at all is proof enough that we are spirit—we've outgrown the limits of our physical state—being spirit and body, we've always been in the nonphysical state, even before we "realized" it.

Phil Callahan's statement about the power of our brain waves to encircle the world "40 times" has some profound implications for us and adds a whole new dimension to our reality. Remember how many times we've thrown up our hands in despair to ask:

"But what can I, as one person, do to change the world?" (Again, we've come to realize that the truth is, we're all already doing it now). When frustrated and overwhelmed about problems we see, we often feel "so small" in this big world, and so alone. Sometimes we even wonder if we're the "only ones" who care. Rest assured that we aren't—we share these feelings with one another whether we are consciously aware of it or not. Because we live in such volatile times (nuclear, ecological, etc.), the fact that we are still here at all is no small miracle. One of the things now holding the world together at this very moment (and since the beginning of the nuclear age) is our tremendous collective will to live and to survive (called our deepest, strongest instinct) radiating outward at every moment, crisscrossing the planet over and over again with its messages: we want to live in peace and tranquility. That we are still here is the collective manifestation of the drive within us to evolve to new states of being, to progress and to grow, to explore our universe and minds and spirits. We are tired of wasting our precious time and lives in the futile efforts of war. Hatred, destruction, rebuilding, and starting over at the beginning again and again—we should have learned our lessons many years ago. These energy draining activities only slow us down and keep us from the beautiful, evolved creatures/ spirits of life that we will be when we work together and give peace a chance. We've had enough—we're weary of having shadows of doom and gloom looming in the back of our minds, and concerned when our children say they don't even know if they'll grow up.

We must never underestimate the power of our thoughts. Remember, just as with the atom, just because we don't see them doesn't mean they have no influence on our world—thoughts carry their own energy too.

Our desire for peace spreads outward like ripples on a pond, renewed with every new thought of peace, being reinforced all over the globe by the network of souls who want to live and let live—ever-gaining strength. We should be very proud to be part of this network of light and of life.

This is why we can't dwell on negative images of our world or future (beyond their imminent warnings), and get lost in our reactions, when it's action we need. In dwelling on the negative, we literally radiate negativity on the negative "wavelength," thus reinforcing the very thing we detest. When we radiate put on the wavelength of life and positive energy, we are joined with all the forces and powers of creation.

There's no tangible profit to be made off higher consciousness—you can't package it or sell it, and it results in people asking all those uncomfortable questions on "product safety" or "company liability for their damaged health," etc. In other words, it seems that one of the last things we hear about these days in the media is nonphysical reality, the evolution of consciousness, and so on (when what could be more relevant and important for those of us who are restless within the limits of our physical reality?). We certainly hear enough about ring-around-the-collar, squeezably soft toilet tissue or being part of the "Pepsi generation." People oriented in physical reality buy physical products. What's more, if they were to become true to their consciences and become their highest, most evolved, most moral selves, with a remarkable code of honor, they might no longer "have a price"—they might begin to care more about life and people than about things—and avoid obsession with material possessions that hinders their "non-material" growth and distracts them from higher pursuits. Why, then they might even refuse to pay for weapons that kill people and destroy life! In other words, "they might just rock the boat."

If we could realize the strength and power—and the incredible positive force of creation and love—that our minds are really capable of, now and at every moment, we would challenge corrupt and unjust systems into which we're locked for our physical survival, and we wouldn't be as easily influenced/manipulated/brainwashed. But as long as we're kept running a treadwheel, trapped like hamsters in a cage, locked in debt just to survive and make ends meet to pay for our physical needs, we'll "stay in our place," and many of us are too busy to find out about all our strength and potential (especially its collective force), or we're just "too tired to care" at the end of another hectic day.

British futurist Peter Russell thinks that we are now moving "from the computer age to the Age of Consciousness, the next step, an epoch when our minds will be linked by common goals, when humans will be creatures without ego, using their large brains to manage the affairs of the planet." He believes that humankind is about to make an unprecedented leap in evolution, a jump beyond petty jealousy, virulent nationalism, unbridled greed. We are to become, Russell says, the nervous system that makes the whole globe tick, a kind of benevolent planetary brain linked by common consciousness. The earth for Russell is a single organism, not just a spinning rock teeming with life, but a life form all by itself, an individual being. And we humans are going to become this organism's brain. We are already the information processors of the planet, says Russell. We collect data, build libraries, museums, and satellites. Information passes through national boundaries as if they didn't exist. In 1944 there were only three computers in the world. "Now look," Russell says. "We moved from the Industrial Age to the Information Age with tremendous speed. Now 40 years after the first computers, we're already starting to go beyond them, to consciousness and awareness." Heightened consciousness, he says, is our inevitable next step. Individual consciousness will become group consciousness, and humankind will interconnect in a single vast cooperative of consciousness. "We are an evolutionary experiment," Russell says. "And the question is, are we a good thing or not? Are we a cancer, a blight destroying the very fiber of life, or will we serve another purpose?"

Peter Russell is not alone in his vision of a living Earth. He studied theoretical physics at Cambridge University but found himself drawn to Eastern philosophies; and when he went to India to pursue those interests, he "experienced a dimension of my consciousness of which I had never dreamed."

Today, doom scenarios are popular, Russell says. "We are in a very dangerous time. But shouldn't our large brains serve some greater purpose than self-destruction?" In his book he quotes1 inventor Buckminster Fuller: "The world now is too dangerous for anything less than Utopia."

101.2.4. The Life Force

We've spent a lot of time discussing health and survival of life and pondered the mysteries of our existence for some time now. What then, do we know about life itself! What is this amazing quality that can come and go, leaving an entity "alive" one moment and "lifeless" the next? Just as we can see and hear, whether we know we have "optic nerves and tympanic membranes" or not, or taste even if we don't know that our taste buds are "small ovoid neuroepithelial structures that lie between the epithelial cells that cover the tongue," so too can we live, once the life force is within us, whether we understand it or not—luckily for us! All of our cellular groupings, organs, bones, and everything down to our Hyoglossus (a muscle that we'd better have between our hyoid bone and tongue if we plan on "pulling the tongue into the floor of our mouths" any time soon), are all part of an incredibly intricate life support system. Ask any car mechanic what's involved in assembling his machine that moves through space—plenty—but well soon see that our bodily machine is infinitely more intricate. If you look at a book on physiology, you'll see how many "parts" our machine has! Being a vessel of the life force is one thing—duplicating it, another. Genetic "engineers" keep trying, and heaven help us, for we're trying to exercise divine power (control life) before we truly understand what divinity is. Yet, as are so many things, I suppose that's "in our nature," too. Whether we knit, garden, build, or tinker, we are all imbued with the passionate urge to create something. In any case, it might be wise if we knew more about the life force before tinkering with it too!

When someone "dies," we say the life force "leaves the body." This is generally agreed upon, although what happens next is still open to discussion after all these years. Perhaps one of the reasons we have a hard time getting past these age-old questions is that we're falling back into that same old trap of "trying too hard" (in this case, thinking too much) once again. Let's face it, we have been wondering about some of these things for a long time now, yet we still seem to get lost somewhere between the question and the answer! What's our problem here? Aside from the fact that we often block our intuitive channels with "logical" reasoning, maybe we'll also see our "abstract" predicament more clearly with a "concrete" example: imagine a primitive person standing in front of a computer, wondering what it is. Whatever the primitive person can conjure up in his mind to explain or comprehend this object, with his limited resources, will still not serve to explain its function. There is a "gap." This primitive person probably has the innate intelligence to operate a computer, but until the gap of understanding is closed, it will remain a mystery. Just as the baby in the car must learn what the gadgets are before they will become "real" to him, so too, the more we learn about our mental abilities, the more meaningful they will be for us.

We often become impatient. Here we are, faced with our human physical mortality, bills due, and a mystery: what happens when we "die"? Like angry children, we demand answers to the mystery of life, but we're still forcing the issue and overlooking the simple. We're already in over our heads when we try to explain "supernatural" phenomena in our human terms and words. If we want to understand the life force, we must begin by realizing that it is "more" than a "human" event—intangible and invisible, it is an event of the spirit, encompassing far more than our limited human reality. Since we can't see the life force in the first place, it would be presumptuous to assume that life dies just because a living entity "becomes lifeless." This is pure speculation on our part. The life force itself doesn't die when the entity "dies."

Mysticism has always included some concept of "eternity", eternal life, infinity. Somewhere along the line, some of our pioneer spirits found something, and began to pass it on: The story of eternity has undergone countless metamorphoses and versions throughout the ages. Some say we "go to heaven" (or, if not so lucky, to the 'big barbecue pit' in the sky?), and some say we're reborn—but, although the accounts differ, enlightened people from all times have clung tenaciously to some common belief in some form of eternal life, or an immortality of the spirit, with absolute certainty that there was life "beyond" the physical form, that the body is like a vehicle that is abandoned after it becomes useless and can't take us any further.

Once upon a time, long ago, someone died, and his friends stood around in sadness and tried to figure out what had happened. One minute he was moving, and the next ... as best they could determine, this person was gone, finished, ended—and the concept or word "dead" was invented to explain this event. Thus came the conclusion that where there is "no life," there is "death." It sounds logical enough, and we've been saying it so long that we've pretty much taken it for granted by now, but one of the main reasons we say there's no life when a person dies is because the person we knew doesn't move anymore and bodily organs have ceased to function. The word "death" may be useful in describing an event, but the notion of death as a finite, final event might have as many flaws in it as our old world-is-flat theory or current germ/contagion theories, held by so many as "absolute" truths. Since we have a profound lack of knowledge (even after all these years) of exactly what happens beyond what is visible to the naked eye when someone dies, we'd be somewhat naive to say that nothing else happens just because we can't see it or don't know what happens! Rather than being an end to life itself, death is just a process of change, a passage, transition, transcendence, metamorphosis, a new journey beyond the physical world of our bodies. Think about it. How can life be dead? How can life not be alive. The pioneer spirits who first spoke of eternal life saw a simple answer to the complex question of what death was: a sort of evolution—life goes on, eternally, forever, endlessly changing form. The first thing we do when we die is change form: our body begins to decay, to "disappear," to break down what it once built up—like a reverse-action film, it's completing the "cycle." The process of cellular decay is one of change, change, change—of metamorphosis as the body fades from the physical world. How can we define what is obvious activity as a "dead" (motionless) process, when this movement of molecular structure from one form to another is obviously a process of change (visible and invisible) and might better be defined as just another part of the life process itself! When the body finally disappears from our visible physical reality, we can't say exactly what has become of its atoms and molecules, for they have rearranged and changed structure from one form into another (or perhaps others). This transformation process of life (called death) is still very much a mystery to us! People already give us "those" looks when we tell them we don't eat meat or cooked food. Wait until we see the looks we get when we say "there's no real death, only eternal life and change and metamorphosis and evolution ..." Here we go again!

So, is that all there is to it? We've been saying this life force weaves its way here and there, as if we could be in the middle of a sentence, and ... poof! We are fortunate enough to have been chosen by the life force as "containers" for its antics, but we too have choices to make. When life asks us to dance with it, we become its partners—we help determine its rhythm within us and the melody of our duet together—life is the voice—we become the words to its song. Studies with terminally ill patients have indicated that the will to live, or the lack of the will to live, do have an effect on the length of our lives, and that a person can literally "turn himself off" at some point, whether consciously or subconsciously. (Another good reason to keep thoughts positive.) If we become too tired or bored, sick, old, etc., to continue the dance, life will understand and move on. If we want to live fully, life will stay with us as long as possible, even until the dawn of our new day.

In each moment, time stands still; in each moment, from whence we came and where we are going are all caught up in an instant of eternity.

Believe in life and its force and you already know eternity. Eternal life is with us forever in this moment.

101.2.5. What Time Is It?

We discussed the concept of time in Lesson 90 and said that it doesn't actually exist exactly as we define it in our human terms! There, and in our above discussion, we mentioned the eternal present: it is always now. Yesterday and tomorrow are actually "abstractions": the only real time is "now." There is no other time we exist in other than "now" (in fact, everyone who ever lived, lived "now").

We say that moments (and time) pass from one to the next, but time isn't moving—it's always now—it is we living beings who move. We form a living chain of beings and we call those who lived before us "from the past" and those who are yet to come "from the future" and the links of this chain of life hold us together. We can assume that everyone was living (or will live) now at the time they lived (or will)—and we who are alive now are living now—so it appears that we're "all living at the same time—now. "Of course, that seems to defy the physical imagination, to say the least, but as much as it defies logical explanation, it is at the same time somehow "logical." It's also interesting to note that this might shed some light on the mystery of the gift of prophecy!

101.2.6. "Time Is of the Essence"

We've talked about some peoples' ability to know things from the "universal mind"— an ability that defies logical explanation and goes beyond our usual "normal" channels for receiving knowledge. Not only that, but our "normal," traditional notion of time is also open to question when we see that some people not only know things or receive information beyond their "normal" physical/mental reality; they are even able to know things (whether from the past or future) beyond the so-called "physical time" in which they exist at that moment. How can this be? How can someone know something that "hasn't happened yet"? What does that do to our "normal" concept of the "future," or of time itself? One of the better-known examples of person with prophetic gifts was Nostradamus, who lived in the 16th century. He is said to have foreseen numerous events that came to pass after his death (which he also saw ahead of time). In 1568, he published the following prophecy:

Century IV, Quatrain 67:

In the year that Saturn and Mars are equally fiery The air is very dry, a long meteor (comet)

By secret fires, many places shall be burnt with heat. There shall be scarcity of rain, hot winds, wars, blood, thirst, and famine (when the comet shall run).

The above quote and the following excerpts are from an article "When Solar Winds Blow Havoc for Mankind" by Jim Cummins, Acres, U.S.A., January 1985, which discusses the return of Halley's comet, due again in our vicinity in November 1985, and to "stay in our backyard" until April 1986. Halley's comet has a well-documented 76-year cycle, with records begun in March 239, B.C. Ever since this sighting, a worldwide three-year drought (and often resultant famine) has followed in its wake each time, (for details—a long list of other climatological, social, and political upheavals throughout history that were on the heels or in the wake of a comet—please get a copy of the above issue.)

"How can all these things be attributed to the passing of a comet? Space probes have sent back data showing that the sun continuously ejects a million tons of gas per second, moving at a radial speed of 250 miles per second, with wind speeds past the earth at some 900,000 miles per hour, and extends to about four times the distance beyond the farthest planet Pluto. (A comet travels in its orbit to several thousand times farther than Pluto.) This solar wind carries chaotic magnetic fields along with it because the gas is ionized. The magnetic fields of the solar wind ruffle the earth's own magnetic field as it passes by, hence, magnetic disturbances affecting communications, etc., at the time of increased solar activity (which is cyclical). Scientists have determined, for instance, a statistical correlation between the accelerations of Halley's Comet and magnetic disturbances on the earth.

"The effects of the solar wind on every earthly activity, from health to markets, weather, and wars, is well-documented. The transverse motion of a comet at many miles per second across the movement of the solar wind blowing radially from the sun results in the i6n tail of the comet interacting with the high velocity of the solar wind in the same way that smoke rising from a smokestack interacts with moving air to produce a graceful billowy arch to the earth.

"Scientists now believe that each interstellar dust grain of comet stuff contains molecules of form aldimine, methyl alcohol, methyl cyanide, hydrogen cyanide or hydrocyanic acid, and some 20 others, including cyanogen and carbon dioxide. (My note here: we have too much CO_2 already.) Many of the radicals they have determined to be the 'smoke' of comets cannot be isolated in a terrestrial laboratory and are probably created by the rapid breakdown of the parent compounds by ultraviolet sunlight. The lingering, billowy arch of smoke falls slowly to the earth in the wake of a comet's passing. Needless to say, no living thing on our tiny planet is made the better for it. We all breathe this cyanide: kings, presidents, common man alike think and act as though we have poison in our system (and we do) ... and we eat the plants and animals which have breathed the same deadly gases ... and the pale settles in for a season."

As we have seen in our studies on ecology and the current world political situation, we're already "teetering on the brink of extinction" in many ways, so we could certainly do without any "pales settling in" because we don't need much pushing, this close to the "edge."

"The advent of two important planets aligning at a crucial astronomical degree from the earth at the precise time that Halley's Comet (with which Nostradamus was familiar) would make as perihelion (closest point of approach to the sun), would be an ominous occurrence, said Nostradamus, warning us in the only way he could, considering the Inquisition under which he lived. Such an event (this planetary configuration at the comet's perihelion) has not happened/or over 1,000 years, but it is due in February 1986, and Nostradamus knew it!"

Here then is a verifiable example of prophecy: the dates of alignment of planets, in this case, Saturn and Mars, can be calculated and determined scientifically; the next such alignment is due in February 1986. How could Nostradamus know, in 1568, that they'd be aligned in a once-in-a-thousand-years configuration at a "crucial astronomical degree from the earth at the precise time (1986) Halley's comet would make its perihelion"?

We do still have a lot to learn about the powers of our minds. Some people apparently "go beyond their physical lifetimes" in their minds or spirits, but in the sense that the eternal present covers all eternity, they really don't even have to "go" anywhere. Apparently it's because it's always now that they can "see it now" if they have that gift of sensitivity.

It is interesting to note that gifts of intelligence, wisdom, insight, vision, enlightenment, clairvoyance, prophecy, and so on, are obviously not limited to people of any particular "time," i.e., they aren't limited to so-called highly-evolved or "civilized" people, nor are they always found in persons with exceptional "conventional" intelligence (ability to learn quickly, etc.). Throughout "the ages," there have been individuals who possessed extraordinary insight, wisdom, or extrasensory perception; such persons are "timeless"—they would stand out and excel in any time period.

One such person was Pythagoras, a Greek philosopher born in 570 B.C. who advocated vegetarianism, among other things, as the key to expanding consciousness and intellect. He was already talking about things Life Scientists believe in now; he was way "ahead of" most people of his day, and even ours. He even taught; that the world was round, long before Copernicus and Galileo came along after the 1400s.

Pythagoras was a mathematical and musical genius, a sage who travelled to many other countries (as far as Egypt and India, rare for people of those times); he was accepted by their wise men, who shared with him secrets often not divulged to their own public, nor to strangers. He accepted women as "thinking beings," and included them in his discussions, being unique in his times in doing so. Space here doesn't permit a detailed account of his life and gifts to humanity; suffice it to say, he was a rare person. Because of his diet, he was said to be in perfect health at all times, and of perfect, calm, harmonious temperament. He had a vision of a changed society with no war, slavery, or violence. Had his communities of followers been left alone in peace and allowed to thrive, we can only imagine where we'd all be today! However, as is so often the case when ignorant people form the "majority," his enemies tried to destroy his books and temples and enslaved his followers! We're still waiting for people to see the light that Pythagoras (and many before and since him) saw already. It seems quite obvious that the "missing link" in the puzzle of our prolonged aggressive tendencies and low-life attitudes up to now is meat-eating. Pythagoras was very specific in his admonitions not to eat meat; he wasn't vegetarian "by coincidence"—he knew exactly what he was doing in avoiding it and said so. Had we listened to his wisdom (and others') we might have avoided another thousand years of human suffering and wars.

101.2.7. Vegetarian Thinkers

A March 1985 newspaper article on Einstein's brain talked about recent studies of its brain cells: nearly 30 years after his death, Marian Diamond was looking at cells taken "from the 20th century's most celebrated clump of human intelligence." Before he died, Albert Einstein stipulated that his brain be preserved and used for research. "When we heard that Einstein's brain was sitting in a cardboard box in Kansas, we saw a chance to study the most highly-evolved brain available in our lifetime," Marian said. Dr.

Janice Stevens, staff psychiatrist at the neuropsychiatry branch of the National Institute of Mental Health, tells a story about the time researchers at Princeton did an electroencephalogram on Einstein. They were measuring the alpha wave, which indicates the brain's "idling activity." Alpha wave activity disappears with arousal or intense brain activity. The researchers started the EEG, and Einstein, so the story goes, was calmly solving quadratic equations in his head. His alpha wave, indicating mental idling, was very high. All of a sudden, the alpha wave went flat. Alarmed, the researchers rushed in and asked Einstein what was wrong. "I hear it's raining outside," said the world's greatest scientist, "and I've left my rubbers at home."

I wanted to include these excerpts (italics above are mine) to show how esteemed Einstein is in the scientific world, even though the article itself was going into details on his "glial cells" and so on (he had a higher ratio of glial cells to neurons compared with 11 other brains tested, with the most significant difference found in the sample from the left lower parietal lobe, the part of the brain most involved with higher mathematical and language abilities).

Einstein is considered a great genius, and he was also a vegetarian. Literature on vegetarians includes the following great thinkers from our history: Pythagoras, Socrates, Plato, Aristotle, Alexander the Great, Epicurus, Apollonius of Tyana, Plutarch, Seneca, Porphyry, Iamblichus, Proclus, Ovid, Tolstoy, the poet Ralph Waldo Emerson, Benjamin Franklin, Sir Isaac Newton, Gandhi, Buddha, Voltaire, Charles Darwin, Albert Schweitzer, and others; the artist Leonardo da Vinci was also a vegetarian— this list is but a sampling.

If we are interested in observing the mind and philosophy and the things of the universe, well do well to observe that some of the world's most "famous" historical figures, those whose names came down to us from the past because they were such outstanding persons in their day, were also vegetarians.

"Truly man is the king of beasts, for his brutality exceeds them. We live by the death of others. We are burial places! I have since an early age abjured the use of meat, and the time will come when men will look upon the murder of animals as they now look upon the murder of men."

—Leonardo da Vinci

"While we ourselves are the living graves of murdered animals, how can we expect any ideal conditions on the earth?"

—Leo Tolstoy

"Only living, fresh foods can enable man to apprehend the truth."

—Pythagoras

"It is my view that the vegetarian manner of living, by its purely physical effect on the human temperament, would most beneficially influence a lot of mankind."

—Albert Einstein

"Animals are my friends... and I don't eat my friends. Man suppresses in himself, unnecessarily, the highest spiritual capacity—that of sympathy and pity toward living creatures like himself—and by violating his own feelings, becomes cruel."

—George Bernard Shaw

"World peace, or any other kind of peace, depends greatly on the attitude of the mind. Vegetarianism can bring about the right mental attitude for peace... it holds forth a better way of life, which, if practiced universally, can lead to a better, more just, and more peaceful community of nations."

—U Nu, former Prime Minister of Burma

By changing our diets and lifestyles, we've already seen how closely they're related to "who we are." Very often the "personality" we think we are totally different after these changes are made in our lives. The sum total of our diet/ life becomes us, talks through us. As we unburden ourselves more and more, we replace our former resentment of ignorant people and our contempt for their wrongful actions with understanding, even forgiveness. We have no place in our minds for wasted thoughts; they distract us and clutter our heads with more useless negativity. We have no time for holding grudges or making judgments, for our time and our lives are precious. We've said it a dozen times, but it bears repeating: if we truly want to free ourselves, we'll replace all our negative thoughts with inner peace and tranquility. People who become trapped in their emotions don't see the diet/lifestyle connection; we know we don't have to be slaves to our emotions.

101.3. Liberty

101.3.1. It's a Gift to Be Simple, It's a Gift to Be Free

101.3.2. We Shall Overcome

101.3.3. "Reaching out to touch someone"

101.3.4. Economic Freedom: A Penny Saved Is a Penny Earned?

101.3.1. It's a Gift to Be Simple, It's a Gift to Be Free

If we have optimism, humor, understanding, faith, hope, love, self-control, and the ability to step outside ourselves into a universal, collective consciousness and into concern for others as well as ourselves; and if we have the desire and willingness to change (not just intent to change or idle talk about changing)—we will become filled with creative energy and vibrant life force, and yes, we will be free. We will free not only our bodies, but also our minds and spirits. The more positive energy that emanates from us into the world, the more healing that will take place in the world. It keeps boiling down to the same thing: what the world needs now (and always) is love. Our positive healing energy is needed everywhere, especially in these trying times.

So, we should ask ourselves, are our world leaders working to lead us toward Utopia or not? The answer is obvious.

Are we told the truth about the link between our food and lifestyle and our state of health? No. We're told to drink Coke, eat sugared cereals, and spray poisonous chemicals on ourselves to "keep bugs off." Let's not expect to be enlightened by our "system," for it is to the system's advantage that the sheep stay in the herd, and not be "carried away" with wild ideas of freedom or notions of exceptional mental clarity or abilities, thus realizing their full potential as human beings. The system of centralized wealth prefers to homogenize its people into a nice, workable "arrangement" that best ensures the continued survival of its authority and power to keep things "under control."

Funny, I was under the impression that the founding fathers (and mothers) of this country intended to govern themselves. What was that they said about government by the people, for the people, and so on?

Those of us of the technological age who've been spared certain survival necessities, such as having to walk miles to a well for water just to live, still have our own special challenges to meet. Our education and the media have given us more opportunity to view the broad spectrum of events and their consequences; "knowing" more, we have a deeper responsibility to truth and to life. The more we receive from life, the more we should give back in return. And, as the saying goes, "somebody has to do it."

It is evident that each of us must explore our own mental capacities and strengths, and find the truths that are to be revealed, for we aren't getting enough support from our world leaders in evolving to a consciousness of world peace and harmony. It is we, the people of this planet, who must demand a release from the bondage of weapons and war and insist that production of instruments of death be stopped, once and for all.

The slaveholders of the past didn't just wake up one day (until forced to do so) and tell the slaves: "Okay, you're free now." We can't wait for our "leaders" to "free" us. We must be free now. We are supposed to be free already, but who are the real slaves today? Every living being that is bound by the chains of war and hostility and who lives under the shadow of potential nuclear destruction—every living being on this planet, to be exact. We are being held back from our true work and kept from evolving toward our higher destiny. Ironically, here is an unusual situation in which even the slave master is enslaved—from now on, what happens to the slaves will happen to the slave "masters" as well. They now risk becoming victims of their own mistakes. While our "leaders" have at their "disposal" thousands of human hands ready (if not willing) for action, capable of making something immense in the spirit of cooperation, what do they do? They use our energy to create a system that could destroy us all, themselves included. Now does that make any sense?

We have years of struggle, suffering, joy, birth, and creation behind us already. Let's not throw it all way! We are free to choose life. What are we waiting for?

Just as fresh air, sunshine and healthy food are necessary for nourishing our physical bodies, freedom is one of our most precious treasures to be preserved in safeguarding our minds and Spirits. We need freedom for our mental health and well-being, as much as we need air to breathe. Although we've made progress in some areas, human rights in the world today cannot be taken for granted by most people. Just as physical illness reflects some imbalance in the body, the sad state of affairs in human rights reflects the moral decay so prevalent today. We are told we live in a democracy, but we must be ever-watchful and vigilant of what freedom we do have and hold on to it with all our strength. It could even use some improvement. Now that the computer age is here, we must be especially cautious of "world systems" and being numbered, catalogued, and filed. The world economy is shaky; if transitions are made to a "cashless" system, necessitating numbering of citizens, a word to the wise ... freedom as we know it could all but disappear in the "ultimate" system. Computers, like all our inventions, are tools—as useful or destructive as we make them.

There are three principal groups in the United States dedicated to ending human rights abuses: Amnesty International, Helsinki Watch and Americas Watch. Amnesty International won the Nobel Peace Prize in 1977 and has 150,000 members here and 500,000 worldwide. It also watches out for political prisoners, for the countless people suffering in jail whose only "crime" was to speak out against injustice—nonviolent people of conscience who tried to better the lives of others. A 1984 report from Amnesty International ("Torture in the Eighties") carried meticulously-detailed accounts of inhumane treatment of prisoners in 96 countries, from Afghanistan to Zimbabwe. Amnesty tries to publicize abuses and pressure governments guilty of human rights violations. Now that the world is so small, we all have a vested interest in global human rights, in staying awake — the fox will come when the chickens are sleeping ...

101.3.2. We Shall Overcome

More and more sanctuary movements have begun to take an active role in reaching out to refugees from other countries who are fleeing political persecution and violence at home, and they must often defy official disapproval (and, or risk imprisonment) in order to shelter these people. Even church members are getting involved, saying that what they are doing is providing sanctuary, a historical and religious tradition dating from the Middle Ages. Court trials have already resulted. A statement issued by Austin Quakers said: "There is a law that binds us as one within the spirit, which cannot be made subject to laws constructed in response to national interests. We declare our willingness to provide sanctuary for these, our sisters, and brothers, to hold them within the boundaries of our spiritual community, safe from pursuit and prosecution by the authorities." Another group made this statement:

"We implore immigration officials and the court system to cease in their persecution of innocent people fulfilling their duty as Christians and are proud of those who lay their reputations and lives on the line to protect, nourish, and care for the poor of other nations who seek nothing more than the same opportunity our refugee forefathers sought and obtained during the past two and more centuries."

Matthew 10:16... "Behold, I send you forth as sheep in the midst of wolves be ye therefore wise as serpents, and harmless as doves."

26: "Fear them not therefore: for there is nothing covered, that shall not be revealed; and hid, that shall not be known."

101.3.3. "Reaching out to touch someone"

With the growth of technology and industry worldwide, our world cultures have been brought from the "dawn of time" to "modern civilization," sometimes almost literally overnight, in a single jump from "primitive" times to the 20th century. Just like the pizza people, we deliver, alright—for a price. There's a trade-off, and many souls have been "sold" along the way.

But while our businesses are arriving in faraway lands to look for a good deal on cheap labor, less safety restrictions perhaps, and so on, and arrive to buy and sell weapons and war, there's a parallel movement going on—one most of us have been part of at one time or another: the "world traveler's association"—the real diplomats-on-the street of this planet. The next time we're gazing from a hammock in a tiny, relaxed terrace nestled among lush vegetation in a tropical country, sipping fresh-squeezed orange juice, be assured that we are actually hard-at-work, as members of the real international Peace Corps, bringing ourselves to others, drawing the world closer. People are travelling internationally as never before and that's had a profound impact on world society as a whole: more and more people see each other now. Even the goatherder in Morocco gazes face-to-face into the eyes of the American family from Kansas—two worlds meet again. The more we see each other, the less we can be "strangers."

Not only does this ever-broadening circle of international friends accelerate the quantum leap humanity is now making into collective consciousness; it also strengthens our chances globally to learn the truth more often. Whereas national leaders, newspapers or TV can (and do) lie or censor news, say what they want and try to shape everyone's reality and conform society's members, the fact remains that nowadays, many more people everywhere are also picking up the phone just to talk to a good old buddy or business associate on the other side of the world and they'll ask, "what's new?". So, stories come out here and there— much news is still shared in the "old-fashioned" way—by word of-mouth. This international grapevine is unlike any there's every been before in our recorded history—even gossip has gone international!

Much truth can leak through, because if there's one thing people are famous for, it's their ability to talk. Now that folks are chatting from Germany to Thailand to Timbuktu, a lot of truth can even leak through today's "sophisticated" totalitarian efforts around the world to control what can be heard in the media! The net thrown out by our dictators now has many holes in it, and as fast as they can "fix" them, we can make new ones! This international network of friends protects all of us because it keeps real channels of communication open; it exists beyond the formal rhetoric of world leaders who communicate to us (and each other) only what they want us to hear. This real communication network functions on a global level and yet is still unstructured—it exists and is thriving outside "government control and regulation"—a loose network of individuals with no control from specific, visible leaders—independent.

The world community is apparently healing itself despite—not because of—government, which is the "drug" in this case that's supposed to "cure" society. If the people "can't take care of themselves," they look to the government to play the role of doctor, to decide "what's best for them," to take the responsibility out of their hands, and the government is more than happy to do so. But even today's tyrants will find that truth will still pop up "in the strangest places." Just as some weeds are much harder than domesticated hybrid plants, luckily for us, truth is one of the strongest weeds of all—stubborn and tenacious. No matter how hard a ruler might try to keep people ignorant (and thus dependent) and uninformed, light still penetrates the darkness again and again. Trying to keep truth a secret is harder than trying to stop the tide of water at the ocean's edge with your bare hands! Truth will surface again and again—that's the beauty of it. Like a blade of grass that clings stubbornly to life in a crack in the cement of a hot city sidewalk, truth clings to us in hope of survival.

And the truth shall set us free.

We've already taken a bit of "license" in speaking freely of phenomena of the mind which we're only beginning to experience, let alone understand. But lest the skeptical among us question the reality of anything in nonphysical "reality" too hastily, let's refer to the following excerpts on the CIA's interest and dabbling in these phenomena. It is becoming increasingly apparent that we have to guard not only the freedom we expect for our physical bodies, but also the nonphysical freedom that is our heritage as spiritual beings.

Omni (10/80) reports: Declassified documents obtained under the Freedom of Information Act (one worth all our effort protecting) by the American Citizens for Honesty in Government revealed a 20-year CIA mind-control operation that experimented with everything from hypnosis and behavior modification to psychoactive drugs (such as LSD) and electroshock, all well-documented. "Less noticed among the esoterica included in the so-called Project Bluebird (later renamed Project Artichoke, still later MKULTRA) was another possible secret weapon: extrasensory perception." The agency's dream was spelled out in an April 1952, memo: "If a number of individuals could be found in the U.S. who have a very high ESP capacity, these talented individuals could be assigned to intelligence problems. Such a problem as whether or not the (deleted) had a submarine pen could be attacked by ESP."

It might be worth noting here that the media In the last few years has also given more attention to incidents of police departments using "psychics" to solve crimes, often with amazing success. If there were "nothing at all" to extrasensory perception, it is highly doubtful that such conventional organizations as the police department (or the CIA) would even consider such angles in the first place. Phenomena occurring out of our physical realities have been given little public attention in the media, but obviously some people know something that hasn't been generally publicized, for evidence does exist that these phenomena are not only real, but being recognized more often, and as with everything else, are capable of being used for us or against us. This is another good reason to be ever vigilant.

Of note is the fact that, after the early fifties, CIA documents are "mum" about ESP and PK (psychokinesis): "Perhaps the CIA dropped the idea. But perhaps it actually implemented an ESP cryptocracy, and perhaps the documents detailing it are classified. The latter possibility is raised (along with a few eyebrows) by this January 1952, statement: 'If we are to undertake to push this research as far and as fast as we can ... it would be necessary to be exceedingly careful about thorough cloaking of the undertaking. The CIA has declined comment."

A later newspaper article (4/18/85) announced that the "Supreme Court recently gave the CIA absolute power to keep sources of information secret, even if the sources are not confidential and the information itself is not classified." Congress in 1947 gave the director of central "intelligence" very broad authority to protect all sources of intelligence information from disclosure. The 1985 decision overturned a ruling by a federal appeals court in Washington—the CIA had said that ruling would "cripple its ability to gather intelligence because the agency would be forced to reveal sources." The case involves a 1977 suit filed under the Freedom of Information Act by lawyer John Sims and Sidney Wolfe, director of Public Citizen Health Research Group. They sought the names of individuals and institutions involved in research under the CIA's MKULTRA project (financed from 1953 to 1966 "to counter Soviet and Chinese brainwashing techniques"). It included "experiments in which researchers administered LSD and other psychoactive drugs to unwitting persons. At least two persons died as a result of the experiments. The agency had refused to reveal names of researchers of many of the institutions involved, citing the 1947 law."

We need to keep a watchful eye on the activities of such groups designed to "protect" our interests, for just as parents can become guilty of Mild abuse, such organizations can easily become guilty of freedom abuse! The reality that we are faced with is every day we're told that such things as vitamins, drugs, weapons, the government, and so on "protect us," but we're becoming increasingly aware of the fact that what really protects us are such things as truth and freedom. Most of the other nonsense we can do much better without!

Here are more excerpts on CIA-sponsored experiments MKULTRA, from Psychology Today, "Mind Control in 1984," by Philip Zimbardo (psychology professor at Stanford University) 1/84:

"MKULTRA was its most notorious covert program designed to develop operational technologies for disrupting and then reprogramming an individual's habitual patterns of perception, thought and action. Government research funds were funneled through universities and mental hospitals to encourage the experimental testing of LSD and other psychoactive drugs, as well as electroshock treatment, hypnosis, and other exotic types of direct intervention in functioning of the human mind. The program was halted not because of the outrage of the citizenry (few knew of its existence) or the ethical concerns of turning American citizens into vegetables, but because it didn't do the job. These potent gadgets and gimmicks could surely scramble anyone's brain, but they could not direct a person's action in pre-determined ways."

One of the major discoveries of modern social psychology is that, under specified conditions, less social pressure can produce more attitude changes:

"The most profound and enduring changes in attitudes occur under two conditions: when people perceive they have free choice in deciding to believe in ways that are against their values, beliefs, or motives, and when the force applied is just strong enough to accomplish the task. The pressure may be as innocuous as having the experimenter in an authoritative white coat say, 'This is an important experiment...' or touch the person's shoulder and say confidingly, 'do me a favor.' People want to be good sports and team players. When people can be subtly induced or seduced into publicly behaving in ways contrary to their needs or usual standards, it produces an uncomfortable state of cognitive dissonance. The tension is particularly great when people believe that they chose the alien action freely, without external pressure. To reduce their feelings of discomfort, they become their own agents of self-persuasion. Since they can't attribute the discrepant behavior to something outside themselves, they explain it in terms of self-generated processes. 'If I chose to do it without promise of reward or threat of punishment,' they rationalize, 'I must have unknowingly liked it or wanted it.' In hundreds of studies, when intelligent subjects were induced, through means of which they were not aware, to lie, cheat, suffer or hurt someone else, they invented personal reasons to account for this atypical behavior. People devise such personal attributions to make sense of apparently irrational actions, such as eating fried grasshoppers after saying they dislike them or accepting powerful electric shocks.

Although behavior can be controlled by powerful external rewards or threats, the person controlled will not also automatically believe in the trainer's ideology; coercion creates conformists, but not true believers. When people think an external force is powerful enough to make them act as it wishes, they often yield to the power, but do not internalize the force's ideology. Without at least an illusion of free choice, they become passive re-actors; they take no responsibility for their actions but attribute them to outside forces."

When Orwell wrote 1984 (in 1948), he saw the potential power and can be wielded by professionals "who intervene in people's lives 'for their own good.'" But, Zimbardo continues, "he did not foresee the extent and depth of that power, which is so evident in our 1984. When control is cloaked as cure, surveillance as a security service and repression as a rehabilitation program, civil liberties can be set aside, and cherished freedoms put on hold without arousing resistance or rebellion. When something is being done for you and not to you, it is difficult to complain without feeling the guilt of the ungrateful. Would-be mind controllers are springing up everywhere, unconstrained by Party allegiance. They pose more of a threat because their tactics are more subtle, their strategies more insidious and their influence more pervasive. They sell us, educate us, treat us, service us and minister to us—after first persuading us of the need to pay willingly and dearly for their product." Let the buyer beware.

"In the end," concludes Zimbardo, "we must individually and collectively challenge the Party line: There is indeed something called human nature that will be outraged by what is done to the least of our kind and will turn us against despots and dictators, demonic or benevolent. We defy Big Brother."

101.3.4. Economic Freedom: A Penny Saved Is a Penny Earned?

"When the whole property of this universe has been inherited by all creatures, how then can there by any justification for a system in which someone receives a flow of huge excess, while others die for lack of a handful of grains."

—P. R. Sankar

Excerpts from John Hamaker's Survival of Civilization, "Taxes, Freedom and the Constitution":

"Fundamental change is required to save this nation from becoming a totalitarian state. Decay is evident in every facet of our society, but few understand the cause. Rightists simply blame it all on 'communism,' and Liberals frantically search their first-aid kits for palliatives to treat the most painful effects of the underlying cause. This essay tells why the rich get richer and the poor get poorer, and why centralization of wealth occurs.

"In the matter of economics, an exponential equation similar to population growth is destroying our economy and our democracy. It is the rot that runs through the forest. Benjamin Franklin willed $100 to the city of Philadelphia. It was to be kept at compound interest until it reached $1,000,000. The inheritance paid off in a little less than 200 years. If the million were kept at 6% compounded annually for 20 years, it would reach 3.2. million; in 40 years, 10.3. million; and in 60 years it would reach 33 million. At 3% it would be only 5.9. million in 60 years; but at 7% it would be 57.9. million. Long before Franklin's time many people made business investments of much more than $100 and realized more than 6%. Those investments which were invested in the steady money-making businesses, and passed on through inheritance, now are valued in the hundreds of millions. Today these fortunes control capital now measured in hundreds of billions. Applying the 20-, 40-, or 60-year factors shows by inspection that the rate of increase of such vast sums has far exceeded the potential rate of growth of the economy. The growth rate of the centralized pools of wealth has exceeded the finite limits of the capacity of the economy to support it. This is particularly so now, because the growth of population is the primary basis for the growth of the economy. The population growth must be stopped.

"One dollar can be plotted as a series of curves using a different rate of interest compounded annually for each curve and plotting time on the abscissa against fund increase on the ordinate. The result is the accumulation of a single dollar—the factor to be multiplied by the amount of the initial fund to find its present value. It will be noted that the curves bend gently upward until half to one million dollars is reached. Then in a 50to 100-year period, the curve breaks upward toward infinitely large numbers. The number of years it takes to reach the break-point depends on the rate of interest (or profit). At 3% it takes about 450 years, at 6% about 220 years, and at 10% about 125 years to reach the break-point. After that point is reached, the rate of increase in funds reaches absurdly large rates of increase which have no relation to the rate of increase of real values in the economy. Therefore, the only way such fortunes can continue to increase is to expand ownership over everything in the economy which makes money. Because of the power of large fortunes to buy out or freeze out competition, they take control of the most stable and lucrative businesses. The theoretical end result is one fortune in possession of everything in the country. In practice, when a majority of people have been impoverished, there is a revolt and a wiping out of all debts. Historically, this has occurred every few hundred years, i.e., when the large fortunes in a country have reached the breakpoint in the curve and have transferred much of the ownership from the people to the pools of wealth. They then have the power to reach out for every real value in the economy. The more they take, the faster the process works until they have it all. "One does not argue with the laws of nature. One either conforms or pays the penalty. The mathematics of compound interest is natural law. We are in the self-destruct stage. Our economy is at the breakpoint in the curve. If we continue to permit funds to accumulate, we are certain to have our economy destroyed and our people in revolt. Money, like everything else in the environment, must be recycled to prevent destructive pollution of the economic environment.

"Specifically, there is now about one and one-half trillion dollars in public and private debts. Most of these debts are owed to pools of money which annually grow by the amount of the interest (or profit) added to it. In 60 years, at an average of 7% interest, the value of the funds would be 58 times their present value. The total growth rate has far exceeded the real growth rate of the economy. The best-protected funds have passed the breakpoint. They are well on the way to owning the entire country. Senator Phillip Hart said, '200 decision makers control two-thirds of all production.' Senator Fred Harris said that centralization of wealth and the question of how to redistribute it will be the major issue of this decade. It had better be, because the claims to ownership by those funds are going to try to double in ten years' time. An awful lot of people and small businesses are going bankrupt. Inflation and government and personal debt will continue at high rates of increase. Super-wealth has a counterfeiting machine and a government to legalize its product. It can buy us all.

"The excessive rate of growth of large pools of money according to an exponential equation is responsible for virtually all the deficiencies of the present capitalistic system as follows:

1. The constant growth of large pools of money in excess of real growth in the economy is highly inflationary. The avidity with which the holders of great wealth seek to multiply it leads to overexpansion of industrial capacity, overextension of credit to consumers, and vicious competition for ownership of all income-producing values.

2. The inflationary 'boom' is turned into a 'bust' when a significant number of people have used up their credit, and when competition caused by overproduction has closed out the least competitive companies, further depleting consumer demand. Small savings are robbed by inflation. So great is the ever-ready inflationary capacity of large pools of wealth, that the cycle of boom and bust has occurred roughly every 10 years since 1840. In each one there is a transfer of ownership from those who fail to those who have larger funds subsidizing them at an exponential rate. Example: In 1935 there were 750 breweries, in 1970 only 140. The rate of bankruptcy and conglomeration insure that there will be a lot fewer breweries after this bust period. The power of the major funds now dominates the economy. Production has become centralized, leaving behind centers of poverty.

3. Charity and government pick up the bill to feed people left destitute. If all present government and private debts were collected from the people tomorrow, most of us would be penniless or in debt. Almost everything in the country would be owned by about one-half of one percent of the people or the businesses in which they hold a controlling interest. Most of the people are broke. The wealth has become highly centralized. Inflation eats up the savings of older people, and they're forced on welfare or social security. They've relied on fund growth for security. Insurance and private pension funds pay off about 40% and 10% respectively, and they pay off in inflated dollars. Social security isn't an insurance fund. It's a tax on present producers to feed older, less productive workers forced off the job by the fixed wage, fixed 8-hour day, maximum benefits concept. If social security tax payments had been funded at compound interest, inflation of the dollar would be far worse than it is, and the government would be well on the way toward ownership of the entire country. The $153 billion in private pension plans doesn't help the 90% of contributors who get nothing back, but it sure helps the big corporations with their conglomeration plans.

4. Because the people of this country have been largely separated from ownership of the real wealth, the pressure of the rapidly multiplying huge pools of wealth has moved toward exploitation of the people and their resources in less developed countries. To insure those investments, large sums have been spent since WWII to insure 'friendly' national legislators and administrators. The result has been the absurdly hopeless policy of 'Containment of Communism.' Meanwhile, the revolt grows within our nation.

5. The forced flow of wealth from the people to the funds (directly and indirectly through taxation) reduces large numbers of people to poverty and the majority of the

working force to the insecurity of having only the job (and in most cases one paycheck) between themselves and poverty. These demoralizing stresses induce crime, alcoholism, drug addiction, and other escape mechanisms to alleviate the pains, needs and wants that attend poverty.

"Poverty provides little market demand. The total national product must therefore shrink relative to actual need. This contraction means that more people enter the ranks of poverty: the rich get richer, and the poor get poorer. Those who still work are heavily taxed to sustain the poor. Ultimately, it's the taxpayers who revolt. "We are ruled by an exponential equation. Either we control it, or we'll join the two-thirds of the world's population which have yielded to dictatorship for survival. Right now, is the time to protect ourselves from the rule of centralized pools of wealth if we are to save our political freedom.

"The rich get richer and the poor get poorer because money 'earns' money at an exponential rate, whereas the economy expands directly with population and the technical ingenuity of the people. The difference between the two rates is the margin of power by which the owners of wealth impose poverty on everyone else.

"In the broad sense, taxes are government-enforced demands for a share of the consumer goods. Nothing has monetary value until human labor is applied to it. Thus, a tax is forced human labor. Whether or not equal goods and services are given in exchange for the tax determines whether it's a service institution or a means of enslaving the people."

Hamaker says we can simplify taxes and increase our freedom by:

"Outlawing all taxes ahead of the sales tax (taxes collected ahead of the consumer goods sales tax are added to the cost of goods sold and are therefore sales taxes, i.e., claims for a share of consumer goods). The burden of taxation can't be shifted from consumer goods. A frugal person can more easily accumulate funds to start a business if taxation is deferred to the point of consumption of goods. Only when this freedom to use our national fund of ingenuity and initiative is established can we expect to eliminate the welfare rolls and withdraw workers from government into the productive economy. Then our tax burden will be lowered accordingly and this, too, is an increment of freedom. Also, if taxes were eliminated at the production level, politicians could no longer sell loopholes in exchange for campaign support. This practice has resulted in establishing economic advantages for the highest bidders— farmers, for example, can't compete with agribusiness (which can lose money on farming and make it up elsewhere in the conglomeration where tax loopholes support it). Thus, the big corporations would be less powerful and the government less corrupt. These are important increments of freedom for the people. "Within the broad definition of taxes, there are three included in the cost of consumer goods which government says are lawful, but which are collected by individuals. When the inheritor of wealth goes to the marketplace for a yacht or a mansion, he brings no products or labor to exchange. The same thing is true of a land speculator who does nothing to increase the value of land, but whom the government allows to collect the increased value. The same is true of the stockholder, who by the grace of government and a stock split, finds himself in possession of a share of several years of company surplus earned by the ingenuity and effort of a good working force. He brings to the consumer marketplace no value which he's earned if it's profit above the true market value (rightful interest) of his original investment. These government-sanctioned private taxes have the same effect as government taxes: they increase demand without increasing supply and therefore inflate he price. They take units of labor without giving units of labor, which is slavery. "This element of slavery is what makes possible the rapid conglomeration of companies and ultimately the centralization of the nation's wealth. Man-hours of labor can be legally expropriated from, each person's paycheck to obtain a pool of wealth with which to buy a new plant from which to hire-people from whom manhours of labor can be expropriated to obtain a new pool of wealth, etc. When slavery is legalized, anti-trust laws have all the effect of a pea shooter against an elephant. It is these three something-for-nothing deals which, by means of the exponential equation, generate sufficient funds so transfer all ownership from the people to the funds. They are taxes collected directly by the property class and enforced by the government it controls.

"Taxes on savings, such as property taxes, can drive older workers with little income out of their homes, which then become properly of mortgage holders. The property tax is an excellent device for transferring ownership from the people to the centralized pools of wealth.

"Savings are stored labor. To take care of ourselves, we must be allowed to accumulate the results of our labor and use it to support ourselves over unproductive periods. The government that collects property or other taxes on stored labor is patently an institution of slavery.

"Another class of taxes are those used to control imports/exports. When we have obtained economic freedom, we're going to be able to work a 4-hour day and have a standard of living and quality of living beyond most people's imagination. Other nations can and will obtain the same results. But it can't be done if we try to compete with technically advanced nations overpopulated with wage slaves. We must therefore control our foreign trade to protect our own progress. As other nations turn toward freedom, we can establish free trade with them and operate as a single economy with a common standard of living. We have yet to establish one peaceful nation.

"Finally, there are special-use taxes based on the principle that if government performs a service for a particular group, they should pay for it. Gasoline taxes pay for roads, but the pressure group that results from pooling such funds has not led to intelligent environmental planning. Special-use taxes are no longer practical.

"One wonders why people have tolerated these burdens for countless centuries. The answer is two-fold: Those who hold power have always been those who have access to the unearned values. They have written the laws to suit themselves. Until very recent times they have kept the people illiterate. Even to this day, all preachers and most schoolteachers fear to discuss the three something-for-nothing deals. It's only because these three causes of the centralization of wealth have brought us to the brink of crisis that the great power of wealth to perpetuate itself is slowly yielding to the force of necessity. For two-thirds of the world's people, these ancient prerogatives of rulers have yielded to the force of bloody revolutions led by ostensibly altruistic dictatorships. Hopefully, an enlightened electorate will bring these institutions down in this country without the loss of political freedom won with so much blood through the centuries.

"What should be done to return these values to those who produced them? Inheritance and land rent value must be collected by the government. This will decrease the sales tax required. The privately-collected tax on the earnings of a working force in excess of interest is composed of increased technical efficiency, human effort, and product demand. Heretofore, this has always accrued to ownership simply because they have hire, fire and bribe control over the management. The unions now contend for this value, while the white-collar workers who had a good deal to do with the increased earnings sit or the sidelines and take whatever is handed out. Instead of the single inflationary force of profit-taking, we now also have an inflationary force from union wage demands. In monopolistic or near-monopolistic necessity industries, the reaching for profit and wages is passed on to consumers as inflated price. Of necessity, less-favored industries and unorganized workers follow along behind. This built-in inflation can be slowed by recession. It might be stopped by depression. But after recovering, it would start up again. The dollar is depreciating at a chaotic rate because we no longer have any semblance of a free-market product evaluation. In order to solve this problem, we're going to have to re-define the commodity called labor as human beings and redefine the investor as one enjoying the privilege of investing his savings at whatever interest rate the market will currently support. We must transfer the management of each company from the ownership board of directors to the working force. This will result in companies whose size rests solely on economic factors. No group of workers will remain in a conglomerate if it costs them money to do so. The better producers will pull out, and the massive pools of wealth that now dictate to government will be dispersed among small companies. We'll have, for the first time since man left the barter economy, free market conditions. Of greatest value is the right of a working force to earn all it can earn. Under this incentive, there will soon be an abundance of goods in the marketplace. Since working hours will no longer be bound by the rigid (most profitable) 8-hour day, they'll work when there is work to do and cut hours back when the demand declines. Technical improvements will be used to shorten hours instead of eliminating people from the payroll. The security (now based on the total payroll) of the individual and the company will both be vastly increased. Interest rates will decline to true market values. Since supply and demand are both relatively constant factors and the rigid artificial factors will be gone from the economy, the economic cycles will cease. Small business initiated and managed by one or two persons must be permitted to operate as they have been. These are some of the creative geese who lay the golden eggs. They probe all the diverse avenues for economic development. They develop products, services, and jobs. Of necessity, they must have full control over their initiative.

"Our economic troubles are man-made. They persist to this late, day in the history of civilization because greed has maintained institutions of enslavement. Even our Constitution contained a provision for the return of run-away slaves. In the intervening 200 years, human populations have covered and been compressed into habitable lands. The means of destruction of human life have been perfected. We are at Armageddon. Either good will triumph over evil or all or most of humanity will be destroyed.

"Every conceivable economic system except economic freedom has been tried without bringing internal peace to any nation, let alone between nations. It is time to test whether or not we, freed of our shackles, can find peace In the United States, the first step toward that end is the establishment of Constitutional basis for constructing a free society."

Hamaker includes a "Proposed General Revision of the Constitution of the United Slates of America" at the end of his book Survival of Civilization. In conclusion he says "the capital goods and personal property must be dispersed among all the people if they're to attain financial security and the independence of action required to initiate an economy of abundance to replace the present hand-to-mouth rat-race economy of scarcity. To accomplish this, 100% of both earnings and savings must be protected by law against the greed of those who hold power. The autocracy of ownership in the corporation must be broken to enable the people who work there to become a flexible unit of production responsive to supply and demand."

"Politicians talk of tax reform as a matter of closing loopholes and/or confiscatory taxes at high levels of income. It's nonsense. If they taxed 100% over $50,000 and closed all the loopholes, it would only accelerate the process of conglomeration of companies. Instead of taking profit, owners would leave it in the corporation where it can be used to buy more companies. The power of wealth, not spending money, is the prize sought. Railroad cars, yachts, airplanes, expense accounts, pseudo-retirement plans—all have been used by corporate ownership as private property exempt from personal income tax. The bill must be paid in the price of goods in the consumer marketplace.

"Politicians talk about inflation as a political argument at election time. Not one of them proposes measures which will get at the cause by stopping the flow of wealth away from the people, and the welfare government that sustains them, to the centralized pools of wealth which new own most of us. When they try to slow the inflation rate of the exploitative economy by arbitrarily raising interest rates, the result is decreasing credit transactions and throwing marginal producers out of work. So great is the inflationary pressure from government debt, national corporations, and national unions that only a serious depression can significantly slow the rate of destruction of the dollar.

"Politicians talk about unemployment at election time (between them they talk of welfare and make-work). Meanwhile, small businesses fall like dominoes at the rate of 10,000 a year. Economists in ivory towers have told politicians that free trade is the ideal international trade system. So, politicians have authorized free trade because this is what their masters (the owners of the centralized pools of wealth) want. The expropriated earned surplus of numerous corporations has been used to ship whole plants and management personnel to countries where labor is cheap. The low-cost goods shipped back to this country have eliminated numerous industries. Even the steel and auto industries are finding they aren't competitive. There's been a large shift from production to service industries. In the process of going out of production, our real unemployment and underemployment has soared. The phony government statistic doesn't give the true figure. The true figure includes the forced retirees over 50 and the 40,000,000 under the poverty level. The government picks up the check for everything, including the price of wars to keep the "free world's" people and resources safe for exploitation by the controllers of our centralized pool of wealth. The government, of course, passes the bill to the people who do the work. This 'free trade' has become one more tool by which rich get richer and poor get poorer.

"Politicians say we can't have a depression again. The fact is that the only thing that has held a depression in check since WWII was an expanding economic system based primarily on electronics, constant war production, and an expanding federal and personal debt load. Environmental costs here, and cheap labor abroad, move industry and capital to foreign lands where the costs can be evaded. We are fed up with the cost of war. Government and personal credit have about run out.

"Politicians have no answers because the exploitative economy doesn't work. As long as history has been recorded, nations have failed every few hundred years. Before the industrial revolution, inheritance and land speculation were primary factors in bringing all the land into the hands of a few people. Those who owned the land had the power to run the government. To protect their ownership, they raised the land rent to raise armies and build castles. When the rent rose above 50% of the crop value, revolt and redistribution of the land always occurred. As trade developed, the profit system was developed and again a share of the labor was confiscated by ownership. As governments became more complex, they, too, learned to take a share of the labor. Thus, the total tax at the point of revolt made up of the personal levies by ownership plus the taxes levied by the government which serves the ownership class. If we add up the total taxes in this country, we have approximately 35% taken by government plus an inexact amount represented by the burden of inheritors, land speculators, and profit in excess of a theoretical free market interest on money. The total tax is probably in excess of 50%.

"In 2 centuries, we've been sorely corrupted by a capitalistic system which included the 3 something-for-nothing deals, which in concert with an irrational exponential equation causes the centralization of wealth and power. By the simple expedient of making our capitalistic system honest, we can gradually disperse the wealth among the people. In the hands of the people, it will support an excellent standard and quality of living. It will never accumulate to sums whose rate of increase reaches toward infinite quantity and infinite power—and arrives at infinite weakness in that the whole system can be destroyed by a single dollar accumulating its interest for a long period of time.

"All the industrialized 'free nations' which now contain large fortunes and funds operating at high rates of interest have the same problem. The bonanza of productivity resulting from widespread public education has peaked. The ever-present ability of the pools of wealth to accumulate ownership is now the dominant force. Within 10 to 20 years the industrialized "free nations" will all either establish economic freedom under law or they'll be under dictatorship. The something-for nothing deals have brought the funds of wealth in this country to the point where they've caused a 60% inflation in the last 15 years. If given our economic freedom, we can work our way out of this mess. Without economic freedom, we're going to lose our political freedom to some form of dictatorship because the economy doesn't work.

"It is pure fantasy to believe that this economy can last for more than a few years without redistribution of wealth. About 15 U.S. manufacturers receive a total of 88% of all business profits. About the only money-making property left to take is the land, and they are gobbling it up. We mere mortals can't compete with fortunes which enjoy the luxury of perpetual life. Nor can the monetary system withstand the inflation of funds increasing exponentially to become so powerful that they can fix profits and prices of necessities. Taxes must inevitably keep rising to pay for the palliatives used to soften the impact of the ever-more numerous problems which arise as our nation and its environment degenerate. The working taxpayers, who inevitably pay for everything, will eventually want to demand radical change.

"People of rank who are saying they know nothing about carbon dioxide and acid rain aren't stupid. They're either lying or using evasive language. Such a massive conspiracy of silence is understandable when one realizes that 'official' announcement of our situation would plunge the world into a financial debacle. They would no doubt like to have more time to prepare an alternate financial system to replace the international banking system. The trouble is, they've been wringing their hands over this for a half dozen years; meanwhile our chance of survival gets weaker and weaker."

In defending their desires for "more studies of the problems," our leaders are stalling for time; no one wants to tell the public the truth, so by stalling, and "not looking for evidence," they just won't "have to admit" that evidence exists.

101.4. And the Pursuit of Happiness

101.4.1. Human Interaction: It Takes Two to Tango

101.4.2. Peace on Earth, Good Will to All . . .

101.4.3. "Where never was heard a discouraging word, and the skies were not cloudy all day. . ."

Excerpts on the Nuclear Winter, by Carl Sagan (10/30/83):

101.4.1. Human Interaction: It Takes Two to Tango

Survival has a twin called Need, and they're always together. We learn from the start that we need more than air, water, and food—we need others. Very early on, people depend on each other for survival; in fact, we're all born completely dependent, as infants, upon someone. In Western society, a conflict often arises between our natural human need for others and our "quest for independence." We have self-sufficiency, self-fulfillment, self-knowledge, self-mastery, self-control, self-indulgence, self-confidence, self-esteem, self-assurance, self-consciousness, self-defense, self-government, self-help, self-improvement, self-interest, self-pity, self-preservation, self-reliance, self-satisfaction, and self-respect. We are self-centered, self-contained, self-evident, self-righteous, self-supporting, self-sustained and self-motivated!

In our world of human interaction, of Give and Take, closely related to our twins Survival and Need are the triplets Power, Submission, and Opposition, although those of us who know Creativity prefer her companionship to that of the triplets. Most human interaction is related to survival/need, give/take, power/submission/opposition, friendship and/or creativity. We learn by trial-and-error to assert our individuality and begin to use our "power" as soon as we realize it's there. Along with our needs, we develop wants and expectations.

Like fire and all forms of energy and tools known to us, our pride can be either a constructive or destructive force, depending upon how it's used. Pride can be our incentive and motivating passion to do our best, to excel and to reach our highest possible achievements—or it can consume us and destroy us—it can become the biggest obstacle of all on our path to our higher selves, if we let it. If we can control it and use its powerful energy for good, we will be able to harness its tremendous force to our advantage and it will work with us—if not, it will control us (as with anger and all other emotions) and work against us, because pride without wisdom and insight is like a boat without a sail or a car without steering. We have but to look at human history to see what pride without direction, guidance and conscience has done to us—or, more aptly—undone for us. We can either indulge in our anger, false pride, and other emotions, and let them grow, or we can find something better to do with our time.

Because we reap what we sow, we'd do well to spend our time in positive pursuits. When we let go of false pride, or anger, we free ourselves to do something that can help us. Negative emotions are like a big, huge wave that hits us at the ocean's edge. If we've ever romped in the surf at the seaside, we know that the best strategy is to "duck and let the wave pass over us" so that it crashes onto the shore, where its force is shattered.

On the other hand, fueling our negative emotions (as with concentrating on symptoms of a healing crisis) lends strength to them, reinforces their control factor over our lives, making us less free. When we find ourselves thinking "so and so (or such and such) makes me so mad," we must remember that it is we ourselves who make the decision on what to do with our anger. It's ironic that we so often find ourselves thinking we don't have "enough" time for this or that, but we'll turn around and burn up twice the vital life energy in anger or other negative emotions—most illogical! Only positive action will help us to change things for the positive. We should use our emotions for fuel, not our life energy itself.

101.4.2. Peace on Earth, Good Will to All . . .

We've reached a point of stagnation on a planetary level, where international relations are concerned. We're all posed and "ready," weapons-in-hand, all trying to act tough and scare each other into peace (or whatever) by threat of possible force. If you've ever watched two tomcats nose-to-nose, making their growling, siren-type sounds, you'll notice that neither one wants to be the first to back down at that point; they're now stuck at this crucial point of a "final confrontation."

We're like these cats, making our most impressive, mean, scary threats, and we're so deep into it that we're afraid to trust one another. We've heard all the threats and made our own, and we've defined ourselves as "enemies," when the reality is that we'd still be better off in the kitchen of a Russian family than with our local mugger here at home. The enemies we fail to recognize are often more dangerous to us in the everyday sense than those we've been told to fear. In any case, we've built the wall between us, and built elaborate "defense" mechanisms for self-"protection"; in fact, as we've said, we've done such a thorough job of building weapons that our self-"defense" now threatens self-destruction as well. We've built the wall by a lack of understanding and lack of cooperation, by fear, mistrust, and refusal to communicate honestly. When we do communicate, our messages are often confusing: we stand with a loaded gun (so to speak) pointed at each other's noses, and our voices are saying, "hey, let's be friends and talk this over." No one dares to be first to put the gun down, and our history of war and violence certainly doesn't help to allay our fears. As long as we can't believe each other and trust each other, the tension persists.

We've arrived at the last stop on this bus, as it were—the end of the line. It's gone round and round in circles, and each time we've found ourselves back where we started; this route has had little to offer for our spiritual evolution as creatures of light. It's time now to decide whether to get off the bus and make a transfer to a new journey, or whether to head once again for the "terminal." A 1984 news item said, "the world will spend $1 trillion for weapons other military purposes by next year," (according to the U.S. Arms Control and Disarmament Agency). From "less" than $300,000,000,000 in 1972, spending rose to $820,000,000,000 in 1982, and was expected to reach $970,000,000,000 in 1984, thus heading for the $1,000,000,000,000 mark (I'm purposely writing these figures out with 0' s because they make more of a visual impression than the respective terms "million, billion, trillion," and so on). The weapons industry is obviously doing a booming business (if you can pardon a bad pun) in an age where funds for positive human endeavors are so often said to be "dwindling, lacking, unavailable, or whatever." Economies in every nation are involved in sales and purchases of these instruments of death, certainly not a wholesome foundation on which to base our economies. With nuclear, chemical, environmental and/or biological war now possible, what we're seeing is global weapons pollution of the highest order, and the world's increasing violence and power struggles are symptomatic of ailing minds and spirits that result from pollution of our human values of love and cooperation, worldwide.

Studies indicate that testing of these weapons has already taken its toll on innocent victims everywhere. Thousands of civilians have filed suits in Nevada and other areas, citing that they've been exposed to deadly radioactive fallout. Hundreds of atmospheric and underground tests have taken place (not all even announced)—we've been told not to trust "foreigners," but it becomes obvious that we can't even trust our health, lives, and safety to our own government either. As just one example of the magnitude of potential and real danger of such tests, consider the following excerpt from Hamaker's Survival of Civilization, page 75:

"In 1972 the Atomic Commission tested a 5-megaton bomb a mile below sea level on the Aleutian island of Amchitka. The Aleutian chain is a continental heater, and the Bering Sea is slowly being raised to plateau status. The underground bomb test had the ingredients for a total change in the world's weather. Fortunately, a group of senators headed by Senator Phillip Hart persuaded the AEC to stop the testing."

An underground test in Nevada (2/81) was the "568th reported at the Yucca Flats" (northwest of Las Vegas) and the "353rd announced since atmospheric testing was stopped (by the U.S.) in 1963." Where does all this radiation go? A May 1984 news article talks of suits by Nevada residents who say the government knew or should have known the fallout was dangerous (atomic tests from 1951-1962) and was negligent in not protecting people downwind from the Nevada Test Site.

A January 1984 news article says, "the Reagan administration has been concealing an unknown number of nuclear explosions at the underground test site in Nevada, signifying a break with a 1975 policy of announcing all explosions."

Hold on to your seats for this one: An official at the Energy Department said "the policy of announcing only the larger tests was adopted a year ago for convenience. There was simply no reason to announce them all. The size of some of the tests was such that they didn't even create a ripple. Nobody could feel them off the test site. It takes a lot of work to announce each of those tests. And it was information that was not germane to the general public." There you have it folks. Don't fret— "what you don't know can't hurt you," right? A ripple? (Just because a person doesn't "feel" those little old cancer cells start to work in his body, doesn't make them any less dangerous.) The article concludes in saying that since Reagan administration took office, the federal budget for nuclear ting has almost doubled, going to $388,000,000 (1984) from 201,000,000 in 1981." Pacific islanders have borne much of the brunt of the nuclear age; over 200 weapons tests have been conducted in the region, and people exposed to the fallout have been plagued with high rates of thyroid cancer, miscarriage, stillbirth, leukemia, and other health problems. When the U.S. conducted its largest hydrogen bomb explosion at Bikini Atoll in the Marshall Islands (March 1, 1954), hundreds of islanders, 28

American meteorologists, and 23 Japanese fishermen were exposed to high amounts of radioactive fallout.

Our weapons aren't merely stockpiled in "safe little cubbyholes for some future use"—some have already killed victims. Physicians and others have banded together to warn the superpowers of the dangers of even "limited" nuclear wars: uncountable burn victims, too many to handle, and so on. We've all heard the details and are well aware of the dangers. Now we hear talk of "space" stations and "star wars," of studies to determine feasibility of dumping nuclear waste in space—when and where will the madness end?

101.4.3. "Where never was heard a discouraging word, and the skies were not cloudy all day. . ."

Scientists have now alerted the world to the latest nuclear danger: that of a "nuclear winter," with many of the negative consequences from increased cloud cover that we've already discussed in reference to potential global climate changes towards colder conditions due to excessive CO_2 and other factors.

News of March 3, 1985, was that "the Pentagon has accepted as valid a theory that nuclear war could generate enough smoke and dust to blot out the sun and cause severe climatic cooling." The 17-page report was the military's first assessment of the theory that detonation of nuclear bombs could cause: "a devastating nuclear winter around the planet and drop temperatures as much as 75 degrees, first in the Northern Hemisphere and then southward as the smoke spread with the wind. Land and water would freeze and cause harsh global effects unrelated to radiation hazards. The upshot, they argued, would be the extinction of a significant proportion of the Earth's animals and plants, possibly including the human race."

An earlier news article (1/20/85) compares the cloud cover with those of past volcanic eruptions known to cause climate changes:

"We have established that volcanic eruptions have an effect on the climate, and enough of them happening at the same time, like exploding nuclear bombs, could have a significant effect. The most famous example of the effect of a volcano on climate was the eruption in 1815 of an Indonesian volcano (Tambora) which lasted three months, the largest eruption in historical times, producing huge quantities of ash and dust that were carried around the world in the stratosphere. The particles sufficiently deflected sunlight to produce what historians later called the year without a summer in 1816. In New England that year, there was widespread snow in June and frosts every month through the summer. Throughout the world it was unusually cold. Crop failures caused food shortages in Ireland and Wales; that's the most famous example. It was the first time a relationship was shown between volcanoes and weather." (Fred Bullard, geology professor, University of Texas.)

"Average annual temperatures in the Northern Hemisphere could be lowered to well below freezing for a month or longer," is another description of potential climatic change. Other studies think extended periods of freezing would be unlikely. Again, everyone has a slightly varying opinion in these matters, but it should be obvious after our lengthy discussion in the last lesson on carbon dioxide excesses and their relation to the Ice Age cycles—plus indications of climatic extremes worldwide—that such cloud covers (added to our current excess CO2-generated clouds) could indeed produce dramatic changes. Here's another description: "dust generated by nuclear explosions still could block enough sunlight to drop summer temperatures to near freezing and destroy food crops for survivors of the initial blast and radiation effects." Bullard said recent volcanic activity hasn't produced anything like the Tambora eruption but has "continued a general world cooling trend that started with the eruption of a West Indies volcano in 1902. Dust and ash from the eruption of Mount St. Helens in Washington in 1980 didn't rise high enough to enter the stratosphere or have much effect on world climate, although the dust still is circulating in the upper atmosphere. But dust from the eruption of El Chicon in Mexico in April 1982, did enter the stratosphere and is adding to the cooling," he said. "It means," he continues, "that frosts could come earlier than usual." The news source then says, "Carbon dioxide from auto pollution in the upper atmosphere often is cited as producing a warming 'greenhouse effect' by intensifying sunlight. But Bullard said the Earth actually is in a cooling trend because of volcanic eruptions throughout this century, generated by dust from the volcanoes in the stratosphere, and there've been a significant number of eruptions in the past few years to help it along. It's really only since scientists began using computers to analyze the changes that we've noticed the effects."

Calculations of the nuclear winter concept have been made independently by several groups of scientists in the U.S. and the Soviet Union, and by now, the theory (if not its details) is probably agreed upon by scientists in other countries as well.

"Into the eternal darkness, into fire, into ice."

—Dante, The Inferno

Excerpts on the Nuclear Winter, by Carl Sagan (10/30/83):

"The results of our calculations astonished us. The amount of sunlight at the ground was reduced to a few percent of normal—much darker, in daylight, than in a heavy overcast and too dark for plants to make a living from photosynthesis. At least in the Northern Hemisphere, where the great preponderance of strategic targets lies, an unbroken and deadly gloom would persist for weeks. Even more unexpected were the temperatures calculated. In the baseline case, land temperatures, except for narrow strips of coastline, dropped to minus 25 degrees Celsius (-13 degrees F) and stayed below freezing for months—even for a summer war. (Because the atmospheric structure becomes much more stable as the upper atmosphere is heated and the lower air is cooled, we may have severely underestimated how long the cold and dark would last.) The oceans, a significant heat reservoir, would not freeze, however, but because temperatures would drop so catastrophically, virtually all crops and farm animals, at least in the Northern Hemisphere, would be destroyed, as would most varieties of uncultivated or undomesticated food supplies. Most of the human survivors would starve. In addition, the amount of radioactive fallout is much more than expected; in long-term fallout, fine radioactive particles lofted into the stratosphere would descend about a year later, after most of the immediate, shorter-lived radioactivity had decayed. However, the radioactivity carried into the upper atmosphere (but not as high as the stratosphere) seems to have been largely forgotten, etc. Carrying of dust and soot from the Northern to the Southern Hemisphere would thin the clouds some over the North, but then only making things worse in the Southern Hemisphere.

"In summary, the overall conclusion seems to be agreed upon: there are severe and previously unanticipated global consequences of nuclear war—subfreezing temperatures in a twilit radioactive gloom lasting for months or longer. If scientists have underestimated the effects and amounts of fallout, didn't know fireballs from high-yield thermonuclear explosions could deplete the ozone layer and missed altogether the possible climatic effects of nuclear dust and smoke, what else have we overlooked? Nuclear war is now a theoretical problem for us, for it certainly isn't amenable to experimentation! It is highly likely that there are even further adverse effects that no one has yet been wise enough to anticipate or recognize. With billions of lives at stake, where does conservatism lie—in assuming that the results will be better than we calculate, or worse? Many species of plants and animals would become extinct. Vast numbers of surviving humans would starve to death. The delicate ecological relations that bind together organisms on Earth in a fabric of mutual dependency would be torn, perhaps irreparably. There is little question that our global civilization would be destroyed. The human population would be reduced to prehistoric levels, or less. Life for any survivors would be extremely hard. And there seems to be a real possibility of the extinction of the human species. It is now almost 40 years since the invention of nuclear weapons ... men and machines are fallible, and fools and madmen can exist and rise to power. Concentrating always on the near future, we have ignored the long-term consequences of our actions ... fortunately it is not yet too late. We can safeguard the planetary civilization and the human family if we so choose."

So, if we don't already have enough reasons for not embarking into a nuclear war of any proportion, here we have another. Nature will insist that we see the truth that what we do to her, or to others, we do to ourselves: we could literally destroy ourselves in seeking to destroy another in any size nuclear war.

War is. indeed, hell—whereas peace is heaven on earth. Ever since time immemorial it has been our dream. Now peace is more than a necessity for survival: it has become a reality that is just within our reach. With just one more burst of evolution of human consciousness, we will grasp it and hold on to it for dear life. Our most precious treasure—world peace—will become a reality. In protecting everyone, we protect ourselves best of all, and the best protection comes in the form of peace. Because we are all one and interconnected, we are beginning to realize that in destroying anyone, we destroy ourselves.

Einstein: 'The bomb changed everything but the way we think. "

Our old ways of thinking of ourselves as separate and divided have become obsolete, and if we don't change our tune soon, we'll risk becoming obsolete with them. Our weapons systems are somewhat like a vicious watchdog that we've chained up to "protect" us, one that's become so mean since it was full-grown, that we've begun to fear it ourselves, and don't dare let it loose or touch it for fear of its bite. As long as it's chained, we try our best to keep out of its way and ignore it, but we know it would attack an innocent person, or ourselves, if it were let off the chain. Some people might feel comfortable with such a dog, while others would see that we've created a monster.

War is our last link with the barbarism of our past. It is "the highest form of criminal acts, grave offenses against morality and social behavior" (David Stry); "when an individual kills another, the legal systems bitterly condemn such acts, but if done in a wholesale fashion by nations (artificial, political units), accompanied by marching bands, flags, uniforms, and propaganda, then medals and decorations are given out for bravery

..." War is the ultimate use of force. Perhaps our outmoded belief that it can "solve" any of our problems is as foolish as our belief that medical drugs can force ("cure") our bodies into health. Just as health alone produces healthful living, so too does peace alone (not war and weapons) produce harmony and cooperation, an environment in which life and all its creatures may flourish.

As long as our world "leaders" keep us separate and divided, as long as they encourage us to remain at odds with one another, they will succeed in holding us captive in warlike thoughts or endeavors. Only we can remove the final obstacle that keeps us from peaceful coexistence: this separation of human beings worldwide that keeps us from seeing one another as human. Once we see each other as human, we will do unto others as we would do unto ourselves. Pacifism isn't a new idea. Although we've reached a crisis point in international world relations, in Psychology Today, June 1983, Erikson says:

"If you study the lives of very creative people, you'll find that at times they all have a terrible sense of stagnation. And the interaction of such opposites is characteristic of every stage of the life cycle ... I cannot help thinking of how nuclear weapons have done away with the boundaries of whole continents, and how, with their threat of global destruction, they call for the recognition of man's indivisible 'species hood.'

Gandhi's pacifists marched unarmed toward their attackers.

... In order for nonviolent behavior to be effective it must be shocking—it has to shake up the violent opponent peacefully. In that situation, what is more important: That you are an Indian? That you are a soldier? That you are an officer? That you are a human being? It has to come to the point where suddenly these other people become human to you. Then you can no longer keep hitting them. Incidentally, it's amazing how American audiences are taking to the (Gandhi) movie, and these are not intellectuals. The movie about a great man's use of nonviolent resistance reaches people who do not belong to special peace organizations, and it makes them thoughtful. That's why it's such an important film. I honestly believe that it focuses on something our Judeo-Christian culture has not yet quite understood and has not used and will probably have to face: the invention of nonviolent tactics to get out of the nuclear dilemma.

"Human beings spend an awful lot of their imagination on defining just what others they don't care for. The danger in rejectivity, that is, the rejecting of other people, other groups, or other nations, is that it leads to what I have called 'pseudo speciation.' People lose the sense of being one species and try to make other kinds of people into a different and mortally dangerous species, one that doesn't count, one that isn't human. Other groups are considered to be a different species, and you can kill them without feeling that you have killed your own kind. People aren't conscious of doing this, and that's why it's so dangerous. The paradox is that pseudospecieshood as a sense of representing the best in humankind binds a group together and inspires loyalty, heroism and discipline, and the very existence of humanity depends on the solution of that paradox. What's important now is a conviction that one's culture and 'system' can go on living in a world that includes one's former enemies."

When asked if he thinks our odds of developing an identity that encompasses the whole species are any better than they were 15 years ago, Erikson replies: "Absolutely. After all, we are one species."

Years ago, someone used force to get his way, and so began a long history of people getting what they could, when they could, if they could, because they could, no matter how they did. We could philosophize endlessly on the moral aspects involved, but the fact remains: we're long overdue for a change in attitude. When Christopher Columbus set sail into the unknown, he had to take a chance. Every explorer, inventor and challenger of traditions has to take some risks. The Wright Brothers had to get up the nerve to take that first flight—how many of us would have found that courage? As our world shrinks in size, there are fewer new horizons left to discover, yet we've seen in our discussions of the mind and consciousness (to say nothing of outer space), that there are many dimensions of reality left to explore, albeit intangible or distant ones. One such reality is that we can live together in peace if we make the combined commitment to such a world. We've never even tried to explore this incredible dimension of human reality, so largely unknown to us in our history, and yet so fondly dreamed of and hoped for and sought after by so many! It's time to really give peace a chance, to explore the unknown territory of working out differences in a new way. We have everything to gain in doing so, and everything to lose if we don't.

Let's finish our discussion of peace with a short story:

Once upon a time there was a big boy and a little boy. The big boy figured that he could do whatever he wanted since he was the big one. One day a little boy was walking down the road, and the big boy called out to him, saying, "who do you think you are walking down my road?"

"The same person who walks down every road," replied the little boy, without even slowing his pace.

Well, this was too much for the big boy, of course, because people didn't just walk down his road, especially not if they were little, because they knew what that would mean. It made the big boy angry just to think about it. In fact, the more he thought about it, the angrier he got. Every angry thought was a brick being laid in a wall just behind the big boy, but he was so busy looking at the object of his anger—the little boy on the road—that he did not see the wall that he would have to face when he would finally turn around, nor imagine how long it would take to climb over this wall once he had built it. His angry thoughts seemed like endless fuel for the fire burning within him, and he. stood in front of the little boy and refused to let him pass. "No one walks on my road," he said.

"This is my road too," replied the little boy. The big boy could not believe what he was hearing. He figured he'd just have to show that little boy whose road it was.

The little boy was thinking the same thing! Then he looked at the big boy, at the wall behind him, and at the look in the big boy's eyes. Maybe there were bigger boys, boys bigger than this big boy, boys who could walk on this road without fear, boys who would challenge bigger boys. But he also saw that the anger became stronger, every time they all let it grow.

He knew laughter. Even the big boys liked to laugh, after all. He wondered what was funny to this big boy, the one whose eyes were empty of life, whose voice echoed bitterness, whose face was etched in lines of hardness, and whose very being seemed to defy all happiness.

"I choose to be your friend," said the little boy, for long ago he'd chosen to become a peacemaker. Perhaps this would be a good joke for the big boy, and he would laugh.

"What would I do with a little friend? sneered the big boy.

"I am a mirror," said the little boy, "and whoever looks into me will see himself," for lack of anything better to say. Maybe this would be funny to the big boy—surely, he knew that all roads went to the same place. Surely, he knew that they were the "same person." Maybe he would see the wall behind him when he looked into the mirror in the little boy's eyes. Or maybe not.

Maybe the little boy could say, "look behind you!" and run by real fast when the big boy looked, well, true, it's an old trick. A big boy might expect to see something big, though—perhaps his fears were bigger too!

While the little boy was busy pondering what strategy to use, the big boy was beginning to get a little bored. It wasn't easy to fight with someone who had no intention of fighting, but he wanted the little boy to get what was coming to him—and with this last angry thought, the final brick was laid on the wall. They had now reached the moment of truth.

The little boy grasped it in an instant and ran forward toward the light. The big boy was close behind, but he ran headlong into his wall!

"Hell is truth seen too late."

—John Locke

Article #1: "Who Is at Fault?"

Freedom Includes Our Right to a Pure Environment

Freedom Includes Our Right to a Pure Environment

Living creatures have a right to a clean environment, and everyone who pollutes it is violating this sacred right. It's time to insist on quality, worldwide. We will all benefit if we "clean up our act." We will all suffer if we don't.

In scanning our environmental problems quickly, the common thread noticed is that it is impossible to "blame" illness on any one particular factor or hazard, because some side effects take years to manifest and because all bodily conditions represent the sum total of the individual's diet and lifestyle habits. In other words, it's as if a young child who's blindfolded in the game hide-and-seek suddenly gets a swift kick in the behind from one of his playmates, but he doesn't know which one. He has only a sore bottom to show for the experience. This is the ultimate legal loophole, and a rather convenient situation for all the thousands of manufacturers of chemical products and other toxic substances, because finger-pointing years down the line is virtually impossible. It's a shame that what this boils down to is that some people are only honest if they "have" to be, for example if they'll be "caught," otherwise there's no guarantee. Whenever you meet a person, you can really trust, treasure this person, for honor is a precious human quality, and people who don't have a price are special in our money-oriented times.

We all want security, safety, guarantees, and assurances nowadays, but the fact is that real security involves more than money, the roof over our heads, and so on—real security is ours when we are healthy, then we have access to the truth and to freedom, when we have lends and people we can trust around us, when we have hope ... there are no price tags or monetary values to be put on real security, when you get right down to it. Security also means a clean environment, which brings us back to our question of who is responsible. Not only is blame difficult to place, but another thing we'll soon notice is that when researchers or doctors are at a loss to explain a problem or "cure" an illness, they often seek, at least, to fix the blame somewhere (or elsewhere). Patients expect answers from doctors, and the public demands results from researchers. Remember when you were in school and you didn't know the answer to one of those essay questions, but you managed to fill 20 lines of paper anyway with something less than the pertinent details and with much imagination? No one wants to come up empty-handed— if they don't know, they'll make something up on short notice. With all the misinformation given us, blame is even harder still to come by.

Because any bodily condition is caused by factors too numerous for our doctors or "experts" to know or mention, we never get the whole story from them anyway. We're always left with the task of synthesizing the information one way or the other.

All this vagueness also raises some serious questions about our personal freedom to have a pure environment. It's obvious that "blaming" and "suing" aren't enough (they don't always change the situation), and we can't even know who to blame or sue most of the time. We can't bring every unseen housewife to court for spraying with an ozone-depleting aerosol can, we can't sue the sun for ultraviolet skin cancer rays, nor can we sue all the motorists for increasing our CO2 levels. We can't afford the time it takes to blame all the people responsible for the state of our world today, and even if we could spare several lifetimes to make a list of guilty persons, it wouldn't remedy our ailing earth. So, what exactly are we free to do? We're free to do what we can.

Article #2: Radiation Hazards

"The hazards of Everyday Radiation," by Elisabeth Rosenthal (Science Digest, 4/84): "There is no doubt that radiation can trigger cancer. Today, Americans are exposed to more low-level radiation than ever before. We get it from X rays or while traveling in an airplane. It seeps from nuclear power plants, from the homes we live in. It rises from the ground beneath us and descends from the sky above. Some scientists say this isn't a serious threat, but others say that if we don't guard against further radiation exposure, we may be saddled with a cancer rate of epidemic proportions. All agree there is no such thing as 'safe' radiation. Many radiation-induced tumors don't appear until 35 to 40 years after exposure; evidence suggests cumulative lifetime exposure also affects tumor growth.

"The loudest voice crying disaster belongs to John Gofman, professor emeritus at the University of California. Gofman discovered uranium 233 with Glenn Seaborg in 1941; he isolated the world's first workable quantity of plutonium for the Manhattan Project; and so on. 1983 had an updated version of his 908-page analysis of radiation risks, Radiation and Human Health (New York, Pantheon books). It contains some terrifying predictions. For example, Gofman estimates that if, in the U.S., we were to produce our energy fully from plutonium and could contain the substance with 99.99%

effectiveness, we'd still produce tens of thousands of deaths from cancer annually. He predicts that 20% of workers in nuclear plants exposed to only one rad a year for 20 years will die prematurely from cancer. He also estimates that plutonium fallout from all the nuclear weapons testing to date will produce 950,000 deaths from lung cancer worldwide. (Italics mine. Imagine what a "surprise lottery" that amounts to for so many of us.) Gorman bases his conclusions on a variety of studies, beginning with those made on the 82,000 survivors of the 1945 Hiroshima and Nagasaki. Among those survivors, at first, there seemed to be no signs of cancer. But in the early 1950s, there was a rise in leukemia among the survivors and in birth defects among their children. In the early 1960s, there was a slight rise in the number of tumors, not all of them cancerous. In 1974, the U.S. National Cancer Institute calculated that only 100 of the 82,000 survivors had died from cancer caused by radiation exposure—not a very impressive number. But, in the past decade, the cancer rate among survivors has continued to rise. It is now believed that the survivors received an average of 25-30 rads of radiation, or a mean of 28 rads, and, says Gofman, many are surprised to find that the average dose of the exposed Japanese atom bomb survivors is comparable to that received during some common diagnostic exams in American medicine." (Keep in mind that today's weapons are much stronger too, but it's still interesting to note how quickly we could accumulate doses like the Japanese in our day-to-day life.) Remember, again, this is our purpose of discussing another unpleasant item from our Pandora's Box: because we live in these times, we, as "healers," must be aware of how all factors interrelate to influence life on earth, and that certainly includes radiation and its effects. Again, our lesson's space cannot cover what is a whole topic in itself, but this serves to remind us to keep our eyes open (in working with people to attain good health) for the things we can't see, such as radiation or other exposure to toxins or chemicals, as well as looking out for dietary factors in physical symptoms and manifestations of the body's healing process. This is obviously difficult work—to assess a person's state of health in terms of so many possible types of (invisible) exposure-it requires a good strong sense of intuition and understanding. There is no one concrete, definitive way to "compute" a person's total lifestyle impacts—this skill can't really be taught—although much information can be shared, and much knowledge can be taught/ learned, we must still develop this in ourselves, as best we can. If we are sensitive and sincere, we can tune ourselves in to the nonphysical world "beyond" our bodies. (Remember, too, the admonition to heal thyself.)

Gofman continues: "In light of these numbers, and given the rising cancer rate among the survivors, the dosage of radiation given to most Americans in diagnostic x-ray exams is unnecessarily high, and if the dosage were cut by one-third, we'd avoid 1,000,000 deaths over the next 30 years." Some scientists think he overestimated risks, but common sense tells me I'd rather overestimate a risk and be more cautious than to take chances, since no one seems to agree on definite risk factors. I for one would prefer not to become a guinea pig or a future statistic. Any figure given for "the number of deaths possible in 30 years" is bound to be somewhat arbitrary, whether low or high, because unpredictable factors can enter into our predictions later. More important than the exact numbers of "nameless victims" counted is the remedying of problems before more victims are found.

One of the common things said by people faced with life-threatening health crises is "that you never think it'll happen to you" or "you never realize what it's like till it's happened to you, or someone you know" ... Something has to "bring it all home" before most of us realize (and or admit) it's time to do some changing. When the roulette wheel in this "surprise" lottery spins, and you're holding your breath that your number won't come up, it becomes more and more evident that the statistics are not nameless or faceless anymore. We all have a chance in this one, whether we like it or not, so we may as well learn how to really play the game, instead of letting someone else spin the wheel while we wait for our number to come up "before our time."

It's better to be alert, awake and ever watchful of our earth's rhythms, sensitive to her very heartbeat itself. When "experts" disagree on a problem's details, the advantage is that we then question their opinions. No truths are finite and stationary—everything is in the process of change, subject to constant alteration. Vigilance on our part also helps us to see through patronizing assurances lightly tossed our way by the no-risk and low risk radiation salespersons who'd rather not rock the boat, and whose sources of funding often encourage low-risk assessments that protect manufacturers and their investments.

Gofman writes, "in a fully developed 'nuclear economy,' radon gas coming from the refuse left over after mining uranium should lead to 3.9. lung-cancer deaths per year in an equilibrium population of 250 million, acknowledging that this is one-thousandth the death rate caused by naturally occurring radon," but he also notes that the damaging material has a half-life of 80,000 years, which means it can kill for 115,400 years. Therefore, he says, a fully operational nuclear power industry would eventually cause 115,400 times 3.9. deaths—or 450,060. But these would "occur over a time frame more than 20 times longer than that of recorded history." X rays and gamma rays are electromagnetic and are simply packets of energy. Alpha and beta rays are streams of charged, subatomic particles. When they rip into our bodies, they dislodge particles of atoms in our cells that carom about with enormous energy; these hopped-up particles behave like the proverbial bull in a china shop; they tear around, breaking bonds and chromosomes and disrupting cell reproduction—such damage may well be the initiating event in cancer.

"It took years for doctors to realize that radiation is dangerous, and there are many old horror stories as a result of this lack of understanding. Fifty years ago, when dentists began x-raying teeth, they would often use their hands to hold the film in their patients' mouths. Many of these dentists contracted skin and bone cancer that began with lesions on their fingers. It is more difficult to collect accurate data on low-dose exposures, of course. Background radiation of all kinds exists nowadays." One estimate says most Americans are exposed to an average of 0.2. rads a year, or 210 millirads. (Remember this figure is an "average" and is arbitrary.) Of this typical individual exposure, about 28 millirads come from outer space in the form of cosmic rays (that's at sea level—at higher elevations, where the thinning atmosphere deflects fewer rays, the number rises;

estimates range from 2 millirads extra at 1000 feet to 70 extra per year at 9000 feet. Perhaps 50 millirads come from the natural decay of radioactive elements in the Earth. Certain areas have measurably more than others. (Leadville, Colorado, residents, more than 1.5. miles up, absorb 125 millirads of cosmic rays per year.) "Your home could be radioactive, too. Contractors occasionally purchase debris from uranium mines to use as filler in construction materials. Alternatively, the rock from which your house is constructed could have been mined from a quarry with naturally-high radiation. The Department of Energy is beginning a 3-year survey of 8,000 buildings that are believed to deliver excessive radiation. And if you live in an area rich in radioactive elements, your water could be radioactive as well. Such water spraying out of shower heads gives an ambient concentration that can approach occupational limits. Fallout from all the nuclear weapons testing to date is said to give us each about 4.4. millirads per year (in 1963, when testing was above ground, it was 13 millirads per year). Nuclear power plants give us each about another millirad. Add almost 3 millirads of cosmic radiation for each hour you fly, because the atmosphere is thinner up there. (A flight attendant on the Boston-New York shuttle, for example, gets an extra 250 millirads per year.) Then, if you sleep next to a radio luminescent clock, add another 9 millirads per year. And some dentures are coated with a uranium-and-cirium glaze to make them sparkle. One estimate figure this gives your mouth about 3 rads annually, localized. Color TVs are said to give about 0.48 millirads per year (if you watch 24 hours a day, otherwise proportionately less). The display screens on personal computers are the same kind of so-called 'safe" cathode-ray tubes. Some occupations increase your risks; you absorb a-lot more radiation if you're a uranium miner, a radiologist, or a worker in a nuclear plant." (I think we can assume most of our students aren't.) "But the biggest radioactive boost most of us get comes from diagnostic X rays. A 1970 survey found 65% of the U.S. population had 'at least one x-ray exam that year.' Collectively we receive about 240 million x-ray exams annually. Ordinary chest X rays require about 30 millirads, and a single dental X ray needs 300 millirads. Unfortunately, there is no such thing as a standard X ray. One radiological physicist says national studies of x-ray trends have shown, factors of variation greater than a hundred: 'it's extremely worrying.' Mammography tests have been found with exposures as 'low' as 300 millirads and high as 3,000. A range of dental x-ray machines was found in a Department of Health, Education and Welfare study in 1976 to deliver 100 to 5,000 millirads. The average was one rad, or more than three times the 'necessary' exposure. The largest x-ray doses come from fluoroscopies, commonly used to find ulcers, tumors, and other abnormalities in the gastrointestinal tract. In a GI series, a patient drinks a solution containing barium (which X rays can't penetrate) or gets the barium in an enema, and an x-ray machine takes series of photos amounting to as much as 10 minutes of radiation. Compared to chest films, Gofman says, barium meals are a horror show—if the doctor is particularly solicitous, the patient could have his ulcer checked every 6 months—that's a lot of radiation.

"Few doctors or dentists even know exactly how much radiation their machines deliver. Then, x-ray doses can be increased for other reasons; the overworked technician might juice up the radiation dose to 'save the time' required to mix a new batch of developer."

We must also question schemes to "dump toxic and nuclear wastes at sea," because leaking barrels have been found (and so on—space here doesn't permit a detailed account of problems in this area, and most of us are aware of them by now). The radioactivity in the sea, if it works its way into the ecosystem there, will become a part of the chain from lower to higher life forms, as each larger fish (etc.) ingests a more concentrated dose than the one before it. We already have a problem controlling toxic substances on land, and an even bigger problem with ethics on land or sea—when "there's no one looking" who knows who will dump what where?

Natural hot springs can be another source of radiation. Several hundred of the world's geothermal springs are radioactive (their waters flow through radioactive rocks), and many of these are popular "health" spas. "Visitors to Luchon, France, drink the water and inhale gas that can be 15,000 times more radioactive than normal air." In the U.S., radioactive springs include Hot Springs, Arkansas ("low" levels), and Alhambra Hot Springs, Montana, "with high levels that could constitute potential hazards to health," says the U.S. Geological Survey.

The news of May 19, 1985, carries a story of "a natural environmental hazard of uncertain but grave dimensions discovered beneath the meadows of eastern Pennsylvania: state and federal investigators have found that many houses are contaminated with radon, a radioactive gas that causes lung cancer after prolonged exposure. Levels in some houses were the highest ever recorded in the U.S.—in one eastern county, nearly 40% had unsafe levels of radon. But the risk may be spread far beyond this semirural county. The radon is seeping up through the soil from uranium deposits in the earth below. Officials believe the radioactive contamination varies from place to place, depending on the permeability of the soil and other factors. Parts of New Jersey and New York are also part of the Reading Prong, a geologic formation with uranium in it. Pennsylvania officials are telling residents that the radon does not constitute an immediate health risk, although it may pose serious long-term problems." More houses still need to be examined; one New Jersey Environmental Protection spokesman described the situation as

"An entirely new area of concern that nobody even guessed at six months ago." A University of Pittsburgh professor of physics says virtually every state has areas of radon contamination that might pose a health threat. "It is really a worldwide problem," he said.

Sheldon Meyers, director of the office of radiation at the federal Environmental Protection Agency, agreed that "there was no doubt radon caused cancer," but (as usual) the exact dangers are still "not certain." One family's living room had the "highest radiation level found in the U.S. from radon contamination; at that level, the chances of contracting lung cancer over a lifetime of exposure are 100%, experts say. They moved, but a nearby neighbor was told that her house showed 2.12. working levels of radon, and that the level was "equivalent to smoking 22 packs of cigarettes a day! At twenty-two packs, "hazardous to your health" becomes quite an understatement!

Who is T.C. Fry

From 1970 to 1996, T.C. Fry went from a half-Cherokee man with an 11th-grade education to a popularizer of Natural Hygiene for "The Suffering Masses" under the name of "Life Science".

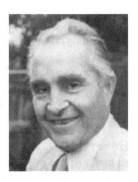

1T.C Fry

He achieved this by writing free and low-cost leaflets, booklets, and books, which he sent out through bulk mail and as non-profit establishments, reaching millions of people.

Although Dr. Shelton's books offered a more scientific and technical approach to superior health through strict hygienic living, Fry's works were popular due to their low cost, simple language, and sensationalized promises.

Fry's works inspired and educated countless Americans who were in need of the truth and wanted to take the Hygienic Road Less Traveled with a leader who was within their humble, grassroots grasp.

In the late 1970s to 1994, T.C. Fry started various newsletters and publications such as Total Well-Being, The Health Crusader, and Better Life Journal, which all folded. He founded the Life Science Institute in 1982, which later became Health Excellence in 1991, putting out two ephemeral newsletters.

For six years, Fry published Healthful Living, which was his most impressive and long-lived publication. This magazine offered useful articles and education through The Life Science Library, which had over 100 Hygienic and near-Hygienic materials and goods.

Although it was advertised to the public as a monthly, it was only published as funds allowed. After the establishment of Health Excellence and the third bankruptcy, Fry turned to sporadically publishing two less costly newsletters, The Health Scene Newsletter and The Healthway Advisor.

In addition to his publications, Fry also offered a course for those who wanted to become "students" of Natural Hygiene. The Life Science Health System was a 106-lesson, $1475.oo, correspondence course with around 4,000 students enrolled as of the end of 2000. Some controversy has surrounded the course, with many maintaining that it could not adequately prepare a student to become a "Hygienic practitioner" in the professional sense.

However, Fry's course was praised for being the only comprehensive course on Natural Hygiene, suitable for self-education or to prepare the student to become a teacher of Natural Hygiene.

From 1994 to 1999, Bob Szucs and associates took over "The Big Course" and renamed it "Feeling Fit for Life". They continued to make the course available under this name.

However, the fate of Fry's publications and course after 1999 is unclear.T.C. Fry emphasized that Natural Hygiene was more than just a dietary approach.

In Part 1 of the 'Life Sciences' instruction materials, he also highlighted the importance of emotional balance, rest, and sleep as essential factors for a healthy life. T.C. believed that by following the laws of Natural Hygiene, one could achieve a long and healthy life.

However, T.C. Fry passed away at the age of 69, in poor health. This came as a shock to many of his followers, who were left disappointed, disillusioned, and confused. Some people tend to follow the man rather than the message, which made Natural Hygiene a soft target for those who opposed its dietary principles, namely a diet high in fruit, vegetables, nuts, and seeds without supplementation.

As a result, many Natural Hygiene students have come across this issue in their research and find it challenging to reconcile the apparent discrepancy between T.C. Fry's message and his untimely death.

TC's initial state before embracing Natural Hygiene

At the age of 45, he was overweight, had digestive problems, a heart condition, gum disease, multiple abscesses, bone degeneration, and possibly a lung condition as indicated by an X-ray at autopsy.

Although there are conflicting reports on whether he had been a smoker, the presence of lymph nodes containing carbon and scar tissue in his autopsy suggests that he might have smoked at some point.

Some sources claim that he was stabbed while working as a detective in New York and injured during World War II, although the latter is unlikely as he would have been too young.

Dr. Doug Graham describes him as being on the brink of death due to an excessively abusive lifestyle, but his decision to adopt Natural Hygiene allowed him to live another 25 years.

While TC's adoption of Natural Hygiene had a profound impact on his health, it's worth considering whether he could have extended his life and reduced his suffering by paying more attention to the "other necessities of healthful living."

The Years of Natural Hygiene

During his lifetime, TC Fry had a number of personal and business struggles that took a toll on his health. One significant incident involved a dispute with a former lover, which resulted in her shooting him in the back of the head at close range. This event not only had an immediate impact on his health, but also caused long-term damage, resulting in blackouts.

After being cleared to drive again, TC was involved in a serious car accident that left him with crushed chest, broken ribs, and damaged lungs. Despite being discharged from the hospital shortly after the accident, he refused to eat for two weeks in order to give his body time to focus on healing. While this approach may have aided his recovery, it's also possible that his quick return to work after the accident contributed to a sense of invincibility that had negative consequences later in life.

Before discovering Natural Hygiene, TC's poor diet had already resulted in damage to his teeth. He did not have the necessary dental work done, which caused him to experience pain and fever from bacterial toxins in abscesses over the years. This likely resulted in a buildup of toxins in his body, leading to septicemia.

Considering all of these factors, it's clear that TC was in poor health before discovering Natural Hygiene. His various injuries and health issues made it challenging for his body to recover and heal from the damage it had sustained over the years.

Was TC as a teacher of healthy lifestyle following Natural Hygiene principles?

Let's examine whether TC adhered to the Natural Hygiene principles of healthful living, including diet, emotional balance, rest, and sleep to improve his health.

At the outset, we can assume that TC must have initially followed the Natural Hygiene lifestyle to some degree, leading to remarkable improvements in his health. His passion and commitment to spreading the Natural Hygiene message attest to this fact.

However, as he became increasingly involved in promoting the movement, certain aspects of his own healthful living were overlooked, creating an ironic situation.

Diet

Not many people, whether they follow an all-raw diet or not, can claim to be perfect in their eating habits. I empathize with those who feel it's unfair to criticize TC for deviating from the ideal. However, since some have used TC's death to discredit the Natural Hygiene and fruitarian diets, and even to sell supplements, what TC actually ate and how he ate is highly relevant.

At the beginning of his Natural Hygiene journey, TC appeared to adhere strictly to the diet. However, as he began to spread the message, his lifestyle began to neglect certain aspects of healthful living. Chet Day and others reported that TC would often eat nothing during the day and then binge-eat in the evening, consuming large meals that mixed various fruits, vegetables, and nuts. Late-night overeating, particularly when stressed, is a recipe for indigestion, according to Dr. Herbert Shelton. This pattern of eating would have only worsened TC's pre-existing gastric problems.

The typical Natural Hygiene diet consists mainly of fruits, both sweet and non-sweet, vegetables, and a small amount of nuts and seeds. Did TC always follow this diet? No. TC's diet sometimes included foods like shop-bought coleslaw with vinegar and mayonnaise, desserts like ice cream, pie, cake, macaroni, cheese, and canned food. However, TC had switched from the standard American diet to 100% Natural Hygiene/raw overnight, which was a tough transition, and occasional slips are understandable. TC's friend notes that he did not come to Natural Hygiene via a cooked vegan diet, so it's understandable that he would revert to what he knew when he relapsed. Unfortunately, TC's departures from the Natural Hygiene diet included the exact types of foods that would exacerbate his pre-existing heart problems and might have partially reversed the remarkable health gains he initially achieved when he discovered Natural Hygiene.

Moreover, it must be noted that TC did not follow the traditional Natural Hygiene diet. He promoted a diet of almost exclusively sweet fruit and excluded nuts from a healthy diet, contrary to the teachings of his mentor Herbert Shelton.

Emotional equilibrium

TC faced constant financial problems and frequent run-ins with the IRS, which put him under considerable stress. His business possessions were confiscated several times, and according to health writer Ric Lambert, "Terry... was under unrelenting stress and never got out of one legal battle or confrontation before he was engaged in a new one."

Rest

When TC discovered Natural Hygiene, his health was in a poor state due to his head and chest injuries. These injuries required an extended period of rest to allow his body to heal. However, TC was a workaholic who refused to rest. Despite needing rest to recover, he worked harder than ever and neglected his own health while spreading the message of Natural Hygiene and helping others.

Sleep

Dr. Vetrano noted that TC slept very little and often got up in the middle of the night to work. TC would wake up feeling groggy at 4 am and go for a run to wake himself up, using exercise as a stimulant. Moreover, TC's habit of eating large amounts of food at night, combined with his chronic gastroenteritis, made it difficult for him to sleep. As a result, TC Fry could not obtain the restorative sleep necessary for his damaged body to heal, let alone support his stressful lifestyle, and must have been seriously enervated.

The Decline

Had TC lived a quiet life, adhering to the principles of Natural Hygiene upon discovering it, his body might have had a chance to heal from the decades of unhealthy living and subsequent traumas.

Perhaps retiring and simplifying his life could have extended his life. However, TC's early success with Natural Hygiene drove him to tirelessly spread its message, leading to unhelpful eating patterns, stress, and lack of rest and sleep that continuously depleted his energy.

Consequently, his body struggled not only to heal pre-existing conditions and injuries but also to eliminate toxins.

During busy and stressful times, TC likely resorted to processed sugary foods, which depleted the vital B vitamins necessary for a healthy nervous system and required during times of stress.

Dr. Vetrano notes that TC suffered from chronic lung problems for at least five years before his death, which likely caused his shortness of breath.

Dr. Ralph Cinque reported oedema (swollen ankles) due to TC's pre-existing heart condition, and TC continued to suffer from digestive problems, including bloating and flatulence with almost every meal.

In the Year of TC's death

In the year leading up to TC's death, he was in a weakened and sickly state. Six months before he passed away, he struggled to walk and breathe and had swollen legs and a pale complexion. He often had a low-grade fever, and Dr. Ralph Cinque noted that he was too frail and undernourished to fast.

According to Natural Hygiene principles, TC should have eliminated the causes of his poor health, rested, and focused on rebuilding his health. Raw fruits, vegetables, nuts, and seeds would have been an essential part of his diet at this time. However, despite his worsening condition, TC felt obligated to continue working towards his mission of establishing a Natural Hygiene college, which may have been driven by financial concerns. Although the retreat owner suggested he extend his short break for his health, TC refused.

Unfortunately, TC's diet during this period included cooked food, which was not in line with Natural Hygiene principles. He also did not seek conventional medical treatment, which some may argue could have helped in crisis management.

Instead, he opted for ozone therapy, a treatment that goes against Natural Hygiene principles. TC reported feeling very ill after the treatments and claimed that he was talked into them. As he grew weaker, TC lost confidence in the principles he had previously advocated for, resulting in a vicious circle of declining health and departure from Natural Hygiene principles.

In the year before his death, TC had 17 ozone treatments, which Dr. Vetrano believes contributed to the acceleration of his pre-existing degenerative conditions and lung damage caused by free radicals generated by the ozone. Dr. Vetrano argues in her book that, had it not been for these treatments, TC may have been able to recover. She describes them as the "coup de grace that killed him."

Events at Death

TC experienced a range of health problems before his death, including oedema, atherosclerosis, emphysema, lung lesions, breathing difficulties, bronchitis, pneumonia, gastritis, gingivitis, and anemia due to B12 deficiency. The cause of death was recorded as a pulmonary embolus, which Dr. Vetrano believes was caused by deep venous thrombosis in the lungs, likely caused by the ozone treatments TC received. Dr. Fuhrmann, however, believes that the B12 deficiency was the cause of death and that TC's failure to supplement his diet with B12 was the reason for the deficiency. Dr. Vetrano disagreed with this, stating that TC's chronic gastritis prevented him from absorbing enough intrinsic factor to obtain B12 from his diet, and that raw vegans don't need supplementation.

Dr. Vetrano also believed that TC's diet was lacking in concentrated proteins, which he needed due to his weakened constitution and stressful lifestyle, and that his fruit-only diet did not provide enough protein for his body's repair and function. However, TC had difficulty digesting nuts, which Dr. Vetrano believed could be remedied by building up tolerance through proper combination with other foods.

While TC's death cannot be solely attributed to his natural hygiene lifestyle, it was a contributing factor. He worked tirelessly to spread the message of natural hygiene and was a mentor to many, including Dr. Doug Graham. Dr. Graham believes that TC's intensity led to his death, as he worked himself too hard to spread the health message. Dr. Vetrano also notes that those who strive to achieve their goals often forget about themselves and their health, leading to their premature demise.

Conclusion

The story of T C Fry reminds us just how important it is to attend to the non-diet factors that can affect our health. Those educating others in health (and, really, that includes all of you reading, unless you never talk to others about your lifestyle) have a responsibility to practice what we preach.

We must work hard (as it were...) to reduce stress and get sufficient rest and sleep. And, by that, I mean 'lying outside in the sun for 30 minutes doing nothing' should be on our 'to-do' lists that's as much part of our jobs just as surely as finishing that article or preparing that demo!

The story of T.C. Fry highlights the importance of addressing non-diet factors that can impact our health. Those who educate others about health have a responsibility to practice what they preach and prioritize reducing stress and getting adequate rest and sleep.

This includes taking time to relax in the sun for 30 minutes, just as we prioritize work tasks. If we do neglect our health, we should be honest about it, so we can still make a positive impact while minimizing confusion to our followers if we become ill.

Even if we generally live a healthy lifestyle, occasional lapses in diet and neglecting non-diet factors can have consequences.

We cannot consider ourselves immune to illness, particularly if our bodies have experienced abuse from an unhealthy lifestyle. Despite our best efforts, there will always be toxins beyond our control, such as those in the air we breathe.

Therefore, prioritizing non-diet health factors like fresh air, rest, and sleep can help us maintain sufficient energy to combat these toxins. If we prioritize other aspects of our lives, such as our career, at the expense of our health, we may become ill due to reduced energy levels.

TC Fry's life and death serves as a reminder that we need to practice what we preach if we want to live a long and healthy life and become a beacon of health. Even if we do not become a renowned health expert, we should aim to live a long and healthy life as a testament to our lifestyle.

Table of contents - Detailed

Made in United States
Troutdale, OR
03/03/2024

18142191R10452